Mastering Structural Heart Disease

Mastering Structural Heart Disease

Edited by

Eduardo J. de Marchena, MD
Professor of Medicine and Surgery
Director of Eberhard Grube International Structural Heart Disease
Training Program at the University of Miami Miller School of Medicine
United States

Camilo A. Gomez, MD
Interventional Cardiologist at the Jackson Memorial Health System
and a Voluntary Assistant Professor, Department of Medicine
University of Miami Miller School of Medicine
United States

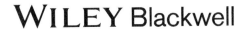

Registered Offices
John Wiley & Sons, Inc., 111 River Street, Hoboken, NJ 07030, USA
John Wiley & Sons Ltd, The Atrium, Southern Gate, Chichester, West Sussex, PO19 8SQ, UK

For details of our global editorial offices, customer services, and more information about Wiley products visit us at www.wiley.com.

Wiley also publishes its books in a variety of electronic formats and by print-on-demand. Some content that appears in standard print versions of this book may not be available in other formats.

Library of Congress Cataloging-in-Publication Data

Names: De Marchena, Eduardo, editor. | Gomez, Camilo A. (Camilo Andres),
  1984- editor.
Title: Mastering structural heart disease / edited by Eduardo J. de
  Marchena, Camilo A. Gomez.
Description: First edition. | Hoboken, NJ : Wiley, 2023. | Includes
  bibliographical references and index.
Identifiers: LCCN 2022030845 (print) | LCCN 2022030846 (ebook) | ISBN
  9781119807810 (cloth) | ISBN 9781119807827 (adobe pdf) | ISBN
  9781119807834 (epub)
Subjects: MESH: Heart Diseases—therapy | Heart Diseases—physiopathology
Classification: LCC RC682 (print) | LCC RC682 (ebook) | NLM WG 210 | DDC
  616.1/2—dc23/eng/20220907
LC record available at https://lccn.loc.gov/2022030845
LC ebook record available at https://lccn.loc.gov/2022030846

Cover Design and Image: Manuela Echeverri

Set in 9.5/12.5pt STIXTwoText by Straive™, Chennai, India

SKY10049645_062223

To my parents for their guidance, support and encouragement; to my teachers for their knowledge, inspiration and patience; to my patients for their confidence; and to my wife Melanie, children and grandchildren for keeping life fun and exciting.

Eduardo J. de Marchena

To God, for all the blessings; to my parents, for their guidance and constant support; to my wife, for her love and encouragement; to my son, for the inspiration and joy he has brought to us; and to my teachers, for their knowledge, mentorship, and opportunities.

Camilo A. Gomez

Acknowledgements

We would like to thank Julissa Gutierrez for her meticulous, untiring support during preparation of this textbook.

We would also like to thank Manuela Echeverri for her inspirational, masterful artwork in the preparation of the book cover.

Cover Design Artist Statement

Manuela Echeverri

Manuela is a renowned Colombian artist, internationally recognized for her work with hearts. Her art includes a variety of colorful heart sculptures and paintings.

Artist Statement

"A piece of color, a piece of life"

I don't recall a specific moment in my life when I began taking an interest in art. On the contrary, I feel that art has always been a part of me, like small shapes that when put together create a larger puzzle full of color. Art gives a greater sense of purpose to my days and fills my life with laughter, joy, and gratitude, knowing that every moment is unique and unrepeatable.

Through art, I have learned things that are not taught in any academy.

My work is full nuances and techniques but always defined by the use of COLOR – driven by my understanding of the world. Through my art, and through color, I have learned to be more human, more sensitive: to create from the HEART.

And as I create, inspired by love, I have always sought to develop artistic projects with people who give meaning to what I do, supporting the causes and perspectives that I hold dear in my life. My art has enabled me to connect with and grow in the company of beautiful people who continue to inspire me to create an impact through my work.

 @MANUECHEVERRI

 manuelaecheverri.com.co

 arte@manuelaecheverri.com

Brief Contents

List of Contributors   *xlv*

Preface   *lv*

About the Companion Website   *lvii*

Part I   Structural Interventions for the Aortic Valve   *1*

1   The Natural History and Hemodynamic Assessment of Aortic Valve Disease   *3*

2   Pathology Insights of Aortic Valve Disease   *11*

3   The Top Ten Clinical Trials in Patients Undergoing Transcatheter Aortic Valve Implantation
The Evolution of a Transformative Therapy into Clinical Practice   *19*

4   Present and Future Generations of Transcatheter Aortic Valves   *31*

5   Computed Tomography for Transcatheter Aortic Valve Replacement Planning
Current Perspectives and Future Directions   *39*

6   Optimal Selection of TAVR Devices   *51*

7   Transcatheter Aortic Valve Replacement
Step-by-Step Approach   *59*

8   Balloon Aortic Valvuloplasty
Current Clinical Role and Technical Aspects   *69*

9   Challenging Anatomy Scenarios in TAVR   *75*

10   TAVR for Bicuspid Aortic Valve   *83*

11   TAVR for Pure Native Valve Aortic Regurgitation   *89*

12   Aortic Valve-in-Valve Interventions   *95*

13   Prevention and Management of Coronary Artery Obstruction in TAVR   *103*

14 Coronary Artery Disease and Transcatheter Aortic Valve Replacement
Timing and Patient Selection for Coronary Intervention in Patients Planned for TAVR *109*

15 Conduction Disturbances Associated with TAVR
Clinical Impact and Techniques to Minimize *115*

16 Management of Conduction Disturbances Post-TAVR *123*

17 TAVR Mechanical Complications Prevention and Management *131*

18 Pathological Insights of TAVR Degeneration and Thrombosis *139*

19 Clinical Implications of Valve Thrombosis and Early Thickening
Management of Antiplatelets and Anticoagulation Post TAVI *151*

20 TAVR and Stroke *155*

21 Current Evidence of Neuroprotection in TAVR *163*

22 Difficult Transfemoral Access for TAVR and Bailout Techniques *169*

23 Alternative Access for TAVR *175*

24 Vascular Access and Closure Options for TAVR *183*

Part II   Structural Interventions for the Mitral Valve   *191*

25 The Natural History of Mitral Valve Disease *193*

26 Hemodynamic Assessment of the Mitral Valve *203*

27 Echocardiographic Assessment Prior to Mitral Valve Edge-to-Edge Repair *211*

28 Intra-procedural Transesophageal Echocardiography for Mitral Valve Structural Interventions *217*

29 Surgical Trials in Mitral Valvular Disease *227*

30 Surgical Techniques for Mitral Valve Repair *233*

31 Structural Interventions for Mitral Stenosis *239*

32 Transcatheter Edge-to-Edge Repair Trials
The EVEREST and COAPT Trials *251*

33 Mitral Valve TEER
The MitraClip Procedure *257*

34 TEER Challenging Anatomy and MitraClip Tips and Tricks *273*

35 MitraClip Complications
Prevention and Management *281*

36 CT Imaging for TMVR *291*

37 Transcatheter Mitral Valve Replacement
Transcatheter Mitral Valve-in-Valve (ViV), Valve-in-Ring (ViR), and Valve-in-MAC (ViMAC) *301*

38 Transseptal Transcatheter Mitral Valve-in-Valve Replacement (TS MViV)
Technical Considerations and Step-by-Step Procedure *311*

39 Transseptal Systems for TMVR and Transcatheter Devices for Mitral Annuloplasty *317*

40 Transcatheter Mitral Valve Replacement
The Tendyne System *325*

41 Self-Expanding Transcatheter Mitral Valve Replacement Systems
Medtronic Intrepid Valve *331*

Part III   Structural Interventions for the Tricuspid Valve *335*

42 Natural History and Hemodynamic Assessment of Tricuspid Valve Diseases *337*

43 Indications and Outcomes for Surgical Tricuspid Valve Repair *343*

44 Intra-Procedural Imaging of Tricuspid Valve Edge-to-Edge Interventions *347*

45 Transcatheter Tricuspid Valve Device Landscape *353*

46 Progress in Transcatheter Tricuspid Valve Repair and Replacement *363*

47 Tricuspid Valve-in-Valve and Valve-in-Ring *383*

48 Caval Valve Implantation (CAVI) for the Treatment of Severe Tricuspid Regurgitation *391*

Part IV   Structural Interventions for Management of Paravalvular Leaks *395*

49 Aortic Paravalvular Leak Closure
Techniques and Devices for Surgical and Transcatheter Prostheses *397*

50 Mitral Paravalvular Leak: Imaging and Interventional Approaches *403*

Part V   Left Atrial Appendage Closure *415*

51 Current Indications for Percutaneous Left Atrial Appendage Occlusion *417*

52 Imaging for LAA Interventions *425*

53 Devices for Left Atrial Appendage Closure *433*

54 LAA Occlusion Technique and Challenging Scenarios *441*

55 Preventing and Managing Complications of LAA Closure *449*

Part VI   Selected Structural Interventions for Cardiomyopathies *457*

56 The Natural History of Hypertrophic Cardiomyopathy *459*

57 Alcohol Septal Ablation in Hypertrophic Cardiomyopathy *463*

58 Transcatheter Edge-to-Edge Repair for Hypertrophic Cardiomyopathy *467*

59 Interatrial Shunt Creation *471*

Part VII   Selected Adult Congenital Structural Interventions *475*

60 Shunt Hemodynamics and Calculations *477*

61 Persistent Foramen Ovale Closure
Technical Considerations *485*

62 Atrial Septal Defects Closure *493*

63 Ventricular Septal Defects Closure *499*

64 Percutaneous Treatment of Aortic Coarctation *505*

65 Percutaneous Pulmonary Valve Replacement (PPVR) *515*

Part VIII   Miscellaneous *523*

66 Hemodynamic Pearls in Adult Structural Heart Disease *525*

67 Percutaneous Closure of Coronary Artery Fistulas *535*

68 Renal Denervation Therapy
Available Evidence, Catheters, and Techniques *541*

69 Acute Pulmonary Embolism Interventions: Data and Indications *547*

70 Acute Pulmonary Embolism Intervention: Devices and Techniques *553*

71 Transseptal Puncture Technique in the ERA of Structural Heart Disease *561*

72 ECMO for Structural Interventions *567*

73 Best Practices for Mechanical Circulatory Support with Impella for Acute Myocardial Infarction Cardiogenic Shock and Selected Structural Interventions *571*

74 Transcatheter Interventions for Aortic Valve Insufficiency in Patients with Left Ventricular Assist Devices *585*

Index *589*

Contents

List of Contributors *xlv*
Preface *lv*
About the Companion Website *lvii*

Part I Structural Interventions for the Aortic Valve *1*

1 The Natural History and Hemodynamic Assessment of Aortic Valve Disease *3*

Aortic Stenosis *3*
  1. What are the causes of aortic stenosis (AS)? *3*
  2. How is AS severity graded? *3*
  3. What are the hemodynamic consequences of AS? *3*
  4. How are the hemodynamics of AS translated into symptoms? *3*
  5. How are the hemodynamics of AS translated into physical exam findings? *4*
  6. How is AS diagnosed (imaging and invasive hemodynamics)? *5*
  7. What is low-flow AS? *5*
  8. What are the indications for medical therapy of AS, and what do those therapies consist of? *6*
  9. What are the indications for mechanical therapy of AS, and what do those therapies consist of? *6*
  10. What is the prognosis for AS? *6*

Aortic Regurgitation *6*
  11. What are the major etiologies of aortic regurgitation (AR)? *6*
  12. How is severe AR defined? *7*

Chronic AR *7*
  13. What are the hemodynamics of chronic AR? *7*
  14. How are chronic AR hemodynamics translated into symptoms? *7*
  15. How are chronic AR hemodynamics translated into physical signs? *7*
  16. How is AR diagnosed (imaging and invasive hemodynamics)? *7*
  17. What are the indications for medical therapy in AR and of what do Those therapies consist? *8*
  18. What are the indications for mechanical therapy of AR and of what do Those therapies consist? *8*
  19. What is the prognosis following treatment *8*

Severe Acute AR *8*
Bibliography *9*

2 Pathology Insights of Aortic Valve Disease *11*

Introduction *11*
  1. What is the normal anatomy of the aortic valve? *11*
  2. What are the etiologies of aortic valve diseases? *11*
  3. What is the epidemiology of aortic valve disease? *11*

4. What is the pathology of tricuspid calcific aortic stenosis?   *12*

5. What is the etiology of bicuspid aortic valve?   *14*

6. What is the classification of bicuspid aortic valves?   *14*

7. What are the pathologic findings of a bicuspid aortic valve?   *15*

8. What are the classification and pathology of the unicuspid aortic valve (UAV)?   *15*

9. What are the differences between the pathological findings in tricuspid vs. bicuspid vs. unicuspid aortic valves?   *15*

10. What are the risk factors for calcific aortic stenosis?   *16*

11. What are the underlying mechanisms of aortic valve calcification?   *16*

Conclusion   *17*

Bibliography   *17*

3   The Top Ten Clinical Trials in Patients Undergoing Transcatheter Aortic Valve Implantation
The Evolution of a Transformative Therapy into Clinical Practice   *19*

1. Who invented TAVI, and where were the early studies performed?   *19*

2. How was TAVI evaluated in the United States?   *19*

Leon, M.B., Smith, C.R., Mack, M. et al. (2010). Transcatheter aortic-valve implantation for aortic stenosis in patients who cannot undergo surgery. *N. Engl. J. Med.* 363 (17): 1597–1607.   *20*

3. Did PARTNER B affect "clinical equipoise" for randomized trials in non-operable patients?   *20*

Popma, J.J., Adams, D.H., Reardon, M.J. et al. (2014). Transcatheter aortic valve replacement using a self-expanding bioprosthesis in patients with severe aortic stenosis at extreme risk for surgery. *J. Am. Coll. Cardiol.* 63 (19): 1972–1981.   *20*

4. When did the Heart Team develop, and what has it meant to TAVI decision-making?   *20*

Smith, C.R., Leon, M.B., Mack, M.J. et al. (2011). Transcatheter versus surgical aortic-valve replacement in high-risk patients. *N. Engl. J. Med.* 364 (23): 2187–2198.   *21*

5. Were the initial concerns about stroke with TAVI justified?   *21*

Adams, D.H., Popma, J.J., Reardon, M.J. et al. (2014). Transcatheter aortic-valve replacement with a self-expanding prosthesis. *N. Engl. J. Med.* 370 (19): 1790–1798.   *21*

6. What contributed to the differences in one-year mortality between TAVI and surgery patients?   *21*

Leon, M.B., Smith, C.R., Mack, M.J. et al. (2016). Transcatheter or surgical aortic-valve replacement in intermediate-risk patients. *N. Engl. J. Med.* 374 (17): 1609–1620.   *22*

Reardon, M.J., Van Mieghem, N.M., Popma, J.J. et al. (2017). Surgical or transcatheter aortic-valve replacement in intermediate-risk patients. *N. Engl. J. Med.* 376 (14): 1321–1331.   *22*

7. What have we learned about the assessment of valve durability?   *22*

Feldman, T.E., Reardon, M.J., Rajagopal, V. et al. (2018). Effect of mechanically expanded vs self-expanding transcatheter aortic valve replacement on mortality and major adverse clinical events in high-risk patients with aortic stenosis: the REPRISE III randomized clinical trial. *J. Am. Med. Assoc.* 319 (1): 27–37.   *23*

Mack, M.J., Leon, M.B., Thourani, V.H. et al. (2019). Transcatheter aortic-valve replacement with a balloon-expandable valve in low-risk patients. *N. Engl. J. Med.* 380 (18): 1695–1705.   *24*

Popma, J.J., Deeb, G.M., Yakubov, S.J. et al. (2019). Transcatheter aortic-valve replacement with a self-expanding valve in low-risk patients. *N. Engl. J. Med.* 380 (18): 1706–1715.   *25*

Makkar, R.R., Cheng, W., Waksman, R. et al. (2020). Self-expanding intra-annular versus commercially available transcatheter heart valves in high and extreme risk patients with severe aortic stenosis (PORTICO IDE): a randomised, controlled, non-inferiority trial. *Lancet* 396 (10252): 669–683.   *25*

8. What did we learn about subclinical leaflet thrombosis from this study?   *25*

9. What are other areas of improvement for TAVI?   *26*

10. What should be considered for the lifetime management of patients undergoing TAVI?   *26*

11. What patient subsets have yet to be studied?   *27*

Moderate Aortic Stenosis   *27*

Asymptomatic Aortic Stenosis   *27*

Aortic Insufficiency   *27*

Conclusions   *28*

Bibliography   *28*

4   Present and Future Generations of Transcatheter Aortic Valves   *31*

   1. What life-long management is required for patients undergoing TAVR   *31*

   2. How is TAVR used for low-surgical-risk patients?   *31*

   3. Describe the hemodynamics after TAVR   *32*

   4. How durable is TAVR?   *32*

   5. Describe coronary access after TAVR.   *33*

   6. Describe pacemaker implantation after TAVR   *33*

   7. What is the present generation of transcatheter valves?   *33*

      SAPIEN 3 Ultra Valve   *33*

      Evolut PRO+ Valve   *34*

      ACURATE *neo2* Valve   *34*

      JenaValve   *34*

      ALLEGRA Valve   *34*

   8. What is the future generation of transcatheter valves?   *35*

      Colibri Valve   *35*

      DurAVR Valve   *35*

      Navitor   *35*

      Triskele UCL Valve   *35*

Conclusions   *35*

Bibliography   *36*

5   Computed Tomography for Transcatheter Aortic Valve Replacement Planning
Current Perspectives and Future Directions   *39*

Introduction   *39*

   1. What Is the best way to approach pre-procedural CT assessment, patient preparation, contrast administration, scanning protocol, and data-reconstruction techniques in patients undergoing CT evaluation prior to TAVR?   *39*

   2. What is the best way to analyze aortic valve calcium extension, scoring, and its clinical significance?   *39*

   3. What is the best approach for aortic valve annular evaluation and sizing?   *40*

   4. What is the best way to evaluate the aorta on CT scan prior to TAVR, and what is the evaluation's clinical significance?   *41*

      Ascending Aorta   *41*

      Coronary Ostium, Sinus of Valsalva, and Sinotubular Junction Measurements   *42*

   5. What are the TAVR access sites, and how are they evaluated on a CT scan?   *42*

      Transfemoral Access   *43*

      Alternative Access   *43*

   6. What is the importance of assessing the suitability of carotid embolic protection devices prior to TAVR?   *44*

   7. What is the best way to evaluate coronary arteries and coronary bypass grafts using CT scan?   *44*

   8. What is the importance of reporting the CT scan functional assessment, and what is the significance of cardiac and non-cardiac incidental findings?   *45*

   9. What is the best way to use myocardial extracellular volume (ECV) as a potential screening for cardiac amyloidosis and myocardial fibrosis?   *45*

  10. What is the best way to perform CT evaluation of valve-in-valve TAVR?   *45*

      Sizing   *46*

      Risk of Coronary Artery Obstruction   *46*

  11. What are the CT assessments in patients with bicuspid aortic valve prior to TAVR?   *47*

      Morphology   *47*

      High-Risk Features   *47*

      Annulus Size   *48*

Bibliography   *48*

6   Optimal Selection of TAVR Devices   *51*
   1. What types of transcatheter aortic valve replacement devices are commercially available?   *51*
   2. Are other TAVR devices under clinical investigation?   *51*
   3. Is there evidence to claim superiority of one type of TAVR device over the others?   *51*
   4. Are there situations in which one valve should be considered over another?   *52*
   5. Does annular size affect the choice of valve?   *53*
   6. What type of valve should be chosen based on aortic valve calcification?   *53*
   7. How does the risk of conduction abnormalities influence the choice of the TAVR device?   *54*
   8. Why are the risk of coronary occlusion and the need to reaccess the coronaries are important?   *55*
   9. What is the impact of aortic angulation on TAVR outcomes?   *56*
  10. What about bicuspid aortic valves?   *56*
  11. Should any other factors be considered for optimal selection of TAVR device?   *56*
   Clinical Vignette   *57*
   Bibliography   *58*

7   Transcatheter Aortic Valve Replacement
Step-by-Step Approach   *59*
   1. What is transcatheter aortic valve replacement (TAVR)?   *59*
   Patient Evaluation   *59*
   2. What are the current indications for TAVR?   *59*
   3. Are there any absolute contraindications to TAVR?   *59*
   Step-By-Step TAVR Approach   *59*
   4. What are the pre-procedural approach to and planning for successful TAVR?   *59*
   5. What are the steps during the TAVR procedure?   *60*
   Vascular Access   *60*
   6. What is the approach for vascular access during TAVR?   *60*
   7. What is the current best practice to establish femoral access safely?   *61*
   8. For patients with inadequate femoral access, what are the potential options for alternative arterial access for transcatheter valve delivery?   *61*
   9. What is the approach to axillary/subclavian artery access?   *62*
  10. What is the approach to carotid artery access?   *62*
  11. What is the approach for transaortic access for TAVR?   *62*
  12. What is the approach to transcaval access for TAVR?   *62*
  13. What is the approach to antegrade, transapical access?   *62*
  14. What is the approach to antegrade, transseptal access?   *62*
  15. What are the optimal vascular closure techniques for large-bore vascular access during TAVR?   *63*
   Balloon-Expandable Transcatheter Aortic Valve Replacement   *63*
  16. What are the components of the Edwards SAPIEN balloon-expandable valve?   *63*
  17. What are the essential considerations during balloon-expandable TAVR?   *64*
   Self-Expanding Transcatheter Aortic Valve Replacement   *65*
  18. What are the components of the self-expanding valve and catheter system?   *65*
  19. What are the essential considerations during self-expandable TAVR?   *66*
  20. Can the Evolut valve be repositioned during deployment?   *67*
  21. After valve implantation, how is adequate valve position confirmed?   *67*
   Conclusion   *67*
   Bibliography   *67*

8   Balloon Aortic Valvuloplasty
Current Clinical Role and Technical Aspects   *69*
   1. What are the guideline recommended indications for aortic balloon valvuloplasty (BAV)?   *69*
   2. What are the contra-indications to aortic balloon valvuloplasty?   *69*
   3. What are the goals of BAV and what defines a successful BAV?   *69*

4. What is the incidence of complications in BAV?   *70*

5. What are the balloon sizing considerations for BAV?   *70*

6. Which types of balloons are available for BAV?   *70*

7. What is the technique used to cross stenotic aortic valve?   *70*

8. How is the valvuloplasty balloon stabilized across the aortic valve during inflation?   *71*

9. What is the role of valvuloplasty in patients undergoing TAVR?   *71*

10. What is the role of BAV in patients with low-flow, low-gradient aortic stenosis?   *71*

11. What is the role of BAV to reduce cardiac complications of patients requiring non-cardiac surgery?   *71*

12. What is the post-procedure care of BAV patients?   *72*

13. What are the options for hemodynamically assisted aortic valvuloplasty?   *72*

Bibliography   *72*

9 Challenging Anatomy Scenarios in TAVR   *75*

Aortic Root   *75*

1. During transcatheter aortic valve replacement (TAVR), what are important principles for patients with severe aortic leaflet and annular calcification?   *75*

2. What unique risks exist during TAVR when there is minimal aortic leaflet and annular calcium?   *75*

3. How does sinotubular junction (STJ) calcification affect valve deployment?   *76*

4. What does "horizontal aorta" refer to during TAVR, and what techniques are required in this situation?   *76*

5. How should LVOT calcification affect valve deployment?   *76*

6. What is the role of TAVR in patients with bicuspid aortic valve disease?   *76*

7. What can be done for patients with a small aortic annulus?   *77*

8. How should a valve be correctly sized in an extremely large annulus?   *77*

9. What are the options for annular sizing in patients who cannot receive computer tomography (CT) with contrast?   *77*

Coronary Arteries   *78*

10. For what patient anatomy should you consider protecting the left main coronary artery?   *78*

11. How should you perform TAVR if a patient will likely need a future percutaneous coronary intervention (PCI)?   *78*

Aorta   *79*

12. Is it possible to perform a TAVR in a patient with an ascending aortic aneurysm?   *79*

13. What techniques allow transfemoral access for patients with a tortuous descending aorta?   *79*

14. Does the presence of a bovine arch prevent the placement of a cerebral embolic protection device?   *80*

Femoral Arterial Access   *80*

15. How can transfemoral TAVR be performed if there is significant iliac artery calcification?   *80*

16. How can transfemoral TAVR be performed if there is significant femoral artery calcification?   *80*

17. What can be done if there is only one patent iliofemoral artery?   *80*

18. If iliofemoral access is not feasible, what are different options for alternate access?   *80*

Valve-in-Valve (ViV)   *81*

19. When performing ViV TAVR, how do you choose the correct transcatheter valve?   *81*

20. What are the relevant considerations when potentially fracturing an existing surgical valve prior to ViV implantation?   *81*

21. What can be done if there is a high risk of coronary artery obstruction with ViV TAVR?   *81*

Bibliography   *82*

10 TAVR for Bicuspid Aortic Valve   *83*

Epidemiology   *83*

1. What is the prevalence of bicuspid aortic valves?   *83*

2. How is BAV identified?   *83*

3. How do patients with bicuspid AS undergoing transcatheter aortic valve replacement compare to patients with tricuspid AS?   *83*

Bicuspid Valve Morphology *83*

4. Match the illustrated valve morphologies to the correct bicuspid phenotypes according to the conventional Sievers classification and the newly derived CT classification (see figure 10.1). *83*

5. What anatomical characteristics commonly associated with BAVs may complicate TAVR? *84*

Procedural Planning *84*

6. What considerations should be taken into account when choosing a THV type (annular/supra-annular; balloon-expandable/self-expanding)? *84*

7. Can computer simulation complement pre-procedural TAVR planning? *85*

8. What sizing strategies exist for selecting THV size in bicuspid AS? *85*

9. What is recommended for pre-dilatation and post-dilatation? *86*

Outcomes *86*

10. How do outcomes of TAVR in bicuspid AS compare with tricuspid AS? *86*

11. Describe how the different bicuspid phenotypes (see question 4) impact outcome after TAVR. *86*

12. What features of the newer-generation THVs significantly improved the outcome of TAVR? *86*

Bibliography *87*

11 **TAVR for Pure Native Valve Aortic Regurgitation** *89*

1. How common is aortic regurgitation (AR)? *89*

2. What are the most common causes of NAVR? *89*

3. What are the natural history and prognosis of AR? *89*

4. What are the indications and the best timing for intervention of the aortic valve in AR? *89*

5. What is the recommended therapy for patients with severe NAVR and indication for intervention? *90*

6. What are the challenges of TAVR in pure NAVR? *90*

7. What is the available evidence evaluating TAVR for pure NAVR? *90*

8. What is the preferred type of THV for TAVR in pure NAVR? *91*

9. What are some critical technical considerations? *91*

Bibliography *93*

12 **Aortic Valve-in-Valve Interventions** *95*

1. Why are aortic valve-in-valve procedures needed? *95*

2. Why are ViV TAVR outcomes better than native valve TAVR? *95*

3. What are the primary limitations of aortic ViV TAVR? *95*

4. Why does the mechanism of bioprosthetic valve failure matter? *96*

5. How do you plan for a ViV procedure? *97*

6. How do you avoid PPM in aortic ViV procedures? *97*

Supra-Annular vs. Intra-Annular Design *98*

Implantation Technique (High vs. Low) *98*

High-Pressure Post-Dilation and Balloon Valve Fracture *98*

7. How do you prevent and treat coronary obstruction? *99*

BASILICA Procedure *99*

Chimney Technique *100*

8. How important is adjunct pharmacology after ViV-TAVI? *100*

Bibliography *101*

13 **Prevention and Management of Coronary Artery Obstruction in TAVR** *103*

1. What is the incidence of coronary artery obstruction in transcatheter aortic valve replacement (TAVR)? *103*

2. What is the mechanism of coronary artery obstruction in TAVR? *103*

3. Which coronary artery is most commonly obstructed during TAVR? *103*

4. What is delayed coronary obstruction after TAVR? *103*

5. What are the symptoms of coronary artery obstruction in TAVR?   *104*

6. What are the outcomes for patients that have coronary artery obstruction with TAVR?   *104*

7. What are risk factors for coronary artery obstruction with TAVR?   *104*

8. How do you prevent coronary artery obstruction with TAVR?   *105*

9. What is the treatment for coronary artery obstruction with TAVR?   *105*

10. What is preparatory coronary protection?   *106*

11. Explain the BASILICA procedure.   *106*

Bibliography   *107*

14 Coronary Artery Disease and Transcatheter Aortic Valve Replacement
Timing and Patient Selection for Coronary Intervention in Patients Planned for TAVR   *109*

1. How common is coronary artery disease (CAD) in patients with severe aortic stenosis (AS)?   *109*

2. What is the clinical impact of CAD on TAVR outcomes?   *109*

3. How do you assess for CAD prior to TAVR?   *109*

4. Can you use the instantaneous wave-free ratio (iFR) in patients with severe AS?   *109*

5. What is the role of percutaneous revascularization in TAVR?   *110*

6. What is the recommendation for the management of left main (LM) disease prior to TAVR?   *111*

7. What is the optimal timing for revascularization in patients being evaluated for TAVR?   *111*

8. What about completeness of revascularization in patients undergoing TAVR?   *111*

9. Are there technical considerations in patients undergoing PCI post-TAVR?   *112*

10. What is the current guideline for revascularization in patients undergoing TAVR?   *113*

Bibliography   *113*

15 Conduction Disturbances Associated with TAVR
Clinical Impact and Techniques to Minimize   *115*

1. What is the relationship between the aortic valve structures and the conduction system?   *115*

2. What is the incidence of conduction disturbances associated with TAVR?   *115*

3. What is the clinical impact of conduction disturbances after TAVR?   *116*

4. What are the predictors of conduction disturbances and PPI associated with TAVR?   *117*

5. What strategies can be implemented to prevent or minimize conduction disturbances associated with TAVR?   *117*

MIDAS Approach   *118*
Cusp Overlap Technique   *118*
Advantages of the Cusp Overlap Technique   *119*
Disadvantages of the Cusp Overlap View   *119*
High-implantation Technique for the Balloon-Expandable SAPIEN 3 Valve   *119*

6. Describe post-procedural monitoring and electrophysiological assessment after TAVR.   *120*

Bibliography   *120*

16 Management of Conduction Disturbances Post-TAVR   *123*

1. What are the components of normal conduction from sinus node to ventricular tissue?   *123*

2. Match the components of the conduction system to the following intervals   *123*

3. What components of the conduction system are susceptible to injury during transcatheter aortic valve replacement (TAVR) implantation?   *123*

4. At what operative stage can AV conduction abnormalities be encountered?   *124*

5. What changes to the EKG can be anticipated after TAVR?   *124*

6. What pre-operative EKG finding is the strongest predictor of post-TAVR conduction disturbances and pacemaker requirement? Why?   *124*

7. What procedural factors have been associated with higher risk of post-TAVR conduction disturbances?   *124*

8. At what point should a 12-lead EKG be performed to determine the duration of temporary pacing wire and post-operative telemetry?   *125*

9. A patient with the pre-operative EKG shown here undergoes TAVR. No change in EKG is seen at the end of the procedure. What is recommended for the duration of temporary pacing and telemetry monitoring? *125*

10. What is the likelihood that a patient with this EKG will require a pacemaker implant after TAVR? *125*

11. The patient in question 10 has no change in the 12-lead EKG at the end of the procedure. How long after the TAVR procedure is temporary pacing recommended? *126*

12. A patient who undergoes TAVR has the pre-operative EKG shown in (a) and the post-procedure EKG shown in (b). What management decisions are recommended for this scenario? *126*

13. The patient from question 12 develops the following EKG 10 hours after LBBB was noticed after TAVR. What pacemaker configuration will maintain atrioventricular synchrony? *126*

14. A patient with severe aortic stenosis and moderately reduced systolic function receives TAVR and develops the rhythm shown here, associated with dizziness, post-TAVR. What kind of pacing configuration is less likely to result in persistent systolic dysfunction? *127*

15. Pre-operatively, an 88-year-old man has the EKG shown in (a); 48 hours after TAVR, he has the EKG shown in (b). An electrophysiology study is performed. The intra-cardiac electrocardiograms are shown in (c). Does this patient require a pacemaker? *128*

Bibliography *129*

17 TAVR Mechanical Complications Prevention and Management *131*

Annular Rupture *131*
1. What constitutes annular rupture in TAVR? *131*
2. How do you classify annular rupture after TAVR? *131*
3. How often does annular rupture occur? *131*
4. Why does annular rupture happen with TAVR? *131*
5. What are the risk factors for annular rupture with TAVR? *131*
6. What are the outcomes of annular rupture? *132*
7. How do you diagnose annular rupture? *132*
8. How do you treat annular rupture? *132*
9. How do you prevent annular rupture? *133*

Perforation and Tamponade *133*
10. How does cardiac tamponade occur in TAVR? *133*
11. Why does ventricular perforation occur? *133*
12. How common is ventricular perforation in TAVR? *133*
13. How do you diagnose and manage perforation? *133*
14. What are the outcomes after perforation? *133*
15. How can you prevent cardiac perforations in TAVR? *134*

Bioprosthetic Valve Infolding *134*
16. What is prosthetic valve infolding? *134*
17. What are the consequences of prosthetic valve infolding? *134*
18. Why does valve infolding occur? *134*
19. What are risk factors for valve infolding? *134*
20. How common is valve infolding? *134*
21. How can you diagnose valve infolding? *134*
22. How do you treat valve infolding? *134*

Valve Embolization *135*
23. What is transcatheter valve embolization? *135*
24. How common is valve embolization? *135*
25. What is the cause of TVEM? *136*
26. How do you treat TVEM? *136*
27. How can you prevent TVEM? *137*

Bibliography *137*

18 Pathological Insights of TAVR Degeneration and Thrombosis *139*

Introduction *139*

Bioprosthetic Valve Failure (BVF) *139*
  1. What types of valve failure modes are observed in TAVR bioprostheses? *139*

Infective Endocarditis *139*
  2. What are the incidence and causative microorganisms of IE after TAVR? *139*
  3. What are the pathological findings of IE? *140*

Leaflet Thrombosis *140*
  4. What are the clinical relevancies of leaflet thrombosis? *140*
  5. What are the pathological findings of valve thrombosis? *141*

Neointimal Coverage and Pannus Formation *141*
  6. Is pannus formation seen in the TAVR valve? *141*
  7. What are the pathological findings of pannus formation and leaflet endothelialization in TAVR bioprostheses? *141*

Leaflet Calcification *142*
  8. What is the cause of leaflet calcification? *142*
  9. When is leaflet calcification seen after implantation? *143*
  10. What are the pathological findings of leaflet calcification? *143*

Structural Changes (Non-calcific Structural Valve Deterioration) *145*
  11. What are the other causes of SVD besides calcification? *145*

Durability of Bioprosthetic Valves *146*
  12. Is the durability of TAVR bioprostheses similar to that of SAVR bioprostheses? *146*
  13. Is the long-term durability the same in both TAVR and SAVR bioprostheses? *147*

Conclusion *147*
Bibliography *147*

19 Clinical Implications of Valve Thrombosis and Early Thickening
Management of Antiplatelets and Anticoagulation Post TAVI *151*
  1. What are the risk factors for transcatheter heart valve (THV) thrombosis? *151*
  2. What is the role of the routine use of anticoagulation post-transcatheter aortic valve implantation (TAVI) in the absence and a concurrent anticoagulation indication (such as atrial fibrillation)? *151*
  3. For bioprosthetic TAVI patients who do not have other indications for anticoagulation, is it appropriate to use a single antiplatelet agent, or is dual antiplatelet always necessary? *151*
  4. In the setting of bioprosthetic TAVI, for whom would dual antiplatelet therapy be indicated? *151*
  5. For bioprosthetic TAVI patients who have a stroke while on antiplatelet therapy, would it be reasonable to start on oral anticoagulation in place of antiplatelet therapy? *152*
  6. For bioprosthetic TAVI patients who have suspected valve thrombosis and are clinically stable, what would be the initial anticoagulation choice? *152*
  7. In the setting of bioprosthetic TAVI, what regimen would be indicated for a patient with concurrent atrial fibrillation and a CHA_2DS_2-Vasc Score of 4, but no other indication for antiplatelet therapy? *152*
  8. In the setting of bioprosthetic TAVI, what regimen would be indicated for a patient with concurrent atrial fibrillation and a CHA_2DS_2-Vasc Score of 4, as well as a recent coronary artery stent? *152*
  9. Which bioprosthetic TAVI patients should be on concurrent dual antiplatelet therapy as well as anticoagulation (i.e. triple therapy)? *152*
  10. For bioprosthetic TAVI patients with a concurrent indication for anticoagulation, are DOACs a reasonable alternative to VKAs? *152*
  11. What are the clinical implications of subclinical valve thrombosis, also called hypoattenuating leaflet thrombosis (HALT)? *152*

Bibliography *153*

20 TAVR and Stroke *155*

Introduction *155*
  1. Describe the evidence for TAVR. *155*

Stroke Following TAVR *156*
  2. What is the incidence of stroke following TAVR? *156*
  3. What are the predictors and impact of stroke associated with TAVR? *157*

Management of TAVR-Related Stroke *157*
  4. How can you prevent stroke related to TAVR? *157*
  5. What is the best way to treat stroke related to TAVR? *158*

Conclusions *159*
Bibliography *159*

21 Current Evidence of Neuroprotection in TAVR *163*

Peri-Procedural Stroke *163*
  1. Is the occurrence of peri-procedural strokes still the Achilles' heel of TAVR? *163*
  2. What is the underlying mechanism of stroke in TAVR patients? *163*
  3. What are the consequences of debris embolizing to the brain? *163*

The Rationale for Cerebral Embolic Protection Devices *163*
  4. How many TAVR patients are affected by embolized debris? *163*
  5. What kind of EPDs are currently available for TAVR? *164*
  6. Are other technologies in the pipeline? *164*

Characteristics of Dislodged Debris *164*
  7. What kind of debris may embolize toward the brain? *164*
  8. What is the captured debris size? *165*
  9. Are there any predicting factors for the dislodgement of debris? *165*
10. Who might benefit most from protected TAVR? *165*

Clinical Evidence of Neuroprotection In TAVR *165*
11. Is there a proven clinical benefit from randomized controlled trials (RCTs) to underpin the systematic use of cerebral embolic protection in **TAVR**? *165*
12. What will the future bring? *167*

Bibliography *167*

22 Difficult Transfemoral Access for TAVR and Bailout Techniques *169*
  1. What are the benefits of transfemoral access? *169*
  2. What is considered "high-risk" vascular anatomy for transfemoral TAVR? *169*
  3. How common is severe peripheral arterial disease in severe aortic stenosis patients? *169*
  4. How do you plan for a successful transfemoral TAVR procedure? *170*
  5. What are the most important technology developments for TF access success? *170*
      Size and Design of TAVR Delivery Systems *170*
      Ultrasound-Guided Vascular Access *170*
      Shockwave Intravascular Lithotripsy *171*

How to Approach High-Risk Vascular Anatomies *171*
  6. How do you approach small vessels? *171*
  7. Can endovascular pretreatment of Illofemoral atherosclerotic disease be performed? *172*
  8. How do you approach significant calcific peripheral disease? *172*
  9. How do you approach severe vascular tortuosity? *172*
10. Can TF TAVR be performed in patients with abdominal aortic aneurysms? *173*

Bibliography *173*

23 **Alternative Access for TAVR** *175*
   1. Why is TF access the gold standard for TAVR? *175*
   2. How are transapical and direct aortic access performed? *175*
   3. What are the important considerations when selecting transaxillary (TAx) access for TAVR? *176*
   4. How is TAx TAVR performed? *176*
   5. What are the advantages and important considerations of transcarotid (TC) access? *177*
   6. What is the physiology that allows for transcaval (TCV) access and prevents a life-threatening retroperitoneal bleed? *178*
   7. How is TCV access for TAVR performed? *178*
   8. How is TCV access closure performed? *179*

   Conclusion *180*
   Bibliography *181*

24 **Vascular Access and Closure Options for TAVR** *183*
   1. What constitutes pre-procedural vascular access evaluation? *183*
   2. What is the gold standard imaging technique for the anatomic evaluation of arterial access sites before TAVR? *183*
   3. What is the optimal arterial puncture technique for common femoral artery access? *183*
   4. What is the best technique for fluoroscopic confirmation of vascular sheath insertion in the common femoral artery? *184*
   5. What are the technical considerations to obtain optimal carotid and axillary artery access? *184*
   6. What are the technical considerations to obtain optimal transcaval access, and what techniques are helpful to achieve hemostasis after removal of large-caliber sheaths following transcaval approach? *185*
   7. What vascular closure devices are currently recommended after transfemoral interventions with large-caliber vascular sheaths? *185*
   8. What accounts for vascular access-site and access-related complications? *185*
   9. What is the incidence of vascular access complications? *187*
   10. What is the most appropriate management of an arterial dissection? *187*
   11. What is the most appropriate management of an arterial perforation? *187*
   12. What is the most appropriate management of retroperitoneal bleeding? *187*
   13. What is the most appropriate management of acute limb ischemia? *187*
   14. What methods can be used to prevent ischemic limbs when large bore access is occlusive? *188*

   Bibliography *188*

   Part II   **Structural Interventions for the Mitral Valve** *191*

25 **The Natural History of Mitral Valve Disease** *193*

   Mitral Stenosis *193*
   1. What are the causes of mitral stenosis (MS)? *193*
   2. What are the hemodynamic consequences of MS? *193*
   3. How are the hemodynamics of MS translated into symptoms? *193*
   4. How are the hemodynamics of MS translated into physical exam findings? *193*
   5. How is MS diagnosed (imaging and invasive hemodynamics)? *194*
   6. What are the indications for medical therapy of MS, and what do those therapies consist of? *195*
   7. What are the indications for mechanical therapy of MS, and what do those therapies consist of? *195*
   8. What is the prognosis of MS? *195*

Mitral Regurgitation 195

  9. What are the two major classes of MR? How do they differ in prognosis and therapy? 195

Primary Mitral Regurgitation 196

10. What are the major etiologies of PMR? 196

11. What are the hemodynamics of PMR? 196

12. How are PMR hemodynamics translated into symptoms? 197

13. How are PMR hemodynamics translated into physical signs? 197

14. How is PMR diagnosed (imaging and invasive hemodynamics)? 197

15. What are the indications for medical therapy in PMR, and what do those therapies consist of? 198

16. What are the indications for mechanical therapy of PMR, and what do those therapies consist of? What is the prognosis following treatment? 198

Secondary Mitral Regurgitation 198

17. What are the major etiologies of SMR? 198

18. What are the hemodynamics of SMR? 199

19. What are common myths about the hemodynamics of SMR? 199

20. How are SMR hemodynamics translated into symptoms? 199

21. How are SMR hemodynamics translated into physical signs? 199

22. How is SMR diagnosed (imaging and invasive hemodynamics)? 199

23. What are the indications for medical therapy in SMR, and what do those therapies consist of? 199

24. What are the indications for mechanical therapy of SMR, and what do those therapies consist of? 199

25. What is the prognosis of SMR? 200

Bibliography 200

26 Hemodynamic Assessment of the Mitral Valve 203

Mitral Stenosis 203

1. Why is it important to distinguish between rheumatic and nonrheumatic calcific mitral stenosis? 203

  2. What is the pathophysiology leading to the hemodynamic consequences of MS? 203

  3. When is it reasonable to consider intervention for MS? 203

  4. What are the findings on invasive hemodynamic assessment to suggest severe MS? 203

  5. What are the pitfalls of using PCWP as surrogate for LA pressure? 204

  6. What can cause an elevated transmitral gradient? 204

  7. What are the expected hemodynamics before and after PMBV? 205

  8. What is a dreaded immediate complication to monitor for during PMBV? 206

Mitral Regurgitation 206

  9. What are the common causes of primary and secondary MR? 206

10. What is the difference in pathophysiology leading to the hemodynamic consequences of acute vs. chronic MR? 206

11. What are mimickers that lead to a prominent *v* wave on PCWP or LA pressure tracings? 206

12. When is it reasonable to consider percutaneous intervention for MR? 206

13. What is the concept of *proportionately* and *disproportionately* severe secondary MR? 207

14. Alternatively, what is the difference between atrial and ventricular functional MR (AFMR vs. VFMR)? 207

15. What are the percutaneous MV interventions currently available and under investigation? 208

16. What are the expected hemodynamic changes after the most common percutaneous edge-to-edge repair with MitraClip? 208

Bibliography 208

27 Echocardiographic Assessment Prior to Mitral Valve Edge-to-Edge Repair 211

1. What is edge-to-edge mitral valve repair? 211

2. What is the role of pre-procedural transthoracic echocardiography (TTE) prior to edge-to-edge mitral valve repair? 211

3. How is MR classified? *211*
4. Which patients with primary MR would benefit the most from percutaneous edge-to-edge repair? *211*
5. Which patients with secondary MR would benefit the most from percutaneous edge-to-edge repair? *211*
6. Which are the most important views in the pre-procedural TTE? *212*
7. Why is pre-procedure transesophageal echocardiography (TEE) important? *212*
8. Which are the most important pre-procedural TEE views to assess for edge-to-edge mitral valve repair? *213*
9. What are the applications of 3D pre-procedural TEE for edge-to-edge repair? *213*
10. What are the differences between real-time 3D and multi-beat 3D acquisition, and how does this affect edge-to-edge mitral valve repair? *213*
11. Does 3D TEE add any information to the quantification of MR? *213*
12. From the EVEREST trial, which anatomy is considered suitable? *214*
13. Pair the figures with the appropriate measurements: (a) coaptation length, (b) coaptation depth, (c) flail gap, and (d) flail width. *215*
14. Which is the appropriate location for transseptal puncture? *215*

Bibliography *215*

28 Intra-procedural Transesophageal Echocardiography for Mitral Valve Structural Interventions *217*
1. Who is "qualified" to perform intra-procedural transesophageal echocardiography (TEE) for structural interventions on the mitral valve (MV)? *217*
2. Which structural mitral interventions is TEE most used for? *217*
3. What are the major views in 2D TEE used for MV structural interventions? *217*
4. Are there any advanced 2D imaging techniques that are useful in guiding structural heart interventions? *218*
5. What are the major views in 3D TEE used for MV structural interventions? *219*
6. Which 3D imaging modalities are most used in structural mitral interventions? *219*

Septal Puncture *220*
7. How is TEE used to guide TSP? *220*
8. What are the procedural-specific considerations for the echocardiographer during TSP? *220*

Edge-to-Edge Repair *220*
9. What measurements are commonly made by echocardiography prior to an edge-to-edge repair? *220*
10. What are the steps and imaging considerations for edge-to-edge repair? *221*
11. What are the unique features of the different generations of MitraClip devices that echocardiographers should be familiar with? *222*
12. What are some common "tricks" that can be used to help with leaflet grasp during the clip procedure? *222*
13. What are the key complications during MitraClip that echocardiographers need to consider? *222*

TMVR *222*
14. What is the role of the echocardiographer in TMVR? *222*
15. How do echocardiographers assist in sizing a valve during valve-in-valve and native valve TMVR? *223*
16. How do echocardiographers aid in valve deployment? *223*
17. Which echocardiographic parameters can predict LVOTO in native valve TMVR? *223*

Balloon Valvuloplasty *223*
18. Are there any special considerations the echocardiographer should be aware of during balloon valvuloplasty? *223*
19. What echocardiographic guided procedures are on the horizon? *224*
20. What are the health system implications of a growing field of structural heart interventions, as it relates to echocardiography? *224*

Paravalvular Leak Closure *225*
Bibliography *225*

29 Surgical Trials in Mitral Valvular Disease *227*

1. Describe the surgical therapy for acute MR. *227*
2. Discuss recent publications on mitral valve reconstruction being superior to replacement in chronic structural MR. *227*
3. Discuss recent publications about MV replacement having similar and non-inferior results in patients with secondary MR. *228*
4. Describe two published randomized trials assessing the outcome of percutaneous MV repair using the MitraClip for therapy of secondary MR. *228*
5. What are the surgical indications for MV repair? *228*
6. Describe the "double-orifice" surgical repair technique described by Alfieri et al. *228*
7. What are the surgical details of performing mitral ring annuloplasty? *229*
8. Should you resect the entire leaflet when replacing the valve? *229*
9. What is the ideal vascular access for VA extracorporeal membrane oxygenation (ECMO) implantation in patients undergoing mitral clip implantation? *229*
10. What are the possible surgical complications during and/or post surgical MV insertion? *229*
11. What size of surgical MV prosthesis placement enables later valve-in-valve implantation? *229*
12. Is persistent MR a negative predictive factor for patients requiring left ventricular assist device (LVAD) insertion? *229*
13. Why should the Heart Team discuss structural cases in detail before the procedure? *230*
14. The Heart Team is consulted on a case with persistent atrial septal defect (ASD) and a left-to-right shunt following mitral clip placement. What is the therapeutic intervention? *230*

Bibliography *230*

30 Surgical Techniques for Mitral Valve Repair *233*

1. What are the stages of primary mitral regurgitation (MR)? *233*
2. When should patients be considered for surgical repair of their MR? *233*
3. Should mitral valves (MVs) be repaired or replaced? What are the advantages? *233*
4. What is SAM, and what are the risk factors for developing it? *233*
5. What is the best initial step when SAM is identified while coming off cardiopulmonary bypass? *234*
6. What should a surgeon do if SAM is still present after initial conservative measures to slow the heart rate and reduce inotropic support? *234*
7. Describe standard surgical approaches to the MV *234*
8. Which patients should be considered for MitraClip or other transcatheter edge-to-edge repair? *235*
9. When should a surgeon consider a MV replacement? What techniques should be used? *235*
10. What is a papillary muscle sling, and when may it be of benefit? *235*
11. How much MR is acceptable following a mitral repair? *235*
12. When is the appropriate time to assess the success of MV repair? *236*
13. What are the advantages of a Heart Team and center of excellence? *236*

Bibliography *236*

31 Structural Interventions for Mitral Stenosis *239*

1. What are the current classification criteria for mitral stenosis (MS)? *239*
2. What are the current indications and contraindications for percutaneous MV intervention in rheumatic MS? *239*
3. What are the predictors of successful/failed PMV? *239*
4. What are the techniques for PMV? *240*

Mitral Balloon Valvuloplasty *242*
5. What are the steps to perform PMV with the Inoue technique? *242*

Equipment List *242*
Balloon Selection *242*
Procedure Detail *242*
6. What are the steps to perform PMV with the antegrade double-balloon technique? *244*

Balloon Selection *244*

Procedure Detail *244*

7. What is the follow-up protocol after PMV? *244*

8. What are the potential complications of PMV? *244*

Hemopericardium *246*

Mitral Regurgitation *246*

Iatrogenic Interatrial Septal Defect *246*

9. What is the role of transcatheter therapy for rheumatic MS in women who are pregnant or contemplating pregnancy? *246*

Before Pregnancy *246*

During Pregnancy *246*

10. What is the role of PMV in patients with aortic regurgitation? *246*

11. What is the role of PMV in patients with concomitant severe tricuspid regurgitation? *246*

12. Should PMV be attempted in patients with MV calcification? *247*

13. Can PMV be done in patients with previous PMV? *247*

14. What are the roles of transcatheter intervention in patients with nonrheumatic calcific MS? *247*

15. What are the current and future transcatheter therapies for nonrheumatic MS? *247*

Transcatheter Mitral Valve Replacement (TMVR) Using Balloon-Expandable Transcatheter Aortic Valves in Mitral Position *247*

Future Directions of TMVR in Non-rheumatic MS *248*

Bibliography *248*

32 Transcatheter Edge-to-Edge Repair Trials
The EVEREST and COAPT Trials *251*

Edge-to-Edge Mitral Valve Repair (EVEREST Trials) *251*

1. What is the difference between primary and secondary mitral regurgitation? *251*

2. What is the basis of edge-to-edge mitral valve (MV) repair? *251*

3. What was the purpose of the EVEREST Phase I clinical trial? *251*

4. What were the results of EVEREST Phase 1? *251*

5. What was the basis of the EVEREST II trial? *253*

6. Describe the patient population in EVEREST II *253*

7. What were the endpoints for comparison used in EVEREST II? *253*

8. What were the results of EVEREST II? *253*

9. What are the takeaway messages of EVEREST II? *253*

Secondary MR and Transcatheter Repair (COAPT Trial) *253*

10. What was the purpose of the COAPT trial? *253*

11. Describe the patient population of the COAPT trial. *254*

12. What were the endpoints of the COAPT trial? *254*

13. What were the results of the COAPT trial? *254*

14. What are the takeaway messages from the COAPT trial? *255*

15. What are the guidelines for transcatheter MV repair in secondary MR? *255*

Bibliography *255*

33 Mitral Valve TEER
The MitraClip Procedure *257*

Introduction *257*

1. What are the anatomical and pathophysiologic considerations of the mitral valve in evaluating patients for TEER? *257*

2. What is the difference between primary mitral valve insufficiency related to degenerative mitral valve disease and secondary functional mitral insufficiency? *258*

3. What is the Heart Team approach to evaluation for mitral valve therapies? *258*
4. What patients are appropriate to consider for surgical mitral valve repair vs. the TEER procedure using the MitraClip device? *259*
5. What are the current indications for the TEER procedure using the MitraClip device? *259*
6. Are there any absolute contraindications to TEER? *259*
7. Aside from the absolute contraindications, what are the relative contraindications to be aware of for TEER? *259*
8. Is the presence of a transcatheter atrial septal defect (ASD) occlusion device a contraindication for TEER? *259*
9. What are the important aspects and key questions in the pre-procedural imaging during the pre-operative evaluation for TEER? *259*
10. In degenerative valve disease including mitral valve prolapse and/or flail mitral valve leaflets, what are the important aspects to assess during the pre-procedural TEE? *260*
11. What are the anatomical considerations for percutaneous TEER? *260*
12. What are the minimal MVA requirements for TEER? *260*
13. What are the important aspects in the assessment of the atrial septum for adequate transseptal access? *260*
14. What are the current literature and trial results using TEER for the treatment of degenerative mitral valve insufficiency? *260*
15. What are the current data for the treatment of functional mitral valve insufficiency? *261*
16. Why do the results from the MITRA-FR and COAPT studies differ so significantly? *261*
17. What are the real-world experience and outcomes using the MitraClip for TEER? *262*

The MitraClip Device *262*
18. What are the components of the MitraClip catheter system? *262*
19. What are the differences between the currently available clips? *262*
20. Are there any evidence-based recommendations for using the NTR vs. XTR clips? *262*

Echocardiographic Imaging *263*
21. What is the role of echocardiography and TEE during TEER? *263*
22. What are the essential TEE views to obtain during TEER? *263*

Procedure *263*
23. What are the steps involved in TEER? *263*
24. What are the preferred access site and vascular closure approaches during TEER? *263*
25. What equipment is necessary for transseptal puncture for TEER? *264*
26. What is the procedure for transseptal puncture for TEER? *264*
27. What are the optimal TEE views during transseptal puncture? *264*
28. What is the optimal positioning for transseptal puncture for TEER? *264*
29. How is the delivery system advanced into the LA? *265*
30. How is the delivery system advanced into the LA and directed toward the mitral valve leaflets? *265*
31. What are the steps for grasping the leaflets with the MitraClip? *266*
32. Prior to deployment, how is the MitraClip assessed to ensure adequate position, grasp, and results? *266*
33. How do you assess mitral valve stenosis during clip deployment? *266*
34. What should you do if the device becomes entrapped in the chordal apparatus during TEER? *266*
35. After deployment, how is the adequacy of the edge-to-edge repair assessed? *266*
36. If there is residual MR after the initial MitraClip, can additional clips be placed? How does the operator decide when and how to deliver additional clips during TEER? *269*

Special Patient Subgroups and Considerations *269*
37. Can TEER still be used in patients with complex mitral valve pathology? *269*
38. Can TEER still be used in patients with mitral valve and/or mitral annular calcification? *270*
39. What are the applications and limitations of TEER in patients with restricted posterior mitral valves, mitral valve clefts, and/or flail mitral valve leaflets? *270*

Conclusion *270*
Bibliography *270*

34 TEER Challenging Anatomy and MitraClip Tips and Tricks *273*

Introduction *273*
  1. What are the Alfieri stitch and transcatheter edge-to-edge repair techniques? *273*
  2. What is the MitraClip system? *273*

MitraClip for the Myxomatous Mitral Valve *273*
  3. What are the anatomical findings of myxomatous mitral valve disease? *273*
  4. Where are some key strategies to increase success in TEER treatment of DMD? *274*
  5. When should an additional clip be placed? *275*

MitraClip for Wide Flail Leaflets *276*
  6. What is considered a wide flail MV prolapse? *276*
  7. What are the technical considerations when treating wide flail mitral leaflets? *276*

Noncentral and Commissural Lesions *276*
  8. How common is noncentral MR, and can it be treated using TEER? *276*
  9. Where should the transseptal puncture be positioned for medial mitral regurgitant lesions? *276*
  10. How is the optimal MitraClip arm angle determined? *277*
  11. What are the strategies to avoid and deal with entanglement? *277*
  12. How can vascular plugs and cardiac occluders be used to treat commissural lesions? *277*

Calcified Mitral Valve *277*
  13. Did the EVEREST and COAPT trials include patients with calcification of the MV? *277*
  14. Is TEER feasible in patients with calcified MV apparatus? *277*

Secondary Mitral Regurgitation *278*
  15. What are the anatomical considerations of secondary MR? *278*
  16. What are the key strategies to success in treating secondary MR? *278*
  17. When should an additional clip be placed? *278*

Bibliography *279*

35 MitraClip Complications
Prevention and Management *281*

Introduction *281*
  1. What is the incidence of vascular complications from the MitraClip procedure? *281*
  2. How can you prevent vascular complications during the MitraClip procedure? *282*

Transseptal Puncture Complications *282*
  3. What are the complications of a transseptal puncture during the MitraClip procedure? *282*

Complications from Device Navigation in the Left Atrium: Air Embolism and Thrombus Formation *283*
  4. What are the complications of device navigation in the LA? *283*

Complications from Leaflet Grasping *284*
  5. What complications may occur during leaflet grasping? *284*
  6. What is a single leaflet device attachment? *284*
  7. How is SLDA treated? *285*
  8. How is SLDA prevented? *286*
  9. What is the incidence of MitraClip embolization? *286*
  10. How can you manage clip embolization? *286*

Complications from Device Deployment *286*
  11. What is the incidence of residual MR after the MitraClip procedure? *286*
  12. How is residual MR treated? *287*
  13. What is the incidence of iatrogenic MS after MitraClip implantation? *287*
  14. What are the complications of elevated mean MV gradients post-MitraClip implantation? *288*

15. How can you prevent iatrogenic MS? *288*

16. What is the incidence of iatrogenic atrial septal defects post-MitraClip procedure? *288*

17. What are the clinical implications of persistent iASD? *288*

18. What are the indications for device closure of persistent iASD? *288*

Bibliography *289*

36 CT Imaging for TMVR *291*

1. What are the important components of the mitral valve apparatus that are important to know for TMVR planning? *291*

2. What is the role of echocardiography in TMVR? *291*

3. What are the advantages of utilizing multi-detector computed tomography (MDCT) in TMVR planning? *292*

4. What are the basic CT scanner image acquisition concepts and technical protocols required for obtaining a usable mitral CT? *293*

5. How is the TMVR landing zone sized and evaluated? *294*

6. What is the neo-LVOT? *294*

7. How can neo-LVOT be predicted? *295*

8. What factors make neo-LVOT prediction modeling complex? *295*

9. Which type of TMVR is at greatest risk of LVOT obstruction: valve-in-valve, valve-in-ring, or valve-in-MAC? *297*

10. How can CT imaging estimate the coplanar fluoroscopic angle? *297*

11. What are other relevant adjacent structures to consider in CT planning for TMVR? *298*

12. What are the important measurements and characteristics to define prior to the transseptal approach for TMVR? *298*

13. What are the important measurements and characteristics to define prior to the transapical approach for TMVR? *299*

14. What is the role of CT in post-procedural imaging? *299*

Conclusion *300*

Bibliography *300*

37 Transcatheter Mitral Valve Replacement

Transcatheter Mitral Valve-in-Valve (ViV), Valve-in-Ring (ViR), and Valve-in-MAC (ViMAC) *301*

1. What is the best way to approach a patient with a failing bioprosthetic mitral valve? *301*

2. What are the important anatomic variables on cardiac computerized tomography to consider when evaluating a patient for TMVR suitability? *302*

3. What is the best way to approach and evaluate a patient with a failing mitral ring in preparation for a ViR procedure? *302*

4. What are the ideal rings in the market for ViR procedures? *303*

5. What fluoroscopic landmarks are important for positioning THVs for ViV and ViR procedures? *303*

6. What are the available treatment options for severe mitral annular calcification? *303*

7. What are favorable characteristics for transcatheter valve anchoring in severe mitral annular calcification? *303*

8. What is the ideal location for a transseptal puncture for TMVR? *304*

9. What are the indications to close the transseptal septostomy site after TMVR? *304*

10. What are the steps taken to perform the procedure? *304*

11. What are potential complications associated with TMVR and the solutions to managing them? *304*

12. What are the contraindications for ViV or ViR procedures? *305*

13. What are the procedural success rates and complications associated with TMVR? *305*

14. What factors are responsible for left ventricular outflow tract obstruction (LVOTO) after ViV and ViR? *305*

15. What is the anticoagulation/antiplatelet strategy after TMVR? *306*

16. What cases are better performed transseptal vs transapical? *307*

Conclusion *308*

Bibliography *308*

38 Transseptal Transcatheter Mitral Valve-in-Valve Replacement (TS MViV)
Technical Considerations and Step-by-Step Procedure *311*
   1. What are the important pre-procedural considerations in transseptal mitral valve-in-valve replacement ? *311*
   2. What are the important recommendations for patient preparation and the room setting for the TS MViV procedure? *311*
   3. What steps should be followed for a successful TS MViV procedure? *311*
   4. What is important for vascular access during TS MViV? *311*
   5. Should the femoral vein access be pre-closed? *311*
   6. How do you obtain baseline LVOT hemodynamics during TS MViV? *312*
   7. How do you perform a safe transseptal puncture at an optimal location for TS MViV? *312*
   8. When do you insert the Edwards E sheath? *312*
   9. How do you cross the surgical mitral valve into the LV? *312*
   10. How do you perform atrial septostomy dilation? *312*
   11. How do you prepare the transcatheter valve for the TS MViV? *313*
   12. Should the surgical mitral valve be pre-dilated? *314*
   13. How do you advance and position the delivery system? *314*
   14. How do you cross the septum and the mitral valve with the delivery system and THV? *314*
   15. How do you position and implant the THV during TS MViV? *314*
   16. What is important in the post–valve deployment assessment? *314*
   17. When should atrial septostomy closure be considered? *314*
   18. How do you obtain adequate hemostasis at the vascular access site? *315*

   Potential Obstacles and Bailout Strategies *315*
   19. What can be done if the THV is not crossing the septum? *315*
   20. What can be done if the THV is not crossing the mitral orifice? *315*

   Bibliography *315*

39 Transseptal Systems for TMVR and Transcatheter Devices for Mitral Annuloplasty *317*
   1. Is there any role for percutaneous treatment of mitral valve disease? *317*
   2. What are the different transcatheter MV techniques? *317*
   3. What is transcatheter mitral valve replacement (TMVR), and how does it differ from transcatheter aortic valve replacement (TAVR)? *318*
   4. What TMVR devices are available? *319*
   5. What is transcatheter MV repair? *320*
   6. What is transcatheter MV annuloplasty? *320*
   7. What are some devices for transcatheter indirect MV annuloplasty? *321*
   8. What are some devices for transcatheter direct MV annuloplasty? *322*
   9. What are some other devices for transcatheter MV repair? *323*
   10. What is the future of transcatheter treatment of MV disease? *323*

   Bibliography *324*

40 Transcatheter Mitral Valve Replacement
The Tendyne System *325*
   1. What is the rationale for the Tendyne transcatheter mitral valve replacement system? *325*
   2. What are the indications and contraindications for considering TMVR with the Tendyne system? *327*
   3. What are the anatomic variables to consider on pre-operative imaging when evaluating a patient for TMVR using Tendyne? *327*
   4. What is the approach to Tendyne valve implantation, and what are the unique features? *327*
   5. What are specific challenges and potential complications of TMVR with the Tendyne system? *328*

   Conclusions *329*
   Acknowledgments *329*
   Bibliography *329*

41 Self-Expanding Transcatheter Mitral Valve Replacement Systems

Medtronic Intrepid Valve *331*

1. What are the key features of the Medtronic Intrepid transcatheter mitral valve replacement (TMVR) valve? *331*
2. How does the Medtronic Intrepid valve achieve fixation and sealing? *331*
3. How does the Medtronic Intrepid valve heal in the heart? *331*
4. What are the available delivery systems for the Medtronic Intrepid valve? *332*
5. How is the Medtronic Intrepid valve deployed via transapical delivery? *332*
6. What has been the experience with the Medtronic Intrepid transapical delivery system? *332*
7. What has been the experience with the Medtronic Intrepid transseptal delivery system? *333*

Conclusions *334*
Bibliography *334*

Part III   Structural Interventions for the Tricuspid Valve *335*

42 Natural History and Hemodynamic Assessment of Tricuspid Valve Diseases *337*

Epidemiology, Natural History, and Prognosis *337*
1. How prevalent is tricuspid regurgitation? *337*
2. What is the significance of TR? *337*

Anatomy *337*
3. What are the four components of the tricuspid valve? *337*
4. How do we classify TR, and what diseases fall into each category? *337*
5. What are the signs and symptoms of TR? *338*

Evaluation/Diagnosis *338*
6. What are the major imaging modalities used to assess the tricuspid valve? *338*
7. What are the advantages of each of these imaging modalities? *338*
8. How is the tricuspid valve evaluated with echocardiography? *339*
9. What are the characteristics of severe TR? *339*

Management *340*
10. What are the broad categories of TR management? *340*
11. When is surgery considered the preferred option? *340*
12. What are the surgical methods for TR management? *340*
13. Which patients are considered for TTVI? *340*
14. What challenges are associated with TTVI? *340*
15. What are the major categories of TTVI? *340*

Bibliography *340*

43 Indications and Outcomes for Surgical Tricuspid Valve Repair *343*

Tricuspid Regurgitation (Tricuspid Valve Insufficiency) *343*
1. What are known etiologies associated with TR? *343*
2. What is the reported mortality rate for surgical repair of TR? *343*
3. Are there better clinical results using transcatheter tricuspid valve intervention (TTVI)? *343*
4. Describe a surgical assessment and repair technique to repair a tricuspid valve *344*
5. Which transcatheter annuloplasty technique resembles the surgical DeVega and Kay techniques? *345*
6. What are some of the most frequently described surgical annuloplasty systems in the literature? *345*
7. What is the outcome of TR repair and LVAD implantation in patients not responding to advanced medical heart failure therapy? *345*

Bibliography *345*

44 Intra-Procedural Imaging of Tricuspid Valve Edge-to-Edge Interventions *347*

Introduction *347*
  1. Is it important to understand the structures adjacent to the tricuspid valve? *348*
  2. What should the transesophageal imaging protocol be? *348*
  3. Why is Tricuspid valve imaging challenging? *349*
  4. What are the steps in TV imaging? *349*
  5. How is TR graded? *350*
  6. How should post-procedural imaging be graded? *351*

Bibliography *352*

45 Transcatheter Tricuspid Valve Device Landscape *353*
  1. What is the magnitude of tricuspid regurgitation disease and its impact on patient outcomes? *353*
  2. What is the pathophysiology of TR? *353*
  3. What are the current medical and surgical recommendations for managing TR? *353*
  4. What are the main surgical TV repair techniques? *354*
  5. What are the main challenges associated with transcatheter TV interventions? *354*
  6. What transcatheter repair and replacement options are available? *354*

Leaflet-Directed Therapies *355*
Annular-Reshaping Therapies *357*
Direct Ring Annuloplasty Therapies *357*
Indirect Ring Annuloplasty Therapies *358*
Direct Suture Annuloplasty Therapies *358*
Heterotopic Caval Valve Implantation (CAVI) *359*
Bibliography *359*

46 Progress in Transcatheter Tricuspid Valve Repair and Replacement *363*
  1. Describe the anatomy of the tricuspid valve. *363*
  2. What are the causes and pathophysiology of tricuspid regurgitation? *363*
  3. What are the signs and symptoms of TR? *364*
  4. What are the indications of treatment of TR in the current guidelines? *365*
  5. What constitutes the pre-procedural planning for tricuspid valve intervention? *365*
    Echocardiography *365*
    Multi-detector Computed Tomography *367*
  6. What are the indications of transcatheter tricuspid valve replacement? *368*
  7. What are different types, outcomes, and complications of transcatheter tricuspid valve replacement devices? *370*
    Coaptation Devices *370*
    Suture Annuloplasty Systems *371*
    Ring Annuloplasty Systems *372*
    Heterotopic Devices *373*
    Orthotopic Devices *373*
    Complications *374*
    Future Development of Devices *374*
  8. What are the limitations of transcatheter tricuspid valve replacement? *374*

Bibliography *379*

47 Tricuspid Valve-in-Valve and Valve-in-Ring *383*

Tricuspid Regurgitation *383*
  1. How is tricuspid regurgitation classified? *383*
  2. When should TR be treated? *383*

Surgical TV Annuloplasty *383*

  3. What is the rationale behind TV annuloplasty? *383*

  4. What are the most common suture-based annuloplasty techniques? *384*

  5. What are the properties of prosthetic rings? *384*

  6. What are the outcomes of TV annuloplasty? *384*

  7. How can the results of TV annuloplasty be predicted? *384*

  8. What is the role of imaging after a failed surgical TV annuloplasty? *385*

  9. What information can be obtained from computed tomography? *385*

  10. How do you manage a failed tricuspid annuloplasty? *385*

Transcatheter Tricuspid Valve-in-Ring Procedure *386*

11. Can you always perform a TTViR? *386*

12. What does the literature say about TTViR procedures? *386*

Transcatheter Tricuspid Valve-In-Valve Procedure *387*

13. What is the rate of bioprosthetic TV failure? *387*

14. What does the literature say about TTViV procedures? *387*

Conclusions *387*

Bibliography *388*

48 Caval Valve Implantation (CAVI) for the Treatment of Severe Tricuspid Regurgitation *391*

  1. What is the concept behind caval valve implantation (CAVI)? *391*

  2. What is the initial data to support CAVI as a treatment for TR? *391*

  3. Who is a candidate for CAVI? *391*

  4. What information is needed to perform CAVI? *391*

  5. What are the steps in CAVI? *391*

  6. What are the current data with CAVI? *392*

  7. What is the future of CAVI? *393*

  8. What are the unknowns of CAVI? *393*

Bibliography *393*

Part IV Structural Interventions for Management of Paravalvular Leaks *395*

49 Aortic Paravalvular Leak Closure

Techniques and Devices for Surgical and Transcatheter Prostheses *397*

  1. What are the indications for percutaneous aortic paravalvular leak (PVL) closure? *397*

  2. What are the contraindications for percutaneous aortic PVL closure? *397*

  3. How do you plan an aortic PVL closure procedure? *397*

  4. How do you cross the aortic PVL defect? *397*

  5. What are the techniques to deliver occluder devices? *397*

  6. How to negotiate an uncrossable defect? *399*

  7. What are the device choices for aortic PVL closure? *399*

  8. What are the mechanisms and treatments for post-transcatheter aortic valve replacement (TAVR) PVL? *399*

  9. What are the specific anatomical challenges to close post-transcatheter aortic valve PVLs? *399*

10. What are some tips and tricks while closing post-TAVR PVLs? *399*

11. What are the potential complications of aortic PVL closure? *400*

Bibliography *400*

50 Mitral Paravalvular Leak: Imaging and Interventional Approaches *403*

Imaging *403*

Echocardiography *403*

  1. What imaging modality should be considered first with suspicion of mitral PVL following repair? *403*

2. What are the limitations of TTE in assessing mitral PVL? What are adjunctive quantitative measures used to ascertain mitral PVL? *403*

3. What is the next study considered after screening TTE for better visualization of the MV? *403*

4. What nomenclature is used to anatomically define the PVL location? Where are severe mitral PVLs most often found? *404*

5. What echocardiographic parameters exist for grading the severity of mitral PVLs? *404*

6. What role does 3D TEE play in evaluating mitral PVLs? *406*

7. What role does cardiac MRI play in evaluating mitral PVLs? *406*

8. What role does cardiac CT play in evaluating mitral PVLs? What are some of its limitations? *407*

9. What are the potential benefits of using intracardiac echocardiography in percutaneous leak closure? *407*

10. What combination imaging modalities are useful when evaluating and intervening in mitral PVLs? *408*

Transcatheter Closure of Mitral PVLs *408*

11. What is the most common approach to mitral PVL closure? *408*

    Anterograde Transseptal Approach *408*

    Transseptal Puncture *408*

12. Describe the approach an interventionalist should take with transseptal puncture. How does this change with (a) posterior defects, (b) anterior defects, and (c) medial defects? *408*

13. In what position should the fluoroscopic gantries be oriented for transseptal puncture? What techniques or equipment should be considered when performing transseptal puncture? *409*

14. Describe the retrograde transapical approach to mitral PVL closure *410*

15. Describe the retrograde femoral approach to mitral PVL closure *411*

    Retrograde Femoral Approach *411*

    Hybrid Anterograde-Retrograde Approach *411*

Defect Crossing and Telescoping Catheters *411*

16. Describe the steps required to cross a mitral PVL *411*

17. Describe the concept of telescoping catheters for mitral PVL closure *412*

Device Selection *412*

18. What are common devices used for mitral PVL closure? *412*

Device Deployment *413*

19. What technique should be used for single-device deployment? *413*

20. What techniques should be considered with multiple-device deployment? *413*

    Simultaneous Deployment Technique (Double Wire) *413*

    Sequential Deployment Technique (Anchor Wire) *413*

21. What technique can be used to increase stability for catheter passage across a serpiginous defect that is difficult to cross? *413*

    Sequential Deployment Technique Using Arteriovenoous or Transapical Rail *413*

Conclusion *413*

Bibliography *414*

Part V   Left Atrial Appendage Closure *415*

51 Current Indications for Percutaneous Left Atrial Appendage Occlusion *417*

1. Is there a rationale for left atrial appendage occlusion (LAAO)? *417*

2. Left atrial appendage occlusion: why percutaneous? *418*

3. What is the level of evidence supporting percutaneous LAAO? *418*

RCTs for Percutaneous LAAO *418*

Registries for Percutaneous Left Atrial Occlusion *418*

4. What are the current US society recommendations for percutaneous LAAO? *420*

5. Are there additional considerations related to LAAO? *420*

Bibliography *421*

52 Imaging for LAA Interventions *425*

Cardiac CT Pre-procedural Planning *425*
1. What are the main objectives of pre-procedural cardiac tomography in left atrium appendage occlusion? *425*
2. How should the patient be prepared before CT? *425*
3. What is the technical protocol for imaging acquisition? *425*
4. Explain how to exclude the presence of thrombus in the LAA with CT *426*
5. How is anatomic feasibility of LAAO assessed by CT? *426*

TEE Pre-procedural Planning *427*
6. What is the role of transthoracic echocardiography (TTE) before LAA closure procedure? *427*
7. What are the objectives of TEE in pre-procedural planning for LAAO? *427*
8. How should the measurements of the LAA be performed during pre-procedural TEE? *427*
9. What is the advantage of using 3D TEE compared with 2D TEE? *427*
10. Apart from LAA sizing, what other information is relevant during pre-procedural planning with TEE? *427*
11. Which imaging technique is preferred for pre-procedural planning for LAAO? *427*

Intra-procedural TEE and ICE Guided Intervention *428*
12. Which imaging modalities can be used for intra-procedural guidance in LAA closure? *428*
13. What are the main objectives of intra-procedural TEE during LAAO? *428*
14. What are the best perspectives for each of the steps of the procedure? *429*
15. Explain how transseptal puncture is guided with TEE *429*
16. When is the device considered to be correctly placed within the LAA? *430*
17. When intracardiac echocardiography is used to guide TEE, where should the probe be placed? *430*
18. What are the advantages of double transseptal puncture for ICE probe transseptal crossing? *431*
19. Is ICE a safe and effective alternative to TEE for intra-procedural LAAO guidance? *431*

Bibliography *431*

53 Devices for Left Atrial Appendage Closure *433*
1. LAA occlusion: does one device fit all? *433*
2. What are the main differences among LAA occlusion device designs? *433*
3. What are the characteristic of the WATCHMAN FLX device? *434*
4. What are the characteristics of the Amulet device? *435*
5. What are the characteristic of the LAmbre device? *436*
6. Lobe and disc vs. plug: is one approach superior to the other? *436*
7. What is in the pipeline? *437*

Bibliography *438*

54 LAA Occlusion Technique and Challenging Scenarios *441*
1. What are the main prerequisites for left atrial appendage occlusion (LAAO)? *441*
2. What are the main imaging techniques employed to guide LAAO? *441*
3. What are the mains steps of LAAO? *441*
4. What features of femoral venous access are most relevant for LAAO? *441*
5. What are the keys steps for TSP? *441*
6. Can LAAO be performed through a patent foramen oval (PFO) or atrial septum defect (ASD)? *443*
7. What steps are required to position the delivery system at the LAA? *443*
8. How is device sizing performed? *443*
9. What are the anatomical landmarks for LAAO device implantation? *444*
Device Deployment *444*
10. What specific considerations must be taken into account with each dedicated LAAO device? *444*
WATCHMAN FLX *444*
Amulet *445*
LAmbre *446*

Ultraseal *446*

11. What are the main steps to perform a "sandwich technique"? *446*
12. What other LAA anatomies can pose a challenge for LAAO? *447*
13. Can LAAO be performed in the presence of LAA thrombus? *447*

References *447*

55 Preventing and Managing Complications of LAA Closure *449*

1. What is the relevance of this topic? *449*

Pericardial Effusion (PE) *449*

2. What is the current incidence of PE? *449*
3. What are the causes of PE, and how can they be prevented? *449*
4. How do you manage a LAAC-related PE? *450*

Device Embolization *450*

5. What is the current incidence of device embolization (DE)? *450*
6. What are the causes of DE, and how can it be prevented? *450*
7. What can be clinical manifestations of DE? *450*
8. How can you perform a device retrieval? *450*

Air Embolism (AE) *451*

9. What are the manifestations of AE? *451*
10. What are the causes of AE, and how can it be prevented? *451*
11. How do you treat AE? *451*

Periprocedural Ischemic Stroke *451*

12. What is the current incidence of periprocedural ischemic stroke (PIS)? *451*
13. What are the causes of PIS, and how can it be prevented? *451*

Complications Related to Vascular Access *452*

14. What are the complications related to access, and how can they be prevented? *452*

Peri-device Leaks (PDLs) *452*

15. What are the clinical relevance and incidence of PDLs? *452*
16. What are the related factors or mechanisms? *452*
17. What are the treatment options for PDL? *452*

Device-Related Thrombus (DRT) *452*

18. What are the incidence and clinical relevance of DRT? *452*
19. What factors predispose patients to DRT, and how can it be prevented? *452*
20. How do you diagnose DRTs? *453*
21. How do you treat DRTs? *453*
22. What other complications have been described? *454*

Bibliography *454*

Part VI Selected Structural Interventions for Cardiomyopathies *457*

56 The Natural History of Hypertrophic Cardiomyopathy *459*

1. What is hypertrophic cardiomyopathy? *459*
2. What is the prevalence of HCM? *459*
3. Is left ventricular outflow tract obstruction a common occurrence in patients with HCM? *459*
4. What is the prognosis of an individual with HCM? *459*
5. Are there predictors of sudden cardiac death? *459*
6. How is a diagnosis of HCM made? *459*
7. Is genetic testing helpful? *460*

8. Are there multiple HCM-related genes? *460*

9. Are all individuals with HCM affected similarly? *460*

10. What kind of symptoms does HCM cause? *460*

11. Are there measures that should be undertaken in all individuals with HCM, even those with no symptoms? *460*

12. What treatment is available for individuals with symptoms? *460*

13. What medical therapy is recommended? *460*

14. Does medical therapy "cure" the problem of HCM? *461*

15. What is alcohol septal ablation? *461*

16. What is septal myectomy? *461*

17. What is permanent pacing, and how is it helpful to the symptomatic HCM patient? *461*

Bibliography *461*

57 Alcohol Septal Ablation in Hypertrophic Cardiomyopathy *463*

1. In the group of patients with hypertrophic cardiomyopathy (HCM) who fail medical therapy, what proportion are candidates for alcohol septal ablation? *463*

2. Are there patients with drug-refractory obstructive HCM who are not excellent candidates for alcohol ablation? *463*

3. What specific baseline conduction system abnormalities are a problem, and why? *463*

4. Are there other conduction system abnormalities that are caused by alcohol septal ablation? *463*

5. What is the time interval for which patients who developed procedural-related conduction system abnormalities must be observed to avoid unnecessary permanent pacemaker insertion? *463*

6. Did the European group reporting AV block with alcohol ablation have a recommendation regarding the length of time patients should be observed before inserting a permanent pacemaker? *464*

7. Are there strategies that may reduce the rate of occurrence of AV block? *464*

8. What complications can be expected in patients undergoing alcohol septal ablation? *464*

9. Subsequently, have long-term studies been reported? *464*

10. What is the first step that the operator takes in performing alcohol ablation? *464*

11. Does this arterial branch always originate from the LAD? *464*

12. Must the septal artery selected for alcohol ablation be of a certain size? *464*

13. How does the operator confirm that the septal artery selected is the correct one? *464*

14. Describe how the proper size of the balloon catheter is determined. *465*

15. What is the consequence of alcohol being injected into the LAD? *465*

16. Is the usual contrast media suitable for alcohol septal ablation? *465*

17. How does the operator determine when the procedure has been successful and should be terminated? *465*

18. Is reduction of LVOT pressure gradient to <20 mm Hg a reliable indicator of a "successful" alcohol ablation procedure? *466*

Bibliography *466*

58 Transcatheter Edge-to-Edge Repair for Hypertrophic Cardiomyopathy *467*

1. Why is the mitral valve important in hypertrophic cardiomyopathy? *467*

2. Are mitral valve abnormalities in HCM a primary or secondary phenomenon, or is there primary mitral valve pathology? *467*

3. What are the options for treatment of patients with HCM who fail medical therapy? *467*

4. Is percutaneous mitral valve repair with the MitraClip an option in HCM? *468*

5. What are the potential benefits of percutaneous mitral valve repair compared to traditional techniques used in HCM? *468*

6. What are the technical considerations if the MitraClip is selected as therapy for HCM? *469*

7. What are future venues for the percutaneous treatment and repair of the mitral valve with the MitraClip or other technologies in HCM? *470*

Bibliography *470*

59 Interatrial Shunt Creation   *471*
   1. What is the rationale for the creation of interatrial shunts?   *471*
   2. Which populations may benefit from interatrial shunt devices?   *471*
   3. How is net shunt volume quantified?   *471*
   4. What is the role of shunt creation via atrial septostomy for patients with refractory cardiogenic shock?   *471*
   5. What are the principal steps in performing bedside AS?   *471*
   6. What are the primary interatrial shunt devices currently under investigation?   *472*
   7. Outline the steps involved in atrial shunt device implantation   *472*
   8. Do interatrial shunt devices increase PA pressure and the risk of RV overload?   *472*
   9. What are other long-term concerns with interatrial shunt devices?   *472*
   10. What is the recommended antithrombotic therapy after implantation?   *473*
   11. What are shunt devices that do not create an ASD?   *473*

   Bibliography   *473*

   Part VII   Selected Adult Congenital Structural Interventions   *475*

60 Shunt Hemodynamics and Calculations   *477*
   1. What is a shunt, and how do we classify shunts?   *477*
   2. What is a diagnostic shunt study?   *477*
   3. During a routine left- or right-heart catheterization, what should prompt an interventional cardiologist to look for an intracardiac shunt?   *478*
   4. Does it matter if the patient is on oxygen while doing a diagnostic shunt study in the catheterization laboratory?   *478*
   5. What are the basic principles and equations required for shunt hemodynamics calculation?   *479*
   6. How does right-heart catheterization (RHC) data help in the decision-making for ASD closure?   *479*
   7. What are the criteria for a significant step up to diagnose a left-to-right shunt (assuming $Q_S = 3L/min/m^2$)?   *480*
   8. What are the criteria for a significant step up to diagnose a right-to-left shunt, and how do you localize it?   *480*
   9. What is a bidirectional shunt, and how do you calculate it?   *481*
   10. What are the implications of peripheral AV shunts like an AV fistula (AVF) for dialysis access?   *482*
   11. How can you differentiate between high-output heart failure and other types of heart failure?   *482*
   12. What is Nicoladoni-Branham sign?   *482*

   Bibliography   *482*

61 Persistent Foramen Ovale Closure
   Technical Considerations   *485*

   Devices and Techniques   *485*
   1. What is the rationale behind the closure of a patent foramen ovale (PFO)?   *485*
   2. What devices are available in the United States for the closure of PFOs?   *485*
   3. What is the appropriate technique for crossing the PFO?   *486*
   4. Are there differences in technique for PFO closure between both approved devices?   *486*
   5. What is the technique for device retrieval?   *488*
   6. What is the goal of anticoagulation throughout the procedure?   *488*
   7. How do you size the device?   *488*
   8. How should multiple shunts associated with a PFO be approached?   *488*
   9. Should the device size be modified in the presence of an atrial septal aneurysm?   *489*
   10. Should transseptal puncture be considered when negotiating difficult anatomies?   *489*
   11. Are there special considerations when closing a PFO associated with a lipomatous atrial septum?   *489*
   12. Can the PFO closure be performed in the presence of an inferior vena cava (IVC) filter?   *489*
   13. Can the procedure be performed from other access sites if the femoral access cannot be used?   *489*

Complication Prevention and Management   *489*

14. Are there complications related to device preparation?   *489*

15. How should you manage a device migration?   *490*

16. What types of complications can you encounter when treating a PFO in association with multiple atrial septal defects?   *490*

17. How can device thrombosis be prevented?   *490*

18. Are there any electrical complications from PFO closure?   *490*

Bibliography   *490*

62 Atrial Septal Defects Closure   *493*

1. What are the indications to close an atrial septal defect (ASD)?   *493*

2. What are the contraindications to close ASD?   *493*

3. What kind of occluding devices are there?   *493*

Self-Centering Devices   *493*

Non-self-Centering Devices   *494*

4. What imaging tests should be done before the procedure?   *494*

5. What are the steps in a conventional procedure?   *495*

6. What can you do if you cannot get a proper device orientation in relation to the IAS?   *496*

7. What should you do when there is more than one defect?   *497*

8. What should you do when the device embolizes? When should you try to remove it percutaneously, and when should you send the patient to the operating room?   *497*

9. What late complications may occur?   *498*

Bibliography   *498*

63 Ventricular Septal Defects Closure   *499*

Muscular VSDs   *499*

1. What muscular ventricular septal defects (MVSD) patients should you think about closing percutaneously?   *499*

2. What are the contraindications for percutaneous closure of MVSDs?   *499*

3. What devices are available?   *499*

4. What are the steps during the procedure?   *500*

5. What are the possible complications of percutaneous closure of MVSDs?   *501*

Perimembranous VSDs (PMVSDs)   *501*

6. In which patients is percutaneous closure of PMVSDs indicated?   *501*

7. What types of devices can be used to close PMVSDs?   *502*

8. What are the steps of the procedure?   *502*

9. What complications may occur in the closure of PMVSDs?   *503*

Bibliography   *503*

64 Percutaneous Treatment of Aortic Coarctation   *505*

1. What is coarctation of the aorta?   *505*

2. What other conditions is coarctation of the aorta associated with?   *505*

3. What is the clinical presentation?   *505*

4. What diagnostic imaging is recommended?   *505*

5. What are the types of transcatheter interventions in a patient with coarctation?   *506*

6. How is balloon angioplasty performed?   *508*

7. Should a low-pressure balloon or high-pressure balloon be used?   *509*

8. How is stent implantation performed?   *509*

9. Should a bare-metal or covered stent be used?   *511*

10. What are the most common complications?   *512*

11. What is the follow-up for patients who undergo percutaneous intervention? *512*

12. What are the short- and long-term results? *513*

Conclusion *513*

Bibliography *513*

65 Percutaneous Pulmonary Valve Replacement (PPVR) *515*

1. In what anatomical settings can we perform percutaneous pulmonic valve replacement (PPVR)? *515*
2. When is PPVR indicated? *516*
3. What diagnostic tests should be performed before doing the PPRV? *516*
4. What kind of valves are available? *516*
5. How is the procedure performed? *517*
6. What technical differences do you have to consider depending on the type of dysfunctional RVOT? *519*

PPVR in Dysfunctional Prosthetic Conduits *519*

PPVR in Dysfunctional Native RVOT *519*

PPVR in Dysfunctional Biological Valves *519*

7. What do you do if you cannot advance the prosthesis to the implant area? *519*
8. What complications are associated with the procedure? *520*
9. What is the result of PPVR during follow-up? *520*
10. What technical innovations in PPVR are available in clinical practice? *520*

Bibliography *522*

Part VIII   Miscellaneous *523*

66 Hemodynamic Pearls in Adult Structural Heart Disease *525*

Hemodynamic Assessment of the Aortic Valve *525*

1. When is an invasive hemodynamic assessment required? *525*
2. How do you calculate the aortic valve area using invasive hemodynamics? *525*
3. Does the Hakki formula accurately estimate the valve area when compared to the more complex Gorlin formula? *525*
4. How do you accurately measure cardiac output? *525*
5. How do you appropriately measure the transvalvular gradient? *526*
6. How do you assess the transvalvular aortic valve gradient in atrial fibrillation? *526*
7. Can a single-catheter pullback from the LV into the aorta be used to assess the transvalvular gradient? *526*
8. Can the left ventricular and femoral pressures be used to evaluate the gradient? *526*
9. How can you use the pressure waveforms to better understand the degree of aortic valve stenosis? *527*
10. What other features suggest that the pressure gradient is due to a static or dynamic obstruction? *527*
11. What is low-flow, low-gradient AS? *527*
12. How do you differentiate true low-flow AS from pseudo-AS or a severe cardiomyopathy without contractile reserve? *528*
13. How does hypertension affect the invasive hemodynamic assessment of AS? *528*
14. What are the expected hemodynamic changes that occur post-transcatheter aortic valve replacement? *529*
15. What hemodynamic findings are concerning post-TAVR? *529*

Hemodynamics of the Mitral Valve *529*

16. What are the main hemodynamic principles of the left atrium (LA)? *529*
17. How do you adequately evaluate the pressure across the mitral valve (MV)? *530*
18. Can you use the pulmonary capillary wedge pressure (PCWP) to measure the left atrial pressure and transmitral gradient? *530*
19. How do you correct the phase lag between the LV pressure tracing and PCWP tracing? *530*

Mitral Stenosis   *530*

20. When should you do invasive hemodynamic measurements for MS?   *530*
21. What invasive hemodynamic findings are suggestive of severe MS?   *531*
22. How are the hemodynamics affected in patients with atrial fibrillation?   *531*
23. What is considered a successful percutaneous mitral balloon valvuloplasty (PMBV) via hemodynamic measurements?   *531*
24. How can you detect worsening MR during the procedure if you cannot get an adequate echocardiographic assessment?   *531*

Mitral Regurgitation   *531*

25. How can you differentiate between acute and chronic MR?   *531*
26. What else can cause an elevated *v* wave on PCWP or LA pressure tracings?   *531*
27. How does atrial fibrillation affect the hemodynamics of MR?   *531*
28. How does the MitraClip affect LA pressure, and should continuous pressure measurement be used?   *532*

Hypertrophic Cardiomyopathy and Septal Ablation   *532*

29. What is the adequate way to measure gradient in patients with left ventricular outflow tract (LVOT) obstruction?   *532*
30. The gradient of LVOT obstruction remains <50 mmHg at rest. What should you do next?   *532*
31. How does atrial fibrillation affect the gradient in hypertrophic cardiomyopathy?   *532*
32. How do you determine success after alcohol septal ablation?   *532*
33. There was intra-procedural relief of obstruction after septal ablation, but the echocardiogram two days post-procedure showed an increase in the LVOT gradient. Does this mean the procedure was a failure?   *532*

Bibliography   *533*

67 **Percutaneous Closure of Coronary Artery Fistulas**   *535*

1. What is the incidence of coronary artery fistulas?   *535*
2. Describe how coronary artery fistulas are currently classified   *535*
3. What is the coronary steal phenomenon?   *535*
4. What diagnostic modalities are used in establishing the diagnosis of CAF?   *535*
5. Describe the clinical presentation of hemodynamically significant CAFs   *536*
6. What are the indications and contraindications for device closure of a CAF?   *536*
7. Describe the devices currently available for occlusion of CAF   *536*
8. Describe the technical principles for device occlusion of CAFs: surgical vs. percutaneous approach   *536*
9. Describe the technical principles for device occlusion of CAFs: retrograde arterial vs. antegrade venous approach   *537*
10. What are the results of device closure of CAFs?   *537*
11. What other coronary problems involving a steal flow phenomenon can be treated using these occlusion devices?   *537*

Bibliography   *538*

68 **Renal Denervation Therapy**
Available Evidence, Catheters, and Techniques   *541*

1. What is renal denervation?   *541*
2. What did first-generation trials on RDN show?   *541*
3. What did second-generation trials on RDN show?   *541*
4. What are other RDN ablation systems?   *542*

RDN Procedure: Technique and Steps   *544*

5. Describe the use of antiplatelet thereapy and anticoagulation   *544*
6. What is the preferred vascular access?   *544*
7. How do you engage the renal artery?   *544*

8. Should you use vasodilators before RDN? *544*

9. What additional medication may be needed? *544*

10. How do you deliver the RDN catheter? *544*

11. How do you deliver the RDN therapy? *544*

12. What are some of the potential complications of RF RDN? *545*

Bibliography *545*

69 Acute Pulmonary Embolism Interventions: Data and Indications *547*

1. How do you risk-stratify patients with acute pulmonary embolism? *547*

2. Is anticoagulation alone enough for patients with high-risk submassive PE? *547*

3. What is the role of catheter-directed thrombolysis in submassive PE? *548*

4. Does CDL-US improve outcomes compared to standard CDL? *548*

5. What is the role of mechanical thrombectomy in patients with submassive PE? *550*

6. What is the role of catheter-directed therapy in massive PE? *550*

7. What is the role of PE response teams in the interventional management of patients with acute PE? *551*

Bibliography *551*

70 Acute Pulmonary Embolism Intervention: Devices and Techniques *553*

1. What devices are currently available to treat acute pulmonary embolism? *553*

2. How do you choose between the different treatment options? *554*

3. Is acute PE treatment similar to chronic PE treatment? *554*

4. How safe is the interventional treatment of acute PE? *555*

5. What patient and what artery do you treat? *555*

6. What is the most efficient technique for catheter placement for directed thrombolysis? *555*

7. How long do you infuse TPA? *556*

8. What are the safe techniques to perform large-bore aspiration? *556*

9. What are the endpoints for percutaneous thrombectomy? *557*

10. How do you manage hemodynamically unstable patients? *557*

11. How do you manage thrombus in transit? *558*

12. How do you manage anticoagulation around treatment? *558*

13. What outpatient follow-up is needed? *558*

Bibliography *559*

71 Transseptal Puncture Technique in the ERA of Structural Heart Disease *561*

Introduction *561*

1. What constitutes the fossa ovalis and the interatrial septum? *561*

2. What are the current indications for accessing the left atrium *561*

3. Why is it relevant to access specific locations of the interatrial septum? *562*

4. What are the typical site-specific locations for the most common procedures requiring transseptal puncture? *562*

5. How is a site-specific transseptal puncture performed? *562*

6. What transseptal needles are commercially available? *564*

7. What recent advances in imaging can assist with transseptal puncture? *565*

8. What are the most common complications associated with transseptal puncture? *565*

9. What is the stitch puncture complication? *566*

10. Is it always required to close the interatrial communication after every transseptal procedure? *566*

11. Is it feasible to cross the interatrial septum in the presence of a percutaneous septal occluder (PFO/ASD)? *566*

Bibliography *566*

72 ECMO for Structural Interventions *567*

1. What is the ideal access strategy to initiate VA-ECMO in TAVR patients? *567*

2. What is the anticoagulation goal following VA-ECMO insertion and initiation? *567*

3. What VA-ECMO flow goal should be maintained in adult patients? *568*

4. Following VA-ECMO insertion, is flow >5.5 liters/min indicated in adult patients? *568*

5. Following balloon aortic valvuloplasty (BAV), the patient goes into extensive cardiogenic shock and requires CPR. How high should VA-ECMO flows be maintained? *568*

6. Will emergency sternotomy and open cardiac massage improve survival in case of cardiac arrest? *568*

7. What is the preferred cannula size used for peripheral ECMO cannulation in CPR patients (ECPR)? *568*

8. What can be done in emergency situations during TAVR when no arterial access is easily available? *568*

9. What is the inotropic management following VA-ECMO insertion? *569*

10. A TAVR patient with patent foramen ovale (PFO) presents with low cardiac output and hypoxia. What should be done? *570*

Bibliography *570*

73 Best Practices for Mechanical Circulatory Support with Impella for Acute Myocardial Infarction Cardiogenic Shock and Selected Structural Interventions *571*

1. What is the historical background of acute myocardial infarction shock intervention? *571*

2. What hemodynamic variables help diagnose and optimize the treatment of cardiogenic shock? *572*

3. What types of Impella devices are available for mechanical circulatory support? *573*

4. What are the hemodynamic benefits of Impella devices? *573*

5. What are the invasive hemodynamic variables to identify right ventricular cardiogenic shock? *574*

6. How is cardiogenic shock with right ventricular infarction and failure clinically managed? *575*

7. Is mechanical circulatory support an option for cardiogenic shock related to right ventricular failure? *575*

8. What is the role of right-heart catheterization in the management of cardiogenic shock? *576*

9. What is the optimal approach for a cardiogenic shock patient in the emergency room? *577*

10. What is the optimal approach for a cardiogenic shock patient in the cardiac catheterization laboratory? *577*

11. What is the optimal approach for a cardiogenic shock patient in the ICU? *577*

12. What is the survival of cardiogenic shock? *577*

13. What is the impact on survival of vasopressors for cardiogenic shock? *579*

14. Describe the National Cardiogenic Shock Initiative. *580*

15. What is the role of multivessel PCI in cardiogenic shock? *580*

16. What is the SCAI classification of cardiogenic shock? *581*

17. What is the role of the Impella during aortic balloon valvuloplasty? *581*

18. What is the utility of the Impella in transcatheter aortic valve replacement (TAVR)? *581*

19. What is the utility of the Impella in transcatheter edge-to-edge mitral valve repair (TEER)? *582*

Bibliography *582*

74 Transcatheter Interventions for Aortic Valve Insufficiency in Patients with Left Ventricular Assist Devices *585*

1. Describe LVADs and the current devices encountered in clinical practice *585*

2. What is the underlying mechanism for AI in patients with LVAD, and how often is it seen? *585*

3. Is post-LVAD AI preventable? *586*

4. What interventions are available for LVAD-related AI? *586*

5. Which percutaneous interventions are available? *586*

6. What technical considerations are important and differ from non-LVAD TAVR? *587*

Bibliography *588*

Index *589*

List of Contributors

Corinne Aberle
Division of Cardiothoracic Surgery,
The DeWitt Daughtry Department of Surgery,
University of Miami Miller School of Medicine,
Miami,
FL USA

Rik Adrichem
Department of Interventional Cardiology,
Thoraxcenter,
Erasmus University Medical Center,
Rotterdam,
The Netherlands

Ankit Agrawal
Department of Cardiovascular Medicine,
Heart Vascular and Thoracic Institute,
Cleveland Clinic,
Cleveland,
OH USA

Felipe N. Albuquerque
Division of Interventional Cardiology and Structural
Heart Diseases,
Holy Cross Hospital,
Fort Lauderdale,
FL USA

Fahad Alfares
Division of Pediatric Cardiology,
Department of Pediatrics,
University of Miami Miller School of Medicine,
Miami,
FL USA

Carlos E. Alfonso
Department of Medicine,
Division of Cardiovascular Medicine,
University of Miami Miller School of Medicine,
Miami,
FL USA

Ahmed Alnajar
Division of Cardiothoracic Surgery,
The DeWitt Daughtry Department of Surgery,
University of Miami Miller School of Medicine,
Miami,
FL USA

Diana Anghel
Medtronic,
Minneapolis,
MN USA

Aditya Bakhshi
Department of Cardiology,
Albert Einstein Medical Center,
Philadelphia,
PA USA

Giselle A. Baquero
John Burns School of Medicine,
University of Hawaii,
Honolulu,
HI USA

Manuel Barreiro-Perez
University Hospital of Salamanca,
Salamanca,
Spain

Kelley N. Benck
Department of Medicine,
Division of Cardiovascular Medicine,
University of Miami Miller School of Medicine,
Miami,
FL USA

Martin Bilsker
Division of Cardiology,
University of Miami,
Miami,
FL USA

Joao Braghiroli
Department of Cardiology,
Jackson Memorial Health System,
Miami,
FL USA

Guilherme Bratz
Structural Heart Disease Intervention,
Interventional Cardiology Department at Heart Institute
(InCor),
University of São Paulo,
São Paulo,
São Paulo,
Brazil

Jonatan D. Nunez
Division of Cardiology,
University of Miami,
Miami,
FL USA

Sharon Bruoha
Montefiore-Einstein Center for Heart and Vascular Care,
Montefiore Medical Center,
Albert Einstein College of Medicine,
Bronx,
NY USA

Blase A. Carabello
East Carolina Heart Institute,
Brody School of Medicine,
and Vidant Medical Center,
East Carolina University,
Greenville,
NC USA

João L. Cavalcante
Minneapolis Heart Institute Foundation – Cardiovascular
Imaging Research Center and Core Lab; Minneapolis
Heart Institute at Abbott Northwestern Hospital,
Minneapolis,
MN USA

Diego Celli
Department of Cardiology,
Jackson Memorial Health System,
Miami,
FL USA

Ying-Hwa Chen
Division of Cardiology,
Taipei Veterans General Hospital,

Taiwan; National Yang-Ming Chiao-Tung University,
Taiwan

Yashasvi Chugh
Valve Science Center at the Minneapolis Heart Institute
Foundation,
Abbott Northwestern Hospital,
Minneapolis,
MN USA

Mauricio G. Cohen
Cardiovascular Division,
Department of Medicine,
University of Miami Miller School of Medicine; Cardiac
Catheterization Laboratory,
UHealth Tower,
University of Miami Hospitals and Clinics,
Miami,
FL USA

Ignacio Cruz-Gonzalez
University Hospital of Salamanca,
Salamanca,
Spain

Robert J. Cubeddu
Department of Interventional Cardiology,
Naples Heart Institute,
Naples,
FL USA

Antonio Dager
Angiografia de Occidente SA,
Clinica de Occidente,
Cali,
Colombia

Michael Dangl
Department of Cardiology,
Jackson Memorial Health System,
Miami,
FL USA

Tawseef Dar
Cardiovascular Division,
Department of Medicine,
University of Miami Miller School of Medicine,
Miami,
FL USA

Fábio S. de Brito
Structural Heart Disease Intervention,
Interventional Cardiology Department at Heart Institute
(InCor),
University of São Paulo; Interventional Cardiology,
Hospital Sírio Libanês,
São Paulo,
Brazil

Eduardo J. de Marchena
Division of Cardiovascular Medicine,
University of Miami Miller School of Medicine,
University of Miami Hospital,
Miami,
FL USA

Shashvat M. Desai
Department of Neuroscience,
HonorHealth Research Institute,
Scottsdale,
AZ USA

Adam A. Dmytriw
Harvard Medical School,
Neuroradiology and Neurointervention Service,
Brigham & Women's Hospital,
Boston,
MA USA

Creighton W. Don
Department of Interventional Cardiology at University of
Washington,
Seattle,
WA USA

John S. Douglas Jr.
Interventional Cardiology,
Emory University School of Medicine,
Emory University Hospital,
Atlanta,
GA USA

Michael D. Dyal
Cardiovascular Division,
Department of Medicine,
University of Miami Miller School of Medicine;
Department of Veterans Affairs,
Miami,
FL USA

Michael Fabbro II
Department of Anesthesiology,
University of Miami Miller School of Medicine,
Miami,
FL USA

Alexandre C. Ferreira
Department of Cardiology,
Jackson Memorial Health System,
Miami,
FL USA

Tiberio Frisoli
Division of Cardiology,
Center for Structural Heart Disease,
Henry Ford Hospital,
Detroit,
MI USA

Miho Fukui
Minneapolis Heart Institute Foundation – Cardiovascular
Imaging Research Center and Core Lab,
Minneapolis,
MN USA

Santiago Garcia
Structural Heart Program and Harold C. Schott
Foundation Endowed Chair for Structural and Valvular
Heart Disease
The Carl and Edyth Lindner Center for Research and
Education at The Christ Hospital,
Cincinnati,
OH

Ali Ghodsizad
Miami Transplant Institute,
University of Miami Miller School of Medicine,
Miami,
FL USA

Camilo A. Gomez
Department of Cardiology,
Jackson Memorial Health System,
Miami,
FL USA

Pedro Engel Gonzalez
Division of Cardiology,
Center for Structural Heart Disease,
Henry Ford Hospital,
Detroit,
MI USA

Jelani K. Grant
Department of Cardiology,
Jackson Memorial Health System,
Miami,
FL USA

Eberhard Grube
Center of Innovative Interventions in Cardiology (CIIC),
University Hospital Bonn,
Bonn,
Germany; Division of Cardiovascular Medicine,
Stanford University School of Medicine,
Stanford,
CA USA; Interventional Cardiology Department at Heart
Institute (InCor),
University of São Paulo,
São Paulo,
São Paulo,
Brazil

Raviteja R. Guddeti
Valve Science Center at the Minneapolis Heart Institute
Foundation,
Abbott Northwestern Hospital,
Minneapolis,
MN USA

Serge Harb
Department of Cardiovascular Medicine,
Cleveland Clinic,
Cleveland,
OH USA

Gabriel A. Hernandez
Cardiovascular Division,
Department of Medicine,
University of Mississippi Medical Center,
Jackson,
MI USA

Edwin Ho
Montefiore-Einstein Center for Heart and Vascular Care,
Montefiore Medical Center,
Albert Einstein College of Medicine,
Bronx,
NY USA

Amr Idris
Department of Cardiovascular Medicine,
Baylor Scott & White The Heart Hospital,
Plano,
TX USA

Ignacio Inglessis-Azuaje
Structural Heart Disease Program,
Massachusetts General Hospital;
Harvard Medical School,
Boston,
MA USA

Toshiaki Isogai
Department of Cardiovascular Medicine,
Heart Vascular and Thoracic Institute,
Cleveland Clinic,
Cleveland,
OH USA

Wissam A. Jaber
Emory University School of Medicine,
Interventional Cardiology,
Grady Memorial Hospital;
Emory University Hospital,
Interventional Cardiology,
Atlanta,
GA USA

Pankaj Jain
Department of Anesthesiology,
University of Miami Miller School of Medicine,
Miami,
FL USA

Napatt Kanjanahattakij
Department of Cardiology,
Albert Einstein Medical Center,
Philadelphia,
PA USA

Samir R. Kapadia
Department of Cardiovascular Medicine,
Heart Vascular and Thoracic Institute,
Cleveland Clinic,
Cleveland,
OH USA

Houman Khalili
Department of Cardiovascular Diseases,
Florida Atlantic University,
Boca Raton,
FL USA; Cardiology,
Delray Medical Center,
Delray Beach,
FL USA

Priyank Khandelwal
Department of Neurological Surgery,
New Jersey Medical School,
Rutgers,
University Hospital Newark,
Newark,
NJ USA

Sibi Krishnamurthy
Department of Medicine,
Division of Cardiovascular Medicine,
University of Miami Miller School of Medicine,
Miami,
FL USA

Herbert G. Kroon
Department of Interventional Cardiology,
Thoraxcenter,
Erasmus University Medical Center,
Rotterdam,
The Netherlands

Toshiki Kuno
Montefiore-Einstein Center for Heart and Vascular Care,
Montefiore Medical Center,
Albert Einstein College of Medicine,
Bronx,
NY USA

Ana E. Laffond
University Hospital of Salamanca,
Salamanca,
Spain

Joseph Lamelas
Division of Cardiothoracic Surgery,
The DeWitt Daughtry Department of Surgery,
University of Miami Miller School of Medicine,
Miami,
FL USA

John M. Lasala
Cardiovascular Division,
Department of Medicine,
Washington University School of Medicine,
St. Louis,
MO USA

Azeem Latib
Montefiore-Einstein Center for Heart and Vascular Care,
Montefiore Medical Center,
Albert Einstein College of Medicine,
Bronx,
NY USA

James C. Lee
Division of Cardiology,
Center for Structural Heart Disease,
Henry Ford Hospital,
Detroit,
MI USA

Timothy Lee
Department of Cardiovascular Surgery,
Mount Sinai Medical Center,
New York,
NY USA

JoAnn Lindenfeld
Cardiovascular Division,
Department of Medicine,
University of Mississippi Medical Center,
Jackson,
MI USA

Hamza Lodhi
Department of Cardiovascular Diseases,
Florida Atlantic University,
Boca Raton,
FL USA; Cardiology,
Delray Medical Center,
Delray Beach,
FL USA

Matthias Loebe
Miami Transplant Institute,
University of Miami Miller School of Medicine,
Miami,
FL USA

Juan G. Lopez
Cardiovascular Division,
Department of Medicine,
University of Miami Miller School of Medicine,
Miami,
FL USA

Lucian Lozonschi
Division of Cardiothoracic Surgery,
Department of Surgery,
University of South Florida Morsani College of Medicine,
Tampa,
FL USA

Brijeshwar Maini
Department of Cardiovascular Diseases,
Florida Atlantic University,
Boca Raton,

FL USA; Cardiology,
Delray Medical Center,
Delray Beach,
FL USA; Tenet Healthcare Corporation,
Delray Beach,
FL USA

Antonio Mangieri
Department of Biomedical Sciences,
Humanitas University; Humanitas Research
Hospital IRCCS,
Rozzano,
Milan,
Italy

Adithya Mathews
Department of Cardiovascular Diseases,
Florida Atlantic University,
Boca Raton,
FL USA; Cardiology,
Delray Medical Center,
Delray Beach,
FL USA

Michael McDaniel
Emory University School of Medicine,
Interventional Cardiology,
Grady Memorial Hospital;
Emory University Hospital,
Interventional Cardiology,
Atlanta,
GA USA

Cesar E. Mendoza
Department of Cardiology,
Jackson Memorial Health System,
Miami,
FL USA

Nestor F. Mercado
University of New Mexico Health Sciences Center,
Albuquerque,
NM USA

Raul Mitrani
Division of Cardiology,
University of Miami,
Miami,
FL USA

Christian McNeely
Cardiovascular Division,
Department of Medicine,

Washington University School of Medicine,
St. Louis,
MO USA

Vinayak Nagaraja
Department of Cardiovascular Medicine,
Heart Vascular and Thoracic Institute,
Cleveland Clinic,
Cleveland,
OH USA

Pedro F. Gomes Nicz
Structural Heart Disease Intervention,
Interventional Cardiology Department at Heart Institute
(InCor),
University of São Paulo; Interventional Cardiology,
Hospital Sírio Libanês,
São Paulo,
São Paulo,
Brazil

Jean C. Núñez García
University Hospital of Salamanca,
Salamanca,
Spain

Brian P. O'Neill
Division of Cardiology,
Center for Structural Heart Disease,
Henry Ford Hospital,
Detroit,
MI USA

William W. O'Neill
Division of Cardiology,
Center for Structural Heart Disease,
Henry Ford Hospital,
Detroit,
MI USA

Igor F. Palacios
Cardiology,
Massachusetts General Hospital,
Harvard Medical School,
Boston,
MA USA

Sankalp P. Patel
Naples Community Hospital,
Naples,
FL USA

Sergio A. Perez
Cardiovascular Service,
Baptist Health Medical Center,
Montgomery,
AL USA

Jeffrey J. Popma
Medtronic,
Minneapolis,
MN USA

Tannavi Prakash
Department of Neurological Surgery,
New Jersey Medical School,
Rutgers,
University Hospital Newark,
Newark,
NJ USA

Pablo Rengifo-Moreno
Tallahassee Memorial Hospital; Florida State University,
Tallahassee,
FL USA

Alejandro Rodríguez Ogando
Gregorio Marañon Hospital. Madrid,
Spain

Michael P. Rogers
Division of Cardiothoracic Surgery,
Department of Surgery,
University of South Florida Morsani College of Medicine,
Tampa,
FL USA

Phillip Rubin
Cardiovascular Division,
Department of Medicine,
University of Miami Miller School of Medicine,
Miami,
FL USA

Shazib Sagheer
University of New Mexico Health Sciences Center,
Albuquerque,
NM USA

Tomas Salerno
Cardiothoracic Surgery,
University of Miami Miller School of Medicine,
Miami,
FL USA

Satinder K. Sandhu
Division of Pediatric Cardiology,
Department of Pediatrics,
University of Miami Miller School of Medicine,
Miami,
FL USA

Rogério Sarmento-Leite
Interventional Cardiology,
Heart Institute,
Fundação Universitária de Cardiologia (IC – FUC);
Interventional Cardiology,
Hospital Moinhos de Vento,
Porto Alegre,
Rio Grande do Sul,
Brazil

Yu Sato
CVPath Institute,
Gaithersburg,
MD USA

Andrea Scotti
Montefiore-Einstein Center for Heart and
Vascular Care,
Montefiore Medical Center,
Albert Einstein College of Medicine,
Bronx,
NY USA

Solomon A. Seifu
Department of Medicine,
Division of Cardiovascular Medicine,
University of Miami Miller School of Medicine,
Miami,
FL USA

Balaji Shanmugam
Cardiovascular Division, Department of Medicine,
University of Miami Miller School of Medicine,
Miami,
FL USA

Abhishek Sharma
Department of Cardiology,
New Jersey Medical School,
Rutgers,
University Hospital Newark,
Newark,
NJ USA

Calvin C. Sheng
Department of Cardiovascular Medicine,
Cleveland Clinic,
Cleveland,
OH USA

Ryan M. Smith
Hawaii Heart Associates,
Kaneohe,
HI USA

Chak-yu So
Division of Cardiology,
Department of Medicine and Therapeutics,
Prince of Wales Hospital,
Chinese University of Hong Kong,
HKSAR,
China

Ruth Solana
Infanta Leonor Hospital,
Madrid,
Spain

David "Chip" Sosa
University of New Mexico Health Sciences Center,
Albuquerque,
NM USA

Nicholas Sturla
Department of Internal Medicine,
Henry Ford Hospital,
Detroit,
MI USA

Atsushi Sugiura
Department of Cardiology,
Heart Center Bonn,
University Hospital Bonn,
Germany

Gilbert H.L. Tang
Department of Cardiovascular Surgery,
Mount Sinai Medical Center,
New York,
NY USA

Catalin Toma
Interventional Cardiology,
University of Pittsburg Medical Center,
Pittsburgh,
PA USA

Blanca Trejo Velasco
University Hospital of Salamanca,
Salamanca,
Spain

Nicolas M. Van Mieghem
Department of Interventional Cardiology,
Thoraxcenter,
Erasmus University Medical Center,
Rotterdam,
The Netherlands

Alex H. Velasquez
Division of Cardiology,
University of Miami,
Miami,
FL USA

Pedro Villablanca
Division of Cardiology,
Center for Structural Heart Disease,
Henry Ford Hospital,
Detroit,
MI USA

Renu Virmani
CVPath Institute,
Gaithersburg,
MD USA

Dee Dee Wang
Division of Cardiology,
Center for Structural Heart Disease,
Henry Ford Hospital,
Detroit,
MI USA

Christian Witzke
Department of Cardiology,
Albert Einstein Medical Center,
Philadelphia,
PA USA

Jonathan D. Wolfe
Cardiovascular Division,
Department of Medicine,
Washington University School of Medicine,
St. Louis,
MO USA

Matthew S. Wu
University of Washington,
Seattle,
WA USA

Yuen Yee Lo Yau Leung
Division of Pediatric Cardiology,
Department of Pediatrics,
University of Miami Miller School of Medicine,
Miami,
FL USA

Dileep R. Yavagal
Department of Neurology and Neurological
Surgery,
University of Miami Miller School of Medicine and
Jackson Health System,
Miami,
FL USA

Ashvin Zachariah
Division of Internal Medicine,
Holy Cross Hospital,
Fort Lauderdale,
FL USA

Sandip Zalawadiya
Cardiovascular Division,
Department of Medicine,
University of Mississippi Medical Center,
Jackson,
MI USA

Sebastian Zimmer
Department of Cardiology,
Heart Center Bonn,
University Hospital Bonn,
Germany

Jose Luis Zunzunegui
Gregorio Marañon Hospital,
Madrid,
Spain

Preface

April 2022 marks the 20th anniversary of the first patient treated with transcatheter aortic valve replacement. Since this time, countless patients have been treated by thousands of physicians at multiple sites throughout the world. The last 10 years have seen the rapid development of the entire field of structural heart disease and new device innovations. Well-designed clinical trials have shown the value of these new devices and their clinical limitations. At the time of the writing of this book, all valvular diseases, and most cardiac structural abnormalities, are either currently treated or being studied for treatment. New device developments and modifications are amplifying at a mind-boggling pace.

Mastering Structural Heart Disease, using the time-proven Socratic tool of questions and answers, aims to cover nearly all present-day structural heart disease devices, their appropriate use, and technical tricks to help ensure treatment success. We have achieved this by assembling, as authors, some of the leading thought leaders and expert educators in the field. In this comprehensive textbook, we hope to be able to offer knowledge, clinical wisdom, and practical pearls for structural interventionalists and trainees.

Eduardo J. de Marchena, MD
Camilo A. Gomez, MD

About the Companion Website

The book is accompanied by a website:

 www.wiley.com/go/deMarchena/Mastering-Structural-Heart-Disease

The website features contains:

- Case studies 'Clinical Cases and Vignettes'

Part I

Structural Interventions for the Aortic Valve

1

The Natural History and Hemodynamic Assessment of Aortic Valve Disease

Blase A. Carabello

East Carolina Heart Institute, Brody School of Medicine, and Vidant Medical Center, East Carolina University, Greenville, NC, USA

Aortic Stenosis

1. What are the causes of aortic stenosis (AS)?

In the developed world, calcification of the aortic leaflets is the most common cause of aortic stenosis (AS). Once thought to be a degenerative process, it is now clear that AS is due to active inflammation, with increased temperature of the areas affected. Those same areas demonstrate lymphocyte infiltration that leads to a calcified plaque similar to that of atherosclerosis. Indeed, the development of AS has many of the same risk factors associated with coronary disease. About 1% of the population is born with a bicuspid rather than a tricuspid aortic valve. When such patients develop AS, it occurs about 10–15 years earlier than in patients with tricuspid aortic valves. Earlier onset of disease may occur due to increased valve leaflet shear stress or to genetic abnormalities that lead to earlier calcification. The bicuspid valve may also be associated with proximal aortic root dilatation. Because calcific AS is an inflammatory process, it is also a progressive one. The rate of AS progression is remarkably variable, ranging from little progression year to year in some patients to an increase in aortic gradient by as much as 15 mmHg/yr in others.

Worldwide, rheumatic heart disease is still a major cause of AS. Congenital AS, chest irradiation, exposure to serotonergic drugs, and/or carcinoid disease and ochronosis are rarer causes of AS.

2. How is AS severity graded?

AS is graded as mild, moderate, or severe based upon the aortic valve area (AVA), aortic jet velocity, mean transvalvular gradient, and AVA indexed for body surface area (Table 1.1). Most importantly, the assessment of AS severity should not be based upon a single criterion. Rather, physical exam findings, the echocardiographic appearance of the aortic valve, jet velocity, gradient, valve calcium score, and valve area should be integrated into the overall assessment. This is especially true in low flow conditions, which reduce the gradient and jet velocity, making valve area, a calculated instead of directly measured value, more important but potentially less reliable.

3. What are the hemodynamic consequences of AS?

The normal AVA is about $3\,cm^2$. Reducing AVA to half its normal orifice creates little obstruction to flow, resulting in only a 10 mmHg gradient transvalvular at rest. However, further reductions in AVA cause a progressively greater LV pressure increase needed to drive blood past the obstruction. Thus for a valve area of $1.0\,cm^2$, the usual resting gradient is 25 mmHg; for an AVA of $0.75\,cm^2$, the gradient is about 50 mmHg; and for an AVA of $0.5\,cm^2$, the gradient could reach 100 mmHg. The increased gradient increases LV afterload, resulting in the development of concentric left ventricular hypertrophy, which results in both compensatory and pathologic consequences.

4. How are the hemodynamics of AS translated into symptoms?

The classic symptoms of AS are angina, syncope, and dyspnea on exertion (or other symptoms of heart failure). The onset of symptoms dramatically changes the prognosis of the disease, from a nearly normal mortality rate to a

Mastering Structural Heart Disease, First Edition. Edited by Eduardo J. de Marchena and Camilo A. Gomez.
© 2023 John Wiley & Sons Ltd. Published 2023 by John Wiley & Sons Ltd.
Companion website: www.wiley.com/go/deMarchena/Mastering-Structural-Heart-Disease

Table 1.1 Decision-making in patients with severe aortic stenosis (AS).

Class I indications for aortic valve replacement

1) Severe symptomatic AS

"Severe" defined as an integration of the following criteria (not all need to be present).

   A. Transaortic jet velocity of $>/=4\,m/s$

   B. Mean valve gradient of $>/=40\,mmHg$

   C. Aortic valve area (AVA) of $</=1.0\,cm^2$

   D. Aortic valve area index $</=0.6\,cm^2$

    (When criteria are discordant, a valve calcium score may be helpful, with a score of $>/=2000\,au$ for men and $>/=1200\,au$ for women suggesting severe disease.)

    (In low flow (stroke volume $</=35\,cc/m^2$) low ejection fraction (EF) patients, augmentation of stroke volume by dobutamine infusion to calculate AVA at higher flow may be helpful.)

2) Severe asymptomatic AS with LV dysfunction (EF $</=50\%$)

Class IIa indications for AVR

1) Very severe (jet velocity $>/=5\,m/s$ or AVA $</=0.6\,cm^2$) asymptomatic AS

2) Asymptomatic patients with a positive exercise tolerance test (unable to achieve 75% of expected workload or failure of systolic pressure to increase with exercise)

3) Brain natriuretic peptide level $>/=3\times$ normal for patient's age and sex

4) Rapid worsening of AS with AVA reduction of $>/=$ of $0.3\,cm^2/yr$

Transcatheter valve replacement (TAVR) preferred over surgical (SAVR) replacement

1) High risk or inoperable patients

2) Age $>/=80$

Surgical valve replacement preferred over TAVR

1) Age <65 in low risk patients

In all other groups, the decision for TAVR vs. SAVR should be made by a multidisciplinary Heart Team that includes patient preference

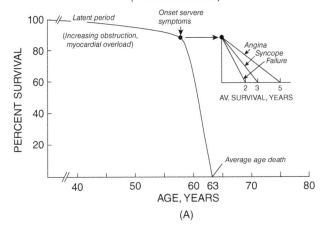

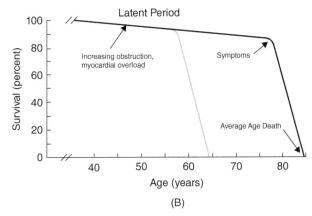

Figure 1.1 The natural history of AS. (a) The original natural history according to symptom onset as compiled by Ross and Braunwald. (b) A more contemporary natural history, reflecting the change in etiology over the past half-century. *Source:* Carabello, B.A. (2013). Compendium: introduction to aortic stenosis. *Circ. Res.* 113 (2): 179–185 / American Heart Association.

mortality rate of about 2%/mo. Thus about 75% of symptomatic patients die from AS in three years unless aortic valve replacement (AVR), the only effective treatment, intervenes (Figure 1.1). All three symptoms are related to the development of left ventricular hypertrophy (LVH).

Wall stress, the afterload on the myocardium, is defined by the formula for Laplacian stress $(\sigma) = P \times R/2h$, where P = LV systolic pressure, R = LV radius, and h = LV thickness. It is generally held that the increased LV pressure caused by the transvalvular gradient in the Laplace numerator is compensated by LVH, which increases thickness in the denominator. Unfortunately, LVH brings with it pathologic consequences despite this compensation. Coronary blood flow is impaired by LVH, as LVH reduces myocardial capillary density, in turn potentiating myocardial ischemia and in part contributing to angina. Concentric hypertrophy reduces LV diastolic volume and LV stroke volume, reducing cardiac output. This potentiates a fall in blood pressure

when peripheral resistance falls during exercise, leading to exercise-induced syncope. Hypertrophy eventually leads to LV systolic dysfunction through several mechanisms including abnormal calcium handling, apoptosis, ischemia, and cytoskeletal proliferation. Hypertrophy also causes increased LV stiffness, leading to diastolic dysfunction.

5. How are the hemodynamics of AS translated into physical exam findings?

AS is often first discovered when the provider auscults a murmur during physical examination. This systolic ejection murmur is typically a harsh raspy sound that radiates to the neck. In some cases, it also radiates to the LV apex, giving the false impression that a second murmur, that of mitral regurgitation (MR), is also present (Gallavardin's phenomenon). If by chance the patient sustains an extra systole during the exam, the murmur intensifies after the pause as stroke volume increases, an increase that does not occur in MR. As AS severity worsens, the murmur peaks progressively later in systole until, in severe AS, peak intensity occurs just before S2. Palpation of the hypertrophied LV finds the LV apex beat sustained and forceful, while at the same time, aortic valve obstruction causes the carotid upstrokes to be delayed and weakened in quality (parvus et tardus). The finding of a forceful apical beat with simultaneously weak carotid upstrokes is an important clue that obstruction, AS, lies between the LV and the carotids. Because the aortic valve motion is reduced, the second heart sound may become single because only the P2 component is heard. However, this finding is less common today because AS is detected earlier in its course when the disease is less severe than it was in the pre-echo era.

6. How is AS diagnosed (imaging and invasive hemodynamics)?

When physical examination has led to suspicion of AS, echocardiography is employed as the key diagnostic tool. Echocardiography with Doppler interrogation of the valve provides data about LVH, LV function, valve movement, and severity of disease. Since the bloodstream must accelerate to maintain flow through the narrowed valve orifice, jet velocity must increase as the orifice becomes narrowed

(Figure 1.2). Flow = area (A)× time-velocity integral (TVI), and flow must be maintained on both sides of the stenotic valve. Thus A_1 (outflow tract)$\times TVI_1 = A_2$ (AVA)$\times VTI_2$. Rearranging the terms, $A_2 = A_1 \times VTI_1/VTI_2$, calculating AVA by this continuity equation. As noted earlier, no single echo parameter should be used to assess AS severity. Rather, all data are taken together to arrive at a final assessment. Because AS is a progressive disease, patients should be followed by a yearly physical exam. For mild AS, echocardiography should be repeated every two to three years; for moderate AS, echocardiography should be performed yearly.

In some cases, the severity of AS is still in doubt following echocardiography. When this occurs, direct invasive gradient measurement is obtained at cardiac catheterization (Figure 1.3) and related to cardiac output to obtain AVA calculated by the Gorlin formula, where AVA = cardiac output/$\sqrt{}$ mean gradient.

7. What is low-flow AS?

The transvalvular gradient is created by the stroke volume passing through the valve. However, two conditions reduce stroke volume, causing the jet velocity and gradient to be reduced, potentially leading to an underestimation of AS severity. Systolic dysfunction reduces ejection fraction (EF) and stroke volume, in turn reducing gradient, a situation often referred to as "classic" low flow, usually defined as stroke volume <35 cc/m^2. In other cases, EF remains normal, but severe LVH reduces LV cavity size, in turn reducing LV stroke volume, often referred to as "paradoxical" low flow AS. Because both conditions reduce gradient and

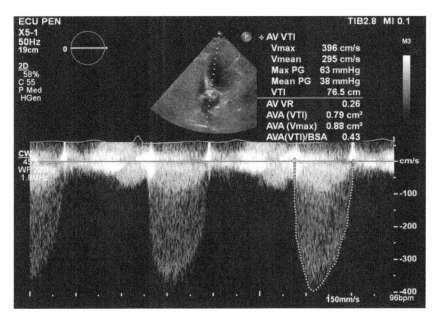

Figure 1.2 The transaortic Doppler jet in a patient with AS. Jet velocity is approaching 4 m/s, a criterion for "severe" AS.

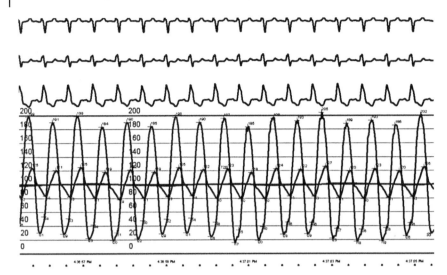

Figure 1.3 The transaortic pressure gradient in a patient with severe AS.

jet velocity, those parameters become unreliable in assessing AS severity, placing more weight on the valve area, itself subject to measurement errors. In such cases, valve calcium scoring adds additional data wherein scores >2000 Agatston units (au) for men and >1200 au for women suggest that AS is severe.

8. What are the indications for medical therapy of AS, and what do those therapies consist of?

There are no known effective therapies for treating AS. Attempts to reduce the progression of the disease with statin drugs have failed. However, as the disease typically occurs in older patients where systemic hypertension is present, hypertension is treated cautiously with standard antihypertensive therapy.

9. What are the indications for mechanical therapy of AS, and what do those therapies consist of?

AVR is indicated when the classic symptoms of angina, syncope, or dyspnea occur in patients with severe disease (Table 1.1). The occurrence of LV dysfunction (EF < 50%) even in asymptomatic patients is also an indication of AVR. Occasionally, patients with borderline moderate/severe AS may develop symptoms although they technically do not meet "severe" criteria. Because symptoms are subjective in nature, corroborating evidence obtained from exercise testing and biomarkers helps tip the decision in favor of AVR if they are abnormal. AVR may be considered in asymptomatic patients with very severe AS, i.e. those

with a jet velocity of >/=5.0 m/s or AVA </=0.6 cm^2 and in patients with a progressive fall in EF toward 50%.

AVR can be performed percutaneously by catheter technique (transcatheter aortic valve replacement [TAVR]) or surgical implantation (surgical aortic valve replacement [SAVR]). TAVR is obviously less invasive and has lower implantation mortality and lower stroke risk than SAVR in most patients. However, because the durability of TAVR is unknown, it is recommended for patients of all risk categories >/=80 years of age and not recommended for low-risk patients </=65 years old, with risk and procedure recommendations for patients aged 65–80 determined by clinical judgment. Surgery is also more apt in cases where additional heart diseases not addressed by TAVR must be considered. In all cases, judgment about which procedure is appropriate should be discussed by a multidisciplinary Heart Team that strongly considers patient preference.

10. What is the prognosis for AS?

As noted earlier, the prognosis for symptomatic patients without AVR is dismal, with only a 25% three-year survival rate. For patients aged 50–65, AVR adds approximately 15 years to their lifespan.

Aortic Regurgitation

11. What are the major etiologies of aortic regurgitation (AR)?

Aortic regurgitation (AR) occurs when the aortic leaflets fail to coapt either due to inherent pathology of the leaflets themselves or due to dilatation of the aortic root, pulling

Table 1.2 Decision-making in patients with severe aortic regurgitation (AR).

Class I indications for aortic valve replacement

1) Severe symptomatic AR
   "Severe" defined as an integration of the following criteria (not all need to be present)
   E. Regurgitant jet fills >/=65% of left ventricular outflow tract
   F. Vena contracta >/=0.6 cm^2
   G. Regurgitant volume >/=60 cc/beat
   H. Holodiastloic reversal of abdominal aortic flow
2) Severe asymptomatic AR with LV dysfunction (EF </=55%)

Class IIa indications for AVR

1) Left ventricular end systolic dimension >/=50 mm

the leaflets away from their coaptation point. Leaflet pathologies include infective endocarditis, rheumatic valve disease, bicuspid aortic valve, myxomatous valve degeneration, serotonergic drugs, carcinoid syndrome, trauma, radiation, collagen vascular disease, and non-infectious endocarditis. Aortic root causes include aortic dissection, hypertension with root dilatation, Marfan syndrome, Ehlers–Danlos syndrome, Loeys Dietz syndrome, ankylosing spondylitis, syphilis, and giant cell arteritis.

12. How is severe AR defined?

Several parameters are incorporated into the assessment of AR severity and are listed in Table 1.2.

Chronic AR

13. What are the hemodynamics of chronic AR?

As AR severity worsens, the LV progressively dilates, increasing total stroke volume, compensating for the volume regurgitated back into the LV during diastole. This produces a hyperdynamic circulation. Because pulse pressure increases with increasing stroke volume, pulse pressure widens; diastolic pressure falls due to diastolic runoff into the LV, while systolic pressure increases caused by the increase in stroke volume. Thus AR is a combined pressure and volume overload, causing both eccentric and concentric LVH. Afterload in AR can be as high as that seen in AS, the more typical pressure overload lesion. In very severe AR, end diastolic aortic pressure and end diastolic LV pressure may become equal (Figure 1.4).

14. How are chronic AR hemodynamics translated into symptoms?

The typical symptoms are those of heart failure, including dyspnea on exertion, orthopnea paroxysmal nocturnal dyspnea. Occasionally, the low systemic diastolic pressure may reduce coronary blood flow, causing angina or reducing cerebral perfusion, leading to syncope. Rare symptoms include flushing, carotid pain, and an uncomfortable awareness of the heartbeat.

15. How are chronic AR hemodynamics translated into physical signs?

The hemodynamics of severe chronic AR produce one of the most dynamic physical exams in cardiology. The enlarged LV that develops to compensate for the regurgitant volume displaces the apical beat downward and to the left. It is often very noticeable upon inspection and easily palpable. The murmur of chronic AR is a diastolic blowing sound best heard with the patient sitting up and leaning forward. In severe AR, the murmur may become holodiastolic. The diastolic jet of AR may impinge upon the mitral valve, partially closing it in diastole and also causing it to vibrate, leading to a rumbling murmur similar to that of mitral stenosis (Austin Flint murmur).

As noted earlier, there is a large total stroke volume and widened pulse pressure that together produce a myriad of clinical signs. There is a rapid, forceful carotid upstroke with a brisk decline (Corrigan's pulse). Compression of the nails finds systolic plethora and diastolic blanching of the nail bed (Quinke's pulse). One may observe bobbing of the head in cadence to the heartbeat (de Musset's sign) or a to-and-fro bruit in the femoral artery when compressed by the bell of the stethoscope (Duroziez' sign). There may be systolic augmentation of the leg blood pressure compared to the arm by >/=40 mmHg (Hill's sign).

16. How is AR diagnosed (imaging and invasive hemodynamics)?

As with all valve lesions, transthoracic echocardiography (TTE) is the mainstay of diagnosis. This tool can visualize the aortic root and valve in helping to define the mechanism for the AR. TTE can quantitate the severity of AR and its effects on LV chamber size as well as LV function (Table 1.2).

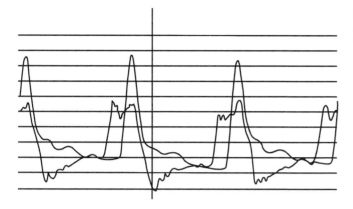

Figure 1.4 Pressure tracing from a patient with severe acute AR, demonstrating the rapid increase in LV diastolic pressure and diastasis between aortic and LV pressures.

TTE is ideal for following the progression of AR longitudinally.

If TTE images are non-diagnostic, cardiac MRI can precisely measure regurgitant volume and regurgitant fraction, LV volume, and LV EF, parameters useful in deciding upon AR therapy.

In some cases, invasive hemodynamics, especially during exercise, may help to clarify discordant resting findings, and aortography may also be helpful in grading AR severity.

17. What are the indications for medical therapy in AR and of what do Those therapies consist?

AR is a mechanical problem, the definitive therapy for which is also mechanical, i.e. AVR. Because afterload is increased in AR, attempts have been made to reduce afterload with vasodilators in the hope of increasing forward flow, in turn decreasing regurgitant flow. These efforts have not produced conclusive results. Currently, the only medical therapy is for standard treatment of systolic hypertension, which often accompanies AR.

18. What are the indications for mechanical therapy of AR and of what do Those therapies consist?

The definitive therapy for AR is AVR. Transcatheter AVR employs the annular calcium present in AS for securing the valve in place. In AR, annular calcium is not dense enough to prevent valve embolization, so the technique is not apt for this lesion. Occasionally, valve repair instead of replacement can be performed by surgeons experienced in this technique.

Because the onset of either symptoms or LV dysfunction worsens prognosis, AVR should be performed at the onset of symptoms or when LV EF Becomes <55% or when end systolic dimension (ESD) >/=50–55 mm. Some authorities would recommend AVR at a smaller ESD if there has been a progressive increase in ESD or a progressive decrease in LV EF.

When AR has been caused by a bicuspid aortic valve, it is often accompanied by dilatation of the aorta itself. Debate continues as to whether this dilatation is due to a genetic abnormality or is due to abnormal turbulent flow impinging on the aorta as the flow exits the valve. In any case, the aortic should be prophylactically replaced at the time of AVR if the aortic diameter exceeds 45–50 mm.

19. What is the prognosis following treatment

Because most patients with AR are in their 50s or 60s when they require AVR, the risks inherent to prosthetic valves reduce life span so that, on average, if AVR has occurred in a timely fashion, the life span is approximately 15 years after implantation.

Severe Acute AR

Severe acute AR as might occur in aortic valve infective endocarditis is often a life-threatening emergency. Unlike in chronic AR, there has been no time in acute AR for compensatory hypertrophy to develop. Accordingly, there is a dramatic fall in forward cardiac output with a concomitant increase in left ventricular (LV) and left atrial (LA) filling pressure, leading potentially to cardiogenic shock and pulmonary edema. Despite these extreme hemodynamic abnormalities, the patient's physical examination may be misleadingly unremarkable. The rapid rise in LV diastolic pressure (Figure 1.4) limits the transaortic pressure gradient driving the AR so that the murmur may become short and unimpressive. High diastolic filling pressure may close the mitral valve prior to systole, causing S1 to be soft in intensity. All of the signs noted in chronic AR are usually absent because the LV volume is not increased so that the increased total stroke volume and wide pulse pressure causing those signs are also absent. Often, subtle changes

in symptoms and vital signs such as mild orthopnea and tachycardia may be the only clues that decompensation is occurring.

Once acute AR is suspected, or if unexplained decompensation occurs in the face of infective endocarditis, TTE is indicated, usually accompanied by transesophageal echocardiography. Severe AR, especially if accompanied by mitral valve pre-closure, is an indication of early AVR. While there may be concern about infection of the AVR, this is in fact rare, occurring in only about 5% of cases.

Bibliography

1 Aggarwal, S.R., Clavel, M.A., Messika-Zeitoun, D. et al. (2013). Sex differences in aortic valve calcification measured by multidetector computed tomography in aortic stenosis. *Circ. Cardiovasc. Imaging* 6 (1): 40–47.

2 Bing, W., Elmariah, S., Kaplan, F.S. et al. (2005). Paradoxical effects of statins on aortic valve myofibroblasts and osteoblasts: implications for end-stage valvular heart disease. *Arterioscler. Thromb. Vasc. Biol.* 25: 592–597.

3 Carabello, B.A. (2013). Compendium: introduction to aortic stenosis. *Circ. Res.* 113 (2): 179–185.

4 Carabello, B.A. (2021). The Pathophysiology of a afterload mismatch and ventricular hypertrophy. *Struct. Heart* 5: 446–456.

5 Carabello, B.A., Ballard, W.L., Gazes, P.C. et al. (1994). *Cardiology Pearls*. Philadelphia: Hanley and Belfus.

6 Clavel, M.A., Malouf, J., Michelena, H.I. et al. (2014). B-type natriuretic peptide clinical activation in aortic stenosis: impact on long-term survival. *J. Am. Coll. Cardiol.* 63 (19): 2016–2025.

7 Clavel, M.A., Messika-Zeitoun, D., Pibarot, P. et al. (2013). The complex nature of discordant severe calcified aortic valve disease grading: new insights from combined Doppler echocardiographic and computed tomographic study. *J. Am. Coll. Cardiol.* 62 (24): 2329–2338.

8 Das, P., Rimington, H., and Chambers, J. (2005). Exercise testing to stratify risk in aortic stenosis. *Eur. Heart J.* 26: 1309–1313. Epub 2005 Apr 8.

9 Funakoshi, S., Kaji, S., Yamamuro, A. et al. (2011). Impact of early surgery in the active phase on long-term outcomes in left-sided native valve infective endocarditis. *Thorac. Cardiovasc. Surg.* 142 (4): 836–842.

10 Gorlin, R. and Gorlin, S.G. (1951). Hydraulic formula for calculation of the area of the stenotic mitral valve, other cardiac valves, and central circulatory shunts. I. *Am. Heart J.* 41 (1): 1–29.

11 Hiratzka, L.F., Bakris, G.L., Beckman, J.A. et al. (2010). ACCF/AHA/AATS/ACR/ASA/SCA/SCAI/SIR/STS/SVM guidelines for the diagnosis and management of patients with thoracic aortic disease. *J. Am. Coll. Cardiol.* 2010: 55.

12 Ikonomidis, J.S., Ruddy, J.M., Benton, S.M. Jr. et al. (2012). Aortic dilatation with bicuspid aortic valves: cusp fusion correlates to matrix metalloproteinases and inhibitors. *Ann. Thorac. Surg.* 93: 457–463.

13 Ito, S., Miranda, W.R., Nkomo, V.T. et al. (2018). Reduced left ventricular ejection fraction in patients with aortic stenosis. *J. Am. Coll. Cardiol.* 2018 (71): 1313–1321.

14 Klein, A.L., Ramchand, J., and Nagueh, S.F. (2020). Aortic stenosis and diastolic dysfunction: partners in crime. *J. Am. Coll. Cardiol.* 76 (25): 2952–2955.

15 Iodas, E., Enriquez-Sarano, M., Tajik, A.J. et al. (1997). Optimizing timing of surgical correction in patients with severe aortic regurgitation: role of symptoms. *J. Am. Coll. Cardiol.* 30: 746–752.

16 Marcus, M.L., Doty, D.B., Hiratzka, L.F. et al. (1982). Decreased coronary reserve: a mechanism for angina pectoris in patients with aortic stenosis and normal coronary arteries. *N. Engl. J. Med.* 307: 1362–1366.

17 Mark, A.L., Abboud, F.M., Schmid, P.G., and Heistad, D.D. (1973). Reflex vascular responses to left ventricular outflow obstruction and activation of ventricular baroreceptors in dogs. *J. Clin. Invest.* 52 (11): 47–53.

18 Mentias, A., Feng, K., Alashi, A. et al. (2016). Long-term outcomes in patients with aortic regurgitation and preserved left ventricular ejection fraction. *J. Am. Coll. Cardiol.* 68 (20): 2144–2153.

19 Minners, J., Allgeier, M., Gohlke-Baerwolf, C. et al. (2008). Inconsistencies of echocardiographic criteria for the grading of aortic valve stenosis. *Eur. Heart J.* 29 (8): 1043–1048.

20 Murashita, T., Schaff, H.V., Suri, R.M. et al. (2017). Impact of left ventricular systolic function on outcome of correction of chronic severe aortic valve regurgitation: implications for timing of surgical intervention. *Ann. Thorac. Surg.* 103: 1222–1228.

21 Otto, C.M., Kuusisto, J., Reichenbach, D.D. et al. (1994). Characterization of the early lesion of 'degenerative' valvular aortic stenosis: histological and immunohistochemical studies. *Circulation* 90: 844–853.

22 Park, S.J., Enriquez-Sarano, M., Chang, S.A. et al. (2013). Hemodynamic patterns for symptomatic presentations of sever aortic stenosis. *J. Am. Coll. Cardiol: Cardiovasc. Imaging* 6: 137–146.

23 Ross, J. Jr. and Braunwald, E. (1968). Aortic stenosis. *Circulation* 38: 61–67.

24 Toutouzas, K., Drakopoulou, M., Synetos, A. et al. (2008). In vivo aortic valve thermal heterogeneity in patients with nonrheumatic aortic valve stenosis the: first in vivo experience in humans. *J. Am. Coll. Cardiol.* 52 (9): 758–763.

25 van Geldorp, M.W.A., Jamieson, W.R.E., Kappetein, A.P. et al. (2009). Patient outcome after aortic valve replacement with a mechanical or biological prosthesis; weighing lifetime anticoagulant-related event risk against reoperation risk. *J. Thorac. Cardiovasc. Surg.* 137 (4): 881–886.

26 Wisenbaugh, T., Spann, J.F., and Carabello, B.A. (1984). Differences in myocardial performance and load between patients with similar amounts of chronic aortic versus chronic mitral regurgitation. *J. Am. Coll. Cardiol.* 3 (4): 916–923.

27 Writing Committee Members, Otto, C.M., Nishimura, R.A. et al. (2021). 2020 ACC/AHA guideline for the management of patients with valvular heart disease: executive summary: a report of the American College of Cardiology/American Heart Association joint committee on clinical practice guidelines. *J. Am. Coll. Cardiol.* 77 (4): 450–500.

2

Pathology Insights of Aortic Valve Disease

Yu Sato and Renu Virmani

CVPath Institute, Gaithersburg, MD, USA

Introduction

The prevalence of valvular heart disease (VHD) is growing worldwide as a result of an aging population and increasing life expectancy. In high-income countries, the greatest burden of VHD referred to hospitals is mainly due to calcific aortic stenosis (AS), accounting for 34% of the total VHD population and 47% of patients who have undergone prior valve interventions. Much of the mortality of VHD is also from AS, accounting for 45% of all deaths from VHD in the United States.

Dramatic improvements in diagnostic imaging techniques available to clinical cardiologists have provided a lifelong understanding of many morphologic aspects of aortic valve disease. However, detailed histologic characteristics cannot be assessed with the current technologies, especially for patients who become symptomatic. Thus, pathologic examination of surgical or autopsy material remains the most definitive method of assessing diseased valves.

This chapter summarizes pathologic findings of aortic valve diseases, especially calcific aortic valve stenosis, and potential mechanisms underlying its pathobiology.

1. What is the normal anatomy of the aortic valve?

The normal aortic valve is composed of three leaflets, and each leaflet has three layers: the fibrosa, the spongiosa, and the ventricularis. The cell populations in those layers are valvular endothelial cells, valvular interstitial cells (VICs), and fibroblasts. Endothelial cells cover the surface of the valve leaflet and work as the interface between the blood and the leaflet. VICs are the major cell type of the valve leaflet and are seen predominantly in the spongiosa; they play an important role in valvular remodeling and regulation of both the synthesis and degradation of the extracellular matrix.

2. What are the etiologies of aortic valve diseases?

Three types of underlying conditions cause AS: calcific AS, formerly known as senile or degenerative AS; congenital abnormalities, including unicuspid or bicuspid (and rarely quadricuspid) valves; and postinflammatory scarring (rheumatic aortic valve diseases). On the other hand, there is a long list of diseases that cause aortic regurgitation (AR). Most AS occurs due to valve pathology, while AR may be caused by abnormalities of either the aortic valve or the aortic root. Common valvular causes of AR are infective endocarditis, inflammatory diseases (e.g. rheumatic disease), calcific degenerative aortic valve (which is usually associated with AS but can be a cause of AR), congenital anomalies (e.g. unicuspid, bicuspid, and quadricuspid), and iatrogenic causes. The aortic causes of AR are aortic dissection, connective tissue disorders (e.g. Marfan syndrome, Ehlers–Danlos syndrome), aortitis (e.g. syphilis, Takayasu's disease), and aortic medial degeneration (e.g. hypertension, age-related change) (Table 2.1). This wide etiologic spectrum of AR causes a marked heterogeneity in the treatment of AR, which hampers the applicability of transcatheter aortic valve replacement for patients with AR.

3. What is the epidemiology of aortic valve disease?

There is a correlation between the age at symptom presentation and underlying pathologic lesions of aortic valve disease.

Mastering Structural Heart Disease, First Edition. Edited by Eduardo J. de Marchena and Camilo A. Gomez.
© 2023 John Wiley & Sons Ltd. Published 2023 by John Wiley & Sons Ltd.
Companion website: www.wiley.com/go/deMarchena/Mastering-Structural-Heart-Disease

Table 2.1 Etiology and mechanisms of aortic regurgitation.

Mechanisms		Specific etiology
Leaflet abnormalities	Congenital	Bicuspid, unicuspid, or quadricuspid aortic valve
		Ventricular septal defect
	Acquired	Senile calcification
		Infective endocarditis
		Rheumatic disease
		Radiation-induced valvulopathy
		Toxin-induced valvulopathy: anorectic drugs, 5-hydroxytryptamine (carcinoid)
Aortic root abnormalities	Congenital	Annuloaortic ectasia
		Connective tissue disease: Loeys–Deitz, Ehlers–Danlos, Marfan syndrome, osteogenesis imperfecta
	Acquired	Idiopathic aortic root dilatation
		Systemic hypertension
		Autoimmune disease: systemic lupus erythematosis, ankylosing spondylitis, Reiter's syndrome
		Aortitis: syphilitic, Takayasu's arteritis
		Aortic dissection
		Trauma

Source: Zoghbi et al 2017 / With permission of Elsevier.

Unicuspid aortic valve (UAV) is found in childhood, adolescence, or early adulthood. The prevalence of UAV is rare and ranges from 0.02% of the population who underwent echocardiography to 4–6% of patients who underwent surgical valve replacement. Bicuspid aortic valve (BAV) is present in 0.5–2% of the general population and is more common in men than women (1.4–4.1). Thirty to 50% of patients with BAV present in their 50s or 60s, and the number of patients with BAV who underwent surgical aortic valve replacement in their 60s was greater than the patients with tricuspid aortic valve (TAV). Calcific AS in TAV is seen in approximately 2–3% of patients older than 65 years and 7% of patients over 80 years old. Calcific AS is more commonly seen in men than women (male:female = 1.6 : 1). Calcific TAV disease results in symptoms in the eighth and ninth decade of life. Quadricuspid valve is the rarest, with an incidence in the general population of 0.0008% (Figure 2.1).

Collins et al. reported a histopathological study from Toronto General Hospital in which they examined 1025 consecutive surgically excised aortic valves. The incidence of TAV, BAV, and UAV was reported as 64.5%, 31.9%, and 3.0% of all patients, respectively (Table 2.2). The incidence of rheumatic heart disease was 11% of all patients, which is lower than in previous reports, suggesting that the prevalence of post-rheumatic AS has decreased over the past half-century in high-income countries (Table 2.2). A decreased number of cusps was associated with an increasing predilection for male gender (83.9% in UAV, 73.4% in BAV) versus 59.2% in TAV and a younger patient age at surgery (41.6 years old, 61.3 years old, vs. 67.5 years old, respectively).

4. What is the pathology of tricuspid calcific aortic stenosis?

Calcific AS is a progressive disease, and pathological findings range from minimal fibrocalcific changes in the early stage of the disease to end-stage lesions characterized by fibrotic thickening and nodular calcification. We have observed a range of calcification in valves removed at surgery as well as at autopsy. Early calcification, assessed by Von Kossa stain, appears as finely stippled calcifications or small nodular concretions, typically in the valve interstitial cells located in the fibrosa of the aortic surface of the leaflet, especially in areas of early atherosclerotic change (Figure 2.2). The "hinge" point of the aortic leaflets near the attachment of the aortic annulus and an area just below the line of valve closure are regions where early calcific deposits are found and may be related to the higher mechanical forces in these regions. Early calcification gradually merges into larger complex nodules and then extends toward the middle portion of the leaflet, sparing the free margin, and may protrude into the aortic surface

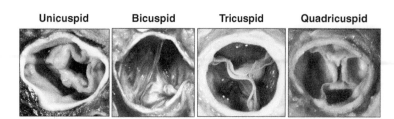

Unicuspid **Bicuspid** **Tricuspid** **Quadricuspid**

Figure 2.1   Images of unicuspid, bicuspid, tricuspid, and quadricuspid aortic valves. *Source:* Reproduced with permission from (2001) Virmani R, Burke AP, Farb A, Atkinson JB (eds): *Cardiovascular Pathology.* Philadelphia, W.B. Saunders Company.

Table 2.2 Etiology of surgically removed aortic valves.

Etiology	Mayo Clinic (1965)	University of Minnesota (1979–1983)	London (1976–1979)	Mayo (1990)	AFIP (1990–1997)	Toronto (2008)
Bicuspid	49%	49%	56%	36%	30%	32%
Post-rheumatic	33%	23%	24%	9%	13%	11%
Tricuspid degenerative	0%	28%	12%	51%	49%	64%
Unicuspid	10%	1%	0%	0%	6%	3%
Other	7%	0%	8%	2%	2%	1%

Source: Ladich E et al.2011 / Future Science Group.

during the progression (Figure 2.2). In later stages, the calcification is often superimposed on a thickened and fibrotic cusp, and there may even be focal bone formation with histologic evidence of bone matrix, osteocytes, and marrow elements (Figure 2.2). In severe calcific AS cases, gross findings of the valve cusps appear markedly thickened and distorted by multiple nodular deposits, often filling the sinuses of the involved cusps and ultimately compromising valve integrity and function (Figure 2.2). Since small calcific nodules are loosely attached to the aortic surface of

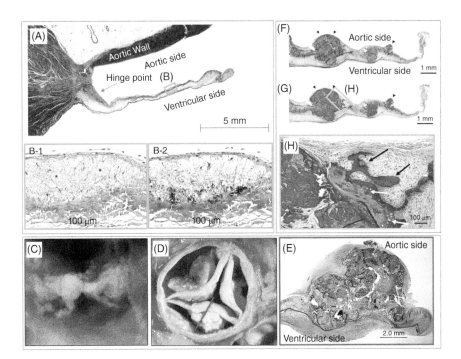

Figure 2.2 Representative histology images of tricuspid aortic valve calcification. (a, b) Early aortic valve calcification resembles atherosclerotic changes. Aortic valve leaflet from a 47-year-old man who died of accidental head trauma. (a) Low-power image of left coronary valve leaflet (Movat Pentachrome stain). (b1 and b2) High-power images from (a) (blue box) at the site of closure of the valve showing lipid insudation (*) (b1; hematoxylin and eosin [H&E]) with calcification as black dots (b2; Von Kossa stain). (c–e) Advanced calcified aortic valve from an 82-year-old female. (c) Radiograph of the aortic valve shows severely calcified leaflets. (d) There is marked nodular calcification of the cusps with bulky deposits filling the sinuses. (e) Histologic section through the cusp shows calcific nodules effacing leaflet architecture. Note fibrotic thickening of the ventricular surface. (f–h) Bone formation within advanced aortic stenosis. Degenerative aortic valve leaflet from a 70-year-old woman who underwent surgical valve replacement for severe aortic valve stenosis. Low-power images of Movat Pentachrome (f) and H&E stain (g) show nodular calcification on the aortic surface (black arrowheads). Top and bottom surface indicate the aortic and ventricular sides, respectively. (h) High-power image of H&E stain from the boxed area in (g). Ossification (black arrows) and cartilaginous metaplasia (white arrows) are found at the edge of nodular calcification. *Sources:* (a–b, f–h) Modified and reproduced with permission from Sakamoto A, et al. *Eur Heart J.* 2019;40:1374-1377; (c–e) Modified and reproduced with permission from Ladich E, et al. *Future Cardiol* 2011;7:629-642.

the leaflet, fragments of calcific nodules may cause calcific emboli during cardiac procedures. A clinical study that evaluated the efficacy of embolic protection filters demonstrated that debris was captured in 99% of patients during transcatheter aortic valve implantation. Calcification was present in 50% of filters. Notably, calcification is usually most pronounced in the non-coronary cusp as compared to the right and the left coronary cusps, which may be due to greater stress during diastole on the non-coronary cusp as compared to the right and left cusps, with less stress on the leaflet from coronary blood flow on the coronary cusps.

5. What is the etiology of bicuspid aortic valve?

BAV is one of the most frequent congenital heart diseases in the general population. The mechanisms of BAV have not been determined yet; however, a genetic basis of the disease is widely accepted, and its heredity within families and the association with other genetic syndromes (e.g. Turner syndrome, Marfan syndrome, and Loeys–Dietz syndrome) have been reported. The BAV works normally at birth and undergoes a similar degenerative process as TAVs. However, rarely, bicuspid valves may be dysplastic and not work normally for long, and become stenotic within the first year of life. Nevertheless, most BAVs become stenotic about 10–15 years earlier than the typical age-related degeneration of TAVs. There is a conjoined

leaflet formed from two underdeveloped leaflets that are separated from one another by what is commonly referred to as "raphe," representing the malformed commissure between two leaflets. The commissure of the aortic valve is the space between the parallel attachments of two adjacent leaflets that normally do not adhere to each other. Obliteration of the two commissures (unicommisural) or a total absence (acommissural) of the commissures is observed in UAV; and when only two commissures and a raphe are present, it is called a BAV.

6. What is the classification of bicuspid aortic valves?

BAV has been classified into three types based on its morphologic features, such as type 0, type 1, and type 2 (Figure 2.3). Sievers et al. described the prevalence of the types of BAV from having examined 304 patients who underwent surgery. The classification is based on (i) the number of raphes, (ii) the spatial position of cusps or raphes, and (iii) the functional status of the valve (i.e. stenosis, regurgitation, or both). Type 0 (when there is no raphe), the prevalence of which was 7%, is thought to be purely "bicuspid," i.e. two leaflets without raphe, and commissures are located anterior/posterior or right/left. Type 1, the commonest type of BAV (88%), has three well-developed cusps with two commissures instead of three and one raphe. The two cusps are unequal in size; the larger is the

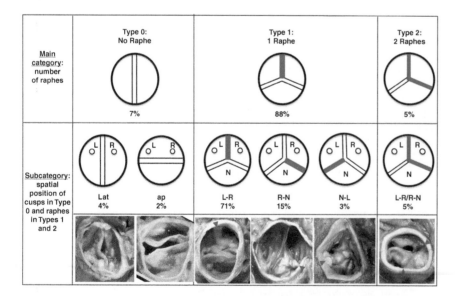

Figure 2.3 Schematic presentation of the classification system of bicuspid aortic valve and corresponding gross images. Red lines in schematic drawings represent a raphe. Three different main categories according to the number of raphes are Type 0, no raphe (7%); Type 1 with one raphe, which is the most common type of configuration (88%); and Type 2 with two raphes (5%). The three types are subcategorized as ap, lat, L-R, R-N, N-L, and L-R/R-N. ap, anterior–posterior; lat, lateral; L, left coronary sinus; R, right coronary sinus; N, non-coronary sinus. *Source:* Modified from Sievers et al. 2007 and Sakamoto et al. 2020.

conjoint cusp that has a raphe in the middle. The size of the conjoint cusp is typically less than 2 times the size of the non-conjoint cusp. Conjoint left coronary cusp (LCC) and right coronary cusp (RCC) are the most dominant type (71%), followed by conjoint non-coronary cusp (NCC) and RCC (15%), and least common is LCC and NCS (3%). In Sievers's classification, BAVs with two raphes are type 2 (5%); however, many others classified them as unicuspid or uni-commissural valves.

7. What are the pathologic findings of a bicuspid aortic valve?

BAVs commonly show signs of calcification before individuals reach their 30s. Calcification usually begins in the raphe, appears as a linear opacity on radiographic examination, and extends into the free margin of the leaflet, largely sparing the true commissures (Figure 2.4). BAV-oriented severe AS is characterized by calcification spreading to the tissue of the conjoint and non-conjoint cusps diffusely within the spongiosa, and calcific nodules may ulcerate the aortic surface (Figure 2.5). The variance of the raphes in BAV sometimes makes it difficult to distinguish a congenital BAV from an acquired BAV (i.e. rheumatic aortic valve disease). The raphe in congenital BAVs is typically rich in elastic fibers, while in acquired BAVs, collagen-rich fibrous tissue is seen in fused-commissures due to inflammatory scarring. Also, the raphe is always below the level of the true commissure. Calcification seen in rheumatic aortic valves is variably present, begins at the fused commissures, and extends into the body of the cusp (Figure 2.5).

8. What are the classification and pathology of the unicuspid aortic valve (UAV)?

UAVs are categorized as two morphologic types: (i) a domed-shaped acommissural valve containing three aborted commissures (or raphes) or (ii) a unicommissural valve with a slit-like opening that reaches the aortic wall with a single intact commissure (Figure 2.6). Unicommissural UAVs account for 60% of AS cases in patients <15 years of age. Leaflet dysplasia is common, and the severity of leaflet calcification is variable; however, dysplasia in UAVs has been reported to be more severe than BAVs and depends on the patient's age.

9. What are the differences between the pathological findings in tricuspid vs. bicuspid vs. unicuspid aortic valves?

A large series of surgically excised aortic valves from Toronto General Hospital showed that pathologic features (e.g. degree of cusp calcification, ossification, cartilaginous

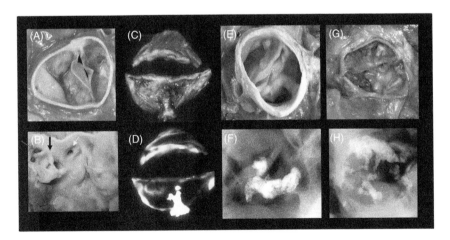

Figure 2.4 Progression of bicuspid aortic valve (BAV) calcification. (a, b) Incidental BAV. (a) Type 0 BAV: no raphe is seen from aortic surface. (b) An image opened at the commissure between the left and right coronary cusps. Raphe (black arrows) is seen in the middle of the cusp, and calcification corresponds to the raphe in the radiographic image. Left and right coronary arterial ostia are seen (yellow and red arrows). (c, d) BAV viewed from the aortic surface (early lesion); gross specimen and X-ray show calcification limited to the raphe. (e, f) A BAV obtained at autopsy from a 49-year-old male who died suddenly (late lesion). (g, h) Severe nodular calcification arising in a bicuspid valve. Note multiple nodules involving the aortic surface and obscuring the raphe. *Sources:* (a–b) Modified and reproduced with permission from (2001) Virmani R, Burke AP, Farb A, Atkinson JB (eds): *Cardiovascular Pathology*. Philadelphia, W.B. Saunders Company; (c–h) Modified and reproduced with permission from Ladich E et al. *Future Cardiol* 2011;7:629-642.

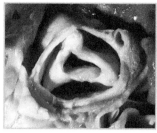
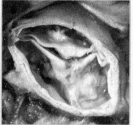
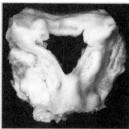

Figure 2.5 Post-inflammatory (rheumatic) aortic valve diseases. Approximately three equal-sized cusps are seen. Fused commissure is an important finding to distinguish rheumatic aortic stenosis from others. Valve cusps are fibrotically thickened. Cusp calcification is variably present and extends out from fused commissures. *Source:* Reproduced with permission from (2001) Virmani R, Burke AP, Farb A, Atkinson JB (eds): *Cardiovascular Pathology*. Philadelphia, W.B. Saunders Company.

metaplasia, and ulceration) were progressively more severe in valves exhibiting congenitally aortic valves (i.e. unicuspid and bicuspid), which may result from abnormal blood flow and stress distribution across the abnormal valve causing accelerated calcification and earlier failures. Patients with congenital UAV and BAV were also associated with increasing replacement of the ascending aorta due to dilatation and aneurysm formation (54.8%, 38.8%, and 16.6% for UAV, BAV, and TAV, respectively) at surgery. In patients with BAV, 78.3% presented with AS, and 15.6% and 4.0% had aortic insufficiencies and both stenosis and insufficiency, respectively. The prevalence of each type of

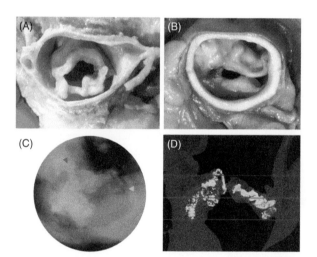

Figure 2.6 Unicuspid aortic valves. (a) Dome-shaped acommissural valve type. (b) Image of unicommissural valve. (c) Radiograph of the same valve showing heavy calcification. Red arrowhead points to rudimentary raphe and blue arrowhead to the true commissure. (d) Sagital microCT image of the valve. *Source:* Reproduced with permission from (2001) Virmani R, Burke AP, Farb A, Atkinson JB (eds): Cardiovascular Pathology. Philadelphia, W.B. Saunders Company, and Sakamoto A, et al. (2020) Basic Pathology of Arterial and Valvular Calcification in Humans. In: Aikawa E., Hutcheson J. (eds) *Cardiovascular Calcification and Bone Mineralization*. Contemporary Cardiology. Humana, Cham.

valve disease is similar to the prevalence in patients with TAV disease. In the patients with UAV, 58.1% were AS, 19.4% were aortic insufficiency, and 19.4% had both stenosis and insufficiency.

10. What are the risk factors for calcific aortic stenosis?

Calcific aortic valve stenosis and coronary atherosclerosis share similar risk factors, such as age, male gender, smoking, elevated cholesterol and lipoprotein(a) level, hypertension, diabetes mellitus, and metabolic syndrome, which has been demonstrated by epidemiological studies. AS is also associated with chronic kidney disease and abnormalities of calcium and phosphate metabolism such as hyperparathyroidism.

11. What are the underlying mechanisms of aortic valve calcification?

Previously, calcific AS was considered a passive age-related degenerative disease. However, recent studies have suggested that calcific aortic valve disease is an active process, similar to atherosclerosis. Kwiecinski et al. reported supporting data for that hypothesis. They demonstrated that 18F-sodium fluoride (18F-NaF) uptake within the native aortic valve in patients who underwent transcatheter aortic valve implantation was higher with a longer duration of implantation, which suggested that disease activity continues despite immobilization of the valve leaflet. Progression of calcific aortic valve degeneration may be related to lipid deposition, oxidative stress, inflammation, osteogenic differentiation of VICs, or the renin-angiotensin-aldosterone system (RAAS). Each of these processes could theoretically be targeted by medical treatment as well as atherosclerosis;

however, no effective pharmacological treatments have been convincingly shown to inhibit the progression of AS and improve prognosis as of today. Thus far, the only treatment for AS is surgical or transcatheter aortic valve replacement.

Conclusion

The dominant underlying cause of AS is calcific AS either in a tricuspid or congenital bicuspid/UAVs, while the prevalence of rheumatic AS has decreased dramatically in high-income countries. Calcific degeneration is the most common cause of AS, and the fewer the number of leaflets, the earlier the calcification and symptoms begin. The calcific aortic disease shares most of the risk factors in common with atherosclerosis; however, no reliable medical treatment has been reported for calcific AS. The treatment for calcific AS has been revolutionized since the introduction of percutaneous aortic transcatheter valves, leading to a decline in the incidence of surgical aortic valve replacement. Nevertheless, surgery remains an important armamentarium for the treatment of bicuspid and unicuspid aortic valve disease. Pathological studies of surgically excised valves still play an important role in elucidating the pathophysiology and mechanisms of aortic valve calcification while we continue to search for novel medical therapies.

Bibliography

1 Anderson, R.H. (2003). Understanding the structure of the unicuspid and unicommissural aortic valve. *J. Heart Valve Dis.* 12: 670–673.

2 Briand, M., Lemieux, I., Dumesnil, J.G. et al. (2006). Metabolic syndrome negatively influences disease progression and prognosis in aortic stenosis. *J. Am. Coll. Cardiol.* 47: 2229–2236.

3 Coffey, S., Cox, B., and Williams, M.J. (2014). Lack of progress in valvular heart disease in the pre-transcatheter aortic valve replacement era: increasing deaths and minimal change in mortality rate over the past three decades. *Am. Heart J.* 167: 562–567.e2.

4 Collins, M.J., Butany, J., Borger, M.A. et al. (2008). Implications of a congenitally abnormal valve: a study of 1025 consecutively excised aortic valves. *J. Clin. Pathol.* 61: 530–536.

5 Cripe, L., Andelfinger, G., Martin, L.J. et al. (2004). Bicuspid aortic valve is heritable. *J. Am. Coll. Cardiol.* 44: 138–143.

6 Danielsen, R., Aspelund, T., Harris, T.B., and Gudnason, V. (2014). The prevalence of aortic stenosis in the elderly in Iceland and predictions for the coming decades: the AGES-Reykjavík study. *Int. J. Cardiol.* 176: 916–922.

7 Edwards, J.E. (1965). Pathology of left ventricular outflow tract obstruction. *Circulation* 31: 586–599.

8 Eveborn, G.W., Schirmer, H., Heggelund, G. et al. (2013). The evolving epidemiology of valvular aortic stenosis. The Tromsø study. *Heart* 99: 396–400.

9 Falcone, M.W., Roberts, W.C., Morrow, A.G., and Perloff, J.K. (1971). Congenital aortic stenosis resulting from a unicommisssural valve. Clinical and anatomic features in twenty-one adult patients. *Circulation* 44: 272–280.

10 Fedak, P.W., Verma, S., David, T.E. et al. (2002). Clinical and pathophysiological implications of a bicuspid aortic valve. *Circulation* 106: 900–904.

11 Gotoh, T., Kuroda, T., Yamasawa, M. et al. (1995). Correlation between lipoprotein(a) and aortic valve sclerosis assessed by echocardiography (the JMS cardiac echo and cohort study). *Am. J. Cardiol.* 76: 928–932.

12 Isner, J.M., Chokshi, S.K., Defranco, A. et al. (1990). Contrasting histoarchitecture of calcified leaflets from stenotic bicuspid versus stenotic tricuspid aortic valves. *J. Am. Coll. Cardiol.* 15: 1104–1108.

13 Iung, B., Baron, G., Butchart, E.G. et al. (2003). A prospective survey of patients with valvular heart disease in Europe: the euro heart survey on valvular heart disease. *Eur. Heart J.* 24: 1231–1243.

14 Kahlert, P., Knipp, S.C., Schlamann, M. et al. (2010). Silent and apparent cerebral ischemia after percutaneous transfemoral aortic valve implantation: a diffusion-weighted magnetic resonance imaging study. *Circulation* 121: 870–878.

15 Kapadia, S.R., Kodali, S., Makkar, R. et al. (2017). Protection against cerebral embolism during transcatheter aortic valve replacement. *J. Am. Coll. Cardiol.* 69: 367–377.

16 Krepp, J.M., Roman, M.J., Devereux, R.B. et al. (2017). Bicuspid and unicuspid aortic valves: different phenotypes of the same disease? Insight from the GenTAC registry. *Congenit. Heart Dis.* 12: 740–745.

17 Kwiecinski, J., Tzolos, E., Cartlidge, T.R.G. et al. (2021). Native aortic valve disease progression and bioprosthetic valve degeneration in patients with transcatheter aortic valve implantation. *Circulation* 144: 1396–1408.

18 Marquis-Gravel, G., Redfors, B., Leon, M.B., and Généreux, P. (2016). Medical treatment of aortic stenosis. *Circulation* 134: 1766–1784.

19 Mckay, R., Smith, A., Leung, M.P. et al. (1992). Morphology of the ventriculoaortic junction in critical aortic stenosis. Implications for hemodynamic function and clinical management. *J. Thorac. Cardiovasc. Surg.* 104: 434–442.

20 Mohler, E.R. 3rd, Gannon, F., Reynolds, C. et al. (2001). Bone formation and inflammation in cardiac valves. *Circulation* 103: 1522–1528.

21 Nkomo, V.T., Gardin, J.M., Skelton, T.N. et al. (2006). Burden of valvular heart diseases: a population-based study. *Lancet* 368: 1005–1011.

22 Owens, D.S., Katz, R., Takasu, J. et al. (2010). Incidence and progression of aortic valve calcium in the multi-ethnic study of atherosclerosis (MESA). *Am. J. Cardiol.* 105: 701–708.

23 Prakash, S.K., Bossé, Y., Muehlschlegel, J.D. et al. (2014). A roadmap to investigate the genetic basis of bicuspid aortic valve and its complications: insights from the international BAVCon (bicuspid aortic valve consortium). *J. Am. Coll. Cardiol.* 64: 832–839.

24 Roberts, W.C. (1970). The structure of the aortic valve in clinically isolated aortic stenosis: an autopsy study of 162 patients over 15 years of age. *Circulation* 42: 91–97.

25 Roberts, W.C. (1992). Morphologic aspects of cardiac valve dysfunction. *Am. Heart J.* 123: 1610–1632.

26 Roberts, W.C. and Ko, J.M. (2005). Frequency by decades of unicuspid, bicuspid, and tricuspid aortic valves in adults having isolated aortic valve replacement for aortic stenosis, with or without associated aortic regurgitation. *Circulation* 111: 920–925.

27 Sievers, H.H. and Schmidtke, C. (2007). A classification system for the bicuspid aortic valve from 304 surgical specimens. *J. Thorac. Cardiovasc. Surg.* 133: 1226–1233.

28 Stewart, B.F., Siscovick, D., Lind, B.K. et al. (1997). Clinical factors associated with calcific aortic valve disease. Cardiovascular health study. *J. Am. Coll. Cardiol.* 29: 630–634.

29 Thanassoulis, G., Massaro, J.M., Cury, R. et al. (2010). Associations of long-term and early adult atherosclerosis risk factors with aortic and mitral valve calcium. *J. Am. Coll. Cardiol.* 55: 2491–2498.

30 Wilmshurst, P.T., Stevenson, R.N., Griffiths, H., and Lord, J.R. (1997). A case-control investigation of the relation between hyperlipidaemia and calcific aortic valve stenosis. *Heart* 78: 475–479.

31 Yener, N., Oktar, G.L., Erer, D. et al. (2002). Bicuspid aortic valve. *Ann. Thorac. Cardiovasc. Surg.* 8: 264–267.

3

The Top Ten Clinical Trials in Patients Undergoing Transcatheter Aortic Valve Implantation

The Evolution of a Transformative Therapy into Clinical Practice

Ying-Hwa Chen[1,2], Diana Anghel[3] and Jeffrey J. Popma[3]

[1] *Division of Cardiology, Taipei Veterans General Hospital, Taiwan*
[2] *National Yang-Ming Chiao-Tung University, Taiwan*
[3] *Medtronic, Minneapolis, MN, USA*

Few therapies in medicine have had such an impact on patient prognosis as the use of transcatheter aortic valve implantation (TAVI) in patients with symptomatic severe aortic stenosis (AS). With an expanding evidence base, TAVI has now been established as superior to medical therapy in patients deemed extreme risk ("inoperable") and as an alternative to surgery in high-risk, intermediate-risk, and low-risk surgical patients. Following an extensive Heart Team discussion about the risks and benefits of surgery and TAVI, TAVI has been endorsed by Societal Guidelines for many patients with symptomatic AS.

This chapter will review the top 10 clinical trials in TAVI and the supportive studies that have formed the foundation for these landmark trials. Between these trials, questions about the mindset of physicians in the early and later experience of TAVI are addressed. The trials are listed in near chronological order rather than by importance, to reflect the evolving evidence for TAVI over the past decade. Evidence generation is continuing in ongoing studies for new bioprostheses and expanded indications, and this evidence will inform our decisions about patient care in the future.

1. Who invented TAVI, and where were the early studies performed?

The experimental inception of TAVI was first described by the Danish cardiologist Henning Rud Anderson, who designed a foldable stent with valve leaflets and implanted it in animal models. The first human implantation of a balloon-expandable TAVI bioprosthesis was performed by Alain Cribier in 2002. Using an antegrade transseptal approach in a 57-year-old man with calcific AS and subacute leg ischemia complicated by cardiogenic shock who was deemed inoperable, the balloon-expandable transcatheter valve was successfully implanted with stable bioprosthesis position, no impairment of the coronary artery blood flow or the mitral valve function, and a mild paravalvular aortic regurgitation (AR). By 2006, the initial first-in-man series of a self-expanding, supra-annular bioprosthesis was reported by Grube et al. In this series of 25 patients with symptomatic AS and multiple co-morbidities precluding surgery, device success and procedural success were achieved in 22 (88%) and 21 (84%) patients, respectively. Successful device implantation resulted in a marked reduction in the aortic valve gradients (mean gradient after implantation, 12.4 ± 3.0 mmHg; $P < 0.0001$). Major in-hospital cardiovascular and cerebral events occurred in eight patients (32%), including mortality in five patients (20%). Remarkably, these TAVI series with first-generation devices successfully relieved the symptoms of AS, albeit with higher but addressable complications with the early procedures.

The self-expanding, supra-annular, porcine pericardial CoreValve bioprosthesis received Conformité Européene (CE Mark) approval in March 2007, and the balloon-expandable, intra-annular, bovine pericardial SAPIEN valve received CE Mark approval on 5 September 2007.

2. How was TAVI evaluated in the United States?

Regulations for approval for CE Mark in the early 2000s required demonstration of feasibility and safety, and often, only 30-day outcomes were required for European regulatory approval. In contrast, the US Food and Drug Administration (FDA) required a "reasonable assurance of safety and

Mastering Structural Heart Disease, First Edition. Edited by Eduardo J. de Marchena and Camilo A. Gomez.
© 2023 John Wiley & Sons Ltd. Published 2023 by John Wiley & Sons Ltd.
Companion website: www.wiley.com/go/deMarchena/Mastering-Structural-Heart-Disease

efficacy in the intended population," prompting the need for randomized clinical trials against conventional therapy.

Based on the studies that follow, the FDA granted approval for US commercial use for the SAPIEN transcatheter valve in inoperable patients on 3 November 2011 and granted approval for US commercial use for the CoreValve bioprosthesis in patients with extreme surgical risk on 12 June 2014.

Leon, M.B., Smith, C.R., Mack, M. et al. (2010). Transcatheter aortic-valve implantation for aortic stenosis in patients who cannot undergo surgery. *N. Engl. J. Med.* 363 (17): 1597–1607.

The Placement of Aortic Transcatheter Valves (PARTNER) B trial was likely one of the most difficult TAVI trials to perform as it evaluated patients with severe AS and coexisting conditions who were not candidates for surgical replacement of the aortic valve. The dismal prognosis of patients with untreated AS was well recognized, and randomization to medical therapy was challenging for investigators, clinicians, and patients. Accordingly, this study randomly assigned 358 patients to standard therapy (including balloon aortic valvuloplasty) or transfemoral transcatheter implantation of a balloon-expandable bovine pericardial valve and assessed one-year all-cause mortality. The results of this study were profound: a one-year rate of death from any cause of 30.7% with TAVI as compared with 50.7% with standard therapy (hazard ratio with TAVI, 0.55; P < 0.001). This translated into 20 lives saved per 100 patients treated, and a number needed to treat prevention mortality of five patients. Similarly, the rate of the composite end point of death from any cause or repeated hospitalization was 42.5% with TAVI as compared with 71.6% with standard therapy (hazard ratio, 0.46; P < 0.001). At 30 days, patients undergoing TAVI experienced a 5% stroke rate vs. 1.1% in patients treated with medical therapy (P = 0.06); major vascular complications developed in 16.2% of TAVI patients vs. 1.1% of medically treated patients (P < 0.001). The importance of this landmark clinical study in patients with AS who are deemed unsuitable for surgery cannot be overstated, and these results foreshadowed the impact of TAVI in other clinical subsets.

3. Did PARTNER B affect "clinical equipoise" for randomized trials in non-operable patients?

With the results of PARTNER B being so profound in non-operable patients, it quickly became apparent that physicians no longer felt that randomization to medical therapy

was an ethical pathway for the evaluation of additional transcatheter valves in this patient population. This set the stage for the trial design for the CoreValve clinical studies, in which patients who were deemed at extreme risk for surgery treated in a consecutive nonrandomized study were evaluated compared with a carefully conducted performance goal, and the "gatekeeper" function of a screening committee chaired by heart surgeons was used to ensure that patients assigned to the nonrandomized cohort were truly not suitable for surgery.

Popma, J.J., Adams, D.H., Reardon, M.J. et al. (2014). Transcatheter aortic valve replacement using a self-expanding bioprosthesis in patients with severe aortic stenosis at extreme risk for surgery. *J. Am. Coll. Cardiol.* 63 (19): 1972–1981.

The CoreValve Extreme Risk was a prospective, multicenter, nonrandomized investigation that evaluated the safety and efficacy of self-expanding TAVI in 506 patients with symptomatic severe AS with prohibitive risks for surgery at 41 clinical sites in the United States; of these, 489 underwent attempted treatment with the CoreValve bioprosthesis. The rate of one-year all-cause mortality or major stroke at 12 months was 26.0% vs. 43.0%, with the optimal performance goal used to estimate the outcome with medical therapy (p < 0.0001). Individual 30-day and 12-month events included all-cause mortality (8.4% and 24.3%, respectively) and major stroke (2.3% and 4.3%, respectively). Additional outcomes included life-threatening/disabling bleeding (12.7%), major vascular complications (8.2%), and need for permanent pacemaker placement (21.6%). The frequency of moderate or severe paravalvular AR was lower 12 months after self-expanding transcatheter aortic valve replacement (TAVR) (4.2%) than at discharge (10.7%; p = 0.004 for paired analysis).

4. When did the Heart Team develop, and what has it meant to TAVI decision-making?

With the initiation of the TAVI randomized trials, by necessity, a collaboration of heart surgeons, structural cardiologists, non-invasive cardiologists and anesthesiologists, and ancillary geriatric, pulmonary, and nephrology specialists, among others, was needed to provide the best options to the patient about the available procedures for aortic valve replacement. While the recognized Society for Thoracic

Surgery Predictor of Mortality (STS PROM) was developed to assess surgical risk, it was quickly recognized that the STS PROM did not include many important factors that rendered patients high risk for surgery. Factors not included in the STS PROM included frailty, prior radiation or brachytherapy, need for home oxygen therapy, porcelain aorta, horizontal aorta, non-femoral approach, and orthopedic limitation. Accordingly, the surgeon's "eyeball" became critically important in assessing surgical risk, and the Society Guidelines now recommend that the Heart Team is central to evaluating patients indicated for aortic valve replacement. The Heart Team also plays a critical role in determining surgical risk in patients enrolled in all the randomized trials.

Smith, C.R., Leon, M.B., Mack, M.J. et al. (2011). Transcatheter versus surgical aortic-valve replacement in high-risk patients. *N. Engl. J. Med.* 364 (23): 2187–2198.

The PARTNER A was performed at 25 centers and randomly assigned 699 "high-risk" patients with severe AS to undergo either transcatheter aortic-valve replacement with a balloon-expandable bovine pericardial valve (either a transfemoral or a transapical approach) or surgical replacement. The primary end point was death from any cause at one year. The rates of death from any cause were 3.4% in the TAVI group and 6.5% in the surgery group at 30 days (P = 0.07) and 24.2% and 26.8%, respectively, at one year (P = 0.001 for noninferiority). The rates of major stroke were 3.8% in the transcatheter group and 2.1% in the surgical group at 30 days (P = 0.20) and 5.1% and 2.4%, respectively, at one year (P = 0.07). Other risks were balanced, with major vascular complications significantly more frequent with TAVI (11.0% with TAVI vs. 3.2% in surgery patients, P < 0.001) and other events higher with surgery, such as major bleeding (9.3% with TAVI vs. 19.5% with surgery, P < 0.001) and new-onset atrial fibrillation (8.6% vs. 16.0%, P = 0.006) at 30 days. This landmark study demonstrated the clinical parity of TAVI with surgery.

5. Were the initial concerns about stroke with TAVI justified?

In the PARTNER A study, there was a numerical higher frequency of stroke in the TAVI patients, leading to speculation about the higher risk of stroke with TAVI. Routine neurologic evaluation and prospective collection of stroke

occurrence were not part of the PARTNER A study but have been incorporated into all subsequent randomized trials of TAVI. With prospective neurologic evaluations, the frequency of stroke is the same or lower for TAVI compared with surgery, particularly for disabling stroke. Standardized definitions for stroke have been included in the Valve Academic Research Consortia, and novel embolic protection devices have been developed. An ongoing large-scale study, PROTECTED (Periprocedural Embolic Cerebral Protection With the Sentinel Device) TAVR, will enroll 3000 patients undergoing TAVI; patients are randomized to embolic protection device or standard therapy (https://clinicaltrials.gov/ct2/show/NCT04149535).

Adams, D.H., Popma, J.J., Reardon, M.J. et al. (2014). Transcatheter aortic-valve replacement with a self-expanding prosthesis. *N. Engl. J. Med.* 370 (19): 1790–1798.

The CoreValve High Risk Randomized Trial assigned 795 patients deemed high risk for surgery by the multidisciplinary heart team to treatment in a 1 : 1 ratio to TAVI with the self-expanding transcatheter valve (TAVI group) or surgical aortic-valve replacement (surgical group). In the as-treated analysis, the rate of death from any cause at one year was significantly lower in the TAVI group than in the surgical group (14.2% vs. 19.1%), with an absolute reduction in risk of 4.9 percentage points (upper boundary of the 95% confidence interval [CI], −0.4; P < 0.001 for noninferiority; P = 0.04 for superiority). TAVI was noninferior with respect to echocardiographic indexes of valve stenosis, functional status, and quality of life. Exploratory analyses suggested a reduction in the rate of major adverse cardiovascular and cerebrovascular events and no increase in the risk of stroke.

6. What contributed to the differences in one-year mortality between TAVI and surgery patients?

Gaudiani et al. examined the timing in the rate of death after aortic valve replacement. During the recovery period (31–120 days), 15 (4%) patients undergoing TAVI and 27 (7.9%) surgery patients died (P = 0.025). This mortality difference was largely driven by higher rates of technical failure, surgical complications, and lack of recovery following surgery. The causes of death were more technical failures in the TAVI group and lack of recovery in the surgery group within the first 30 days. Late mortality (121–365 days) in both arms was most commonly ascribed to other circumstances, comprising death from medical complications from comorbid disease. These differences were likely related to the lesser invasiveness of the TAVI procedure compared with surgery. The discordance would be less apparent in patients at lower surgical risk in whom the post-operative recovery would be better.

Leon, M.B., Smith, C.R., Mack, M.J. et al. (2016). Transcatheter or surgical aortic-valve replacement in intermediate-risk patients. *N. Engl. J. Med.* 374 (17): 1609–1620.

In a study of 2032 intermediate surgical risk patients with severe AS at 57 centers, patients were assigned to treatment with either balloon-expandable TAVI or surgical replacement. Before randomization, patients were entered into one of two cohorts based on clinical and imaging findings: 76.3% of the patients were included in the transfemoral-access cohort and 23.7% in the transthoracic-access cohort. At two years, the rate of death from any cause or disabling stroke was similar in the TAVI group and the surgery group (P = 0.001 for noninferiority); the Kaplan–Meier event rates were 19.3% in the TAVI group and 21.1% in the surgery group (hazard ratio in the TAVI group, 0.89; 95% CI, 0.73–1.09; P = 0.25). In the transfemoral-access cohort, TAVI resulted in a lower rate of death or disabling stroke than surgery (hazard ratio, 0.79; 95% CI, 0.62–1.00; P = 0.05), whereas in the transthoracic-access cohort, outcomes were similar in the two groups. A trade-off suggested that TAVI resulted in larger aortic-valve areas than did surgery and lower rates of acute kidney injury, severe bleeding, and new-onset atrial fibrillation, whereas surgery resulted in fewer major vascular complications and less paravalvular aortic regurgitation.

The initial PARTNER IIA study included patients treated with the SAPIEN XT device. In the SAPIEN 3 observational study, 1077 intermediate-risk patients were assigned to receive TAVI with the SAPIEN 3 valve. A propensity-matched analysis was performed to compare patients treated with SAPIEN 3 and patients undergoing surgery in the PARTNER IIA study. At one year follow-up of the SAPIEN 3 observational study, patients who initiated the TAVI procedure had an all-cause mortality of 7.4% (6.5% in the transfemoral access subgroup) and disabling strokes had occurred in 24 (2.3%) and aortic valve re-intervention in 6 (0.6%). The propensity-score analysis included 963 patients treated with SAPIEN 3 TAVI and 747 with surgical valve replacement. For the primary composite endpoint of mortality, strokes, and moderate or severe AR, TAVI was both noninferior (pooled weighted proportion difference of −9.2%; 90% CI −12.4 to −6; p < 0.0001) and superior (−9.2%, 95% CI −13.0 to −5.4; p < 0.0001) to surgical valve replacement.

The five-year outcomes related to structural valve deterioration (SVD) were published by Pibarot et al. The five-year rates of SVD and SVD-related bioprosthetic valve failure (BVF) were significantly lower in SAPIEN 3 vs. SAPIEN XT TAVI matched cohorts. Compared with surgery, the second-generation SAPIEN XT balloon-expandable valve has a higher five-year rate of SVD, whereas the third-generation SAPIEN 3 has a rate of SVD that was not different from surgery.

Reardon, M.J., Van Mieghem, N.M., Popma, J.J. et al. (2017). Surgical or transcatheter aortic-valve replacement in intermediate-risk patients. *N. Engl. J. Med.* 376 (14): 1321–1331.

The SURTAVI (Surgical Replacement and Transcatheter Aortic Valve Implantation) study evaluated the clinical outcomes in intermediate-risk patients with severe, symptomatic AS in a randomized trial that compared TAVI (performed using a self-expanding prosthesis) with surgery. A Bayesian analytical method was used to evaluate the noninferiority of TAVI compared with surgical valve replacement. A total of 1746 patients underwent randomization at 87 centers. Of these patients, 1660 underwent an attempted TAVI or surgical procedure. The mean (+/−SD) age of the patients was 79.8+/−6.2 years, and all were at intermediate risk for surgery as determined by the local multidisciplinary heart team. At 24 months, the estimated incidence of the primary end point was 12.6% in the TAVI group and 14.0% in the surgery group (posterior probability of noninferiority, >0.999). Surgery was associated with higher rates of acute kidney injury, atrial fibrillation, and transfusion requirements, whereas TAVI had higher rates of residual AR and need for pacemaker implantation. TAVI resulted in lower mean gradients and larger aortic-valve areas than surgery.

7. What have we learned about the assessment of valve durability?

One of the most important unanswered questions in TAVI is the comparative long-term durability of TAVI and surgery. In the NOTION (Nordic Aortic Valve Intervention

Trial) trial, patients with symptomatic severe aortic valve stenosis were randomized to TAVI using the first-generation self-expanding Medtronic CoreValve or surgical aortic valve replacement (SAVR). At eight-year follow-up, the estimated risks for all-cause mortality (51.8% vs. 52.6%; P = 0.90), stroke (8.3% vs. 9.1%; P = 0.90), or myocardial infarction (6.2% vs. 3.8%; P = 0.33) were similar after TAVI and surgery. The risk of SVD was lower after TAVI than after surgery (13.9% vs. 28.3%; P = 0.0017), whereas the risk of bioprosthetic valve failure (valve-related death, severe hemodynamic SVD, or aortic valve re-intervention) was similar (8.7% vs. 10.5%; P = 0.61).

While most surgical series have used repeat valve replacement as an index for bioprosthetic valve failure, more extensive criteria have now been established to assess the long-term durability of transcatheter bioprosthetic valves. The European Association of Percutaneous Cardiovascular Interventions (EAPCI) endorsed by the European Society of Cardiology (ESC) and the European Association for Cardio-Thoracic Surgery (EACTS) has suggested that bioprosthetic valve dysfunction includes SVD, determined by changes in gradients or central regurgitation; non-SVD, manifested primarily by paravalvular regurgitation or moderate to severe patient-prosthesis mismatch; thrombosis; and endocarditis (Figure 3.1).

The Valve Academic Research Consortium-3 provided further clarification of these criteria (Figure 3.2). Importantly, 10-year follow-up is ongoing for both intermediate-risk and low-risk patients randomized in trials with TAVI bioprostheses and surgery.

Feldman, T.E., Reardon, M.J., Rajagopal, V. et al. (2018). Effect of mechanically expanded vs self-expanding transcatheter aortic valve replacement on mortality and major adverse clinical events in high-risk patients with aortic stenosis: the REPRISE III randomized clinical trial. *J. Am. Med. Assoc.* 319 (1): 27–37.

Following the approval of two transcatheter bioprostheses, novel transcatheter bioprosthesis has a pathway for regulatory evaluation that requires demonstration of noninferiority for commercially approved transcatheter valves rather than surgical valves. A mechanically expanded transcatheter bioprosthesis was evaluated in REPRISE III (Repositionable Percutaneous Replacement of Stenotic Aortic Valve Through Implantation of Lotus Valve System) for noninferiority to an approved self-expanding valve, CoreValve, or Evolut R in 912 high-risk patients with AS undergoing TAVI. Participants were randomized in a 2 : 1 ratio to receive either the mechanically expanded Lotus bioprosthesis (n = 607) or a self-expanding CoreValve (either CoreValve or Evolut R) bioprosthesis (n = 305). Among 912 randomized patients, the primary safety composite end point at 30 days occurred in 20.3% of Lotus patients and 17.2% of CoreValve patients (difference, 3.1%; P = 0.003 for noninferiority). The primary effectiveness composite end point at one year occurred in 15.4% with the

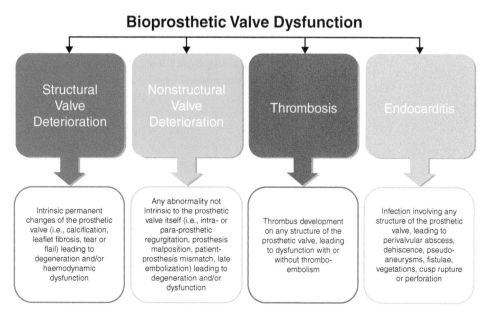

Bioprosthetic Valve Dysfunction

Structural Valve Deterioration	Nonstructural Valve Deterioration	Thrombosis	Endocarditis
Intrinsic permanent changes of the prosthetic valve (i.e., calcification, leaflet fibrosis, tear or flail) leading to degeneration and/or haemodynamic dysfunction	Any abnormality not Intrinsic to the prosthetic valve itself (i.e., intra- or para-prosthetic regurgitation, prosthesis malposition, patient-prosthesis mismatch, late embolization) leading to degeneration and/or dysfunction	Thrombus development on any structure of the prosthetic valve, leading to dysfunction with or without thrombo-embolism	Infection involving any structure of the prosthetic valve, leading to perivalvular abscess, dehiscence, pseudo-aneurysms, fistulae, vegetations, cusp rupture or perforation

Figure 3.1 EAPCI recommendations for bioprosthetic valve dysfunction. *Source:* Reproduced from Capodanno et al. (2017) / Oxford University Press.

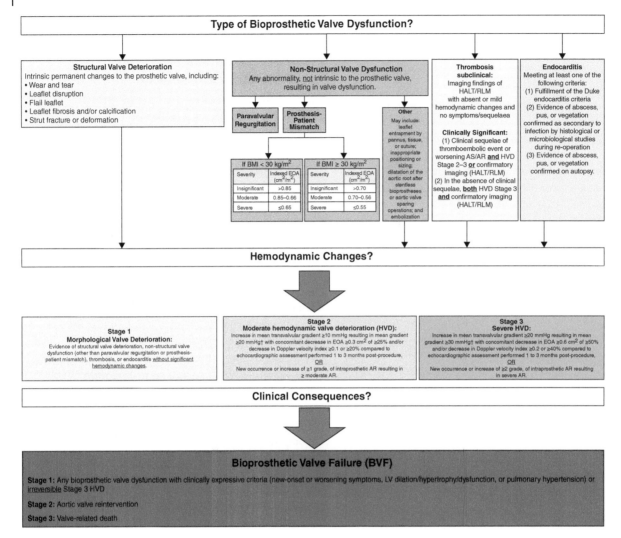

Figure 3.2 VARC-3 criteria for bioprosthetic valve dysfunction. *Source:* From Genereux et al. (2021) / Oxford University Press.

Lotus and 25.5% with the CoreValve (difference, −10.1%; Farrington-Manning 97.5% CI, −infinity to −4.4%; P < 0.001 for noninferiority). The one-year rates of moderate or severe paravalvular leak were 0.9% for the mechanically expandable valve (MEV) and 6.8% for the self expandable valve (SEV; difference, −6.1%; 95% CI, −9.6% to −2.6%; P < 0.001). The superiority analysis for primary effectiveness was statistically significant (difference, −10.2%; 95% CI, −16.3% to −4.0%; P < 0.001). The MEV had higher rates of new pacemaker implants (35.5% vs. 19.6%; P < 0.001) and valve thrombosis (1.5% vs. 0%) but lower rates of repeat procedures (0.2% vs. 2.0%), valve-in-valve deployments (0% vs. 3.7%), and valve malpositioning (0% vs. 2.7%).

A detailed echocardiographic analysis was performed by the MedStar Echocardiographic Core Laboratory. CoreValve demonstrated lower gradients and larger aortic valve area and Doppler velocity index than Lotus at discharge; the difference decreased in subsequent follow-up

at one year (all P < 0.01). Lotus had lower rates of paravalvular leak that persisted over time (P < 0.05). Hemodynamic differences between two valves did not translate into worse clinical outcomes.

While the Lotus transcatheter valve is no longer clinically available, a large randomized clinical trial evaluating the ACURATE *neo2* and commercially available valves is ongoing (https://clinicaltrials.gov/ct2/show/NCT03735667).

Mack, M.J., Leon, M.B., Thourani, V.H. et al. (2019). Transcatheter aortic-valve replacement with a balloon-expandable valve in low-risk patients. *N. Engl. J. Med.* 380 (18): 1695–1705.

The PARTNER III study randomly assigned 1000 patients with severe symptomatic AS at low risk for surgery to treatment with balloon-expandable TAVI or surgery. The mean age of the patients was 73 years, and the mean Society of Thoracic Surgeons risk score was 1.9%. The Kaplan–Meier estimate of the rate of the primary composite end point at one year was significantly lower in the TAVI group than in the surgery group (8.5% vs. 15.1%; absolute difference, −6.6 percentage points; 95% CI, −10.8 to −2.5; $P < 0.001$ for noninferiority; hazard ratio, 0.54; 95% CI, 0.37–0.79; $P = 0.001$ for superiority). At 30 days, TAVI resulted in a lower rate of stroke than surgery ($P = 0.02$) and lower rates of death or stroke ($P = 0.01$) and new-onset atrial fibrillation ($P < 0.001$). TAVI also resulted in a shorter index hospitalization than surgery ($P < 0.001$) and a lower risk of a poor treatment outcome (death or a low Kansas City Cardiomyopathy Questionnaire score) at 30 days ($P < 0.001$). There were no significant between-group differences in major vascular complications, new permanent pacemaker insertions, or moderate or severe paravalvular regurgitation.

Popma, J.J., Deeb, G.M., Yakubov, S.J. et al. (2019). Transcatheter aortic-valve replacement with a self-expanding valve in low-risk patients. *N. Engl. J. Med.* 380 (18): 1706–1715.

The Evolut Low Risk Trial evaluated 1468 patients with severe AS at low risk for surgical valve replacement who were randomly assigned to Evolut TAVI or surgery. When 850 patients had reached 12-month follow-up, we analyzed data regarding the primary end point, a composite of death or disabling stroke at 24 months, using Bayesian methods. The patients' mean age was 74 years. The 24-month estimated incidence of the primary end point was 5.3% in the TAVI group and 6.7% in the surgery group (difference, −1.4 percentage points; posterior probability of noninferiority >0.999). At 30 days, patients who had undergone TAVI, as compared with surgery, had a lower incidence of disabling stroke (0.5% vs. 1.7%), bleeding complications (2.4% vs. 7.5%), acute kidney injury (0.9% vs. 2.8%), and atrial fibrillation (7.7% vs. 35.4%) and a higher incidence of moderate or severe AR (3.5% vs. 0.5%) and pacemaker implantation (17.4% vs. 6.1%). At 12 months, patients in the TAVI group had lower aortic-valve gradients than those in the surgery group (8.6 mmHg vs. 11.2 mmHg) and larger effective orifice areas (2.3 cm^2 vs. 2.0 cm^2).

Makkar, R.R., Cheng, W., Waksman, R. et al. (2020). Self-expanding intra-annular versus commercially available transcatheter heart valves in high and extreme risk patients with severe aortic stenosis (PORTICO IDE): a randomised, controlled, non-inferiority trial. *Lancet* 396 (10252): 669–683.

PORTICO IDE (Portico Re-sheathable Transcatheter Aortic Valve System US IDE Trial) included high and extreme risk patients with severe symptomatic AS who were randomly assigned to TAVI with the first-generation Portico valve and delivery system or a commercially available valve (either an intra-annular balloon-expandable Edwards SAPIEN, SAPIEN XT, or SAPIEN 3 valve; or a supra-annular self-expanding CoreValve, Evolut R, or Evolut PRO valve). A total of 750 patients were randomly assigned to the Portico valve group (n = 381) or the commercially available valve group (n = 369). The mean age was 83 years. For the primary safety endpoint at 30 days, the event rate was higher in the Portico valve group (13.8%) than in the commercial valve group (9.6%). At one year, the rates of the primary efficacy endpoint were similar between the groups (14.8% in the Portico group vs. 13.4% in the commercial valve group). At two years, rates of death (22.3% vs. 20.2% in the commercial valve group) or disabling stroke (3.1% vs. 5.0% in the commercial valve group) were similar between groups. In summary, the Portico valve was associated with similar rates of death or disabling stroke at two years compared with commercial valves but was associated with higher rates of the primary composite safety endpoint, including death at 30 days. A new generation of the Portico valve is currently undergoing randomized clinical studies.

8. What did we learn about subclinical leaflet thrombosis from this study?

PORTICO IDE was the first to shed light on the important finding of subclinical leaflet thrombosis (Figure 3.3). Clinical data was obtained from 55 patients enrolled in the PORTICO clinical trial of TAVI and supplemented from two single-center registries that included 132 patients who were undergoing either TAVI or surgical

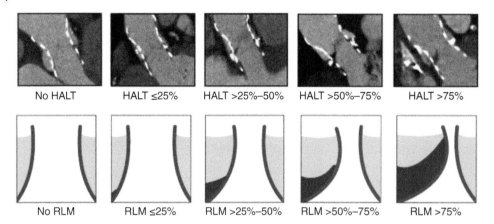

No HALT	HALT ≤25%	HALT >25%–50%	HALT >50%–75%	HALT >75%
No RLM	RLM ≤25%	RLM >25%–50%	RLM >50%–75%	RLM >75%

Figure 3.3   Classification of subclinical leaflet thrombosis. HALT = hypoattenuated leaflet thrombosis; RLM = reduced leaflet motion. *Source:* From Makkar et al. (2015) / With permission of Elsevier.

aortic-valve replacement. Reduced leaflet motion was noted on computed tomography in 40% of patients in the clinical trial and 13% in the two registries, and reduced leaflet motion was detected among patients with multiple bioprosthesis types, including transcatheter and surgical bioprostheses. Importantly, in patients who were reevaluated with follow-up CT, restoration of leaflet motion was noted in all 11 patients who were receiving anticoagulation and in 1 of 10 patients who were not receiving anticoagulation (P < 0.001).

Two high-quality, prospective computed tomographic studies were then performed in low surgical risk patients undergoing TAVI. In the PARTNER 3 substudy, 435 patients with AS at low surgical risk were randomized to undergo TAVI or surgery. The incidence of hypoattenuated leaflet thrombosis (HALT) increased from 10% at 30 days to 24% at one year; spontaneous resolution of 30-day HALT occurred in 54% of patients at one year, whereas new HALT appeared in 21% of patients at one year. HALT was more frequent in transcatheter vs. surgical valves at 30 days (13% vs. 5%; p = 0.03) but not at one year (28% vs. 20%; p = 0.19). The presence of HALT did not significantly affect aortic valve mean gradients at 30 days or one year. Patients with HALT at both 30 days and one year, compared with those with no HALT at 30 days and one year, had significantly increased aortic valve gradients at one year. In the second study of low-risk patients undergoing Evolut TAVI, the frequency of HALT was 17.3% for TAVI and 16.5% for surgery at 30 days. At one year, the frequency of HALT was 30.9% for TAVI and 28.4% for surgery. Aortic valve hemodynamic status was not influenced by the presence or severity of HALT or reduced leaflet motion (RLM) at either time point. The reason for the different HALT frequencies in the surgical groups of these two studies is not known.

Our current understanding is that subclinical leaflet thrombosis can occur with all bioprosthetic valves, and clinically related valve thrombosis should be suspected for a significant (>10 mmHg) change in gradient, the occurrence of a clinical embolic event, or sudden valve deterioration. Use of anticoagulants in these patients is recommended for the treatment of valve thrombosis.

9.   What are other areas of improvement for TAVI?

A number of considerations relating to TAVI will be addressed in the coming years. The 17.4% need for permanent pacemaker implantation in the Evolut Low Risk Trial has been substantially improved with the use of improved procedural techniques, including the cusp overlap technique. In the event that coronary angiography or coronary intervention is required in the future, concern has been raised about the ability to access the coronary arteries with transcatheter bioprostheses, and attention to commissural alignment has improved this. Finally, strategies for redo TAVI for transcatheter bioprosthesis failure are under development.

10.   What should be considered for the lifetime management of patients undergoing TAVI?

The ACC-STS Guidelines for the management of valvular heart disease suggest that patients should be considered first for aortic valve surgery if they are younger than 65 years of age, and the recent European guidelines suggest that patients should be considered first for aortic valve surgery if they are younger than 75 years of age.

While scenarios for initial and later valve selection have been characterized, the most compelling data relates to determine the longevity after aortic valve replacement (Figure 3.4). Ten-year survival after successful surgical aortic valve replacement in patients 65–80 years of age is approximately 50%. It is important to match the life expectancy with the expected duration of the bioprosthetic valve when planning the risk for subsequent aortic valve therapies.

11. What patient subsets have yet to be studied?

Randomized and single-arm studies are ongoing to evaluate additional subsets of patients with aortic valve disease.

Moderate Aortic Stenosis

Patients with moderate AS, defined by an aortic valve area between >1.0 and <1.5 cm², mean gradient 20 mmHg or greater and less than 40 mmHg, and peak aortic valve velocity 3 m/s or greater and less than 4 m/s, may benefit from TAVI, and randomized clinical trials are ongoing with TAVI and guideline-directed medical therapy. The TAVR UNLOAD (Transcatheter Aortic Valve Replacement to UNload the Left Ventricle in Patients With ADvanced Heart Failure) study is evaluating patients with moderate AS and a reduced left ventricular ejection fraction (https://clinicaltrials.gov/ct2/show/NCT02661451), while the PROGRESS Trial (Management of Moderate Aortic Stenosis by Clinical Surveillance or TAVR; https://clinicaltrials.gov/ct2/show/NCT04889872) and the EXPAND TAVR II study ()(https://clinicaltrials.gov/ct2/show/NCT05149755) will evaluate patients with moderate AS without restrictions for the left ventricular ejection fraction.

Asymptomatic Aortic Stenosis

Symptom development, including dyspnea, chest pain, or syncope, is a key factor in determining the prognostic risk in patients with AS. Current guidelines support the use of aortic valve replacement in asymptomatic patients with markedly elevated gradients (i.e. mean aortic valve gradient >60 mmHg or peak velocity > 5 m/s), reduced ventricular function (left ventricular ejection fraction <55%), or a positive exercise test. Other patients with asymptomatic AS are being evaluated in the EARLY TAVR (Evaluation of TAVR Compared to Surveillance for Patients With Asymptomatic Severe Aortic Stenosis) clinical trial (https://clinicaltrials.gov/ct2/show/NCT03042104).

Aortic Insufficiency

Primary aortic insufficiency is much less common than AS. TAVI with a current transcatheter bioprosthesis may be less suitable due to the inability to stabilize the device during deployment. A novel transcatheter bioprosthesis, the JenaValve, is being evaluated in the Align-AR Early Feasibility Study (https://clinicaltrials.gov/ct2/show/NCT02732704).

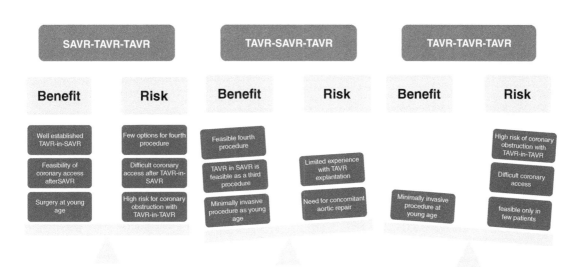

Figure 3.4 Options for lifetime management in patients with aortic stenosis. *Source:* From Yerasi et al. (2021) / With permission of Elsevier.

Conclusions

TAVI has become a well-established alternative to surgical aortic valve replacement. The TAVI procedure continues to improve early and intermediate-term outcomes in patients with symptomatic severe AS. Lifetime management concerns about the need for permanent pacemaker, coronary access, and the long-term durability of TAVI devices, including the treatment of transcatheter heart valve failure due to degeneration or stenosis, are being addressed with design iterations, more clinical studies, and the introduction of novel transcatheter devices. Sound clinical evidence will continue to inform strategies and guidelines for the management of patients with aortic valve disease.

Bibliography

1 Adams, D.H., Popma, J.J., Reardon, M.J. et al. (2014). Transcatheter aortic-valve replacement with a self-expanding prosthesis. *N. Engl. J. Med.* 370 (19): 1790–1798.

2 Asch, F.M., Vannan, M.A., Singh, S. et al. (2018). Hemodynamic and echocardiographic comparison of the Lotus and CoreValve transcatheter aortic valves in patients with high and extreme surgical risk: an analysis from the REPRISE III randomized controlled trial. *Circulation* 137 (24): 2557–2567.

3 Blanke, P., Leipsic, J.A., Popma, J.J. et al. (2020). Bioprosthetic aortic valve leaflet thickening in the Evolut low risk sub-study. *J. Am. Coll. Cardiol.* 75 (19): 2430–2442.

4 Capodanno, D., Petronio, A.S., Prendergast, B. et al. (2017). Standardized definitions of structural deterioration and valve failure in assessing long-term durability of transcatheter and surgical aortic bioprosthetic valves: a consensus statement from the European Association of Percutaneous Cardiovascular Interventions (EAPCI) endorsed by the European Society of Cardiology (ESC) and the European Association for Cardio-Thoracic Surgery (EACTS). *Eur. J. Cardiothorac. Surg.* 52 (3): 408–417.

5 Cribier, A., Eltchaninoff, H., Bash, A. et al. (2002). Percutaneous transcatheter implantation of an aortic valve prosthesis for calcific aortic stenosis: first human case description. *Circulation* 106 (24): 3006–3008.

6 Feldman, T.E., Reardon, M.J., Rajagopal, V. et al. (2018). Effect of mechanically expanded vs self-expanding transcatheter aortic valve replacement on mortality and major adverse clinical events in high-risk patients with aortic stenosis: the REPRISE III randomized clinical trial. *J. Am. Med. Assoc.* 319 (1): 27–37.

7 Gaudiani, V., Deeb, G.M., Popma, J.J. et al. (2017). Causes of death from the randomized CoreValve US pivotal high-risk trial. *J. Thorac. Cardiovasc. Surg.* 153 (6): 1293–301 e1.

8 Genereux, P., Piazza, N., Alu, M.C. et al. (2021). Valve academic research consortium 3: updated endpoint definitions for aortic valve clinical research. *Eur. Heart J.* 42 (19): 1825–1857.

9 Grube, E., Laborde, J.C., Gerckens, U. et al. (2006). Percutaneous implantation of the CoreValve self-expanding valve prosthesis in high-risk patients with aortic valve disease: the Siegburg first-in-man study. *Circulation* 114 (15): 1616–1624.

10 Henrik, H. and Nielsen, M. (2012). Transcatheter aortic valve implantation. *Dan. Med. J.* 59 (19): B4556.

11 Jorgensen, T.H., Thyregod, H.G.H., Ihlemann, N. et al. (2021). Eight-year outcomes for patients with aortic valve stenosis at low surgical risk randomized to transcatheter vs. surgical aortic valve replacement. *Eur. Heart J.* 42 (30): 2912–2919.

12 Kapadia, S.R., Kodali, S., Makkar, R. et al. (2017). Protection against cerebral embolism during transcatheter aortic valve replacement. *J. Am. Coll. Cardiol.* 69 (4): 367–377.

13 Kappetein, A.P., Head, S.J., Genereux, P. et al. (2013). Updated standardized endpoint definitions for transcatheter aortic valve implantation: the valve academic research Consortium-2 consensus document. *J. Thorac. Cardiovasc. Surg.* 145 (1): 6–23.

14 Leon, M.B., Piazza, N., Nikolsky, E. et al. (2011). Standardized endpoint definitions for transcatheter aortic valve implantation clinical trials: a consensus report from the valve academic research consortium. *Eur. Heart J.* 32 (2): 205–217.

15 Leon, M.B., Smith, C.R., Mack, M. et al. (2010). Transcatheter aortic-valve implantation for aortic stenosis in patients who cannot undergo surgery. *N. Engl. J. Med.* 363 (17): 1597–1607.

16 Leon, M.B., Smith, C.R., Mack, M.J. et al. (2016). Transcatheter or surgical aortic-valve replacement in intermediate-risk patients. *N. Engl. J. Med.* 374 (17): 1609–1620.

17 Mack, M.J., Leon, M.B., Thourani, V.H. et al. (2019). Transcatheter aortic-valve replacement with a balloon-expandable valve in low-risk patients. *N. Engl. J. Med.* 380 (18): 1695–1705.

18 Makkar, R.R., Blanke, P., Leipsic, J. et al. (2020). Subclinical leaflet thrombosis in transcatheter and surgical bioprosthetic valves: PARTNER 3 cardiac computed tomography substudy. *J. Am. Coll. Cardiol.* 75 (24): 3003–3015.

19 Makkar, R.R., Cheng, W., Waksman, R. et al. (2020). Self-expanding intra-annular versus commercially available transcatheter heart valves in high and extreme risk patients with severe aortic stenosis (PORTICO IDE): a randomised, controlled, noninferiority trial. *Lancet* 396 (10252): 669–683.

20 Makkar, R.R., Fontana, G., Jilaihawi, H. et al. (2015). Possible subclinical leaflet thrombosis in bioprosthetic aortic valves. *N. Engl. J. Med.* 373 (21): 2015–2024.

21 Mihaljevic, T., Nowicki, E.R., Rajeswaran, J. et al. (2008). Survival after valve replacement for aortic stenosis: implications for decision making. *J. Thorac. Cardiovasc. Surg.* 135 (6): 1270–1278. discussion 8-9.

22 Otto, C.M., Nishimura, R.A., Bonow, R.O. et al. (2021). 2020 ACC/AHA guideline for the management of patients with valvular heart disease: executive summary: a report of the American College of Cardiology/American Heart Association joint committee on clinical practice guidelines. *Circulation* 143 (5): e35–e71.

23 Pibarot, P., Ternacle, J., Jaber, W.A. et al. (2020). Structural deterioration of transcatheter versus surgical aortic valve bioprostheses in the PARTNER-2 trial. *J. Am. Coll. Cardiol.* 76 (16): 1830–1843.

24 Popma, J.J., Adams, D.H., Reardon, M.J. et al. (2014). Transcatheter aortic valve replacement using a self-expanding bioprosthesis in patients with severe aortic stenosis at extreme risk for surgery. *J. Am. Coll. Cardiol.* 63 (19): 1972–1981.

25 Popma, J.J., Deeb, G.M., Yakubov, S.J. et al. (2019). Transcatheter aortic-valve replacement with a self-expanding valve in low-risk patients. *N. Engl. J. Med.* 380 (18): 1706–1715.

26 Reardon, M.J., Van Mieghem, N.M., Popma, J.J. et al. (2017). Surgical or transcatheter aortic-valve replacement in intermediate-risk patients. *N. Engl. J. Med.* 376 (14): 1321–1331.

27 Schaff, H.V. (2011). Transcatheter aortic-valve implantation--at what price? *N. Engl. J. Med.* 364 (23): 2256–2258.

28 Smith, C.R., Leon, M.B., Mack, M.J. et al. (2011). Transcatheter versus surgical aortic-valve replacement in high-risk patients. *N. Engl. J. Med.* 364 (23): 2187–2198.

29 Tang, G.H.L., Zaid, S., Gupta, E. et al. (2019). Impact of initial Evolut transcatheter aortic valve replacement deployment orientation on final valve orientation and coronary reaccess. *Circ. Cardiovasc. Interv.* 12 (7): e008044.

30 Thourani, V.H., Kodali, S., Makkar, R.R. et al. (2016). Transcatheter aortic valve replacement versus surgical valve replacement in intermediate-risk patients: a propensity score analysis. *Lancet* 387 (10034): 2218–2225.

31 Vahanian, A., Beyersdorf, F., Praz, F. et al. (2021). 2021 ESC/EACTS guidelines for the management of valvular heart disease. *Eur. Heart J.* 43: 561–632.

32 Yerasi, C., Rogers, T., Forrestal, B.J. et al. (2021). Transcatheter versus surgical aortic valve replacement in young, low-risk patients with severe aortic stenosis. *JACC Cardiovasc. Interv.* 14 (11): 1169–1180.

33 Yudi, M.B., Sharma, S.K., Tang, G.H.L., and Kini, A. (2018). Coronary angiography and percutaneous coronary intervention after transcatheter aortic valve replacement. *J. Am. Coll. Cardiol.* 71 (12): 1360–1378.

4

Present and Future Generations of Transcatheter Aortic Valves

Atsushi Sugiura[1], Sebastian Zimmer[1], Solomon A. Seifu[2] and Eberhard Grube[1,3]

[1] Department of Cardiology, Heart Center Bonn, University Hospital Bonn, Germany
[2] Department of Medicine, Division of Cardiovascular Medicine, University of Miami Miller School of Medicine, Miami, FL, USA
[3] Center of Innovative Interventions (CIIC) Heart Center, Bonn, Germany

1. What life-long management is required for patients undergoing TAVR

The first transcatheter aortic valve replacement (TAVR) was performed in a patient with aortic valve stenosis by Dr. Alain Cribier in 2002. Since then, multiple studies have validated the safety and efficacy of this novel approach. TAVR was first approved in 2011 for the treatment of severe aortic stenosis (AS) in patients with a prohibitively high surgical risk. Now we are able to use TAVR for patients in all of the risk groups. The field has shifted from extreme-risk and high-risk patients to intermediate-risk patients, where we worry more about procedural outcomes such as procedural risk, an immediate quality-of-life (QOL) benefit, or the risk of vascular complications. Nowadays, we have to think even more broadly to include low-risk patients when making decisions. How long will the patient live? How durable is the valve? And what is the life expectancy of the valve and the patient together? Hemodynamics has become an important consideration, as well as the potential for patient–prosthesis mismatch (PPM). An additional consideration in younger, lower-risk patients is the potential need for future coronary access. Furthermore, as the total number of transcatheter aortic valve implantation (TAVI) procedures has grown exponentially, there is an increasing need to develop new transcatheter heart valve (THV) devices with improved performance, decreased vascular complications and paravalvular leakage (PVL), and a reduced need for pacemaker implantation.

2. How is TAVR used for low-surgical-risk patients?

Three randomized clinical trials and several prospective cohort studies have collectively reported the safety and feasibility of TAVR in low-surgical-risk patients. The risk of adverse outcomes (i.e. mortality, stroke, re-hospitalization due to heart failure) after TAVR was comparable or even lower compared to conventional surgical intervention. TAVR has the advantage of better QOL than the surgical procedure. TAVR patients recovered significantly faster than patients undergoing surgical aortic valve replacement (SAVR), which is especially important in younger, low-risk patients. Furthermore, the hemodynamic outcomes were significantly better after TAVR than SAVR, which should maximize the patient's physical capacity after the procedure.

Also, as we transition into a population with a lower surgical risk, we will encounter more patients with a bicuspid aortic-valve morphology. The pivotal randomized trials for TAVR originally excluded patients with bicuspid aortic-valve pathology due to the anatomic complexity. Despite the feasibility of the procedure as well as comparable device success rate and one-year mortality, the bicuspid aortic valve was associated with cerebral ischemic events and aortic root injury compared to TAVR on the tricuspid aortic valve. Furthermore, moderate to severe PVL after TAVR was more likely to be observed in the bicuspid aortic valve than in the tricuspid aortic valve, which raises concerns about the durability of the replacement valve. These observations underscore the need to develop THV devices that fit specifically to a bicuspid aortic valve.

3. Describe the hemodynamics after TAVR

Ensuring safety and procedural results is important for all patients who receive TAVR, and particularly for patients with low surgical risk and younger age, it is also essential for the valve to be durable. The most crucial factor of durability may be hemodynamics. If patients have a low pressure gradient and large effective orifice area (EOA), we can expect the implanted THV to last longer. Additionally, this point matters even more if patients have a small aortic valve and, therefore, a higher risk of PPM.

The aim is to achieve near-normal hemodynamics following TAVR. Although TAVR has been shown to be associated with superior hemodynamic performance compared to SAVR, severe PPM has been observed in approximately 10% of TAVR patients. PPM occurs when the EOA of the prosthesis is too small relative to the patient's body size. PPM is associated with valve degeneration over time and may be linked to an increased risk of mortality. How do we avoid PPM and thereby increase valve durability? One potential solution is the use of a supra-annular valve design, which allows for a larger EOA and, therefore, may reduce the risk of PPM. The CHOICE-Extend registry compared supra-annular Evolut R and intra-annular SAPIEN 3 THVs and found that the Evolut R THV had a significantly larger EOA than the SAPIEN 3 THV, with the biggest difference seen for the smallest valves. Similarly, a cohort study reported that intra-annular THVs were associated with an increased risk of PPM in patients with a small aortic annulus (i.e. an annular perimeter <72 mm or area <400 mm^2). On the other hand, relatively larger body size (i.e. obesity) may also be linked to the risk of PPM. Okuno et al. reported that a higher body-mass index (BMI) (>1.83 m^2) was associated with an increased risk of PPM. Furthermore, chronological or biological age should be considered for lifelong management of AS. Younger patients are likely to be more active, and normal hemodynamics is even more important to them than to older patients. A holistic approach will need to be taken by the Heart Team to determine the optimal strategy to achieve the largest EOA possible. This decision should be based not only on the type of THV available or aortic valve anatomy but also on patient demographics (i.e. age and BMI).

Another concern may be subclinical leaflet thrombosis after TAVR, which could limit the hemodynamic status of the patient. Recently, a post hoc analysis of the Evolut Low-Risk Trial investigated the frequency, predictors, and clinical correlates of hypoattenuating leaflet thickening and reduced leaflet motion.

4. How durable is TAVR?

In addition to improved hemodynamics, the durability of the implanted valve will become more important as we move the procedure to younger patients. To achieve optimal durability of the TAVR procedure, we need to improve the design of THVs to achieve a larger EOA, have more durable materials for the leaflets, and achieve less PVL after the procedure. As already mentioned, a supra-annular design is more optimal for achieving a larger EOA after TAVR. It is possible that small differences in EOA or the trans-aortic pressure gradient could result in a significant difference in mortality or the need for a repeat aortic-valve intervention in the long run. There is already evidence that a small increase in the pressure gradient may lead to significantly increased mortality over time.

Structural deterioration of the valve is one of the essential factors limiting the durability of a prosthesis. Previous studies have shown that bioprosthetic valves can experience thrombus, fibrosis, and calcification, which can cause the leaflets to malfunction. Anti-platelet therapy can reduce the risk of valve degeneration. Furthermore, using valves with anti-calcification technology may improve the long-term performance of the valve. Patient demographics may also be associated with increased structural valve deterioration. Several studies in SAVR patients have reported that younger age, female sex, chronic kidney disease, and diabetes mellitus were all associated with an increased risk of structural valve deterioration. So far, the incidence of structural valve deterioration or bioprosthetic valve failure after TAVR is comparable to that of the surgical prosthesis within five years. Previous studies have shown that structural valve deterioration and bioprosthetic valve deterioration were rare after TAVR, even in a long-term follow-up. However, caution should be paid to these results as the follow-up rates in these studies were low due to the advanced age of the TAVR cohorts.

PVL is another important factor associated with valve durability after TAVR and is more likely to be observed than with surgery. Given that it is associated with mortality after TAVR, minimizing PVL is an essential factor in patients undergoing TAVR. Moderate/severe PVL has nearly disappeared with the use of contemporary THVs. However, Okuno et al. recently reported that even mild PVL was associated with an increased risk of five-year mortality compared to no PVL or only a trace. This finding is important when considering younger or low-surgical-risk patients, as they are likely to live much longer after TAVR. Also, eliminating PVL might lead to a reduced risk of endocarditis after TAVR. More recently, Wilde et al. reported that the latest iteration of the balloon-expandable system (SAPIEN 3 Ultra), which has a 40% taller polyethylene terephthalate (PET) outer skirt, had less PVL compared to the SAPIEN 3 valve. Similarly, the latest versions of self-expandable THVs with outer skirts have shown favorable outcomes for reducing PVL. Looking at long-term management after TAVR, using a skirt is becoming a standard design feature for THVs.

5. Describe coronary access after TAVR.

Coronary artery access after TAVR is increasingly a concern for younger patients, who might develop future coronary disease and may require an intervention. Similar to the surgical bioprostheses, valve degeneration can occur over time and may result in the need for a repeat intervention. This means good coronary access and the ability to do a valve-in-valve procedure if necessary should not be disregarded. Coronary angiography and percutaneous coronary intervention after the TAVR procedure are usually feasible but may sometimes be challenging, especially for the right coronary artery. Following a TAVR procedure, commissure misalignment was observed in 78% of patients (25% for mild, 22% for moderate, 31% for severe), whereas commissural misalignment was observed in just 3.6% of patients undergoing SAVR. This may be because surgical biological heart valves (BHVs) are sutured to the annulus under direct visual observation and are tested to maintain the geometry of the stent frame. More recently, commissure alignment techniques have been developed with self-expandable THVs, allowing the device to be oriented according to the native commissures or coronary arteries and, therefore, avoid coronary artery overlap. Anatomical and device-related factors, such as a narrow sino-tubular junction, low sinus of Valsalva height, supra-annular design of a prior implanted THV, and high implant position of a prior implanted THV, were linked to either impaired coronary access or acute coronary obstruction after TAVR-in-TAVR. Optimal THV selection and a dedicated strategy are needed for TAVR in younger patients, looking at the long-term perspective. Furthermore, we need a THV that is designed to provide the best hemodynamics as well as optimal coronary access after TAVR.

6. Describe pacemaker implantation after TAVR

According to the 2020 Society of Thoracic Surgeons-American College of Cardiology Transcatheter Valve Therapy Registry (STS-ACC-TVT TAVR registry) data, the incidence of permanent pacemaker implantation at 30 days after TAVR was 10.8%. To reduce the rate of pacemaker implantation, we need to attain higher implant heights without complications, which may also reduce PVL. Minimizing a protrusion of THVs into the left ventricular outflow tract (LVOT) may mitigate the risk of interference with the conduction system. Recently, a cusp-overlap technique was developed to optimize the implantation depth of THVs, which may reduce the need for pacemaker implantation. The basics of the technique involve using computed tomography (CT) and moving away from the traditional three-cusp view, overlapping the insertion points of the left and right coronary cusps on the right-hand side of the screen, translating that into a fluoroscopic image, and using the non-coronary cusp as the lowest part of the annulus. The mechanics of the technique are step-wise and can be used as a reliable, reproducible protocol for most patients, even those with a vertical annulus or horizontal aorta. The cusp-overlap technique allows us to elongate the LVOT and eliminate the calculation of the foreshortening area that was inherent in the three-cusp view. This retains the ability to complement the two views (i.e. cusp-overlap view, three-cusp view) with each other to end up with two to three mm below the lowest point of the annulus.

7. What is the present generation of transcatheter valves?

SAPIEN 3 Ultra Valve

The Edwards SAPIEN valve platform (Edwards Lifesciences) is a balloon-expandable type of transcatheter aortic valve. The valve bioprosthesis is made of bovine pericardial tissue that forms the valve leaflets, polyethylene terephthalate (PET) that forms the outer skirt, and a cobalt–chromium valve frame. The Edwards SAPIEN 3 Ultra valve, which is the most recent edition, has an extended outer sealing skirt to decrease paravalvular leaks (Figure 4.1). The SAPIEN valves have an intra-annular leaflet position and come in 20, 23, 26, and 29 mm sizes. These valves are compatible with a 14 Fr excel sheath, which is expandable to accommodate a THV prosthesis and delivery system. The SAPIEN 3 valve platform can be used for antegrade as well as retrograde TAVR. It is also approved for aortic, mitral, and pulmonary valve-in-valve procedures. The PARTNER (Placement of Aortic Transcatheter Valves) 1B and 1A, 2, and 3 trials are major randomized clinical trials that have proven the clinical efficacy of the SAPIEN valve series in patients with all ranges of surgical risk.

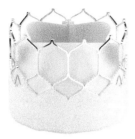

Figure 4.1 Edwards SAPIEN 3 transcatheter heart valve.

Evolut PRO+ Valve

The Medtronic valve platform (Medtronic) is a self-expanding type of transcatheter aortic valve. This valve bioprosthesis is made of porcine tissue that forms the valve leaflets and skirt on a Nitinol self-expanding valve frame (Figure 4.2). The porcine valve leaflets are located at a supra-annular plane, thus achieving a larger EOA and lower transvalvular gradients. The Medtronic aortic valve platform has evolved from the CoreValve to Evolut R to Evolut PRO+. The Evolut PRO+, which is the most recent edition, has porcine tissue that forms a skirt over the inside and outside of the inflow portion of the Nitinol frame to decrease paravalvular leaks. The Medtronic valve bioprostheses come in 23, 26, 29, and 34 mm diameters to cover a range of different annular sizes. The 23–29 mm valves are delivered through a 14 Fr in-line sheath and the 34 mm valve through an 18 Fr in-line sheath. The SURTAVI (CoreValve US Pivotal, Surgical Replacement and Transcatheter Aortic Valve Implantation) and Evolut Low Risk Trials have proven the clinical efficacy of the CoreValve Evolut valve series in patients with all ranges of surgical risk.

ACURATE *neo2* Valve

The ACURATE *neo* valve platform (Boston Scientific) is a self-expanding type of transcatheter aortic valve. The valve bioprosthesis is made of a Nitinol stent frame with leaflets made from porcine pericardium (Figure 4.3). The stent

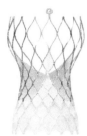

Figure 4.2 Medtronic Evolut PRO+ transcatheter heart valve.

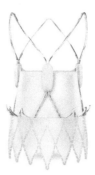

Figure 4.3 ACURATE *neo2* transcatheter heart valve.

frame is covered both externally and internally by a porcine pericardium skirt. The valve leaflets are supra-annular in location. This valve cannot be repositioned or retrieved. The ACURATE *neo* valve comes in three sizes (23, 25, and 27 mm) and uses a 14 Fr sheath for delivery. The SCOPE I and II (Safety and Efficacy Comparison of Two TAVI Systems in a Prospective Randomized Evaluation) randomized controlled trials (RCTs) compared this valve with the SAPIEN valve and did not show superior clinical outcomes.

JenaValve

The JenaValve (JenaValve Technology) is a transcatheter aortic valve that can be implanted in a native valve with no calcification. This valve bioprosthesis is made of porcine valve leaflets mounted on a low-profile, self-expanding Nitinol stent (Figure 4.4). The valve comes in three sizes (23, 25, and 27 mm). The valve leaflets are positioned intra-annularly. This valve is unique among the other aortic prostheses in that it is implanted with active clip fixation to the native aortic leaflets, thus reducing the radial forces on cardiac and aortic structures. This also provides a secure anchoring point even in the absence of calcifications; therefore, JenaValve is indicated for noncalcified aortic regurgitation. It is the only valve type approved for pure aortic insufficiency. The ALIGN-AR (The JenaValve ALIGN-AR Pivotal Trial) RCT, which is currently ongoing, is investigating the clinical efficacy of this valve.

ALLEGRA Valve

The ALLEGRA valve (NVT GmbH) has a self-expanding Nitinol frame; bovine pericardial tissue; 23, 27, and 31 mm sizes; and supra-annular leaflet position. It uses an 18 Fr sheath and is repositionable and fully recapturable. Superior hemodynamic profiles have been seen with this valve platform in small annular sizes, which may be beneficial for a valve-in-valve procedure.

8. What is the future generation of transcatheter valves?

The future generation of valves will have expanded indications and will be able to be used across a large spectrum of anatomy and a broad patient base. Individualized valve shaping and sizing with 3D printing could help achieve same-day discharge, less sedation, higher valve durability, easier deliverability, and better hemodynamics (higher EOA and minimal gradient) and allow use for the extremes of annulus size.

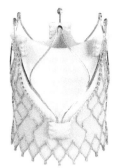

Figure 4.4 Jena Valve transcatheter heart valve.

Colibri Valve

The Colibri valve is composed of cryo-dried porcine tissue, which allows it to be folded and delivered through a 14 Fr delivery system. Using dry tissue technology allows the heart valve to be pre-mounted, pre-crimped, and pre-loaded on a balloon-delivery catheter. The valves range in size from 21 to 30 mm. Currently, the Colibri valve is going through a clinical trial in Europe to assess its safety and performance.

DurAVR Valve

DurAVR (Anteris) is a balloon-expandable valve that has a single-sheet bovine pericardium valve. This one-piece design has fewer suture lines and, therefore, is thought to increase the durability of the valve. Furthermore, the tissue has been treated to fully decellularize it and remove DNA from the valve with anti-calcification technology, which promotes long-lasting durability of the valve. DurAVR is also designed to have a near-normal opening, which can match the hemodynamics of the self-expanding, supra-annular valve. Finally, this system can rotate the prosthesis at the level of the commissure so physicians can align the commissures. Together with the short design of the valve, these features provide optimal accessibility to coronary arteries after TAVR. Currently, the DurAVR is undergoing the first in-human study.

Navitor

The Navitor valve platform (Abbott) builds on the Portico TAVR system, which is an intra-annular, self-expanding transcatheter aortic valve. The new Navitor system features a unique fabric cuff (NaviSeal) that works with the cardiac cycle to eliminate PVL. Exclusive Linx anti-calcification technology is also intended to improve the long-term durability of the valve. The large cell area and annular positioning allow for easy coronary artery access (Figure 4.5). The valve comes in 23, 25, 27, and 29 mm sizes. The Navitor is designed to be recaptured, repositioned, and fully retrievable until it is completely deployed. This valve platform includes a 14 Fr delivery system (FlexNav) with 5.0 mm minimum vessel diameter, which is smaller than the original Portico system. The former version of the device (i.e. Portico) has shown comparable outcomes for mortality and stroke for up to two years follow-up. The Portico NG study, which is a prospective, multi-center, global, investigational study evaluating the safety and effectiveness of the Navitor THV in patients with AS, showed initial safety and feasibility of the device, with only 0.8% of patients experiencing major vascular complications and 0% with PVL of moderate grade or more.

Triskele UCL Valve

The Triskele UCL valve is the only type of transcatheter valve that is free from all biomaterials. It is created from a nanocomposite polymer, which has a lower risk of calcification than bovine or porcine tissue and does not degrade when it is crimped; the theoretical advantage of this type of valve will be better long-term durability.

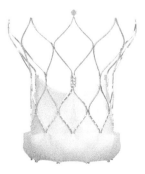

Figure 4.5 Navitor.

Conclusions

Continuing rapid growth of TAVR procedures can be expected in the next decade, with a large amount of evidence for its safety and efficacy and advancing technologies. In 2022, after 20 years in use, TAVR is the predominant therapy for the treatment of AS in all the risk groups. However, the long-term durability of the THV system remains to be proven. Furthermore, normalized hemodynamics, low to no PVL, and maintaining secure coronary access are goals for future THV devices. We are still far from the end of the TAVR journey.

Bibliography

1 Abdelghani, M., Mankerious, N., Allali, A. et al. (2018). Bioprosthetic valve performance after transcatheter aortic valve replacement with self-expanding versus balloon-expandable valves in large versus small aortic valve annuli. *JACC Cardiovasc. Interv.* 11: 2507–2518.

2 Balmforth, D., Dimagli, A., Benedetto, U., and Uppal, R. (2021). Fifty years of the pericardial valve: long-term results in the aortic position. *J. Card. Surg.* 36: 2865–2875.

3 Blanke, P., Leipsic, J.A., Popma, J.J. et al. (2020). Bioprosthetic aortic valve leaflet thickening in the Evolut low risk sub-study. *J. Am. Coll. Cardiol.* 75: 2430–2442.

4 Buzzatti, N., Romano, V., De Backer, O. et al. (2020). Coronary access after repeated transcatheter aortic valve implantation: a glimpse into the future. *JACC Cardiovasc. Imaging* 13: 508–515.

5 Carroll, J.D., Mack, M.J., Vemulapalli, S. et al. (2020). STS-ACC TVT registry of transcatheter aortic valve replacement. *J. Am. Coll. Cardiol.* 76: 2492–2516.

6 Cribier, A., Eltchaninoff, H., Bash, A. et al. (2002). Percutaneous transcatheter implantation of an aortic valve prosthesis for calcific aortic stenosis: first human case description. *Circulation* 106: 3006–3008.

7 Garcia, S., Cubeddu, R.J., Hahn, R.T. et al. (2021). 5-year outcomes comparing surgical versus transcatheter aortic valve replacement in patients with chronic kidney disease. *JACC Cardiovasc. Interv.* 14: 1995–2005.

8 Hansson, N.C., Grove, E.L., Andersen, H.R. et al. (2016). Transcatheter aortic valve thrombosis: incidence, predisposing factors, and clinical implications. *J. Am. Coll. Cardiol.* 68: 2059–2069.

9 Hayashida, K., Lefèvre, T., Chevalier, B. et al. (2012). Impact of post-procedural aortic regurgitation on mortality after transcatheter aortic valve implantation. *JACC Cardiovasc. Interv.* 5: 1247–1256.

10 Johnston, D.R., Soltesz, E.G., Vakil, N. et al. (2015). Long-term durability of bioprosthetic aortic valves: implications from 12,569 implants. *Ann. Thorac. Surg.* 99: 1239–1247.

11 Kim, W.-K., Pellegrini, C., Ludwig, S. et al. (2021). Feasibility of coronary access in patients with acute coronary syndrome and previous TAVR. *JACC Cardiovasc. Interv.* 14: 1578–1590.

12 Leon, M.B., Mack, M.J., Hahn, R.T. et al. (2021). Outcomes 2 years after transcatheter aortic valve replacement in patients at low surgical risk. *J. Am. Coll. Cardiol.* 77: 1149–1161.

13 Leone, P.P., Regazzoli, D., Pagnesi, M. et al. (2021). Predictors and clinical impact of prosthesis-patient mismatch after self-expandable TAVR in small annuli. *JACC Cardiovasc. Interv.* 14: 1218–1228.

14 Liao, Y.-B., Li, Y.-J., Jun-Li, L. et al. (2017). Incidence, predictors and outcome of prosthesis-patient mismatch after transcatheter aortic valve replacement: a systematic review and meta-analysis. *Sci. Rep.* 7: 15014.

15 Long, Y.-X. and Liu, Z.-Z. (2020). Incidence and predictors of structural valve deterioration after transcatheter aortic valve replacement: a systematic review and meta-analysis. *J. Interv. Cardiol.* 2020: 4075792.

16 Lorusso, R., Gelsomino, S., Lucà, F. et al. (2012). Type 2 diabetes mellitus is associated with faster degeneration of bioprosthetic valve: results from a propensity score–matched Italian multicenter study. *Circulation* 125: 604–614.

17 Mack, M.J., Leon, M.B., Thourani, V.H. et al. (2019). Transcatheter aortic-valve replacement with a balloon-expandable valve in low-risk patients. *N. Engl. J. Med.* 380: 1695–1705.

18 Makkar, R.R., Cheng, W., Waksman, R. et al. (2020). Self-expanding intra-annular versus commercially available transcatheter heart valves in high and extreme risk patients with severe aortic stenosis (PORTICO IDE): a randomised, controlled, non-inferiority trial. *Lancet* 396: 669–683.

19 Manoharan, G., Grube, E., Van Mieghem, N.M. et al. (2020). Thirty-day clinical outcomes of the Evolut PRO self-expanding transcatheter aortic valve: the international FORWARD PRO study. *EuroIntervention* 16: 850–857.

20 Mathieu, P. and Boulanger, M.-C. (2019). Autotaxin and lipoprotein metabolism in calcific aortic valve disease. *Front. Cardiovasc. Med.* 6: 18.

21 Mendiz, O.A., Noč, M., Fava, C.M. et al. (2021). Impact of cusp-overlap view for TAVR with self-expandable valves on 30-day conduction disturbances. *J. Interv. Cardiol.* 2021: 1–7.

22 Montalto, C., Sticchi, A., Crimi, G. et al. (2021). Outcomes after transcatheter aortic valve replacement in bicuspid versus tricuspid anatomy: a systematic review and meta-analysis. *JACC Cardiovasc. Interv.* 14: 2144–2155.

23 Ochiai, T., Chakravarty, T., Yoon, S.-H. et al. (2020). Coronary access after TAVR. *JACC Cardiovasc. Interv.* 13: 693–705.

24 Okuno, T., Khan, F., Asami, M. et al. (2019). Prosthesis-patient mismatch following transcatheter aortic valve replacement with supra-annular and intra-annular prostheses. *JACC Cardiovasc. Interv.* 12: 2173–2182.

25 Okuno, T., Tomii, D., Heg, D. et al. (2021). Five-year outcomes of mild paravalvular regurgitation after transcatheter aortic valve implantation. *EuroIntervention* 18 (1): 33–42.

26 Pibarot, P., Ternacle, J., Jaber, W.A. et al. (2020). Structural deterioration of transcatheter versus surgical aortic valve bioprostheses in the PARTNER-2 trial. *J. Am. Coll. Cardiol.* 76: 1830–1843.

27 Popma, J.J., Deeb, G.M., Yakubov, S.J. et al. (2019). Transcatheter aortic-valve replacement with a self-expanding valve in low-risk patients. *N. Engl. J. Med.* 380: 1706–1715.

28 Redondo, A., Baladrón Zorita, C., Tchétché, D. et al. (2022). Commissural versus coronary optimized alignment during transcatheter aortic valve replacement. *JACC Cardiovasc. Interv.* 15: 135–146.

29 Rogers, T., Greenspun, B.C., Weissman, G. et al. (2020). Feasibility of coronary access and aortic valve reintervention in low-risk TAVR patients. *JACC Cardiovasc. Interv.* 13: 726–735.

30 Rück, A., Kim, W.-K., Kawashima, H. et al. (2021). Paravalvular aortic regurgitation severity assessed by quantitative aortography: ACURATE neo2 versus ACURATE neo transcatheter aortic valve implantation. *J. Clin. Med.* 10: 4627.

31 Sá, M.P.B.O., Cavalcanti, L.R.P., Sarargiotto, F.A.S. et al. (2019). Impact of prosthesis-patient mismatch on 1-year outcomes after transcatheter aortic valve implantation: meta-analysis of 71,106 patients. *Braz J Cardiovasc Surg.* 34: 318–326.

32 Sellers, S.L., Gulsin, G.S., Zaminski, D. et al. (2021). Platelets. *JACC: Basic Transl. Sci.* 6: 1007–1020.

33 Strange, G., Stewart, S., Celermajer, D. et al. (2019). Poor long-term survival in patients with moderate aortic stenosis. *J. Am. Coll. Cardiol.* 74: 1851–1863.

34 Tabata, N., Al-Kassou, B., Sugiura, A. et al. (2020). Predictive factors and long-term prognosis of transcatheter aortic valve implantation-associated endocarditis. *Clin. Res. Cardiol.* 109: 1165–1176.

35 Tanaka, A., Jabbour, R.J., Testa, L. et al. (2019). Incidence, technical safety, and feasibility of coronary angiography and intervention following self-expanding transcatheter aortic valve replacement. *Cardiovasc. Revasc. Med.* 20: 371–375.

36 Tang, G.H.L., Zaid, S., Fuchs, A. et al. (2020). Alignment of transcatheter aortic-valve neo-commissures (ALIGN TAVR): impact on final valve orientation and coronary artery overlap. *JACC Cardiovasc. Interv.* 13: 1030–1042.

37 Thyregod, H.G.H., Ihlemann, N., Jørgensen, T.H. et al. (2019). Five-year clinical and echocardiographic outcomes from the NOTION randomized clinical trial in patients at lower surgical risk. *Circulation* 139: 2714–2723.

38 Waksman, R., Torguson, R., Medranda, G.A. et al. (2021). Transcatheter aortic valve replacement in low-risk patients: 2-year results from the LRT trial. *Am. Heart J.* 237: 25–33.

39 Wilde, N., Rogmann, M., Mauri, V. et al. (2022). Haemodynamic differences between two generations of a balloon-expandable transcatheter heart valve. *Heart* 1–7.

40 Yoon, S.-H., Kim, W.-K., Dhoble, A. et al. (2020). Bicuspid aortic valve morphology and outcomes after transcatheter aortic valve replacement. *J. Am. Coll. Cardiol.* 76: 1018–1030.

5

Computed Tomography for Transcatheter Aortic Valve Replacement Planning

Current Perspectives and Future Directions

Amr Idris[1], Miho Fukui[2] and João L. Cavalcante[2,3]

[1] Department of Cardiovascular Medicine, Baylor Scott & White The Heart Hospital, Plano, TX, USA
[2] Minneapolis Heart Institute Foundation – Cardiovascular Imaging Research Center and Core Lab, Minneapolis, MN, USA
[3] Minneapolis Heart Institute at Abbott Northwestern Hospital, Minneapolis, MN, USA

Introduction

The rapid progress over the past decade of transcatheter aortic valve replacement (TAVR) in symptomatic patients with severe aortic stenosis (AS) has expanded to include the entire spectrum of high- to low-surgical-risk patients. Continued improvements in patient selection, device technology, procedure technique, and post-procedural management have contributed to the establishment and adoption of disruptive treatment of AS. In parallel, technological advancements in the field of cardiac computed tomography (CT) angiography with substantial understanding of anatomy, data analysis, and continued improvements in spatial and temporal resolutions have provided incredible value in patient selection and procedural planning to improve outcomes and reduce complications.

1. What Is the best way to approach pre-procedural CT assessment, patient preparation, contrast administration, scanning protocol, and data-reconstruction techniques in patients undergoing CT evaluation prior to TAVR?

It is important to review several aspects of the patient's medical history, medications, and allergies during preparation for the TAVR scan. Protocol details of contrast administration, scanning technique, and data reconstruction are covered in Table 5.1.

2. What is the best way to analyze aortic valve calcium extension, scoring, and its clinical significance?

CT evaluation of the aortic valve (AV) morphology and function prior to TAVR is useful for patients with AS of uncertain severity, such as patients with low-flow, low-gradient AS with normal or reduced left ventricular ejection fraction. The AV calcium score can be obtained with an optional pre-contrast electrocardiogram (ECG)-gated prospective acquisition similar to the coronary artery calcium score (i.e. matrix 512×512, tube voltage: $120\,kV$, slice thickness $3\,mm$). This will be valuable in differentiating true severe AS from moderate AS, especially in patients with no increase in the stroke volume with a low-dose dobutamine ECG or even in the absence of it. AV calcium score thresholds have been identified to characterize AS severity, with $>2000\,AU$ (Agatston units) in men and >1300 in women. In addition to confirming the diagnosis of severe AS in equivocal cases, emerging data links anatomical details as risk factors, such as AV and left ventricular outflow tract (LVOT) calcium for post-TAVR paravalvular regurgitation, annular rupture, atrioventricular block with need for pacemaker implantation, and adverse clinical outcomes for both balloon-expandable and self-expandable TAVR valves that predict a possible need for post-dilation. The TAVR device landing zone comprises the LVOT, aortic annulus, and valve cusps. Therefore, it is essential to detect the presence of AV calcium and quantify it by using the same coronary artery calcium scoring system to characterize the location, extension of the calcium to the LVOT, coronary artery calcification, and symmetry of the calcium on the AV leaflets. At our center, this information is routinely obtained and

Table 5.1 Pre-Procedural computed tomographic (CT) assessment, data acquisition, and reconstruction summary.

Patient preparation:

1. Maintain hydration, and reduce the total amount of iodine contrast to the minimum.
2. Medications:
   A. Metformin suspension for 48 h prior to the exam.
   B. Caution with nitroglycerine usage (relative contraindication).
   C. Beta-blockers are not withheld on the day of the exam.
   D. Additional beta-blockers are not recommended prior to transaortic valve replacement (TAVR) CT examination.
3. Avoid any metal, jewelry, or radio-opaque objects on the patient's clothing by having them change into a hospital gown.
4. Ensure proper ECG lead placement on the lower part of the chest and firm skin contact with the ECG leads.
5. Place the patient in a supine position, centering the patient's heart within the gantry and having the patient raise both arms above the head.
6. Practice the breath-hold maneuver and instructions with the patient.
7. Explain to the patient the steps of CT data acquisition, answer any questions before data acquisition, and remind the patient about the importance of lying still.

Contrast administration:

1. The antecubital vein is the preferred and frequently used intravenous (IV) access site.
2. Dual-head injectors are preferable.
3. Imaging data acquisition timing: test bolus or bolus-tracking techniques.
4. Injection rate: 4–6 ml/s for peripherally inserted IV catheters compared to 1.5–2 ml/s in central venous catheters.
5. Total contrast volume: 50–120 cc, adjusted based on patient characteristics, scan duration, and injection rate.

Scan protocols:

1. Obtain motion-artifact-free images of the aortic root with high contrast to noise using ECG synchronization.
2. Retrospective ECG-gated data acquisition should cover at least the aortic root and ideally encompass the entire cardiac silhouette.
3. Image acquisition matrix: 512×512.
4. Detector collimator width: 0.4–0.625 mm with 0.4 mm slice overlap.

Data reconstruction technique:

1. Image reconstruction for the aortic annulus and AV root complex should be performed for the systolic phases with a slice thickness reconstruction of 0.5–0.6 mm for gated acquisition and 1 mm for non-gated/vascular acquisition.
2. Manual checking of ECG tracing and correction is required. Depending entirely on automatic software is not recommended.
3. 5% reconstruction is recommended to optimize the evaluation of functional images.

incorporated into patient-management decisions regarding additional testing and the type of TAVR device (Figure 5.1).

3. What is the best approach for aortic valve annular evaluation and sizing?

For the purpose of TAVR imaging, the basal attachments of the AV cusps, known as the basal hinge points, form a virtual ring inferior to the anatomic ventricular-aortic junction that is used as the valvular annulus. This virtual ring is used in sizing the AV in patients undergoing TAVR; it is important to identify all three basal attachments of the leaflets. The superior attachments of the AV cusps form a true anatomical ring and demarcate the sinotubular junction (STJ). Since the AV annulus is not circular, 3D imaging is necessary through gated cardiac computed tomography angiography (CTA) and/or transesophageal echocardiography (TEE), which has shown improved prosthesis sizing and outcomes compared to transthoracic echocardiography (TTE) or 2D TEE. Contrast-enhanced ECG-synchronized CT is more commonly used to assess the AV annulus with high inter-reader and intra-reader reproducibility. The geometry of the AV root and annulus changes throughout the cardiac cycle. During systole, there is a stretch of the aortic root anatomic structures compared to diastole; there is also a flattening of the aortic-mitral junction, causing the AV annular dimension to be the largest during systole. Therefore, obtaining TAVR measurements for valve sizing should focus on involving the mid-systolic phase of the cardiac cycle, selecting the phase with the fewest motion/misregistration artifact. Mean annulus diameters are calculated by measuring the long and short axes in addition to the annulus area and perimeter by planimetry.

Because most patients undergoing TAVR have a high AV calcium burden, measuring the annulus should be standardized to avoid measurement errors and post-TAVR complications. The annular contour should be measured along the tissue-blood interface with focused attention while measuring to draw the contour in a consonant fashion regardless of the presence of calcium. One practical tip to improve measurement reproducibility is to draw the annular contour as if the calcification did not exist (Figure 5.2).

Using the spline method with manual placement of segmentation points that are automatically connected by a spline interpolation is the most accurate method compared to freehand, attenuation/Hounsfield-based, or polygon techniques. However, smoothing algorithms in different workflows can be used to increase the accuracy of these

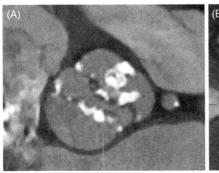
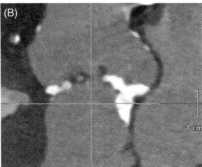

Figure 5.1 Qualitative grading of a bicuspid aortic valve demonstrating (a) severe calcification burden with asymmetric calcifications of the aortic cusps and raphe in the transverse oblique projection (b) that extends into the left ventricular outflow tract in the sagittal oblique projection.

methods. Occasionally, despite optimizing image acquisition and reconstruction, artifacts are unavoidable, and the interpreter should report the image quality.

AV annular rupture is a rare event, but it is catastrophic when it occurs. Risk factors have been identified such as small AV annulus, small aortic root, aggressive prosthesis oversizing, using balloon-expandable TAVR devices compared to self-expandable devices, protruding subannular calcifications (especially non-coronary cusps), and LVOT.

4. What is the best way to evaluate the aorta on CT scan prior to TAVR, and what is the evaluation's clinical significance?

Defining the geometry and anatomic characterization of the aorta is required in severe AS patients undergoing

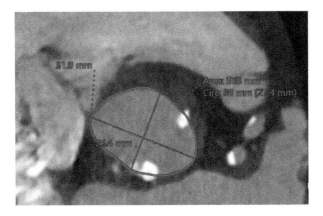

Figure 5.2 The annular contour measurement along the tissue-blood interface with focused attention while measuring to draw the contour in a consonant fashion regardless of the presence of calcium.

TAVR evaluation to prevent serious complications, including coronary artery occlusion, device embolization, or annular rupture.

Ascending Aorta

Measurements of the thoracic aorta dimensions should be made using a double-oblique multiplanar reformat, orthogonal to the vessel centerline. Detection of aortopathy, including dilatation, aneurysm, dissections, extensive plaque, or extensive calcification, may affect the approach for these patients prior to TAVR and the need for possible contemporaneous surgical aortic root replacement or surgical clamping.

3D CTA can also provide two important fluoroscopic angles for TAVR implantation: one that is co-planar and equidistant to the three cusps (non-right–left bisecting the right coronary cusp, and typically left anterior oblique/cranial [LAO/CRA]) and one that overlaps the right and left cusps (cusp overlap angle bisecting the non-coronary cusp, typically right anterior oblique/caudal [RAO/CAU]), which isolates the non-coronary cusp and is important particularly for self-expanding valves (SEVs) to avoid lower implantation and membranous septum contact and the subsequent risk of new pacemaker implantation after the procedure (Figures 5.3 and 5.4). Therefore, in addition to the aortic measurements, CT can help predict the optimal angiographic angle during TAVR. This is accomplished by providing information regarding the angulation of the aortic root axis relative to the body main axis, which can be done manually or automatically using the workflow station (Figure 5.5). Accurate information can be obtained only when the patient is positioned in a similar orientation on both the CT scanner and operation tables. This should be reported using the same catheterization laboratory view terms, such as LAO and RAO, with their corresponding angulation.

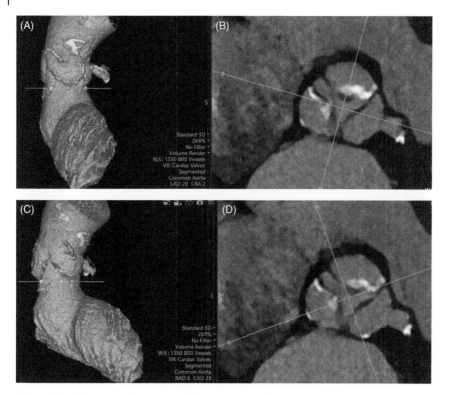

Figure 5.3 3D computed tomographic angiography (CTA) provides two fluoroscopic angles for transcatheter aortic valve replacement (TAVR) implantation. (a, b) Left anterior oblique (LAO) cranial projection for balloon-expandable valves (BEVs) that shows co-planar and equidistant to the three cusps (non-coronary cusp (green), right coronary cusp (red), and left coronary cusp (blue)). (c, d) Right anterior oblique (RAO) caudal projection for self-expanding valves (SEVs) that shows the left and right coronary cusp overlap angle, which isolates the non-coronary cusp.

Coronary Ostium, Sinus of Valsalva, and Sinotubular Junction Measurements

In contrast to surgical aortic valve replacement (SAVR), where the calcified native AV is removed and replaced with a surgical prosthesis valve, in patients undergoing TAVR, the native leaflets are pushed by the TAVR valve, which may lead to coronary artery occlusion. Despite being rare, coronary artery occlusion can be disastrous and has high mortality. Measurements of the coronary ostia height should be standardized by drawing a perpendicular line from the AV annular plane to the lower coronary artery ostium edge (Figure 5.6). The STJ height should be measured by drawing a similar line perpendicular to the AV annulus extending to the lower edge of the junction. Finally, the sinus of Valsalva should be measured parallel to the annular valve plane by measuring the cusp to commissure distance of the three cusps. Note that this cusp-to-commissure measurement is smaller than the cusp-to-cusp measurement typically used to evaluate the aortic root diameter and aortopathy.

Therefore, high-risk anatomy with a low coronary ostial height of <12 mm, sinus of Valsalva diameter of <30 mm, and STJ height of <15 mm, in addition to the length of the AV cusps with the degree of calcification, are important anatomical considerations and ought to be reported prior to the procedure. However, these risk features are not prohibitive for TAVR; the measurements should be used as a tool in determining the risks and benefits of the approach in treating patients using TAVR vs. SAVR.

5. What are the TAVR access sites, and how are they evaluated on a CT scan?

CT scan evaluation prior to TAVR has been extended beyond the cardiac evaluation to include vascular assessment due to its high productive value compared to peripheral angiography. Despite the advancement of TAVR devices' delivery systems with a reduction in their size, vascular complications remain a major source of post-TAVR complications including length of hospital stay, morbidity, and mortality. Therefore, pre-procedural planning and evaluation of the vascular tree are important to aid in choosing the appropriate vascular access and predict the risk of vascular complications.

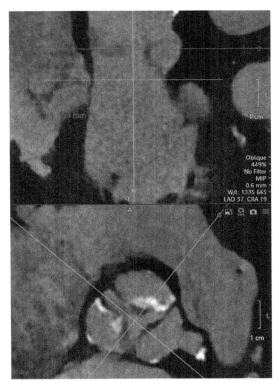

Figure 5.4 The membranous septum measurement is made from the aortic annulus down to the basal interventricular septum, measuring 8 mm in this example. The membranous septum resides between the non and right commissures (green line).

Transfemoral Access

Transfemoral access is the default vascular access route for TAVR. Unfavorable anatomy and risk factors should be identified in advance to avoid unexpected complications. Risk factors in determining suitability for femoral access include significant circumferential/horseshoe-like calcification that, when extensive, causes luminal diameter reduction (<6 mm). Severe vessel tortuosity can be an additional risk factor, especially in heavily calcified arteries. However, due to the lack of a standardized definition, and because *tortuosity* is a subjective term, this should not be used as the sole determinant of the access route and should

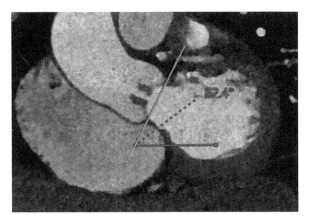

Figure 5.5 Left ventricle-aortic annulus angle measurement. The angle (62.4°) is steep, which may be problematic, especially for self-expanding valves.

instead be addressed in combination with other vascular risk factors. In addition, identifying common femoral artery anatomy such as high bifurcation, anterior wall calcification, or focal stenosis will aid in identifying the access site location for TAVR patients or predicting arterial closure device success (Figure 5.7).

The CT assessment is usually achieved either manually, using multiplanar reformation (MPR), or automatically, with a software-generated centerline. Automatic measurements should always be manually verified by the interpreter. Vascular calcification grading is currently subjective and can range from none or minimal to extensive, severe calcification.

Alternative Access

Peripheral arterial disease is common in patients with severe AS, and transfemoral access may not be feasible in every patient. In these patients, preference has increased for transcarotid, transaxillary, or subclavian access in recent years because multiple observational studies have reported the feasibility of this type of access for TAVR patients who require an alternative access approach. Direct aortic and inferior vena cava access have also emerged as

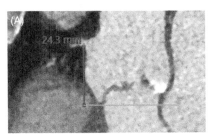 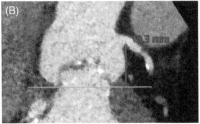

Figure 5.6 (a) Right coronary artery ostial height and (b) left coronary artery ostial height relative to the aortic annular plane.

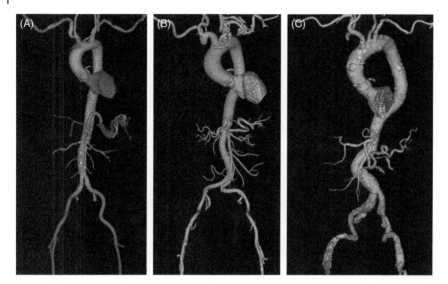

Figure 5.7 Volume-rendered computed tomography (CT). (a) Minimal luminal diameter >6 mm with no calcification or tortuosity. (b) Minimal luminal diameter >6 mm with no calcification but significant tortuosity involving the left common iliac artery. (c) Despite minimal luminal diameter >6 mm, there is severe tortuosity of the abdominal aorta and tortuosity and calcification of the bilateral common and external iliac arteries with diffuse calcification and aneurysmal dilation of both common femoral arteries, making transfemoral access more problematic. In this case, the left carotid artery was chosen instead of transfemoral access.

alternative TAVR accesses. Although in limited series, the stroke rate for some of these alternative types of access might be higher than with the femoral approach, randomized trials comparing different access sites in TAVR patients are still lacking. Thus the use of an alternative TAVR access approach is mostly based on the patient's anatomy and local Heart Team expertise.

6. What is the importance of assessing the suitability of carotid embolic protection devices prior to TAVR?

Stroke remains a concerning complication in TAVR patients, although it has significantly improved from previous experience. While the majority of strokes occur in the peri-procedural time, other sources of cardioembolism are also prevalent in this population. To date, carotid protection devices have not shown a reduction in the low current rates of silent or clinical cerebral ischemic lesions or a decrease in mortality, but studies have shown a reduction in the total cerebral ischemic volumes that could affect long-term outcomes and quality of life, especially for younger patients who are considered low surgical risk. Therefore, suitability for these devices should be assessed, including aortic arch vessel anatomy, vessel diameter, and calcification.

7. What is the best way to evaluate coronary arteries and coronary bypass grafts using CT scan?

Given that nitrate usage has traditionally been relatively contraindicated in severe AS and additional beta-blockers have not commonly been administered prior to TAVR CTA, the quality of the coronary arteries evaluation may be affected in these severe AS patients who typically have a greater burden of coronary calcification and atherosclerotic plaque. Technical advances, particularly with volumetric and dual-source scanners, have reduced breath-holding time, improved z-axis coverage and temporal resolution, allowing for upfront CAD screening by TAVR CTA in the majority of these patients. This upfront screening approach seems to be safe in identifying and selecting patients who will need additional invasive coronary angiography evaluation prior to TAVR.

Furthermore, a recent pilot study using selected patients undergoing pre-TAVR CT examination with the use of nitroglycerin, beta-blockers, and computed tomography-fractional flow reserve (CT-FFR) showed its safety and diagnostic accuracy for CAD. Evaluation of bypass grafts is typically easier because they tend to have less movement and larger caliber. CT scan is also helpful in identifying different coronary artery anomalies that are considered either higher risk or prohibitive for TAVR instead of SAVR.

8. What is the importance of reporting the CT scan functional assessment, and what is the significance of cardiac and non-cardiac incidental findings?

CT scan has a high temporal and spatial resolution that aids in cardiac anatomy and functional assessment, especially in cases of difficult echocardiographic images without prior ventricular assessment. Our group has pioneered the functional evaluation of global longitudinal strain assessment at baseline TAVR CTA and shown it to have an important association with post-TAVR outcomes, despite preserved left ventricular ejection fraction (LVEF) and successful procedure. Identification of right ventricular (RV) dysfunction was found in 1 : 4 patients by a baseline functional TAVR CTA and, importantly, associated with post-TAVR outcomes. Although at this time functional CTA information is not routinely reported and/or leveraged due to demanding post-processing and analysis, it is important to recognize and report additional information regarding left and right ventricular function and annular and subvalvular abnormalities because it may be associated with adverse clinical effects. Equally important is reporting non-cardiac incidental findings, because these could also impact morbidity and mortality and may change the timing of treatment and management in patients undergoing TAVR evaluation.

9. What is the best way to use myocardial extracellular volume (ECV) as a potential screening for cardiac amyloidosis and myocardial fibrosis?

The prevalence of AS increases with age, which is associated with an increased prevalence of other comorbidities including hypertension, diabetes mellitus, renal failure, and even transthyretin cardiac amyloidosis (ATTR). Recent improvements in ATTR diagnostic tools and new therapies have led to increased awareness of this underdiagnosed condition. Clinical implications of ATTR in AS patients are largely unknown, but dual diagnosis can be as high as 16%. It is important to diagnose amyloidosis prior to TAVR: both diseases share common symptoms that could affect survival and treatment approach, so high suspicion is required. Screening starts with ECG, cardiac biomarkers, and noninvasive studies such as echocardiogram with global longitudinal strain, cardiac magnetic resonance, and myocardial technetium-99m stannous pyrophosphate (PYP) or 3,3-diphosphono-1,2-propanodicarboxylic acid (DPD) scintigraphy. Due to the improvement in noninvasive diagnostic methods for ATTR, the need for routine invasive endomyocardial biopsy can be spared, which can miss the diagnosis due to sampling errors. Evidence of the possible benefit of measuring the myocardial extracellular volume (ECV) has grown as an additional tool to screen severe AS patients for ATTR. ECV is obtained by the change of the Hounsfield unit (HU) attenuation pre- and post-contrast using the formula $ECV = (1\text{-hematocrit}) \times (\Delta HU_{myocardium} / \Delta HU_{blood})$. This technique could help detect and even quantify the extension of the infiltration with a minimal increase in CT duration acquisition (Figure 5.8).

10. What is the best way to perform CT evaluation of valve-in-valve TAVR?

Implanting a transcatheter aortic valve (TAV) prosthesis into a failed aortic bioprosthetic valve (also known as *valve-in-valve* [VIV] implantation) has emerged as an alternative therapy for high-risk patients with failed SAVR prostheses. VIV TAVR has been increasingly used in recent years, with high technical success rates and promising patient outcomes. The most common complication of the VIV procedure is coronary occlusion, which is more common than TAVR in native aortic valves (2.3% vs. 0.66%). Pre-procedural CT plays a crucial role in assessing the risk of

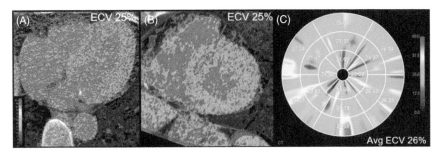

Figure 5.8 Cardiovascular tomography (CT) derived extracellular volume measurement (ECV) with the region of interest contours at the interventricular septum seen in the (a) four-chamber and (b) short-axis views, both measuring 25% (normal value). (c) Entire 3D ECV segmentation is also possible to produce the 17-segment polar map with global myocardial ECV measurement.

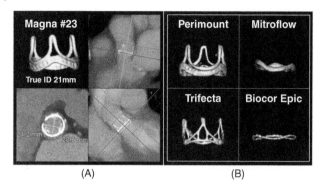

(A)   (B)

Figure 5.9 (a) Example of implanted surgical bioprosthesis seen by computed tomography with (b) different stent frame characteristics that allow for the identification and/or confirmation of operative reports and adequate valve-in-valve TAVR planning.

coronary occlusion in patients undergoing VIV procedures. In this section, we review the planning for TAV in surgical aortic valve (SAV) implantation.

Sizing

First we need to identify the size and type of the implanted surgical bioprosthesis to determine the appropriate TAVR prosthesis to be implanted, to assess the risk of coronary obstruction and the feasibility of bioprosthetic valve fracture. Although surgical information may be available from patient records or the surgical valve card, TAVR CTA reconstruction allows for confirmation, correction, or generation of the SAVR data. The stent frame morphology and measurement of the basal internal diameter of the SAVR prosthesis can be verified (Figure 5.9) by referring to the Valve in Valve app (https://apps.apple.com/us/app/valve-in-valve/id655683780) or published reference charts.

Risk of Coronary Artery Obstruction

The risk assessment for coronary artery obstruction depends on whether the implanted surgical valve is stented or stentless (Figure 5.10). When implanting a TAV into a stented SAV, the relative position of each coronary ostium to the uppermost aspect of the surgical valve struts needs to be assessed first. The final form of TAV in the stented surgical valve is cylindrical, with the TAV frame covered by the surgical prosthesis stent and opened leaflets. When the coronary artery ostium is above the uppermost aspect of the surgical valve, no further assessment is needed because there is no risk of coronary artery occlusion due to sealing by the surgical valve leaflet or strut.

On the other hand, the risk of coronary artery occlusion needs to be considered and further evaluated when the coronary artery ostium is below the uppermost aspect of the surgical valve. The virtual TAV to coronary (valve-to-coronary [VTC]) distance from the anticipated, expanded THV frame to the coronary ostium is the key assessment in this situation. VTC, especially less than 4 mm, was shown to be the only independent predictor of procedure-related coronary obstruction. The concept of VTC is based on the fact that surgical valves are often implanted in a canted position to the aortic root, which may mean close proximity of the TAV to the coronary ostium and subsequent mean at risk of coronary obstruction despite a large aortic root. The conventional measurements of coronary artery height and Valsalva sinus width are inadequate to assess the risk. The VTC should be assessed for each coronary artery using either an advanced post-processing platform capable of simulating a virtual cylinder with a defined diameter and height or a MPR: carefully place the MPR in the orientation of the surgical valve, draw a region of interest (ROI) at the level of the coronary ostium, assess the distance from

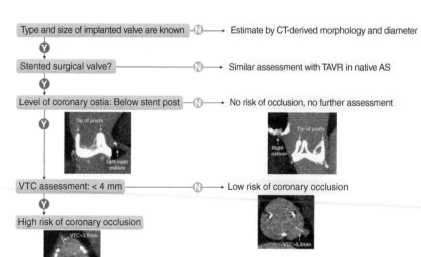

Figure 5.10 Risk assessment for coronary artery obstruction for valve-in-valve transcatheter aortic valve replacement.

the ROI to the coronary ostium with a caliper tool, and report in millimeters. The assessment of VTC needs to be performed at multiple levels, not only at the ostium but also above the coronary ostium, to identify the risk of potential sinus sequestration, since the expanded TAV frame may occupy the entire sinus of Valsalva (deficient sinus) and/or be close to the STJ (sinus sequestration), depending on the shape of the aortic root and the THV-to-STJ distance. Identification of high-risk anatomical features (particularly the combination of VTC <4 mm and average sinus of Valsalva diameter <30 mm) may warrant performing the BASILICA procedure, which can be planned by the CTA but is beyond the scope of this review.

When implanting a TAV into a stentless SAV, the risk assessment should be similar to that of TAVR in native AS as described earlier because of the biomechanical similarity due to the lack of a rigid scaffold. Stentless surgical valves are often implanted in small roots. This, coupled with anatomical distortions, may increase the risk of coronary occlusion and should be considered with caution.

11. What are the CT assessments in patients with bicuspid aortic valve prior to TAVR?

The prevalence of bicuspid aortic valve (BAV) is 1–2%, of whom up to 50% of patients require surgical intervention. The use of the TAVR procedure for BAV has increased, and BAV is seen in up to 3% of patients undergoing TAVR. With current-generation devices, TAVR is a viable treatment option for patients with BAV compared to tricuspid aortic valve or SAVR.

Morphology

The identification and characterization of BAV morphology carry considerable importance, and societal guidelines recommend comprehensive assessments of the valve morphology in TAVR planning for patients with BAV. The Sievers classification has conventionally been used. Recently, a TAVR directed and simplified BAV classification has been proposed, using three morphologies according to the number of commissures and the presence or absence of raphes: (i) tricommissural (one commissure completely fused between two cusps; often referred to as *functional* or *acquired* BAV); (ii) bicommissural raphe-type (two cusps fused by a fibrous or calcified ridge; equivalent to Sievers Type 1); and (iii) bicommissural non-raphe type (two cusps completely fused from their basal origin with no visible seam; equivalent to Sievers Type 0).

High-Risk Features

There are several unfavorable features of BAV anatomy for the TAVR procedure: very elliptical/eccentric annulus, asymmetric calcium distribution, bulky calcification extending into LVOT, low coronary ostia height, short sinus of Valsalva height, and ascending aortic dilatation (Figure 5.11). The extent of calcification on raphe and leaflets should be evaluated using a qualitative scale (mild, moderate, severe) since calcified raphe and excess leaflet calcification may associate with an increased risk

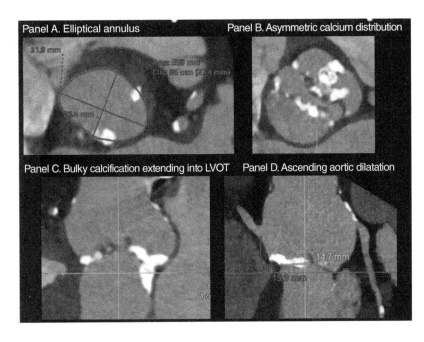

Figure 5.11 Examples of high-risk anatomical features for transcatheter aortic valve replacement. (a) Elliptical annulus. (b) Asymmetric calcium distribution. (c) Bulky calcification extending into the left ventricular outflow tract (LVOT). (d) Ascending aortic dilatation.

of procedural complications (i.e. aortic root injury, moderate to severe paravalvular regurgitation) and mid-term mortality.

Annulus Size

Appropriate measurement of the aortic annulus size is critical for procedure success and to reduce the risk of complications in BAV as well as in tricuspid aortic valves, although it may be challenging. TAV sizing for BAV should be done at the annular level and is no different than in tricuspid AV. The assessment of BAV-related aortopathy (root and/or ascending aorta dilation) should be performed similarly to tricuspid AV.

Bibliography

1 Abbara, S., Blanke, P., Maroules, C.D. et al. (2016). SCCT guidelines for the performance and acquisition of coronary computed tomographic angiography: a report of the society of cardiovascular computed tomography guidelines committee: endorsed by the North American Society for Cardiovascular Imaging (NASCI). *J. Cardiovasc. Comput. Tomogr.* 10 (6): 435–449.

2 Bapat, V. and Attia, R. (2012). Transaortic transcatheter aortic valve implantation: step-by-step guide. *Semin. Thorac. Cardiovasc. Surg.* 24 (3): 206–211.

3 Bapat, V.N., Attia, R., and Thomas, M. (2014). Effect of valve design on the stent internal diameter of a bioprosthetic valve: a concept of true internal diameter and its implications for the valve-in-valve procedure. *JACC Cardiovasc. Interv.* 7: 115–127.

4 Barbanti, M., Yang, T.H., Rodès Cabau, J. et al. (2013). Anatomical and procedural features associated with aortic root rupture during balloon-expandable transcatheter aortic valve replacement. *Circulation* 128 (3): 244–253.

5 Blanke, P., Euringer, W., Baumann, T. et al. (2010). Combined assessment of aortic root anatomy and aortoiliac vasculature with dual-source CT as a screening tool in patients evaluated for transcatheter aortic valve implantation. *Am. J. Roentgenol.* 195 (4): 872–881.

6 Blanke, P., Russe, M., Leipsic, J. et al. (2012). Conformational pulsatile changes of the aortic annulus: impact on prosthesis sizing by computed tomography for transcatheter aortic valve replacement. *J. Am. Coll. Cardiol. Interv.* 5: 984–994.

7 Blanke, P., Schoepf, U.J., and Leipsic, J.A. (2013). CT in transcatheter aortic valve replacement. *Radiology* 269 (3): 650–669.

8 Blanke, P., Weir-McCall, J.R., Achenbach, S. et al. (2019). Computed tomography imaging in the context of transcatheter aortic valve implantation (TAVI)/transcatheter aortic valve replacement (TAVR): an expert consensus document of the Society of Cardiovascular Computed Tomography. *J. Cardiovasc. Comput. Tomogr.* 13 (1): 1–20.

9 Castaño, A., Narotsky, D.L., Hamid, N. et al. (2017). Unveiling transthyretin cardiac amyloidosis and its predictors among elderly patients with severe aortic stenosis undergoing transcatheter aortic valve replacement. *Eur. Heart J.* 38 (38): 2879–2887.

10 Cavalcante, J.L., Rijal, S., Abdelkarim, I. et al. (2017). Cardiac amyloidosis is prevalent in older patients with aortic stenosis and carries worse prognosis. *J. Cardiovasc. Magn. Reson.* 19 (1): 98.

11 Chieffo, A., Giustino, G., Spagnolo, P. et al. (2015). Routine screening of coronary artery disease with computed tomographic coronary angiography in place of invasive coronary angiography in patients undergoing transcatheter aortic valve replacement. *Circ. Cardiovasc. Interv.* 8 (7): e002025.

12 Dahle, T.G., Kaneko, T., and McCabe, J.M. (2019). Outcomes following subclavian and axillary artery access for transcatheter aortic valve replacement: Society of the Thoracic Surgeons/American College of Cardiology TVT registry report. *JACC Cardiovasc. Interv.* 12 (7): 662–669.

13 Elbadawi, A., Saad, M., Elgendy, I.Y. et al. (2019). Temporal trends and outcomes of transcatheter versus surgical aortic valve replacement for bicuspid aortic valve stenosis. *JACC Cardiovasc. Interv.* 12: 1811–1822.

14 Ewe, S.H., Ng, A.C.T., Schuijf, J.D. et al. (2011). Location and severity of aortic valve calcium and implications for aortic regurgitation after transcatheter aortic valve implantation. *Am. J. Cardiol.* 108: 1470–1477.

15 Fujita, B., Kütting, M., Seiffert, M. et al. (2016). Calcium distribution patterns of the aortic valve as a risk factor for the need of permanent pacemaker implantation after transcatheter aortic valve implantation. *Eur. Heart J. Cardiovasc. Imaging* 17 (12): 1385–1393.

16 Fukui, M., Hashimoto, G., Lopes, B.B.C. et al. (2022). Association of baseline and change in global longitudinal strain by computed tomography with post-transcatheter aortic valve replacement outcomes. *Eur. Heart J. Cardiovasc. Imaging* 23 (4): 476–484.

17 Fukui, M., Sorajja, P., Hashimoto, G. et al. (2021). Right ventricular dysfunction by computed tomography associates with outcomes in severe aortic stenosis patients undergoing transcatheter aortic valve replacement. *J. Cardiovasc. Comput. Tomogr.* S1934–5925 (21): 00465–00462.

18 Généreux, P., Webb, J.G., Svensson, L.G. et al. (2012). Vascular complications after transcatheter aortic valve replacement: insights from the PARTNER (Placement of AoRTic TraNscathetER Valve) trial. *J. Am. Coll. Cardiol.* 60 (12): 1043–1052.

19 Gurvitch, R., Wood, D.A., Leipsic, J. et al. (2010). Multislice computed tomography for prediction of optimal angiographic deployment projections during transcatheter aortic valve implantation. *J. Am. Coll. Cardiol. Interv.* 3: 1157–1165.

20 Halabi, M., Ratnayaka, K., Faranesh, A.Z. et al. (2013). Aortic access from the vena cava for large caliber transcatheter cardiovascular interventions: pre-clinical validation. *J. Am. Coll. Cardiol.* 61 (16): 1745–1746.

21 Halim, S.A., Edwards, F.H., Dai, D. et al. (2020). Outcomes of transcatheter aortic valve replacement in patients with bicuspid aortic valve disease: a report from the Society of Thoracic Surgeons/American College of Cardiology Transcatheter Valve Therapy Registry. *Circulation* 141: 1071–1079.

22 Hansson, N.C., Nørgaard, B.L., Barbanti, M. et al. (2015). The impact of calcium volume and distribution in aortic root injury related to balloon-expandable transcatheter aortic valve replacement. *J. Cardiovasc. Comput. Tomogr.* 9 (5): 382–392.

23 Harloff, M.T., Percy, E.D., Hirji, S.A. et al. (2020). A step-by-step guide to trans-axillary transcatheter aortic valve replacement. *Ann. Cardiothorac. Surg.* 9 (6): 510–521.

24 Ibeiro, H.B., Webb, J.G., Makkar, R.R. et al. (2013). Predictive factors, management, and clinical outcomes of coronary obstruction following transcatheter aortic valve implantation: insights from a large multicenter registry. *J. Am. Coll. Cardiol.* 62: 1552–1562.

25 Jilaihawi, H., Chen, M., Webb, J. et al. (2016). A bicuspid aortic valve imaging classification for the TAVR era. *JACC Cardiovasc. Imaging* 9: 1145–1158.

26 Khalique, O.K., Hahn, R.T., Gada, H. et al. (2014). Quantity and location of aortic valve complex calcification predicts severity and location of paravalvular regurgitation and frequency of post-dilation after balloon-expandable transcatheter aortic valve replacement. *J. Am. Coll. Cardiol. Interv.* 7: 885–894.

27 Kittleson, M.M., Maurer, M.S., Ambardekar, A.V. et al. (2020). Cardiac amyloidosis: evolving diagnosis and management: a scientific statement from the American Heart Association. *Circulation* 142 (1): e7–e22.

28 Kurra, V., Kapadia, S.R., Tuzcu, E.M. et al. (2010). Pre-procedural imaging of aortic root orientation and dimensions: comparison between X-ray angiographic planar imaging and 3-dimensional multidetector row computed tomography. *JACC Cardiovasc. Interv.* 3 (1): 105–113.

29 Kurra, V., Schoenhagen, P., Roselli, E.E. et al. (2009). Prevalence of significant peripheral artery disease in patients evaluated for percutaneous aortic valve insertion: preprocedural assessment with multidetector computed tomography. *J. Thorac. Cardiovasc. Surg.* 137 (5): 1258–1264.

30 Lederman, R.J., Babaliaros, V.C., Rogers, T. et al. (2019). Preventing coronary obstruction during transcatheter aortic valve replacement: from computed tomography to BASILICA. *JACC Cardiovasc. Interv.* 12 (13): 1197–1216.

31 Mack, M.J., Leon, M.B., Thourani, V.H. et al. (2019). Transcatheter aortic-valve replacement with a balloon-expandable valve in low-risk patients. *N. Engl. J. Med.* 380 (18): 1695–1705.

32 Majmundar, M., Kumar, A., Doshi, R. et al. (2021). Meta-analysis of transcatheter aortic valve implantation in patients with stenotic bicuspid versus tricuspid aortic valve. *Am. J. Cardiol.* 145: 102–110.

33 Masson, J.B., Kovac, J., Schuler, G. et al. (2009). Transcatheter aortic valve implantation: review of the nature, management, and avoidance of procedural complications. *JACC Cardiovasc. Interv.* 2 (9): 811–820.

34 Mentias, A., Sarrazin, M.V., Desai, M.Y. et al. (2020). Transcatheter versus surgical aortic valve replacement in patients with bicuspid aortic valve stenosis. *J. Am. Coll. Cardiol.* 75: 2518–2519.

35 Michail, M., Ihdayhid, A., Comella, A. et al. (2021). Feasibility and validity of computed tomography-derived fractional flow reserve in patients with severe aortic stenosis: the CAST-FFR study. *Circ. Cardiovasc. Interv.* 14 (1): e009586.

36 Michelena, H.I., Prakash, S.K., Della Corte, A. et al. (2014). Bicuspid aortic valve: identifying knowledge gaps and rising to the challenge from the international bicuspid aortic valve consortium (BAVCon). *Circulation* 129: 2691–2704.

37 Modine, T., Sudre, A., Delhaye, C. et al. (2012). Transcutaneous aortic valve implantation using the left carotid access: feasibility and early clinical outcomes. *Ann. Thorac. Surg.* 93 (5): 1489–1494.

38 Murphy, D.T., Blanke, P., Alaamri, S. et al. (2016). Dynamism of the aortic annulus: effect of diastolic versus systolic CT annular measurements on device selection in transcatheter aortic valve replacement (TAVR). *J. Am. Coll. Cardiol. Interv.* 10: 37–43.

39 Ng, A.C., Delgado, V., van der Kley, F. et al. (2010). Comparison of aortic root dimensions and geometries before and after transcatheter aortic valve implantation by 2- and 3-dimensional transesophageal echocardiography and multislice computed tomography. *Circ. Cardiovasc. Imaging* 3 (1): 94–102.

40 Pasic, M., Unbehaun, A., Buz, S. et al. (2015). Annular rupture during transcatheter aortic valve replacement: classification, pathophysiology, diagnostics, treatment approaches, and prevention. *JACC Cardiovasc. Interv.* 8 (1 Pt A): 1–9.

41 Piazza, N., de Jaegere, P., Schultz, C. et al. (2008). Anatomy of the aortic valvar complex and its implications for transcatheter implantation of the aortic valve. *Circ. Cardiovasc. Interv.* 1 (1): 74–81.

42 Reardon, M.J., Van Mieghem, N.M., Popma, J.J. et al. (2017). Surgical or transcatheter aortic-valve replacement in intermediate-risk patients. *N. Engl. J. Med.* 376 (14): 1321–1331.

43 Ribeiro, H.B., Rodés-Cabau, J., Blanke, P. et al. (2018). Incidence, predictors, and clinical outcomes of coronary obstruction following transcatheter aortic valve replacement for degenerative bioprosthetic surgical valves: insights from the VIVID registry. *Eur. Heart J.* 39: 687–695.

44 Sá, M., Van den Eynde, J., Simonato, M. et al. (2021). Valve-in-valve transcatheter aortic valve replacement versus redo surgical aortic valve replacement: an updated meta-analysis. *JACC Cardiovasc. Interv.* 14: 211–220.

45 Sievers, H.H. and Schmidtke, C. (2007). A classification system for the bicuspid aortic valve from 304 surgical specimens. *J. Thorac. Cardiovasc. Surg.* 133: 1226–1233.

46 Smith, C.R., Leon, M.B., Mack, M.J. et al. (2011). Transcatheter versus surgical aortic-valve replacement in high-risk patients. *N. Engl. J. Med.* 364 (23): 2187–2198.

47 Suchá, D., Daans, C.G., Symersky, P. et al. (2015). Reliability, agreement, and presentation of a reference standard for assessing implanted heart valve sizes by multidetector-row computed tomography. *Am. J. Cardiol.* 116: 112–120.

48 Tops, L.F., Wood, D.A., Delgado, V. et al. (2008). Noninvasive evaluation of the aortic root with multislice computed tomography implications for transcatheter aortic valve replacement. *JACC Cardiovasc. Imaging* 1 (3): 321–330.

49 Treibel, T.A., Fontana, M., Steeden, J.A. et al. (2017). Automatic quantification of the myocardial extracellular volume by cardiac computed tomography: synthetic ECV by CCT. *J. Cardiovasc. Comput. Tomogr.* 11 (3): 221–226.

50 Vlastra, W., Jimenez-Quevedo, P., Tchétché, D. et al. (2019). Predictors, incidence, and outcomes of patients undergoing transfemoral transcatheter aortic valve implantation complicated by stroke. *Circ. Cardiovasc. Interv.* 12 (3): e007546.

51 Writing Committee Members, Otto, C.M., Nishimura, R.A. et al. (2021). 2020 ACC/AHA guideline for the management of patients with valvular heart disease: executive summary: a report of the American College of Cardiology/American Heart Association joint committee on clinical practice guidelines. *J. Am. Coll. Cardiol.* 77 (4): 450–500.

52 Yoon, S.H., Kim, W.K., Dhoble, A. et al. (2020). Bicuspid aortic valve morphology and outcomes after transcatheter aortic valve replacement. *J. Am. Coll. Cardiol.* 76: 1018–1030.

6

Optimal Selection of TAVR Devices

Sergio A. Perez[1] and Eduardo J. de Marchena[2]

[1] Cardiovascular Service, Baptist Health Medical Center, Montgomery, AL, USA
[2] Division of Cardiovascular Medicine, University of Miami Miller School of Medicine, University of Miami Hospital, Miami, FL, USA

1. What types of transcatheter aortic valve replacement devices are commercially available?

Currently, two types of transcatheter aortic valve replacement (TAVR) devices are approved by the US Food and Drug Administration (FDA) for clinical use in the United States: the balloon-expandable (BE) SAPIEN family (Edwards Lifesciences) and the self-expanding (SE) CoreValve family of valves (Medtronic).

The Cribier-Edwards, SAPIEN, and SAPIEN XT are older generations of the SAPIEN family, whereas the current generation, SAPIEN 3 and SAPIEN 3 Ultra, are the only two FDA-approved BE valves. These BE devices have an intra-annular design and consist of bovine pericardium mounted in a cobalt-chromium frame. Similarly, CoreValve, Evolut R, and Evolut PRO are predecessors of the newer Evolut PRO+. These valves have a supra-annular design and consist of porcine pericardium leaflets sewn to a SE nitinol frame.

The LOTUS mechanically expandable valve (Boston Scientific) was recalled and withdrawn from the market due to complexities associated with the delivery system.

2. Are other TAVR devices under clinical investigation?

Since the advent of TAVR, the previously mentioned types of prostheses have dominated the choice of valve. However, a wide range of TAVR devices have now been approved for clinical use outside the US or are undergoing clinical investigation. Most of the diversity is in the field of SE valves. A growing variety of transcatheter heart valves (THVs) will enhance the opportunity to select the most appropriate device in an individualized and patient-centered approach (Figure 6.1).

The ACURATE Neo 2 (Boston Scientific) and Portico (Abbott Structural Heart) SE devices are currently under investigational device exemption, whereas the JenaValve (JenaValve Technology) and the J-Valve (JC Medical) are undergoing early feasibility studies. The ACURATE valve has a supra-annular design and a top-down deployment that allows hemodynamic stability. It also has crowns that assist in capping the displaced native leaflets below the coronary ostia, mitigating the risk of coronary occlusion in cases with low coronary ostia. The Portico valve, also repositionable and retrievable, has an intra annular design. JenaValve is a self-expandable valve with a low-profile stent frame that is individually fixed into the native leaflets using paperclip-like anchors. Similarly, the J-Valve uses U-shaped anchor rings to facilitate self-positioning implantation. The active fixation mechanism makes these valves attractive for use in non-calcified valves with pure aortic regurgitation or mixed aortic stenosis and aortic regurgitation.

3. Is there evidence to claim superiority of one type of TAVR device over the others?

Currently, there is not enough evidence to claim the superiority of one particular type of device over the others. There are very few large-scale randomized trials with head-to-head comparisons. In addition, head-to-head randomized trials are designed with ideal TAVR patients in mind instead of more challenging real-world cases. Direct comparison of outcomes rates from individual regulatory approval trials should be discouraged because of important

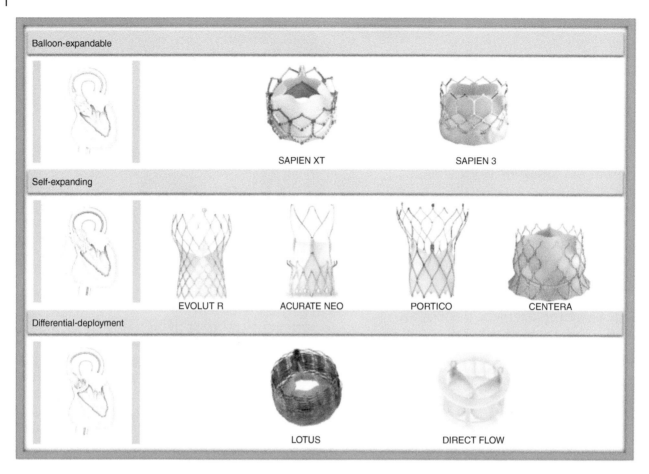

Figure 6.1 TAVR devices. Of the platforms shown in this figure, the only two currently commercially available in the US are the balloon-expandable (BE) SAPIEN family (Edwards Lifesciences), with the SAPIEN 3 and SAPIEN ULTRA as the latest iterations, and the self-expanding (SE) CoreValve family (Medtronic) with the Evolut PRO+ as the newest version. *Source:* Jose et al. (2016) / With permission of Elsevier.

differences in the patient populations' risk profile and the variety in device iterations used.

The CHOICE (Randomized Comparison of Transcatheter Heart Valves in High-Risk Patients with Severe Aortic Stenosis: Medtronic CoreValve Versus Edwards SAPIEN XT) study showed no differences in clinical outcomes five years after TAVR among patients treated with early-generation SE and BE devices. Hemodynamics favored SE valves; and although uncommon, valve deterioration happened more often with BE valves.

The SOLVE-TAVI (The compariSon of secOnd-generation seLf-expandable vs. BE Valves and gEneral vs. local anesthesia in Transcatheter Aortic Valve Implantation) trial compared the newer-generations of BE (Edwards SAPIEN S3) and SE (Medtronic Evolut R) devices and showed that both had equivalent clinical outcomes at 30 days. A primary endpoint composed of all-cause mortality, stroke, significant prosthetic valve regurgitation, and permanent pacemaker implantation (PPI) occurred in 25.9% of the BE group and 28.4% (p for equivalence = 0.04,

p for superiority = 0.83) in the SE group. However, one-year stroke rates were significantly higher with Edwards SAPIEN 3 (6.9 vs. 1%, p = 0.002), while moderate to severe prosthetic valve regurgitation rates were higher with Evolut R (3.4 vs. 1.5%, p = 0.0002). Although these are important findings, the study was underpowered for most individual endpoints.

Long-term outcomes and hemodynamic comparisons between different types of valves in large randomized clinical trials may still be needed. Until then, no type of TAVR device can claim superiority over the others.

4. Are there situations in which one valve should be considered over another?

Although most patients are suitable for any valve, specific patient- and device-related factors may slightly favor one valve over another. These differences may translate into variations in efficacy and safety outcomes in specific patient subgroups. There are many factors that, although not always decisive, may influence the decision in one direction or another (Box 6.1 and Table 6.1). Some of the factors that are carefully considered when selecting a type of TAVR device include the size of the annulus and long-term durability of the THV, the risk of coronary obstruction and the future need to reaccess, the severity and pattern of calcium distribution at an annular/subannular level, the risk of developing conduction abnormalities after TAVR, and the aortic angle (AA).

In theory, an ideal valve should have several properties to fulfill all the clinical needs in different patient populations. Among others, a theoretical ideal valve would have a low profile size, achieve optimal effective orifice area (EOA), have consistent neo-commissural alignment, induce minimal paravalvular leak (PVL) and conduction abnormalities, cover a wide range of annular sizes, be repositionable and retrievable, and be durable. Because there is no ideal valve, specific scenarios may favor one design of the currently available valves.

5. Does annular size affect the choice of valve?

Most available TAVR devices are available in an extensive range of sizes. Both types of commercially available devices in the US cover an annulus with an average diameter from 16 to 30 mm.

In small annuli, the supra-annular design of a SE valve may result in superior hemodynamics: higher indexed EOA, lower prosthetic gradients, and reduced patient-prosthesis mismatch (PPM) rates. Although there has been heterogeneity in the definition of small annuli, a proposed

---

Box 6.1   Factors to Consider in the Selection of TAVR Device

- Annular size
- Risk of patient-prosthesis mismatch
- Percentage of undersizing or oversizing
- Risk of coronary occlusion
- Need to reaccess the coronaries
- Dense annular/subannular calcium
- Angulation of the aorta
- Risk of significant conduction abnormalities
- Prior permanent pacemaker implant
- Valve-in-valve TAVR
- Tolerance of rapid pacing

---

definition is an aortic annulus ≤ 23 mm. In the CHOICE trial, early-generation SE patients had a larger EOA (1.9 ± 0.5 cm^2 vs. 1.6 ± 0.5 cm^2, p = 0.02) and lower prosthetic gradients (6.9 ± 2.7 mmHg vs. 12.2 ± 8.7 mmHg, p = 0.001) compared to BE at five years. In this study, the percentage of patients with a 23 mm THV size was 9.9 and 1.7% in the BE and SE groups. Other patients in whom the hemodynamics of a supra-annular design may be favorable are those at increased risk of severe PPM: patients undergoing valve-in-valve TAVR of small surgical bioprosthesis (21 mm or less) and obese patients with relatively high body weight for their annuli.

The 29 mm SAPIEN 3/Ultra and the 34 mm Evolut R/PRO are the largest sizes available for patients with a large annulus. Use of these valves beyond manufacturer recommendation (area ≥ 683 mm^2 for the SAPIEN 3 and perimeter ≥ 94.2 mm for the Evolut) for the extra-large annulus is considered off-label. However, both devices' specific design elements have allowed successful use of these devices in patients with a very large annulus. The S3 balloon can be overfilled with good results (Figure 6.2). In contrast, the 34 mm Evolut diameter at the inflow allows for oversizing of an annulus with a perimeter up to 100 mm if the valve is implanted high. Most of the published experiences in the very large annulus use the overfilled S3. In the study by Tang et al., the largest annular area was 852 mm^2 with a corresponding perimeter of 105 mm. The S3 has been over-expanded by adding up to five extra milliliters of volume in the balloon. In this study, TAVR with over-expanded S3 was safe, with acceptable PVL and pacemaker rates.

6. What type of valve should be chosen based on aortic valve calcification?

Most THV devices require some degree of landing zone calcification for adequate anchoring; this includes the valve cusps, aortic annulus, and left ventricular outflow tract (LVOT). However, extensive calcification in the landing zone, subannular plane, and sinotubular junction can affect procedural success and safety. Heavy calcification is associated with significant paravalvular leakage (PVL) and annular or aortic root rupture.

Newer-generation BE and SE valves have a circumferential sealing skirt that minimizes the risk of PVL as compared with early-generation devices. There is no significant difference in the rate of significant PVL between new-generation BE and SE prostheses.

Table 6.1 Preference to use a balloon-expandable (BE) or self-expanding (SE) valve in different scenarios.

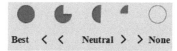

Best < < Neutral > > None

	Balloon-expandable (BE)	Self-expanding (SE)
Small annuli	◖	●
Very large annuli	●	◖
Horizontal aorta	●	◢
Sub annular calcification	◢	◖
Intolerance to rapid pacing	◢	◖
Need to re access coronaries	●	◗
High risk of PPM need	◖	◗
Bicuspid aortic valve	◗	◗
Antegrade or transapical approach	●	○

However, the risk of annular rupture is higher, particularly when using oversized BE valves in the presence of large protruding nodules of calcification. Because of this, most operators recommend using a SE valve if there is extensive, protruding, subannular calcification. In a study by Leipsic et al., patients with LVOT/annular rupture complicating BE TAVR had ≥20% annular area oversizing more frequently.

In patients without significant leaflet calcification, the investigational JenaValve and J-Valve are deployed with an active leaflet fixation mechanism. This feature makes them a potentially good option for off-label use in pure or mixed native leaflet aortic regurgitation or in cases of non-calcific AS such as rheumatic disease.

7. How does the risk of conduction abnormalities influence the choice of the TAVR device?

Conduction disturbances after TAVR are dependent on patient characteristics, deployment technique, and valve type. Despite significant inter-individual variability in the length of the membranous septum, the proximity between the aortic valve and the conduction system explains the origin of post-TAVR conduction abnormalities because of direct mechanical injury.

The SE CoreValve prosthesis has been associated with a higher incidence of new-onset left bundle branch block (LBBB) and PPI than BE valves. The need for PPI among

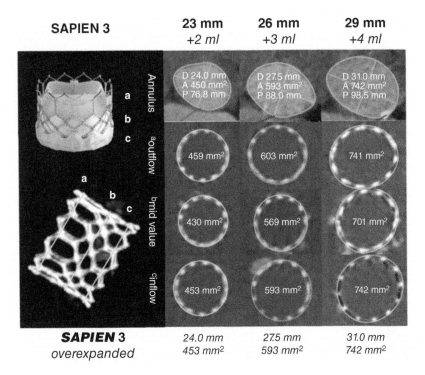

Figure 6.2   Computed tomography images with cross-sectional areas of overexpanded SAPIEN 3 transcatheter heart valves. *Source:* Obtained from Shivaraju et al. Overexpansion of the SAPIEN 3 Transcatheter Heart Valve: A Feasibility Study JACC: *Cardiovascular Interventions,* Volume 8, Issue 15, 2015, Pages 2041–2043, ISSN 1936-8798.

early-generation SE recipients has been reported to be 25–28% compared to 5–7% in patients receiving early-generation BE valves, around five times more frequent. Based on available evidence, the need for a permanent pacemaker has not drastically decreased with new iterations of THV. Overall, the rate of PPI with new-generation devices is highly variable. Despite a reduction in PPI rates with Evolut R compared to CoreValve, the rates remain relatively high for SE prostheses. For BE prostheses, PPI rates with new-generation SAPIEN devices are similar to those with early-generation SAPIEN devices. The difference in the incidence of conduction abnormalities and PPI rates between SE and BE prostheses is probably related to higher radial force on the ventricular side of the prosthesis with an often deeper implant. Other predictors of conduction abnormalities, independent of the type of valve chosen, are valve oversizing and lower implant depth.

8.   Why are the risk of coronary occlusion and the need to reaccess the coronaries are important?

Approximately 30% of patients evaluated for TAVR have concomitant coronary artery disease. Furthermore, as TAVR continues to expand in scope to include younger patients, a significant proportion of patients will need coronary angiography and percutaneous coronary interventions after TAVR.

In addition to anatomical characteristics, several device-related factors can affect the technical complexity of coronary reaccess post TAVR. In general, coronary reaccess after TAVR with the CoreValve family of SE prosthesis can be more challenging than with the SAPIEN family of BE valves because the taller stent frame can be a barrier to the selective engagement of the coronary ostia with regular diagnostic catheters. The height of the Evolut PRO+ is 45 mm, whereas the height of a fully deployed SAPIEN 3 varies between 15.5 and 22.5 mm depending on the diameter. Despite the concave design of the central portion of the Evolut, which avoids contact of the frame with the coronary ostia, and the size of the cell diamonds in the waist designed to accommodate 10 French catheters, the struts of the frame can affect coaxial engagement. Another important aspect is the height of the sealing skirt incorporated in both types of newer-generation devices to minimize the rates of PVL. The circumferential sealing skirt of the Evolut prosthesis is 13–14 mm. For the SAPIEN 3 prosthesis, an inner sealing skirt (maximum height 11.6 mm) covers two-thirds of the frame, and an outer skirt covers the lower third (maximum height 8.1 mm). For both valves, the relationship between final deployment depth, skirt height, and the height of native coronary ostia plays a major role during coronary reaccess.

There has been increasing attention on improving neo-commissural alignment with the native aortic valve commissures to facilitate coronary reaccess. Commissural alignment is critical when the proximal edge of the stent frame of a selected valve will be higher than the coronary ostia. For both valves, techniques to improve new commissural alignment have been described. If alignment is not optimal, a commissure will be positioned directly in front of the coronary ostia, making coaxial engagement almost impossible. In these cases, the coronary ostia can be engaged non-coaxially from diamonds on either side of the ostium.

Coronary occlusion during TAVR can be a fatal complication if it results in frank myocardial infarction. Risk factors for coronary occlusion include low coronary ostia, narrow sinuses of Valsalva, long native leaflets, and undergoing valve-in-valve TAVR. In patients with risk factors for coronary occlusion but within the manufacturers' recommended measurements, SE is recommended because of its capacity to be retrievable and repositionable. Techniques for coronary protection with a coronary guidewire and a non-deployed stent or preemptive bioprosthetic leaflet laceration during valve-in-valve TAVR have been used with SE and BE devices.

9. What is the impact of aortic angulation on TAVR outcomes?

A horizontal aorta poses significant challenges to optimal delivery, positioning, and deployment of the THV during TAVR. Early randomized clinical trials of SE CoreValve excluded patients with AA >70°. Afterward, available data suggested that increased AA adversely affects outcomes when using early-generation SE valves. Because of this data, the BE valve was the preferred choice in patients with high AA. An observational study by Waksman et al. showed that an AA >48° did not influence outcomes in patients undergoing TAVR with new-generation SE or BE valves. Despite this, most operators continue to use BE prostheses in patients with a horizontal aorta. The manufacturer of the CoreValve family of devices continues to recommend their use with AA <70° when using the iliofemoral and left axillary approach, AA <30° with the right axillary approach, and any angle with the direct aortic approach.

A major difference between both platforms in patients with elevated AA is the flexibility capacity of the delivery systems. The delivery system of BE valves (Edwards NovaFlex or Commander) has a flex feature that allows for active flexion and extension during valve delivery, optimizing the coaxial alignment of the THV. Conversely, the operator does not control the flexion of the delivery system of SE valves. In many cases, a non-coaxial approach can create challenges for crossing the native aortic valve and achieving an optimal position before deployment. However, one refinement in recent iterations of the SE delivery system is the addition of two shaft spines, improving strength and 1 : 1 torque response.

Another relevant difference is the length of the stent frame. The longer stent frame of SE valves may result in a less symmetrical position and the incomplete seal of the paravalvular space. The shorter stent frame of BE valves has less interaction with the aorta. However, the addition of sealing skirts in newer generations of both types of valves has significantly reduced the rates of PVLs.

10. What about bicuspid aortic valves?

Bicuspid aortic valve (BAV) is associated with worse outcomes with early generation TAVR devices. Leaflet asymmetry, the presence of a raphe, aortic dilation, and variable distribution of calcium are all factors that increase the risk of PVL. In one of the largest registry-based cohorts, Makkar et al. found no significant difference in mortality but increased 30-day rates of stroke in patients with BAV compared to patients with tricuspid aortic valve undergoing TAVR with BE SAPIEN valves. However, currently, there is no data comparing or supporting the use of a particular type of valve for patients with BAV AS.

11. Should any other factors be considered for optimal selection of TAVR device?

When selecting a TAVR device for a particular patient, additional patient or procedural factors may be considered. For example, in general, BE valves are deployed using rapid pacing to induce cardiac standstill and decrease catheter movement; conversely, SE valves are deployed without pacing or with slow-rapid pacing. Although more of a theoretical concern because there is no data supporting differences in outcomes between both types of devices, some operators recommend the use of a SE device in situations where the patient may be intolerant to rapid pacing, such as severe LV dysfunction or severe non-revascularized coronary artery disease with a large amount of ischemic myocardium.

Although TAVR was initially primarily done via the antegrade transeptal approach with a high success rate, this approach is rarely used today because improvements in technology decreased the profile size of delivery catheters. In addition, techniques were refined to use safe alternative access when needed. The vast majority of TAVR procedures are currently done using a transfemoral retrograde approach, and in a minority of cases, alternative access such as axillary, carotid, apical, direct aortic, or carotid can be used. A BE device can be used with an antegrade transeptal approach because the valve can be mounted and crimped with a reversed orientation on the balloon. However, a SE valve cannot be loaded with a reversed orientation; therefore, in a theoretical case where femoral access is not suitable and there is no adequate alternative access other than the femoral vein, a BE valve with antegrade transeptal approach may be the best option.

Clinical Vignette

An 88-year-old man presented with progressive dyspnea and severe aortic stenosis. He has a history of abdominal aortic aneurysm treated with endovascular aortic repair (EVAR) 4 years ago and coronary artery disease with coronary bypass grafting (CABG) 20 years ago. He was considered high surgical risk due to age and co-morbidities, and transcatheter aortic valve replacement (TAVR) was recommended. Pre-procedural evaluation revealed a couple of challenges: the stent grafts in the iliac arteries and abdominal aorta needed to be traversed, and there was significant calcification extending to the left ventricular outflow tract (LVOT). The aortic angle (AA) was measured at 43° (Figure 6.3). To minimize the risk of annular rupture and perivalvular leak with the extent and pattern of calcification, we decided to implant a self-expanding (SE) transcatheter valve (THV). Although the AA was not considered unfavorable based on the manufacturer's recommendation, we were unable to cross the annular plane with the delivery system because of a non-coaxial position of the catheter favoring the sides of the sinuses of the Valsalva (Figure 6.4a). Gentle push and pull, balloon predilation, use of a stiffer wire, and a snaring technique were unsuccessful at allowing the valve to cross the annular plane. To address this challenge, we decided to change the THV for a balloon-expanding (BE) device. A major benefit of the delivery system is the ability to use active flexion of the distal portion of the catheter that allows a more coaxial orientation and crossing the annular plane (Figure 6.4b,c). After crossing, a 26 mm Edwards S3 device was implanted without complications.

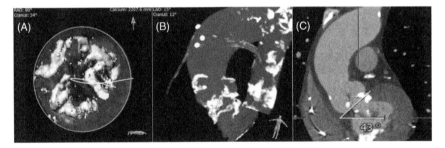

Figure 6.3 A case that demonstrates the utility of the flexion capacity of BE delivery system. Pre-procedural imaging showed an aortic angle of 43°. Initially, a SE valve was selected because of the degree of subannular calcification.

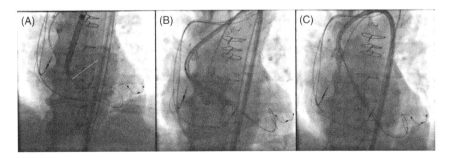

Figure 6.4 A case that demonstrates the utility of the flexion capacity of a BE delivery system. The aortic angle in this patient was measured at 43°. (a) Initially, a SE valve was selected because of the degree of subannular calcification; however, a non-coaxial alignment of the catheter with the aortic valve made it impossible to cross the annular plane. (b) When using a BE valve, we were able to obtain a more coaxial orientation by applying flex to the delivery catheter, and (c) we were able to cross the annular plane and proceed with the procedure.

Bibliography

1 Abdel-Wahab, M., Mehilli, J., Frerker, C. et al. (2014). Comparison of balloon-expandable vs self-expandable valves in patients undergoing transcatheter aortic valve replacement: the CHOICE randomized clinical trial. *JAMA* 311: 1503–1514.

2 Abramowitz, Y., Maeno, Y., Chakravarty, T. et al. (2016). Aortic angulation attenuates procedural success following self-expandable but not balloon-expandable TAVR. *JACC Cardiovasc. Imaging* 9: 964–972.

3 Auffret, V., Puri, R., Urena, M. et al. (2017). Conduction disturbances after transcatheter aortic valve replacement: current status and future perspectives. *Circulation* 136: 1049–1069.

4 Barbanti, M., Yang, T.H., Rodes Cabau, J. et al. (2013). Anatomical and procedural features associated with aortic root rupture during balloon-expandable transcatheter aortic valve replacement. *Circulation* 128: 244–253.

5 Barr, P., Ormiston, J., Stewart, J. et al. (2018). Transcatheter aortic valve implantation in patients with a large aortic annulus. *Heart Lung Circ.* 27: e11–e14.

6 Claessen, B.E., Tang, G.H.L., Kini, A.S., and Sharma, S.K. (2021). Considerations for optimal device selection in transcatheter aortic valve replacement: a review. *JAMA Cardiol.* 6: 102–112.

7 Dvir, D., Webb, J.G., Bleiziffer, S. et al. (2014). Transcatheter aortic valve implantation in failed bioprosthetic surgical valves. *JAMA* 312: 162–170.

8 Freitas-Ferraz, A.B., Tirado-Conte, G., Dagenais, F. et al. (2019). Aortic stenosis and small aortic annulus. *Circulation* 139: 2685–2702.

9 Leon, M.B., Smith, C.R., Mack, M. et al. (2010). Transcatheter aortic-valve implantation for aortic stenosis in patients who cannot undergo surgery. *N. Engl. J. Med.* 363: 1597–1607.

10 Nombela-Franco, L., Ruel, M., Radhakrishnan, S. et al. (2013). Comparison of hemodynamic performance of self-expandable CoreValve versus balloon-expandable Edwards SAPIEN aortic valves inserted by catheter for aortic stenosis. *Am. J. Cardiol.* 111: 1026–1033.

11 Ribeiro, H.B., Webb, J.G., Makkar, R.R. et al. (2013). Predictive factors, management, and clinical outcomes of coronary obstruction following transcatheter aortic valve implantation: insights from a large multicenter registry. *J. Am. Coll. Cardiol.* 62: 1552–1562.

12 Sathananthan, J., Sellers, S., Barlow, A. et al. (2018). Overexpansion of the SAPIEN 3 transcatheter heart valve: an ex vivo bench study. *JACC Cardiovasc. Interv.* 11: 1696–1705.

13 Shivaraju, A., Kodali, S., Thilo, C. et al. (2015). Overexpansion of the SAPIEN 3 transcatheter heart valve: a feasibility study. *JACC Cardiovasc. Interv.* 8: 2041–2043.

14 Siontis, G.C., Juni, P., Pilgrim, T. et al. (2014). Predictors of permanent pacemaker implantation in patients with severe aortic stenosis undergoing TAVR: a meta-analysis. *J. Am. Coll. Cardiol.* 64: 129–140.

15 Tang, G.H.L., Zaid, S., George, I. et al. (2018). Impact of aortic root anatomy and geometry on paravalvular leak in transcatheter aortic valve replacement with extremely large annuli using the Edwards SAPIEN 3 valve. *JACC Cardiovasc. Interv.* 11: 1377–1387.

16 Tang, G.H.L., Zaid, S., Gupta, E. et al. (2019). Impact of initial Evolut transcatheter aortic valve replacement deployment orientation on final valve orientation and coronary Reaccess. *Circ. Cardiovasc. Interv.* 12: e008044.

17 Thiele, H., Kurz, T., Feistritzer, H.J. et al. (2020). Comparison of newer generation self-expandable vs. balloon-expandable valves in transcatheter aortic valve implantation: the randomized SOLVE-TAVI trial. *Eur. Heart J.* 41: 1890–1899.

18 Vlastra, W., Chandrasekhar, J., Munoz-Garcia, A.J. et al. (2019). Comparison of balloon-expandable vs. self-expandable valves in patients undergoing transfemoral transcatheter aortic valve implantation: from the CENTER-collaboration. *Eur. Heart J.* 40: 456–465.

19 Yoon, S.H., Bleiziffer, S., De Backer, O. et al. (2017). Outcomes in transcatheter aortic valve replacement for bicuspid versus tricuspid aortic valve stenosis. *J. Am. Coll. Cardiol.* 69: 2579–2589.

20 Cribier, A., Eltchaninoff, H., Tron, C. et al. (2004). Early experience with percutaneous transcatheter implantation of heart valve prosthesis for the treatment of end-stage inoperable patients with calcific aortic stenosis. *J. Am. Coll. Cardiol.* 43: 698–703.

7

Transcatheter Aortic Valve Replacement

Step-by-Step Approach

Solomon A. Seifu and Carlos E. Alfonso

[1] *Department of Medicine, Division of Cardiovascular Medicine, University of Miami Miller School of Medicine, Miami, FL, USA*

1. What is transcatheter aortic valve replacement (TAVR)?

Transcatheter aortic valve replacement (TAVR) refers to a percutaneous aortic valve implantation technique through a transcatheter approach. Before the development of TAVR, surgical valve replacement was the standard of care and the only approach for treating degenerative aortic valve disease. While different surgical approaches, including minimally invasive surgical valve replacement, have been developed, TAVR remains the only nonsurgical, completely percutaneous approach for aortic valve replacement. The first TAVR valve was implanted in humans in 2002. Since then, multiple studies have validated the safety and efficacy of this novel approach. Based on the results of the PARTNER (Placement of Aortic Transcatheter Valves) and CoreValve trials, TAVR was first approved for the treatment of severe aortic stenosis (AS) in prohibitive surgical risk patients in 2011 and subsequently for patients at high surgical risk in 2012. In 2015, the valve-in-valve procedure for failed surgical bioprosthetic valves was included [4]. The FDA approved TAVR valves for use in patients with severe AS at intermediate risk in 2016 and, in 2019, further expanded the indication for TAVR valves to include low-risk patients.

Patient Evaluation

2. What are the current indications for TAVR?

TAVR is currently indicated for treating degenerative severe aortic valve stenosis across the spectrum of surgical risk from low to inoperable patients. TAVR is FDA approved for the following conditions:

- Low to prohibitive surgical risk patients with symptomatic severe AS
- Valve-in-valve procedures for failed prior bioprosthetic valves

3. Are there any absolute contraindications to TAVR?

There are a few absolute contraindications to TAVR, including:

- Presence of left ventricular (LV) thrombus
- Plaques with mobile thrombi in the ascending aorta
- Comorbidities that limit life expectancy to <1 year
- Comorbidity suggesting a lack of improvement in quality of life
- Inadequate annulus size (<18 mm, >30 mm)
- Active endocarditis
- Large calcific valvular nodules
- Short distance between the annulus and the coronary ostium

Relative contraindications or considerations prior to TAVR include:

- Inadequate vascular access (such patients could be treated from the transapical approach)
- Hemodynamic instability
- Severe LV dysfunction

Step-By-Step TAVR Approach

4. What are the pre-procedural approach to and planning for successful TAVR?

Before a TAVR procedure, the patient should undergo full workup with coronary angiography; CT angiography of the heart, aorta, and peripheral vessels; echocardiography; electrocardiogram; and laboratory investigations (Table 7.1). Initial investigations will help assess the severity of AS, anatomy of the aortic valve and aortic root, aortic valve calcification, annular sinotubular and sinus of Valsalva dimensions, ventricular function, coronary artery disease, height of the coronary ostia from the aortic annulus, iliofemoral vessel size, calcification, and tortuosity. Computed tomography angiography (CTA) has emerged as the best pre-procedural tool for aortic annular sizing.

Table 7.1 Components of the pre-procedural evaluation for transcatheter aortic valve replacement (TAVR).

Clinical evaluation	• Interventional and cardiothoracic surgical evaluation • Additional consultation as warranted • Assess comorbid conditions, frailty • Functional status
Cardiac catheterization	Coronary angiography Left heart catheterization and hemodynamics

Echocardiogram	• Evaluate aortic valve disease
	  ○ Peak velocity, velocity time integral (VTI), gradients, aortic valve area (AVA)
	  ○ Degree of calcification, restricted motion
	• Evaluate other valvular heart disease
	• Evaluate left ventricular systolic function (ejection fraction [EF])
	• Transesophageal echocardiogram (optional)

Cardiac computed tomography angiography (CTA)	• Evaluate iliofemoral anatomy and dimensions:
	  ○ Size and dimensions
	  ○ Tortuosity
	  ○ Degree of calcification
	  ○ Prior iliac stents or grafts
	  ○ Need for adjunctive lithotripsy
	• Evaluate the aorta
	  ○ Abdominal aorta, aneurysm, thrombus
	  ○ Aortic arch plaque
	  ○ Aortic valve annular angle
	  ○ Coplanar angle for valve deployment
	  ○ Great vessels for neuroprotection
	• Evaluate aortic valve anatomy:
	  – Annular dimensions
	    ■ Area and perimeter
	    ■ Maximum, minimum, and average diameter
	  – Sinotubular and sinus of Valsalva dimensions
	  – Coronary height
	  – Calcification in annulus, sinotubular junction, and left ventricular outflow tract (LVOT)
	  – Prior-bioprosthesis dimensions

5. What are the steps during the TAVR procedure?

A stepwise approach can be implemented for successful percutaneous TAVR (Table 7.2). Each step has a few key considerations, skills, and techniques to master. While there was considerable variation in some techniques during the initial worldwide experience of TAVR, some best practices and optimal strategies have emerged over the past decade.

Vascular Access

6. What is the approach for vascular access during TAVR?

Vascular access is the first step. The transfemoral approach is the most widely used access route. With the reduction in delivery sheath dimensions, a majority of patients can be treated via the transfemoral approach, and the incidence of vascular complications has decreased.

Prior to the procedure, an assessment of vascular access is recommended using CTA of the abdomen and pelvic vessels. In patients with advanced chronic kidney disease, a non-contrast CT can sometimes provide sufficient information regarding vessel size, degree of calcification, and tortuosity. A small vessel size of less than 5 mm, circumferential calcium, and extreme vessel tortuosity are contraindications for the transfemoral approach. The two major commercially available valve delivery systems are 14–16 Fr equivalent and compatible with most vessel sizes, making more than 95% of TAVR cases compatible with the transfemoral approach. Access site complications include bleeding, hematoma formation, dissection, pseudoaneurysm, retroperitoneal bleeding, and acute limb ischemia. Reported rates of access site complication range from 6.3 to 30.7%. For patients with severely calcific iliofemoral arteries, intravascular lithotripsy has more recently been shown to be feasible and to facilitate transfemoral large-bore arterial access.

Table 7.2 Stepwise approach to transcatheter aortic valve replacement (TAVR).

Procedural setup	• Anesthesia ○ General vs. MAC or moderate sedation • Room setup ○ Standard for transfemoral approach ○ Alternative access setup: depending on access route, may need an additional table to facilitate positioning
Vascular access	Primary large-bore access US guided access Confirmation angiogram Plan for closure (e.g. pre-close vs. Manta) Secondary access for pigtail, angiography during implant Placement of temporary venous pacemaker. Balloon tipped (best, safest practice) Neuroprotection (optional) Need right radial access for Sentinel* device
Assess coplanar angle	• Angiogram to confirm coplanar angle for deployment ○ Adjust as necessary

Aortic valve crossing	• Use standard guides and wires for crossing
	• Exchange length wire to change catheter for pigtail catheter.
	• Use pigtail catheter to deliver stiff wire in the left ventricular apex:
	 ○ Wires requiring shaping:
	  ▪ Amplatz Extra-Stiff™ wire: preferred for S3
	  ▪ Lunderquist®: stiffest wire on the market
	 ○ Pre-formed wires: Confida™, Safari™

Balloon pre-dilation (optional)	• Aortic valvuloplasty for pre-dilation if needed • Performed with rapid ventricular pacing (180 bpm) • Conservative sizing of BAV balloon size
Valve deployment	• Standard procedure based on selected bio-prosthesis: ○ Balloon expandable: load S3 on the balloon in the aorta, advance, deploy in coplanar angles under rapid ventricular pacing. ○ Self-expanding bio-prosthesis: cusp overlap technique increasingly used for deployment
Post-TAVR assessment	• Completion aortogram • Post-TAVR invasive hemodynamics ○ Transvalvular gradients measurement ○ Diastolic gradient and left ventricular end-diastolic pressure (LVEDP) • Echocardiographic assessment: ○ Transvalvular gradients ○ Assess for perivalvular leaks and aortic insufficiency ○ Assess complications (e.g. pericardial effusion) • Peripheral angiogram after access closure

7. What is the current best practice to establish femoral access safely?

The ideal transfemoral access remains an anterior wall stick of the common femoral artery at the mid-femoral-head level, above the femoral bifurcation and below the inguinal ligament. For large-bore vascular access, it is crucial that fluoroscopy be used initially to identify the appropriate level for vascular access.

It is established best practice to obtain the primary access under ultrasound guidance to confirm an anterior wall stick at the appropriate site. Access can be obtained using a micropuncture system, which can then be exchanged for a 6 Fr sheath. At the time of access, femoral angiography should confirm the appropriate position and can be performed via the micropuncture system.

A secondary arterial access is necessary and can be obtained on either the contralateral common femoral artery or the left radial artery. Venous access is also usually necessary for temporary pacemaker placement and is generally obtained contralateral to the planned large-bore access site in the femoral vein under ultrasound guidance.

8. For patients with inadequate femoral access, what are the potential options for alternative arterial access for transcatheter valve delivery?

Over the past decade, with continued device developments and innovative engineering, catheter delivery system dimensions have continued to decrease. This has led to an increase in the percentage of patients with approachable femoral vascular access for TAVR. Nonetheless, approximately 5% of patients do not have adequate vascular access for transfemoral delivery. The choice of alternative access route is based on the anatomy of the patient, risk factors, operator and institutional experience, and type of valve delivery system used. The potential alternative access approaches include (i) axillary/subclavian artery access, (ii) transaortic access, (iii) carotid artery access, (iv) transcaval access, and (v) antegrade, transseptal access. There may be regional and institutional variations in the preferred alternative access, and each technique has potential benefits and hazards. Irrespective of the vascular access point chosen, best practices should be followed to optimize the results and maximize safety. The pre-procedural planning for alternative access is similar, and a CTA is essential.

9. What is the approach to axillary/subclavian artery access?

Axillary/subclavian access remains the most frequent alternative access route for TAVR and leads to results equivalent to transfemoral access. Arterial access can be obtained by either a surgical cutdown or percutaneous axillary access. The pre-procedural CTA should be assessed to ensure adequate vessel sizing and exclude peripheral artery disease (PAD), significant calcification, or tortuosity that may preclude safe axillary/subclavian access. The left subclavian axillary is generally preferred unless a left internal mammary artery (LIMA) bypass graft is present. In patients with end-stage renal disease (ESRD), consideration should also be given to the presence of AV fistulas/grafts.

Compared to the open surgical subclavian arterial access, percutaneous axillary access for large-bore access for TAVR is feasible with similar 30-day mortality, stroke rates, and major vascular complications and less major bleeding when compared to open surgical cutdown and subclavian access. The step-by-step process for percutaneous axillary large-bore access has been recently summarized. Initial vascular access should be systematically and routinely done under ultrasound guidance using a micropuncture system.

10. What is the approach to carotid artery access?

Trans-Carotid access is gained through a surgical cutdown of the common carotid artery and insertion of the TAVR valve delivery system. Neurologic monitoring by electroencephalogram (EEG), transcranial doppler, and cerebral pulse oximetry is performed during the procedure. Observational studies have found that patients undergoing trans-carotid TAVR have lower transfusion rates and shorter lengths of stay compared with patients undergoing transapical or transaortic access.

11. What is the approach for transaortic access for TAVR?

The transaortic approach (TAO) is a retrograde surgical approach where the sheath for the TAVR valve delivery system is inserted directly into the ascending aorta via an arteriotomy. Access to the aorta can be achieved by either a small median mini-sternotomy or right lateral thoracotomy at the second intercostal space to expose the proximal ascending aorta. A soft spot on the aorta is identified with palpation. Purse string sutures placed directly on the aorta are tightened at the end to maintain hemostasis.

TAVR via the TAO approach is technically feasible and has favorable outcomes compared to other alternative access approaches in high-risk and inoperable patients who are ineligible for transfemoral (TF) TAVR. After the initial experience, the TAO largely supplanted TA access as the intrathoracic approach of choice.

12. What is the approach to transcaval access for TAVR?

The transcaval approach has been shown to be effective for TAVR in non-TF patients.

This approach first gains access to the femoral vein; an electrified guidewire is used to cross from the inferior vena cava to the abdominal aorta, where the wire is caught by a prepositioned snare in the aorta. The valve delivery sheath is advanced after progressive dilatation of the tract. The TAVR valve is then advanced and deployed using a standard retrograde valve placement technique. At the end of the procedure, the aortic hole is sealed using standard cardiac occluder devices. The transcaval approach was shown to be a viable option for patients who are not good candidates for transfemoral and transthoracic approaches, with an acceptable risk of life-threatening bleeding (7%) and overall mortality of 9.6% [6].

13. What is the approach to antegrade, transapical access?

Transapical access is an antegrade approach with direct access to the left ventricular apex through a small anterolateral thoracotomy. The valve delivery system is passed through the small LV apical incision, and an antegrade valve implantation is performed. This approach can be used in patients with severe peripheral artery disease and heavily calcified ascending aorta and arch where other approaches have increased risk of stroke.

14. What is the approach to antegrade, transseptal access?

The initial experience with TAVR by Dr. Cribier et al. was performed via the antegrade femoral vein with a transseptal puncture, and the aortic valve was crossed in an antegrade fashion from the left ventricle to the aorta. While largely abandoned in favor of the simpler femoral arterial access and retrograde aortic valve crossing approach, the antegrade, transseptal approach remains feasible for use with balloon-expandable (BE) valves in patients with no other vascular access. More recently, the procedure has been successfully performed with current-generation S3 BE valves as well.

This approach is performed by first obtaining right femoral venous access, which is the access point for the large delivery sheath and the valve. Contralateral venous access for the transvenous pacer, contralateral arterial access for the externalization wire, and third arterial access for the pigtail for aortic root contrast injections during positioning are also obtained. A standard transseptal atrial puncture is then performed. After the transseptal puncture, a 6–7 Fr balloon-tipped catheter or a diagnostic catheter (e.g. AL1) is advanced through the Mullins sheath, looped in the left ventricle, and used to direct the passage of a guidewire (e.g. a 0.035 in. floppy-tipped Wholey wire or 0.035 in. stiff Glidewire) antegrade across the aortic valve into the ascending aorta and arch. A 6F 125 cm multipurpose catheter is advanced through the TS sheath and around the aortic arch. A stiffer, more supportive exchange-length wire can then be advanced to the descending aorta, snared in the descending aorta from a contralateral femoral artery access, and externalized. A 6Fr MPA1-guiding catheter advanced retrograde over the externalized wire serves a protective role, allowing the operators to maintain control of the wire loop in the left ventricle while reducing the potential for shearing by the wire. Antegrade atrial septostomy is performed using an 8–14 mm peripheral vascular balloon advanced from the venous side. Atrial septostomy facilitates crossing the atrial septum with the BE device. The transcatheter heart valve (THV) is advanced through the venous access sheath and across the interatrial septum and looped through the mitral valve and left ventricle, and up and out the aortic valve. The valve is deployed antegrade during rapid ventricular pacing.

Some technical and procedural considerations need to be remembered. First, the valve needs to be mounted in reverse fashion on the balloon. Additionally, great care should be taken during manipulation of the externalized guidewire, as the wire can sinch the anterior mitral valve leaflet quickly, leading to hemodynamic collapse; this can usually be reversed by relaxing the tension on the wire. Further, the guidewire can induce mitral valve injury and anterior leaflet laceration, resulting in severe mitral regurgitation and cardiogenic shock. While technically challenging, the antegrade transeptal approach for TAVR with BE valves remains feasible for patients with no alternative access.

15. What are the optimal vascular closure techniques for large-bore vascular access during TAVR?

The transfemoral access site is the most widely used for TAVR and is used in more than 95% of cases. Surgical cutdown access was the initial preferred vascular approach for large-bore access.

Percutaneous vascular closure can be obtained with a suture-based pre-closure technique: two ProGlide (Abbott Vascular) devices place perpendicularly oriented sutures (positioned at 10 o'clock and 2 o'clock) at the arteriotomy site. The sutures are placed after initial arterial access is obtained and then deployed at the end of the procedure after removing the large-bore catheters. Newer dedicated plug-based large-bore arteriotomy closure devices such as the Manta closure device (Teleflex) are also safe and effective, with a major access site complication rate of approximately 4%. Comparisons of vascular closure devices (VCDs) suggest that the mechanisms of failure may be different. While suture-based closure often required additional closure devices, Manta needed more covered stents and surgical bailouts.

Balloon-Expandable Transcatheter Aortic Valve Replacement

16. What are the components of the Edwards SAPIEN balloon-expandable valve?

The Edwards SAPIEN valve platform (Edwards Lifesciences) is a BE type of transcatheter aortic valve. The system has two components: the valve bioprosthesis and the valve delivery system [8].

The Edwards SAPIEN valve bioprosthesis (Figure 7.1) is made of bovine pericardial tissue forming the valve leaflets, polyethylene terephthalate (PET) forming the outer skirt, and cobalt-chromium forming the valve frame. The Edwards SAPIEN 3 valve, which is the most recent edition, has an outer sealing skirt to decrease paravalvular leakage (PVL). This valve comes in 20, 23, 26, and 29 mm diameters to cover a range of annular sizes.

The Edwards Commander delivery system (Figure 7.2) components include the following:

- *Flex catheter:* Aids valve alignment to the balloon and tracking and positioning of the valve.
- *Balloon catheter:* Has a tapered tip and radiopaque valve alignment markers to delineate the working length of

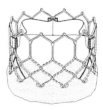

Figure 7.1 Edwards SAPIEN 3 transcatheter heart valve. *Source:* US Food and Drug Administration FDA.

the balloon, a radiopaque center marker to help with valve positioning, and a radiopaque triple marker proximal to the balloon to indicate Flex catheter position during valve deployment.

- *Handle:* Contains a flex wheel to control the flex catheter, a balloon lock, and a fine adjustment wheel to facilitate valve alignment and position the valve within the native annulus.
- *Edwards eSheath introducer:* A low-profile sheath and a dynamic expansion mechanism that expands transiently during the passage of the Edwards SAPIEN valve. It comes in 14 Fr and 16 Fr sizes.

17. What are the essential considerations during balloon-expandable TAVR?

The Edwards eSheath, with the E logo facing up, is advanced through primary arterial access under fluoroscopy guidance, and the tip of the sheath is parked in the distal part of the descending aorta above the iliac bifurcation. Heparin is given to keep the activated clotting time (ACT) above 250 seconds. Then a temporary pacemaker is advanced through the femoral vein access to the right ventricle, and the pacing capture threshold is assessed. A pigtail catheter is then advanced through the secondary arterial access site and placed in the right coronary cusp.

At this point, the coplanar angle should be assessed and determined by root injections (Figure 7.3a).

The aortic valve is crossed using an Amplatz left (AL) catheter and straight-tip wire (Figure 7.3b). Judkins right (JR) or Amplatz right (AR) catheters may also be needed for aortic valve crossing. Once the aortic valve is crossed with the straight wire, the catheter is advanced to the left ventricle. The straight wire is then exchanged for a J-tipped wire, a pigtail is advanced to the left ventricle apex, and the operator confirms no entanglement of the mitral chordae apparatus. Hemodynamic assessment is then performed to assess the baseline systolic gradient as well as the diastolic pressure separations (Figure 7.3c).

A pre-shaped extra-stiff wire is advanced and positioned in the left ventricle. The loader at the tip of the valve delivery system is then inserted into the eSheath. If balloon aortic valvuloplasty for valve pre-dilatation is needed, it is performed at this point with rapid ventricular pacing. Then the Commander valve delivery system follows, with the Edwards logo facing up, through the sheath until the valve exits the sheath. Then the loader is retracted.

Valve alignment to the balloon is performed in the straight part of the descending aorta under fluoroscopy. The balloon lock should be disengaged first, after which the balloon catheter is pulled straight back until part of the warning marker is visible on the balloon catheter. Then the balloon lock is engaged, and the valve is positioned between the valve alignment markers using the fine adjustment wheel.

The valve delivery system is advanced through the descending aorta, aortic arch, and ascending aorta to the aortic valve with a smooth continuous motion while flexing the catheter using the flex wheel. Once the bioprosthetic valve is across the aortic annulus at the appropriate depth, the balloon lock is disengaged, and the flex catheter is retracted to the center of the triple markers. The bioprosthetic valve position is then adjusted as necessary using the flex wheel to adjust the co-axiality of the valve and the fine adjustment wheel to adjust the depth of the valve

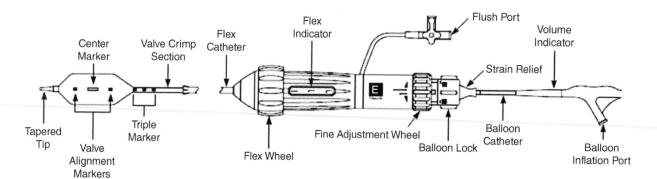

Figure 7.2 Edwards Commander delivery system.

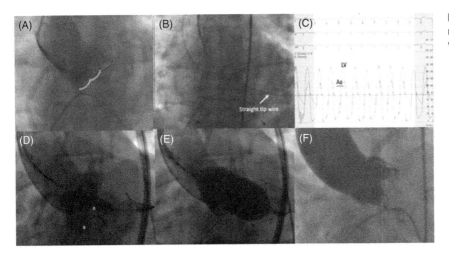

Figure 7.3 Transcatheter aortic valve replacement with a balloon-expandable valve.

(Figure 7.3d). The valve position between the valve alignment markers and the flex catheter tip position over the triple marker should be confirmed before valve delivery.

Valve delivery is performed at the predetermined deployment coplanar angle. It is executed by inflating the delivery balloon under rapid pacing once the systolic blood pressure drops to less than 50 mmHg. The balloon should be inflated with the entire volume in the Inflation device and held for three seconds before deflating (Figure 7.3e). The rapid pacing is stopped once the balloon is fully deflated.

After the valve is successfully deployed, the valve delivery system is slowly withdrawn into the descending aorta while maintaining the guidewire in the left ventricle. Catheter withdrawal is facilitated with unflexing of the delivery system while retracting it. Then the delivery system can be removed from the body.

Post-implantation aortogram should be performed to confirm the bioprosthetic valve location, assess for any aortic insufficiency, and evaluate the patency of the coronary ostia (Figure 7.3f). A pigtail catheter is also advanced into the left ventricle to assess the transvalvular pressure gradient and diastolic pressure separation. Transthoracic echocardiography also should be done to confirm valve function and assess for aortic regurgitation, left ventricular function, and pericardial effusion.

Self-Expanding Transcatheter Aortic Valve Replacement

18. What are the components of the self-expanding valve and catheter system?

The Medtronic valve platform (Medtronic) is a self-expanding type of transcatheter aortic valve. The system has two components: the valve bioprosthesis and the valve delivery system.

The Medtronic valve bioprosthesis (Figure 7.4) is made of a porcine tissue component forming the valve leaflets and skirt on a Nitinol self-expanding valve frame. The porcine valve leaflets are located at a supra-annular plane. The Medtronic aortic valve platform has evolved from the CoreValve to Evolut R to Evolut Pro. The Evolut Pro, which is the most recent edition, has porcine tissue forming a skirt over the inside and outside of the inflow portion of the Nitinol frame to decrease PVL. The Medtronic valve bioprosthesis comes in 23, 26, 29, and 34 mm diameters to cover a range of different annular sizes.

The Medtronic valve delivery system (Figure 7.5) components include the following:

- *Introducer sheath:* A 16 Fr size InLine sheath.
- *Radiopaque catheter tip* (nosecone).
- *Capsule:* Covers the bioprosthetic valve and maintains it in a crimped position. The capsule has a distal flare that enables the bioprosthetic valve to be partially or fully recaptured after partial deployment.
- *Handle/Knob:* Located at the proximal end of the valve delivery catheter and used to load, deploy, recapture, and reposition the bioprosthetic valve.

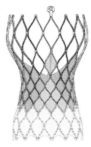

Figure 7.4 Medtronic Evolut PRO+ transcatheter heart valve. *Source:* US Food and Drug Administration FDA.

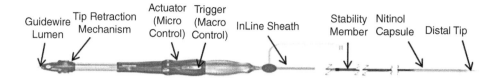

Figure 7.5 EnVeo Medtronic valve delivery system.

19. What are the essential considerations during self-expandable TAVR?

Implantation of the Medtronic CoreValve Evolut biopros-thetic valve should be avoided in patients with aortic root angulation of >30° for right subclavian/axillary access or >70° for femoral and left subclavian/axillary access. In selected cases with horizontal aortic root angle, the CoreValve Evolut system can be used with the help of a snare to facilitate the advancement of the valve system across the aortic root.

Once an optimal femoral access is obtained, as detailed previously (Figure 7.6a), heparin is given to keep the ACT above 250 seconds. Then a temporary pacemaker is advanced through the femoral vein access to the right ven-tricle and the capture threshold is assessed. A pigtail is advanced through the secondary arterial access site and placed in the non-coronary cusp. At this point, the copla-nar or cusp overlap angles should be assessed and deter-mined by root injections (Figure 7.6b).

The aortic valve is crossed using an AL catheter and straight-tip wire. JR or AR catheters may also be needed. Once the aortic valve is crossed with the wire, the catheter is advanced to the left ventricle. The straight wire is then exchanged for a J-tipped wire, a pigtail is advanced to the

left ventricle apex, and the operator confirms no engage-ment of the mitral chordae apparatus. Hemodynamic assessment is performed, assessing the baseline systolic gradient as well as the diastolic pressure separations. Then a pre-shaped coiled stiff wire is advanced and positioned in the left ventricle.

The preloaded valve in the capsule should be evaluated under Cine-fluoroscopy at 30 frames/second. This is per-formed by rotating the valve delivery tip in the fluoroscopy field outside the body (Figure 7.6c). The integrity of the valve, capsule, and paddles should be assessed. If balloon aortic valvuloplasty for valve pre-dilatation is needed, it is performed at this point with rapid ventricular pacing. The valve delivery system is then loaded on the wire and advanced through the iliofemoral arteries, descending aorta, arch, and ascending aorta. The valve is positioned across the native aortic valve, targeting an implant depth of 3–5 mm (Figure 7.6d).

Valve delivery is performed at the predetermined deploy-ment cusp overlap angle via counterclockwise rotation of the valve delivery knob on the handle. There is a one-to-one response between the unsheathing of the capsule and the delivery knob rotation after a couple of rotations. Rapid ventricular pacing at a heart rate of 120–160 beats per min-ute can be used during the initial valve deployment phase until annular contact is achieved. Shortly after annular

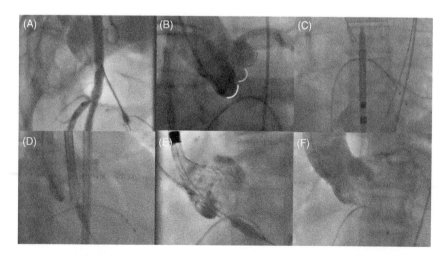

Figure 7.6 Transcatheter aortic valve replacement with a self-expandable valve

contact, the blood pressure is reduced until approximately 60% of the valve is deployed, at which point the bioprosthetic leaflets are exposed and functioning normally. The valve deployment is continued by counterclockwise rotation of the deployment knob until a tactile response is noted. This is a precautionary mark that indicates the point of no recapture is nearing. The point of no recapture is reached once the radiopaque capsule marker band reaches the distal end of the radiopaque paddle attachment (Figure 7.6e). If the valve position and depth are optimal, the valve capsule should then be detached from the radiopaque paddles with the continued counterclockwise rotation of the deployment knob.

After successfully deploying the valve, slowly withdraw the valve delivery catheter tip into the descending aorta while maintaining the guidewire in the left ventricle. Catheter withdrawal should be under fluoroscopic guidance after confirming that the catheter tip is coaxial with the inflow portion of the deployed bioprosthetic valve. The capsule should be closed until it is aligned with the catheter tip by pulling the catheter tip under fluoroscopy. This is accomplished by pulling the gray front grip part with the operator's left hand toward the blue handle while fixing the blue handle with the operator's right hand. Then the delivery system can be removed from the body.

20. Can the Evolut valve be repositioned during deployment?

The Evolut valve allows for partial or full recapture of the valve during deployment. Often, recapture is necessary because the position is either too high or shallow. There may be a concern that more maneuvering of the valve may result in longer dwell time in the body and an increased risk of adverse effects. Repositioning during Evolut R or PRO valve implantation is safe and has no observed difference in death or disabling stroke at 30 days or 1 year based on analysis of data from the SURTAVI (Surgical Replacement and Transcatheter Aortic Valve Implantation) and Evolut Low Risk Trials.

21. After valve implantation, how is adequate valve position confirmed?

Post-implantation aortogram should be performed to confirm the bioprosthetic valve location, assess for any aortic insufficiency, and evaluate the patency of the coronary ostia (Figure 7.6f). A pigtail catheter is also advanced to the left ventricle, and transvalvular pressure gradient and diastolic pressure separation should be assessed. Transthoracic echocardiography also should be done to confirm valve function and assess for aortic regurgitation, left ventricular function, and pericardial effusion.

Conclusion

Over the past decade, best practices have emerged for TAVR. By following a series of steps during TAVR, the procedure becomes easier, with more predictable results and safety outcomes. Following the best established practices is important to improve both the safety and efficacy of the procedure. There are general and device-specific considerations to take into account that operators must become facile with. As the TAVR procedure and valve devices continue to evolve, further modifications to these established best practices may emerge and improve the procedure's overall safety.

Bibliography

1 Adams, D.H., Popma, J., Reardon, M.J. et al. (2014). Transcatheter aortic-valve replacement with a self-expanding prosthesis. *N. Engl. J. Med.* 370 (19): 1790–1798.

2 Allen, K.B., Chhatriwalla, A.K., Saxon, J. et al. (2019). Transcarotid versus transapical and transaortic access for transcatheter aortic valve replacement. *Ann. Thorac. Surg.* 108 (3): 715–722.

3 Attizzani, G.F., Dallan, L.A., Markowitz, A. et al. (2020). Impact of repositioning on outcomes following transcatheter aortic valve replacement with a self-expandable valve. *JACC Cardiovasc. Interv.* 13 (15): 1816–1824.

4 Bapat, V., Thomas, M., Hancock, J. et al. (2010). First successful trans-catheter aortic valve implantation through ascending aorta using Edwards SAPIEN THV system. *Eur. J. Cardiothorac. Surg.* 38 (6): 811–813.

5 Barbanti, M., Binder, R., Freeman, M. et al. (2013). Impact of low-profile sheaths on vascular complications during transfemoral transcatheter aortic valve replacement. *EuroIntervention* 9 (8): 929–935.

6 Bob-Manuel, T., Almusawi, H., Rezan, T. et al. (2020). Efficacy and safety of transcarotid transcatheter aortic valve replacement: a systematic review. *Cardiovasc. Revasc. Med.* 21 (7): 917–926.

7 Cohen, M.G., Singh, V., Martinez, C.A. et al. (2013). Transseptal antegrade transcatheter aortic valve replacement for patients with no other access approach – a contemporary experience. *Catheter. Cardiovasc. Interv.* 82 (6): 987–993.

8 Cribier, A., Eltchaninoff, H., Bash, A. et al. (2002). Percutaneous transcatheter implantation of an aortic valve prosthesis for calcific aortic stenosis: first human case description. *Circulation* 106: 3006.

9 Dahle, T.G., Kaneko, T., and McCabe, J.M. (2019). Outcomes following subclavian and axillary artery access for transcatheter aortic valve replacement: Society of the Thoracic Surgeons/American College of Cardiology TVT registry report. *JACC Cardiovasc. Interv.* 12 (7): 662–669.

10 Damluji, A.A., Murman, M., Byun, S. et al. (2018). Alternative access for transcatheter aortic valve replacement in older adults: a collaborative study from France and United States. *Catheter. Cardiovasc. Interv.* 92 (6): 1182–1193.

11 Dawson, K., Jones, T.L., Kearney, K.E. et al. (2020). Emerging role of large-bore percutaneous axillary vascular access: a step-by-step guide. *Interv. Cardiol.* 15: e07.

12 Gleason, T.G., Schindler, J.T., Hagberg, R.C. et al. (2018). Subclavian/axillary access for self-expanding transcatheter aortic valve replacement renders equivalent outcomes as transfemoral. *Ann. Thorac. Surg.* 105 (2): 477–483.

13 Greenbaum, A.B., Babaliaros, V.C., Chen, M.Y. et al. (2017). Transcaval access and closure for transcatheter aortic valve replacement: a prospective investigation. *J. Am. Coll. Cardiol.* 69 (5): 511–521.

14 Grube, E., Van Mieghem, N., Bleiziffer, S. et al. (2017). Clinical outcomes with a repositionable self-expanding Transcatheter aortic valve prosthesis: the international FORWARD study. *J. Am. Coll. Cardiol.* 70 (7): 845–853.

15 Hanzel, G.S., Harrity, P.J., Schreiber, T.L., and O'Neill, W.W. (2005). Retrograde percutaneous aortic valve implantation for critical aortic stenosis. *Catheter. Cardiovasc. Interv.* 64 (3): 322–326.

16 Kasel, A.M., Cassese, S., Bleiziffer, S. et al. (2013). Standardized imaging for aortic annular sizing: implications for transcatheter valve selection. *JACC Cardiovasc. Imaging* 6 (2): 249–262.

17 Kroon, H.G., Tonino, P.A.L., Savontaus, M. et al. (2021). Dedicated plug based closure for large bore access – the MARVEL prospective registry. *Catheter. Cardiovasc. Interv.* 97 (6): 1270–1278.

18 Lardizabal, J.A., Macon, C.J., O'Neill, B.P. et al. (2015). Long-term outcomes associated with the transaortic approach to transcatheter aortic valve replacement. *Catheter. Cardiovasc. Interv.* 85 (7): 1226–1230.

19 Lardizabal, J.A., O'Neill, B.P., Desai, H. et al. (2013). The transaortic approach for transcatheter aortic valve replacement: initial clinical experience in the United States. *J. Am. Coll. Cardiol.* 61 (23): 2341–2345.

20 Leon, M.B., Smith, C., Mack, M.J. et al. (2016). Transcatheter or surgical aortic-valve replacement in intermediate-risk patients. *N. Engl. J. Med.* 374 (17): 1609–1620.

21 Leon, M.B., Smith, C.R., Mack, M. et al. (2010). Transcatheter aortic-valve implantation for aortic stenosis in patients who cannot undergo surgery. *N. Engl. J. Med.* 363 (17): 1597–1607.

22 Mack, M.J., Martin, L., Thourani, V.H. et al. (2019). Transcatheter aortic-valve replacement with a balloon-expandable valve in low-risk patients. *N. Engl. J. Med.* 380 (18): 1695–1705.

23 Makkar, R.R., Thourani, V., Mack, M.J. et al. (2020). Five-year outcomes of transcatheter or surgical aortic-valve replacement. *N. Engl. J. Med.* 382 (9): 799–809.

24 Misumida, N., Anderson, J.H., Greason, K.L. et al. (2020). Antegrade transseptal transcatheter aortic valve replacement: back to the future? *Catheter. Cardiovasc. Interv.* 96 (5): E552–e556.

25 Popma, J.J. et al. (2019). Transcatheter aortic-valve replacement with a self-expanding valve in low-risk patients. *N. Engl. J. Med.* 380 (18): 1706–1715.

26 Smith, C.R., Martin, L., Mack, M.J. et al. (2011). Transcatheter versus surgical aortic-valve replacement in high-risk patients. *N. Engl. J. Med.* 364 (23): 2187–2198.

27 Southmayd, G., Hoque, A., Kaki, A. et al. (2020). Percutaneous large-bore axillary access is a safe alternative to surgical approach: a systematic review. *Catheter. Cardiovasc. Interv.* 96 (7): 1481–1488.

28 van Wiechen, M.P., Tchetche, D., Ooms, J.F. et al. (2021). Suture- or plug-based large-bore arteriotomy closure: a pilot randomized controlled trial. *JACC Cardiovasc. Interv.* 14 (2): 149–157.

8

Balloon Aortic Valvuloplasty

Current Clinical Role and Technical Aspects

Alexandre C. Ferreira, Joao Braghiroli and Cesar E. Mendoza

[1] *Department of Cardiology, Jackson Memorial Health System, Miami, FL, USA*

1. What are the guideline recommended indications for aortic balloon valvuloplasty (BAV)?

The European Society of Cardiology guidelines gives aortic valvuloplasty a Class IIb indication, level of evidence C, for hemodynamically unstable patients with severe symptomatic aortic stenosis as a bridge to recovery prior to future TAVR or SAVR. It also gives the same level of recommendation for severe symptomatic AS requiring noncardiac surgery. Additionally, it is considered a palliative measure in symptomatic severe AS patients who are not candidates for transcatheter aortic valve replacement (TAVR) or surgical aortic valve replacement (SAVR; Table 8.1).

The American College of Cardiology/American Heart Association (ACC/AHA) Practice Guidelines give aortic valvuloplasty a Class IIb indication, level of evidence C, for severe symptomatic aortic stenosis, as a bridge to recovery prior to future TAVR or SAVR, without mentioning hemodynamic stability. It does not recommend valvuloplasty prior to noncardiac surgery due to lack of evidence that it is beneficial (Table 1).

2. What are the contra-indications to aortic balloon valvuloplasty?

Aortic valvuloplasty is contraindicated in patients with suspected aortic valve endocarditis, metallic aortic valves, or when there is a risk of fragmentation of valve debris. Aortic valvuloplasty should not be performed when there is left ventricle (LV) thrombus, active bleeding, or when the life expectancy or quality of life is not expected to improve. The decision-making for BAV should be made by the Heart Team approach with a multi-disciplinary team. Family discussion and plan should be made prior to BAV regarding patient candidacy for sternotomy and cardio-pulmonary bypass or LV support. BAV should not be performed by operators without experience in structural heart intervention or familiarity with large bore access management.

3. What are the goals of BAV and what defines a successful BAV?

The ultimate goal of BAV is improvement in functional class and clinical symptoms. The primary goal is to reduce gradient and increase the aortic valve area without causing significant valvular regurgitation or any major cardiac or neuro-vascular complications. There are no clinical studies post-BAV that correlated the degree of improvement in the aortic valve area with improvement in functional class; therefore, any definition of success is arbitrary.

It is generally accepted that in a successful valvuloplasty, a reduction in the mean valvular gradient of 50% is achieved. A commensurate increase in cardiac output and valve area is expected. In the largest balloon valvuloplasty registry to date, compiled by the NHLBI, a 674 patient registry from the USA and Canada, the valve area increased only from 0.5 to 0.8 cm^2. A similar improvement in valve area was reported by the 492 patient Mansfield registry.

Although a more complete valvuloplasty, with goals of achieving an aortic valve area (AVA) greater than 1 cm^2, has been advocated by some and may be possible with contemporary BAV technique and better imaging, understanding of valve anatomy and annulus sizing, correlates of improvement in long term outcomes are lacking, and concerns regarding the increasing risk of acute complications remain.

Table 8.1 Indications for balloon valvuloplasty in severe symptomatic aortic stenosis.

Indication for balloon valvuloplasty in severe symptomatic aortic stenosis	ACC/AHA Guidelines 2014	European Society Guidelines 2012
• Bridge to TAVR or SAVR	Yes	Yes
• Prior to noncardiac surgery	No	Yes
• As palliative procedure in patients not candidates for TAVR/SAVR	No	Yes
• Differentiate severe from pseudo-severe AS	No	No

4. What is the incidence of complications in BAV?

The incidence of BAV complications has changed little despite increased operator experience and a substantial increase in BAV procedures in the TAVR era. This might be partly due to an increased patient risk profile. A recent evaluation found that procedural and in-hospital mortality were 1.4 and 8.5%, respectively. Vascular complications occurred in 7.0% of cases, blood transfusion in 17.5%, clinical stroke in 1.8%, and pacemaker implantation in 3.0%. Acute aortic insufficiency, cardiac perforation, and cardiac tamponade remain rare.

5. What are the balloon sizing considerations for BAV?

The size of the balloon for BAV is usually selected based on the annular size obtained on transthoracic echocardiography (TTE). Usually, a 1 : 1 balloon to annulus ratio is selected based on the para-sternal long-axis view of TTE. This may underestimate the true annular size by 1–2 mm. If cardiac computed tomography (CT) is available, mean annular diameter can be selected. Balloon size should not exceed aorta size at the sino-tubular junction and should be smaller, at least 10% of LVOT size.

If balloon valvuloplasty is performed to prepare the annulus prior to TAVR, the minimal annulus diameter is usually used for sizing. Post TAVR BAV is usually performed with a balloon sized to the mean annulus diameter. If a bioprosthetic valve fracture is needed, a balloon sized 2–3 mm greater than the true internal diameter of the bioprosthetic valve is used.

6. Which types of balloons are available for BAV?

BAV balloons are semi-compliant and non-compliant. Balloon sizes range from 16 to 30 mm, and balloon lengths are usually 3–6 cm. Semi-compliant balloons (Tyshak II, NuCLEUS-X, Z-MED and-MED II [Braun Interventional Systems]) have lower profiles and require smaller sheaths. Non-compliant balloons (TRUE Dilatation devices [Bard Peripheral Vascular]) are generally preferred for calcific aortic stenosis and post dilatation of TAVRs. Most BAV balloons are cylindrical, but hour-glass balloons (Nucleus NuMED balloon) are also available without unclear evidence of benefit. True flow balloons (Bard) composed of multiple small balloons are available to allow continuous ventricular ejection, obviating rapid pacing and allowing forward flow in low ejection fraction patients. Bioprosthetic valve ring fracture can be performed with a high-pressure non-compliant balloon (TRUE balloon). For the antegrade procedure, the Inoue-balloon (Toray) is usually selected. With severe peripheral vascular disease, an alternative dual balloon strategy using peripheral balloons and radial or brachial access can be used.

7. What is the technique used to cross stenotic aortic valve?

Crossing calcific stenotic valves can be challenging, particularly for bicuspid valves with extensive calcification of bioprosthetic valves. Amplatz left catheters (usually AL1 curve), Amplatz right catheters (usually AR2 curve), or Judkins right (JR 4.0) are preferred crossing catheters. If the radial approach is used, Judkins right catheters (JR 4.0 curves) or AR 1 catheters are used. A 0.35 standard straight wire is used to cross the valve, but alternatively, a hydrophilic straight wire (Glidewire, Terumo) can be selected if unable to cross.

The catheters are initially pointed toward the left cusp and slowly rotated clockwise or counterclockwise as the wire is advanced to probe the valve. If cardiac CT is available, a coplanar radiographic view with the three cups aligned is used to cross the valve. If CT is not available, a shallow LAO caudal view is selected. Once the wire is across the aortic valve, the catheter is advanced over the wire and rotated clockwise so it can be directed to the apex. Once the catheter is fully across the aortic valve, an exchange J tip wire can be exchanged, and a pigtail catheter can be then advanced across the valve toward the apex of the heart. An RAO view can be used to confirm the position of the pigtail in the apex of the heart. If the catheter fails to advance to the apex, contrast can be injected to assure the catheter is not entrapped under the papillary muscle or mitral valve apparatus.

8. How is the valvuloplasty balloon stabilized across the aortic valve during inflation?

Rapid ventricular pacing has become the routine during balloon valvuloplasty. The idea is to reduce cardiac output and prevent ejection of the balloon during ventricular systole. In theory, it could also prevent left ventricular wire injury and allow more complete valvuloplasty. Clinical consequences and benefits of rapid pacing may be negated by the possibility of transient ischemia or hemodynamic instability. Nevertheless, rapid pacing, heart rate between 180 and 220 bpm, with the goal to reduce BP to less than 60 mmHg, is usually recommended. An intravenous temporary pace-maker wire is used; alternatively, ventricular pacing using the LV guidewire obviates the need for venous access. If rapid ventricular pacing is to be avoided, using a smaller valvuloplasty balloon or a True Flow ® (Bard, USA) balloon to allow ventricular ejection during valvuloplasty can be considered.

9. What is the role of valvuloplasty in patients undergoing TAVR?

BAV is frequently performed as an adjunct to TAVR implant. Potential benefits include to facilitate the advancement of the TAVR valve across the stenosis and allow a more controlled deployment without occluding flow, particularly in severely stenotic valves. BAV can also aid in annulus sizing, particularly when the annulus measures borderline between valve sizes, assess displacement of bulky leaflets, and assess the risk of coronary occlusion during TAVR. Post TAVR, valvuloplasty can be used to further expand the TAVR prosthesis in the case of perivalvular leakage or when the device is partially constrained. The role of valvuloplasty in TAVR continues to evolve as pre-TAVR valvuloplasty may be associated with complications, including the risk for heart block, aortic insufficiency, and cerebrovascular complications.

A direct TAVR approach without BAV has been advocated, which simplifies the procedure. Multiple studies have demonstrated that for most patients, a direct TAVR approach is associated with similar outcomes compared to BAV-facilitated TAVR for both self-expanding and balloon-expandable valves. Despite this, most operators favor BAV-assisted TAVR in patients with bicuspid valves, heavy calcification, and in very critical AS with AVA <0.6 cm^2.

10. What is the role of BAV in patients with low-flow, low-gradient aortic stenosis?

With appropriate technique, BAV can be safely performed in patients with severely reduced LV function. Although approximately half of the patients will improve LV function, predictors of improvement are not uniformly accepted. Baseline gradients, contractile reserve parameters, dobutamine stress testing, valve calcium scores, associated ischemic heart disease, and serum biomarkers have been investigated as possible predictors of improvement. Patients who had improvement in EF detected 30-days post BAV and rapid improvement in serum pro-BMP as early as 24 hours post BAV appears to have better 1-year survival.

11. What is the role of BAV to reduce cardiac complications of patients requiring non-cardiac surgery?

Both the European Society and ACC/AHA guidelines were drafted in 2014. There is still controversy about how to handle severe AS patients who are asymptomatic but require elective noncardiac surgery. In adults who meet the criteria for either TAVR or SAVR, it is reasonable to perform AVR prior to elective noncardiac surgery. There is no uniform agreement on the role of BAV prior to semi-urgent moderate or high-risk surgery. The frequent challenging clinical setting would be a patient who experienced a syncopal event with hip fracture, and is found to have severe aortic stenosis. Options being BAV followed by hip surgery, versus hip surgery with appropriate intraoperative and post-operative hemodynamic monitoring without BAV. Recent improvements in cardiac anesthesia care, better understanding of how to manage hemodynamics of severe AS, and the lack of clear guideline recommendation to the benefits of BAV prior to semi-urgent procedures might explain the trend to use a hemodynamic monitoring strategy without BAV in most patients.

12. What is the post-procedure care of BAV patients?

Post-BAV patients are usually managed in the cardiac ICU or step-down unit for the first 24–48 hours. Close monitoring of vital signs, cardiac monitoring for the risk of complete heart block, late development of cardiac tamponade, and bleeding from large bore access is recommended. Routine neuro checks for early detection of cardio-embolic events allows for stroke team activation as early intervention can be associated with improved outcome. Post-procedure monitoring of blood count to detect silent retroperitoneal blood loss, kidney function to track contrast nephropathy, and measurement of cardiac biomarkers, particularly whether pro-BNP levels are reasonable. Echocardiography should be performed prior to discharge to document new baseline valve velocities and valve area. Follow-up echocardiography after three to six months and one year are generally obtained to monitor cardiac function and to evaluate restenosis of aortic valve.

13. What are the options for hemodynamically assisted aortic valvuloplasty?

Severe aortic stenosis patients in cardiogenic shock can be supported with an intra-aortic balloon pump (IABP). In a cohort of 25 patients, the cardiac index improved from $1.77 \, l/min/m^2$ to 2.18 and $2.36 \, l/min/m^2$ at 6 and 24 hours post-insertion. Systemic vascular resistance was reduced from $1331 \, dyn/s/cm^5$ to 1265 and $1051 \, dyn/s/cm^5$ at 6 and 24 hours. The central venous pressure was also reduced from 14.8 mmHg to 13.2 and 10.9 mmHg at 6 and 24 hours. Impella-assisted BAV is feasible and has been successfully performed. ECMO and tandem heart are also alternative options in extreme risk patients in profound shock who might improve with BAV as a bridge to recovery.

Bibliography

1 Aksoy, O., Yousefzai, R., Singh, D. et al. (2011). Cardiogenic shock in the setting of severe aortic stenosis: role of intra-aortic balloon pump. *Heart* 97 (10): 838–843.

2 Alkhouli, M., Zack, C., Sarraf, M. et al. (2017). Morbidity and mortality associated with balloon aortic valvuloplasty: a national perspective. *Circ. Cardiovasc. Interv.* 10: e004481.

3 Bashore, T.M., Berman, A.D., Davidson, C.J. et al. (1991). Percutaneous balloon aortic valvuloplasty. Acute and 30-day follow-up results in 674 patients from the NHBI balloon valvuloplasty registry. *Circulation* (6): 2383–2397.

4 Dorros, G., Lewin, R.F., Stertzer, S.H. et al. (1990). Percutaneous transluminal aortic valvuloplasty: the acute outcome and follow up of 149 patients who underwent the double balloon technique. *Eur. Heart J.* 11 (5): 429–440. https://doi.org/10.1093/oxfordjournals. eurheartj.a059726.

5 Fleisher, L.A., Fleischmann, K.E., Auerbach, A.D. et al. (2014). 2014 ACC/ AHA guideline on perioperative cardiovascular evaluation and management of patients undergoing noncardiac surgery: a report of the American College of Cardiology/American Heart Association Task Force on practice guidelines. *J. Am. Coll. Cardiol.* 64 (22): e77–e137.

6 Giustino, G., Montorfano, M., Latib, A. et al. (2014). TCT-743 to predilate or to not predilate in transcatheter aortic valve implantation? Single-center experience with self-expandable CoreValve revalving system. *J. Am. Coll. Cardiol.* 64: B217–B218.

7 Keeble, T.R., Khokhar, A., Akhtar, M. et al. (2016). Percutaneous balloon aortic valvuloplasty in the era of transcatheter aortic valve implantation: a narrative review. *Open Heart* 3: e000421.

8 Kefer, J., Gapira, J.M., Pierard, S. et al. (2013). Recovery after balloon aortic valvuloplasty in patients with aortic stenosis and impaired left ventricular function: predictors and prognostic implications. *J. Invasive Cardiol.* 25 (5): 235–241.

9 Kennon, S., Jain, A., Kennon, S. et al. (2011). Circulatory support in severe aortic stenosis. *Heart* 97 (10): 783–784.

10 Kristensen, S.D., Knuuti, J., Saraste, A. et al. (2014). 2014 ESC/ESA guidelines on noncardiac surgery: cardiovascular assessment and management: the Joint Task Force on noncardiac surgery: cardiovascular assessment and management of the European Society of Cardiology (ESC) and the European Society of Anaesthesiology (ESA). *Eur. Heart J.* 35 (35): 2383–2431.

11 Martinez, C.A., Singh, V., Londoño, J.C. et al. (2012). Percutaneous retrograde left ventricular assist support for interventions in patients with aortic stenosis and left ventricular dysfunction. *Catheter. Cardiovasc. Interv.* 80 (7): 1201–1209.

12 Mckay, R.G. (1991). The Mansfield scientific aortic valvuloplasty registry: overview of acute hemodynamic

results and procedural complications. *J. Am. Coll. Cardiol.* 17 (2): 485–491.

13 Möllmann, H., Kim, W.-K., Kempfert, J. et al. (2014). Transfemoral aortic valve implantation of Edwards SAPIEN XT without predilatation is feasible. *Clin. Cardiol.* 37: 667–671.

14 Nishimura, R.A., Otto, C.M., Bonow, R.O. et al. (2014). 2014 ACC/AHA guideline for the management of valvular heart disease: executive summary: a report of the American College of Cardiology/American Heart Association Task Force on Practice Guidelines. *J. Am. Coll. Cardiol.* 63: 2438–2488.

15 Shivaraju, A., Thilo, C., Sawlani, N. et al. (2018). Aortic valve predilatation with a small balloon, without rapid pacing, prior to transfemoral transcatheter aortic valve replacement. *Biomed. Res. Int.* 1–6.

16 Vahanian, A., Alfieri, O., Andreotti, F. et al. (2012). Join Task Force on the management of valvular heart disease of the European Society of Cardiology. Guidelines on the management of valvular heart disease (version 2021). *Eur. Heart J.* 33: 2451–2496.

17 Williams, T. and Hildick-Smith, D.J. (2020). Ballon aortic valvuloplasty: indications, patient eligibility, technique and contemporary outcomes. *Heart* 106: 1102–1110.

9

Challenging Anatomy Scenarios in TAVR

Timothy Lee and Gilbert H.L. Tang

[1] *Department of Cardiovascular Surgery, Mount Sinai Medical Center, New York, NY, USA*

Aortic Root

1. During transcatheter aortic valve replacement (TAVR), what are important principles for patients with severe aortic leaflet and annular calcification?

Severe aortic leaflet calcification is a very common occurrence during transcatheter aortic valve replacement (TAVR), and this situation is associated with an increased risk of complications such as left main coronary obstruction, particularly with a tall and bulky left cusp. In cases of annular and left ventricular outflow tract (LVOT) calcification, there is an increased risk of annular rupture or paravalvular leak (PVL). Cerebral embolic protection is encouraged due to the increased risk of calcific emboli during pre-balloon aortic valvuloplasty (pre-BAV), valve deployment, or balloon post-dilatation. Crossing the native valve can be very difficult, and useful techniques include localizing wire positioning with echocardiography and attempting multiple combinations of catheters and wires. Pre-BAV is utilized to allow the transcatheter valve to cross the native valve, with balloon size based on the minimum annular diameter, as well as to prevent the valve from being constrained post-deployment. Pre-BAV may cause significant aortic regurgitation (AR) and hemodynamic collapse, and in this situation, the team should be prepared to rapidly deploy the transcatheter valve. When using a balloon-expandable valve in the presence of annular or LVOT calcium, one may consider undersizing or true-sizing the device relative to the annular dimensions to reduce the risk of annular injury, and adding balloon volume to optimize the seal and minimize PVL. This is especially important in severely calcified bicuspid aortic

valves. Alternatively, if one wants to oversize relative to the annular dimensions with a balloon-expandable valve, removing volume from the inflation balloon and watching the atmospheric pressure on the pressure gauge during inflation is prudent to avoid annular injury. Finally, post-deployment PVL should be addressed by balloon dilatation, with the balloon size based on the mean annular diameter (or mean annular diameter minus 1 mm if there is significant annular or LVOT calcium). Mild PVL may be acceptable in high or extreme surgical risk patients with hostile annular/LVOT anatomy with high risk of injury with post dilatation.

2. What unique risks exist during TAVR when there is minimal aortic leaflet and annular calcium?

Calcium is helpful for performing TAVR in several ways. First, it provides a visual landmark during valve deployment to aid in the implantation of the prosthesis at the correct depth. Second, calcium provides support to help anchor the valve within the root after deployment. Therefore, a lack of calcium increases the risk of implantation at the incorrect depth as well as valve migration or embolization into the LVOT or aorta.

Implanting the valve at the proper depth is made easier by using visual benchmarks within the aortic root, such as in the coronary arteries, LVOT, or sinotubular junction, by imaging the root under fluoroscopy and with rapid pacing runs (150–180 beats per minute) to minimize prosthesis movement. The risk of valve embolization may be minimized by oversizing the valve relative to the annulus dimensions, with >10% oversizing to allow adequate anchoring of the transcatheter valve

Mastering Structural Heart Disease, First Edition. Edited by Eduardo J. de Marchena and Camilo A. Gomez.
© 2023 John Wiley & Sons Ltd. Published 2023 by John Wiley & Sons Ltd.
Companion website: www.wiley.com/go/deMarchena/Mastering-Structural-Heart-Disease

against the minimally calcified leaflets. Note that oversizing the valve is associated with an increased risk of root rupture and conduction abnormalities (e.g. heart block), so a meticulous analysis of the aortic root complex is essential.

3. How does sinotubular junction (STJ) calcification affect valve deployment?

There are two major risks with STJ calcification. The first is causing dissection or rupture of the STJ. Avoiding STJ rupture involves carefully sizing the prosthesis preoperatively and limiting the oversizing of a balloon-expandable valve if its target height will be higher than the calcified STJ. Intraoperatively, care must be taken to deploy the balloon-expandable valve below the STJ such that the top of the valve does not provide radial outward force onto the calcified portions of the STJ. During deployment of a balloon-expandable valve, it is reasonable to accept implant depths deeper within the LVOT to avoid the valve from interacting with the STJ calcification.

Second, STJ calcification may also interact with the inflation balloon of a balloon-expandable valve during deployment and result in the valve deploying deeper into the LVOT. This must be accounted for when determining the correct starting point for the valve during deployment. STJ calcification is typically not an issue with self-expanding valves, but the outflow of the devices may be constrained by the STJ if it is smaller than the annulus.

4. What does "horizontal aorta" refer to during TAVR, and what techniques are required in this situation?

Horizontal aorta refers to situations in which the aortic angulation, or the degree of angulation between the plane of the aortic valve and the horizontal plane as measured in a coronal image, is large enough to make valve deployment more complicated. Depending on the study, this can be defined as anywhere between 48 and 70°. An initial study found that when the aortic angulation is >=48°, there were worse outcomes among first-generation self-expanding valves than when the angle was <48°, although this was not true of balloon-expandable valves. The mechanism behind this finding is potentially attributable to the self-expanding stent frame being longer and the delivery

catheter not being steerable. However, more recent studies with newer-generation devices that used varying degree thresholds for horizontal aorta have not consistently reproduced this finding.

Techniques to overcome a horizontal aorta include using balloon-expandable devices, stiffer wires to help straighten the aorta, and slow and controlled deployment of devices to ensure that the valve is deployed at the proper depth. Of note, patients with aortic angulation >70° have been excluded from clinical trials of self-expandable valves.

5. How should LVOT calcification affect valve deployment?

Similar to calcification of the aortic annulus and STJ, significant LVOT calcification increases the risk of aortic root rupture and mechanical complications like aorto-atrial/ventricular fistula or ventricular septal defect. In one series with the earlier generation balloon-expandable TAVR, the only significant risk factors for aortic root rupture were LVOT calcification and >20% oversizing of the valve compared to the LVOT dimensions. Therefore, judicious annular and LVOT measurements and valve sizing are the most important steps for avoiding injury.

Current recommendations in balloon-expandable TAVR include true-sizing or undersizing the latest-generation valve relative to the annulus to avoid annular and LVOT complications. In balloon-expandable TAVR, LVOT narrowing may also lead to potential aortic migration of the valve; during valve deployment, the operator charged with positioning the deployment system should be prepared to provide forward tension of the delivery catheter if the valve appears to be migrating in the aortic direction. Slow balloon inflation is key to avoiding annular and LVOT injury. In self-expanding TAVR, LVOT calcium may risk residual PVL, and aggressive balloon post-dilatation has been associated with annular or LVOT injury.

6. What is the role of TAVR in patients with bicuspid aortic valve disease?

Bicuspid patients have been largely excluded from pivotal trials comparing TAVR vs. surgical aortic valve replacement (SAVR) due to concerns about the elliptical shape of the annulus and the younger presenting age of patients with bicuspid disease. Additionally, TAVR for bicuspid anatomy is associated with increased stroke, annular rupture, conversion to open surgery, and pacemaker compared to TAVR for tricuspid anatomy. However, patients with bicuspid anatomy do well overall with TAVR, and outcomes have improved with newer-generation devices. Therefore, it may be reasonable to perform TAVR for patients with bicuspid disease if they are at high or prohibitive risk for SAVR. Cerebral embolic protection should be utilized if possible, given higher rates of stroke among bicuspid patients using either balloon-expandable or self-expanding valves.

In balloon-expandable TAVR, true-sizing or undersizing the valve relative to the annular dimensions, as well as monitoring the inflation pressure on the inflation device during valve deployment, can be done to reduce the risk of aortic root injury. In self-expanding TAVR, balloon pre-dilatation can facilitate the opening of fused raphe, if present, to avoid under-expansion of the valve frame requiring balloon post dilatation. Finally, additional femoral venous access can be placed prophylactically in the event of the need for emergency bypass due to hemodynamic collapse from complications.

7. What can be done for patients with a small aortic annulus?

The main concern is prosthesis-patient mismatch (PPM), defined as the implantation of a prosthesis with an effective orifice area (EOA) that is inadequate for a patient's body surface area. EOA refers to the cross-sectional area of the smallest portion of the valve, and thus a smaller EOA results in decreased maximum flows. If a patient experiences PPM post-deployment, this will present as higher-than-expected gradients and symptoms of aortic stenosis (e.g. shortness of breath, fatigue) despite a normally functioning valve. The main strategy to overcome this is selecting the largest self-expanding valve feasible.

The design of self-expanding valves places the transcatheter valve above the native annulus, referred to as a *supra-annular position*. This design results in a larger EOA than if the valve were placed in an annular position, as is the design for balloon-expandable valves. A second technique to minimize the risk of PPM is attempting higher implantation of the valve within the root to achieve a supra-annular effect with an intra-annular device, but avoiding device pop-out or aortic migration is critical. Third, if it appears the valve is constrained, post-dilatation with BAV may help expand the valve further. However, be very cautious with aggressive balloon post-dilatation, as ballooning a valve within a small aortic

annuls may result in aortic root rupture, particularly in the presence of severe leaflet calcification or annular/LVOT calcification.

8. How should a valve be correctly sized in an extremely large annulus?

All decisions about TAVR valve sizes should be based on the manufacturer's sizing charts, and use of devices beyond the limits of manufacturer guidelines is considered off-label. The largest existing valve sizes are the 29 mm SAPIEN 3 and 34 mm Evolut R. However, patients with an extra-large root may require TAVR, and it is imperative to be able to execute this situation correctly, which is feasible with success rates reaching 95%.

Large series have been reported using the SAPIEN 3 in extra-large annuli; it has both a flexible frame and an outer cuff that allows the valve to function well without significant paravalvular or central AR even in extra-large annuli. Pre-BAV is performed in situations described in this chapter, most commonly due to significant calcification if there is not significant AR. Post-dilatation is commonly performed with 1–3 cc depending on the degree of undersizing of the valve to the native annulus and LVOT and the severity of leaflet, annular, and LVOT calcification. Less data exists for the Evolut R in extra-large roots, and therefore we use the S3 valve in these situations.

9. What are the options for annular sizing in patients who cannot receive computer tomography (CT) with contrast?

Contrast CT in early-mid systole with imaging software reconstruction provides the most accurate sizing of the aortic annulus and root. It also provides valuable information about the coronary anatomy, aortic anatomy and tortuosity, and peripheral vessels for the feasibility of transfemoral or alternative access. However, the typical contrast load of a full-dose contrast CT is 85–100 cc, which may not be feasible for patients with advanced kidney disease. In these situations, a non-contrast CT should be performed, supplemented with another modality such as non-contrast magnetic resonance imaging (MRI) or 3D transesophageal echocardiography (TEE) (Figure 9.1). Each imaging modality has advantages but also limitations, and cross-referencing multiple studies allows more accurate sizing.

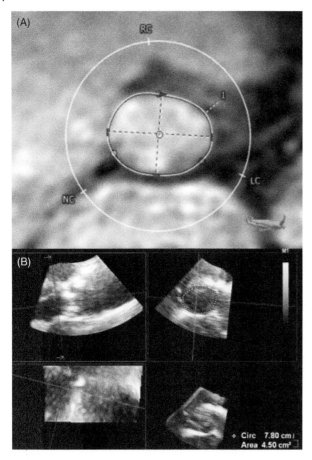

Figure 9.1 Aortic annulus sizing without computed tomography with contrast. This situation requires multi-modality measurements to attempt to accurately size the valve. Options include computer tomography without contrast, (a) magnetic resonance imaging analyzed by imaging software. (b) Echocardiography, which should be measured in long-axis X-plane views.

Coronary Arteries

10. For what patient anatomy should you consider protecting the left main coronary artery?

The risk of left main coronary obstruction is greatest when the ostium height is low (<10mm from the annulus), the left sinus of Valsalva is small, and the left cusp is tall, bulky, and calcified. In these situations, the left main may be protected with a coronary wire placed into the distal left anterior descending artery or left circumflex artery and a coronary guide catheter placed at the ostium of the left main (Figure 9.2). These are typically placed either before or after pre-BAV and before transcatheter valve deployment. If there is a very high risk of coronary obstruction, an un-deployed coronary stent can be loaded onto the wire and

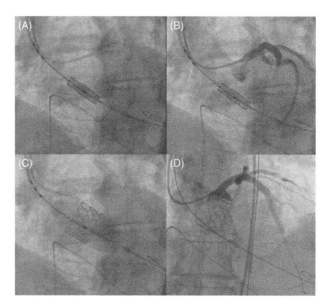

Figure 9.2 Protecting the left main coronary artery. (a, b) Prior to valve deployment, a wire can be passed into the distal left anterior descending artery or left circumflex artery and a guide catheter placed at the left main ostium. (c) This ensures the left main artery will not be obstructed during valve deployment. (d) After valve deployment, contrast should be injected to the left sinus to ensure that there is flow between the aortic root and the left coronary tree. If there are signs of ischemia, a coronary stent should be rapidly deployed.

placed within the left coronary system. This facilitates rapid placement of the stent, should there be signs of ischemia post-deployment. Note that the presence of only one of these risk factors alone may not necessarily require left main protection. For example, it may not be required in a patient with a left main coronary height of 9mm but a large left sinus and minimal calcification of a short left cusp.

11. How should you perform TAVR if a patient will likely need a future percutaneous coronary intervention (PCI)?

Coronary artery disease is present in 50–60% of patients undergoing TAVR. The concern is that the transcatheter valve will create barriers facing the coronary ostium (e.g. stent frame, native leaflet, transcatheter valve commissure) and make it challenging to perform future PCI. This risk may be reduced by selecting a balloon-expandable valve with a shorter frame height or a low-profile self-expanding valve (e.g. ACURATE *neo2*) rather than a tall self-expanding valve. For both balloon-expandable and self-expanding valves, it is important to attempt alignment of transcatheter aortic valve commissures with native commissures to facilitate future coronary access. Evidence suggests that it is currently not feasible to intentionally align the SAPIEN 3 commissures with the native commissures to avoid coronary overlap. For the Evolut system, commissural alignment involves inserting the delivery catheter into the patient's femoral artery with the flush port facing away from the operator (3 o'clock position), which translates to the Evolut "hat" marker aligning on the outer curve of the aortic root and the C-tab aligning on the inner curve of the ascending aorta; see Figure 9.3 for a more detailed explanation. Other patient-specific techniques are currently being studied to improve the commissural alignment of other self-expanding valves.

Aorta

12. Is it possible to perform a TAVR in a patient with an ascending aortic aneurysm?

Yes. For patients with severe aortic stenosis and an ascending aneurysm, surgery to replace the aortic valve and ascending aorta may provide a more durable solution. However, if surgery is contraindicated or not preferred, it is reasonable to proceed with TAVR alone as long as the aortic aneurysm does not meet the criteria for intervention. Of course, extra caution must be taken when passing wires, catheters, and particularly the valve across the ascending aorta to avoid aortic injury and dissection. A flexible delivery system (active or passive) may aid in the safe delivery of the valve across an aneurysmal ascending aorta.

13. What techniques allow transfemoral access for patients with a tortuous descending aorta?

This is a common situation in patients with severe spinal deformities. The aorta can be straightened with an extra-stiff "buddy" wire (e.g. Lunderquist) that is placed as a separate wire adjacent to the valve delivery system with an extra-stiff wire already placed across the native valve into the left ventricle. A second technique is to use a flossing technique by placing a stiff wire from the radial artery

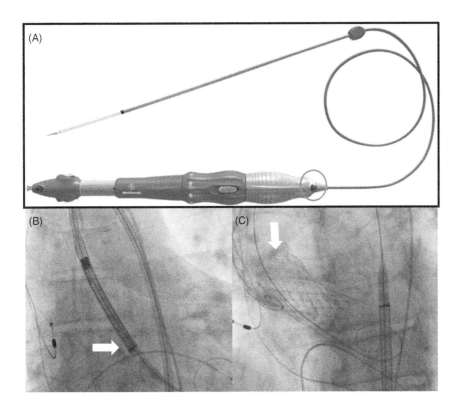

Figure 9.3 Commissural alignment for patients requiring post-TAVR coronary catheterization, using the Evolut PRO+ valve. When inserting the Evolut delivery system into the patient, ensure the gray flush port (a, orange circle) is oriented at the 3 o'clock position (away from the operator). *Source:* Medtronic, Inc. This translates to the Evolut "hat" marker aligning on the outer curve of the aorta (b, white arrow) and the C-tab (one of the commissures) aligning at the inner curve of the ascending aorta (c, white arrow) at the three-cusp coplanar view. This will result in optimizing commissural alignment between the native aortic valve and the transcatheter aortic valve.

and exteriorizing it out to the contralateral femoral artery to help straighten the tortuosity. Finally, a flexible delivery catheter may be easier for navigating tortuous vessels. With a combination of these three approaches, it is possible to navigate very torturous aortas with up to 180° bends, provided the affected aorta is not significantly calcified.

14. Does the presence of a bovine arch prevent the placement of a cerebral embolic protection device?

The evidence for the cerebral protection device is mixed, and randomized trials are currently underway to determine its true benefit. However, in situations in which cerebral protection is desired, such as severely calcified ascending aorta or aortic valve leaflets, the presence of a bovine arch does not necessarily prevent the placement of a cerebral embolic protection device. In addition to normal techniques for placing the device, other techniques include using semi-stiff wires, prewiring the left carotid artery, and reimaging the ostia of the head vessels under fluoroscopy with small contrast loads to guide placement. As a last resort, the proximal filter alone can be deployed either within the brachiocephalic trunk or the bovine trunk to protect significant portions of the cerebral territory, while the distal filter can be placed in the left subclavian artery.

Femoral Arterial Access

15. How can transfemoral TAVR be performed if there is significant iliac artery calcification?

Transfemoral TAVR is associated with improved outcomes compared to alternative access, and transfemoral TAVR is almost always feasible. Preoperative CT angiography provides crucial imaging on the size of peripheral vessels and the presence of calcium or stents. For calcified lesions within the iliofemoral arteries causing a luminal diameter <5 cm, the entire iliofemoral tree can be treated with shockwave lithotripsy (currently up to 7 mm balloon), percutaneous transluminal angioplasty (e.g. 8 mm balloon), and pre-dilatation of the vessel with a large dilator (e.g. 18 Fr) prior to main sheath placement. Collaborating with an endovascular expert or vascular surgeon is recommended, as they are invaluable in assisting in the pretreatment of vessels and in the event of vascular complications.

16. How can transfemoral TAVR be performed if there is significant femoral artery calcification?

The goal for arterial access is to puncture the anterior wall below the inguinal ligament and above the femoral bifurcation, avoiding areas of significant calcification. Preoperative CT imaging is helpful in assessing areas of calcification and the height of the femoral bifurcation. This can be supported with intraoperative ultrasound-guided access, which has the added benefit of ensuring an anterior stick. In the setting of anterior wall calcification of the femoral artery, femoral artery cutdown can be performed to directly palpate soft areas of the non-calcified vessel; and, if needed, an endarterectomy can be performed to remove diseased intima.

17. What can be done if there is only one patent iliofemoral artery?

It is possible to perform TAVR via the single ipsilateral femoral artery. This necessitates the use of a radial artery for a pigtail catheter to visualize the root. Pressure can then be transduced through the contralateral radial artery or the femoral arterial sheath.

18. If iliofemoral access is not feasible, what are different options for alternate access?

While there are at least five options for alternative access besides transfemoral access, no randomized trials have prospectively compared them. Recent large retrospective series have shown transcarotid delivery to have lower mortality and stroke rates than transapical and direct aortic access. Subclavian and transaxillary access, delivered via direct puncture or a sutured Gore-Tex conduit, have better alignment for delivery if performed from the left side as opposed to the right, but reported stroke rates are higher than with the transfemoral approach. Transcaval is another option that creates an aorto-inferior vena cava (IVC) fistula to deliver the valve from the IVC to the abdominal aorta, and the fistula can be closed with an occlusive device. Each center develops a preferred alternate access technique, and operator comfort is likely the most important determinant of safe outcomes when performing alternate access. That being said, in the authors' opinion, transfemoral access is possible in the vast majority of cases, and a true need for alternative access is rare.

Valve-in-Valve (ViV)

19. When performing ViV TAVR, how do you choose the correct transcatheter valve?

The choice of transcatheter valve for ViV TAVR (Figure 9.4) depends on many factors. The existing valve's internal diameter, model, and implant position and whether it is stented or stentless determine whether a transcatheter valve can be implanted into the existing valve without causing severe PPM. Understanding the manufacturer, model, and size of the existing prosthesis is crucial and can be accomplished by gaining the original operative/procedure report, asking the patient for the manufacturer's device card, checking the manufacturer registries, or imaging the valve directly. Multiple publications and mobile phone applications contain valuable information regarding the appearance of different valves on imaging and their internal diameter (e.g. Aortic VIV application). The valve should also always be imaged to measure the internal diameter. Stented valves make it easier to align the valve during deployment, although the frames limit the size of the valves that may be implanted. PPM may be unavoidable but can be minimized by implanting a supra-annular self-expanding valve, implanting valves higher, and possibly fracturing the stented surgical valve (see the next question for more information). In the case of stentless valves, there may be a lack of visual landmarks, and the use of contrast injection will be helpful in determining the correct level during valve deployment.

20. What are the relevant considerations when potentially fracturing an existing surgical valve prior to ViV implantation?

Fracturing the surgical valve frame is an option to increase the internal diameter of existing stented valves. This allows implantation of larger-sized transcatheter valves or improves expansion of a potentially constrained transcatheter valve, thereby decreasing the risk of PPM. Not all valves can be fractured, and the device manufacturer or published literature should be consulted prior to attempting it. Fracturing can also be technically difficult, with a higher rate of complications, and should only be undertaken when severe PPM cannot be avoided.

Patients with a prior Bentall procedure (aortic root replacement) with a stented valve should not undergo balloon fracture, given the high risk of aortic root rupture,

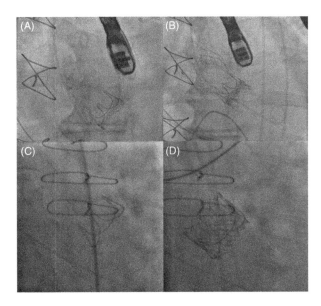

Figure 9.4 Valve-in-valve transcatheter aortic valve replacement. (a, b) Valve-in-valve implantation of a 23 mm Medtronic Evolut PRO+ CoreValve in a 21 mm Carpentier-Edwards Perimount 2800 bioprosthetic valve. (c, d) Placement of a 26 mm Edwards SAPIEN 3 Ultra valve, in a 25 mm Carpentier-Edwards Perimount 2700 bioprosthetic valve.

due to the lack of aorto-ventricular continuity with native tissue. Technically, the valve is fractured with a non-compliant balloon either before or after ViV implantation, each of which has pros and cons. The true balloon can be attached to a pressure monitor, and signs of successful fracturing will include an audible click, a visible break in the surgical valve frame on fluoroscopy, and a sudden decrease in the pressure monitor. If the fracture is performed before VIV implantation, acute prosthetic AR may occur, necessitating rapid valve implantation to avoid prolonged hemodynamic compromise. Note that the team should be prepared for emergency conversion to surgery in the event of a significant complication, such as root rupture.

21. What can be done if there is a high risk of coronary artery obstruction with ViV TAVR?

The BASILICA (Bioprosthetic or native Aortic Scallop Intentional Laceration to prevent Iatrogenic Coronary artery obstruction during TAVR) trial looked at the feasibility of radiofrequency laceration of existing leaflets before ViV TAVR to prevent coronary occlusion. The initial report showed a high success rate with low rates of mortality, disabling stroke, and hemodynamic compromise. However, no long-term data has been reported. Given the overall low rate of obstructive complications and this technique's high procedural complexity, especially when doing the leaflets facing both coronary arteries, it has not been widely adopted. Left main protection can be performed in the standard fashion (as detailed in question 10) as an alternative to BASILICA.

Bibliography

1 Abramowitz, Y., Maeno, Y., and Chakravarty, T. (2016). Aortic angulation attenuates procedural success following self-expandable but not balloon-expandable TAVR. JACC Cardiovasc. Imaging 9 (8): 964–972.

2 Adams, D.H., Popma, J.J., and Reardon, M.J. (2014). Transcatheter aortic-valve replacement with a self-expanding prosthesis. N. Engl. J. Med. 370: 1790–1798.

3 Armijo, G., Tang, G.H.L., and Kooistra, N. (2020). Third-generation balloon and self-expandable valves for aortic stenosis in large and extra-large aortic annuli from the TAVR-LARGE registry. Circ. Cardiovasc. Interv. 13 (8): e009047.

4 Babanti, M., Yang, T.H., Cabau, J.R. et al. (2013). Anatomical and procedural features associated with aortic root rupture during balloon-expandable transcatheter aortic valve replacement. Circulation 128 (3): 244–253.

5 Chandrasekhar, J., Hibbert, B., Ruel, M. et al. (2015). Transfemoral vs non-transfemoral access for transcatheter aortic valve implantation: a systemic review and meta-analysis. Can. J. Cardiol. 31 (12): 1427–1438.

6 Halim, S.A., Edwards, F.H., Dai, D. et al. (2020). Outcomes of transcatheter aortic valve replacement in patients with bicuspid aortic valve disease: a report from the Society of Thoracic Surgeons/American College of Cardiology transcatheter valve therapy registry. Circulation 141 (13): 1071–1079.

7 Khan, J.M., Greenbaum, A.B., Babaliaros, V.C. et al. (2019). The BASILICA trial: prospective multicentered investigation of intentional leaflet laceration to prevent TAVR coronary obstruction. JACC Cardiovasc. Interv. 12 (13): 1240–1252.

8 Makkar, R.R., Yoon, S.H., Leon, M.B. et al. (2019). Association between transcatheter aortic valve replacement for bicuspid vs tricuspid aortic stenosis and mortality or stroke. JAMA 321 (22): 2193–2019.

9 Tang, G.H.L., Zaid, S., Fuchs, A. et al. (2020). Alignment of transcatheter aortic-valve neo-commissures (ALIGN-TAVR): impact on final valve orientation and coronary artery overlap. *JACC Cardiovasc. Interv.* 13 (9): 1030–1042.

10 Tang, G.H.L., Zaid, S., George, I. et al. (2018). Impact of aortic root anatomy and geometry on paravalvular leak in transcatheter aortic valve replacement with extremely large annuli using the Edwards Sapien 3 valve. *JACC Cardiovasc. Interv.* 11 (14): 1377–1387.

11 Yoon, S.H., Bleiziffer, S., Backer, O.D. et al. (2017). Outcomes in transcatheter aortic valve replacement for bicuspid versus tricuspid aortic valve stenosis. *J. Am. Coll. Cardiol.* 69 (21): 2579–2589.

10

TAVR for Bicuspid Aortic Valve

Rik Adrichem, and Nicolas M. Van Mieghem

[1] *Department of Interventional Cardiology, Thoraxcenter, Erasmus University Medical Center, Rotterdam, The Netherlands*

Epidemiology

1. What is the prevalence of bicuspid aortic valves?

Bicuspid aortic valve (BAV) is the most common congenital heart valve abnormality, with a reported prevalence of 2% in the general population and as high as 50% in young patients undergoing aortic valve replacement. But in patients older than 80 years, 20% of symptomatic aortic stenosis (AS) may also be caused by congenital BAV.

2. How is BAV identified?

Echocardiography is the main modality to identify BAV, with sensitivity and specificity of >90% in the presence of adequate image quality. However, heavy aortic root calcification may compromise aortic leaflet identification. In such cases, magnetic resonance imaging (MRI) or computed tomography (CT) may offer higher diagnostic yields.

3. How do patients with bicuspid AS undergoing transcatheter aortic valve replacement compare to patients with tricuspid AS?

The Society of Thoracic Surgeons/American College of Cardiology TVT Registry has shown that BAV patients undergoing transcatheter aortic valve replacement (TAVR) are in general younger and more often male. Traditional cardiovascular risk factors such as diabetes, hypertension, and peripheral artery disease seem less common. BAV patients have a lower Society of Thoracic Surgeons predicted risk of mortality.

Bicuspid Valve Morphology

4. Match the illustrated valve morphologies to the correct bicuspid phenotypes according to the conventional Sievers classification and the newly derived CT classification (see figure 10.1).

The Sievers classification is based on the number of raphes. Sievers 0 is the quintessential bicuspid valve with two commissures and no raphe. Sievers 1 and 2 are tricommissural bicuspid valves with one and two raphes, respectively.

In recent years, a new classification based on CT findings has been published. This classification identifies eight phenotypes (see Figure 10.1) based on three characteristics:

1) The number of commissures
2) The extent of leaflet calcification
3) The presence of a raphe and its extent of calcification – in bicommissural bicuspids only

It can be difficult or even impossible to discern a tricommissural phenotype from a bicommissural phenotype with a raphe. Often the imager will notice the presence of three more or less developed commissures. One can argue that these two phenotypes represent a continuum and that some so-called bicuspid valves were in essence tricuspid valves that over time transitioned to a more bicuspid appearance because of commissural fusion. The clinical consequence of these phenotypes will be explained in response to question 11.

I. Sievers classification

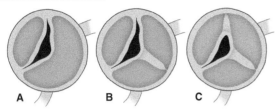

II. TAVR-directed bicuspid aortic valve CT classification

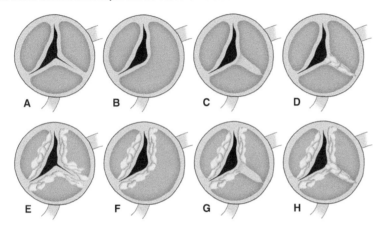

Figure 10.1   Classification of bicuspid aortic valves. (Ia) Sievers type 0; (Ib) Sievers type 1; (Ic) Sievers type 2. (IIa) tricommissural bicuspid; (IIb) bicommissural bicuspid with noncalcified leaflets; (IIc) bicommissural bicuspid with noncalcified leaflets and noncalcified raphe; (IId) bicommissural bicuspid with noncalcified leaflets and calcified raphe; (IIe) tricommissural bicuspid with calcified leaflets; (IIf) bicommissural bicuspid with calcified leaflets; (IIg) bicommissural bicuspid with calcified leaflets and noncalcified raphe; (IIh) bicommissural bicuspid with calcified leaflets and calcified raphe. *Source:* R. Adrichem; N. M. Van Mieghem.

5.   What anatomical characteristics commonly associated with BAVs may complicate TAVR?

The annulus of BAVs is more elliptical in shape, and root calcification is more extensive and irregular. As a result, transcatheter heart valve (THV) frame expansion may be suboptimal or elliptical, resulting in higher rates of para-valvular leakage (PVL). Additionally, BAVs are associated with connective tissue disorders within the aortic wall, potentially resulting in higher rates of aortic root injury. BAVs are also associated with a shorter membranous septum length, increasing the risk of TAVR-related conduction disorders. Concomitant aortic pathology such as thoracic aorta dilatation, aneurysms, horizontal aorta (see Figure 10.2), or coarctation may complicate the transcatheter approach and may sometimes warrant surgical intervention in the absence of prohibitive operative risk.

Procedural Planning

6.   What considerations should be taken into account when choosing a THV type (annular/supra-annular; balloon-expandable/self-expanding)?

Considerable heterogeneity in BAV morphology, calcifications, membranous septum length, and aortic annulus angulation may drive platform selection in favor of a self-expanding or balloon-expandable THV.

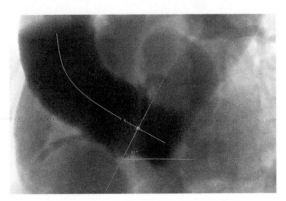

Figure 10.2   Example of horizontal aorta with aortic angle >60°.

To date, no head-to-head comparisons of balloon-expandable vs. self-expanding valves have been conducted in the context of bicuspid AS. Therefore, current practice in THV selection is derived from non-randomized studies focusing on bicuspid AS. A review by Claessen et al. offers considerations for device selection and highlights several important factors in the THV selection process.

Annular size. Annular size may become important at both ends of the sizing matrix. Supra-annular valve functioning devices seem to yield superior hemodynamic valve performance, particularly in small annuli (<21mm). Arguably, a balloon-expandable THV may offer an easier and steadier implant in very large annuli.

Aortic angulation. A horizontal aorta may be easier to negotiate with a flex delivery catheter because it may facilitate coaxial THV alignment with the native aortic valve.

Root calcification. Excessive aortic root calcification, especially in the presence of calcification in the left ventricular outflow tract (LVOT), may be associated with aortic rupture. To minimize this risk, a 1 : 1 sized balloon dilatation should be avoided, and some operators might favor a self-expanding device over a balloon-expandable system.

Pre-existing conduction abnormalities and short membranous septum. Self-expanding valves with a nitinol frame tend to exert continuous pressure on the aortic annulus, LVOT, and membranous septum. This may explain a higher rate of acquired conduction abnormalities and the need for new pacemaker implantation after TAVR. Therefore, a balloon-expandable valve or a self-expanding THV with a top-down mode of deployment (e.g. the ACURATE THV) may be preferred in patients with pre-existent conduction disorders – especially right bundle branch block – or a short membranous septum length. Whether new implantation concepts for self-expanding THVs, such as the cusp overlap technique, may reduce the conduction issues remains unclear and requires further study.

7. Can computer simulation complement pre-procedural TAVR planning?

Based on artificial intelligence and computer learning, a pre-procedural multislice computed tomography (MSCT) scan can help integrate anatomy with tissue and device characteristics. This technique may predict, for any given THV size and implant depth, the extent of calcium displacement, the occurrence of PVL, and device contact

pressures in the LVOT that may be associated with the need for a permanent pacemaker.

8. What sizing strategies exist for selecting THV size in bicuspid AS?

MSCT remains the cornerstone for anatomy and THV sizing in patients with bicuspid AS. A conventional strategy is based on annular sizing and is identical to the sizing algorithm for patients with degenerative tricuspid aortic valve disease. Other sizing concepts promote supra-annular sizing because the most constrained and calcified area will be located at the commissural level, which is typically situated approximately 5mm above the annular plane (see Figure 10.3). However, the potential benefit of supra-annular sizing is still under debate. The BAVARD (Bicuspid Aortic Valve Anatomy and Relationship with Devices) registry demonstrated that in most patients currently undergoing TAVR for bicuspid AS, annular sizing algorithms may be safe because dimensions at the commissural and annular plane are often similar. Still, in the context of bicuspid AS, it seems worthwhile to evaluate and integrate the dimensions at the level of the commissures, annulus, and LVOT to identify sizing mismatch and adjust THV size accordingly.

In tricuspid AS patients, it is shown that three-dimensional transesophageal echocardiography (3D-TEE) may underestimate the aortic annulus area by almost 10% as compared to MSCT measurements. Nevertheless, it seems safe to rely on 3D-TEE for THV sizing in patients with end-stage renal disease who should not undergo contrast MSCT evaluation.

With the balloon sizing technique, contrast is injected into the ascending aorta during undersized balloon inflation. The absence of left ventricular opacification determines the minimum THV size that would fit in a given anatomy. This technique may mitigate the risk of aortic rupture and PVL.

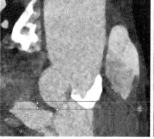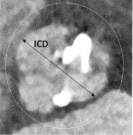

Figure 10.3 Supra-annular sizing method. The intercommissural distance (ICD) is measured at 5mm above the annular plane.

In rotational angiography, contrast is injected in the ascending aorta during rotational fluoroscopy imaging. A 3D reconstruction can then be created for analysis within minutes. Aortic dimensions derived from rotational angiography correspond well with those obtained from MSCT. Both balloon sizing and rotational angiography techniques are limited by their use of contrast but require less logistical planning.

9. What is recommended for pre-dilatation and post-dilatation?

Pre-dilatation. BAV characteristics, including an asymmetrical aortic orifice, excessive and irregular calcium, fusion of cusps, and ascending aorta appearance (e.g. dilated, horizontal), may complicate bicuspid valve crossing. Pre-dilatation with an undersized balloon may facilitate smooth crossing and positioning of the THV. In addition, balloon dilatation may be used for sizing purposes or to evaluate the safety of a more supra-annular/intracommissural THV anchoring. A rule of thumb is to choose a balloon size that equals the smallest diameter of the annulus by MSCT.

Post-dilatation. Post-dilatation may be required in the context of residual gradient, PVL, and/or frame underexpansion. A rule of thumb is to start with a balloon size equal to the area or perimeter derived annulus diameter.

Outcomes

10. How do outcomes of TAVR in bicuspid AS compare with tricuspid AS?

In recent series, hard clinical endpoints (all-cause death and stroke) appeared similar between bicuspid and tricuspid AS, although several large registries have shown numerically increased stroke rate with bicuspid AS. One study by Makkar et al. reported an increased stroke rate at 30 days but not at one-year follow-up. In a propensity-matched cohort, there were no differences in the incidence of new permanent pacemaker implantation, coronary intervention, or life-threatening bleedings. However, bicuspid valve morphology was associated with more aortic valve reinterventions. Additionally, despite the presence of sealing fabric in contemporary THV platforms (see question 12), rates of post-TAVR moderate or severe aortic regurgitation remain higher in patients with BAV morphology.

Procedure duration seems higher in patients with bicuspid AS than in patients with tricuspid AS, probably due to the more challenging anatomical phenotype that requires more maneuvering and manipulations (balloon pre- and post-dilatation, THV repositioning).

11. Describe how the different bicuspid phenotypes (see question 4) impact outcome after TAVR.

Procedural outcome. The highest rates of PVL are reported in patients with bicommissural BAVs with both extensive leaflet calcification and a calcified raphe (Figure 10.1IIh). In patients with this combination, more than mild PVL was present in 37.3% of TAVR cases compared to 19.8% in patients without excess leaflet calcification and/or calcified raphe (Figure 10.1IIb, c).

Mortality. The presence of calcified leaflets or a calcified raphe is associated with higher early and mid-term mortality. A combination of calcified leaflets with a calcified raphe has the worst overall prognosis. Mortality at two years was approximately four times higher in patients with this unfavorable phenotype than in patients with bicuspid morphology and no calcifications (25.7 vs. 5.9%).

Stroke. As stated in the response to question 10, large registries suggest that bicuspid valve morphology may be associated with increased rates of peri-procedural stroke, presumably because of excessive valve calcifications. Intuitively, cerebral embolic protection devices may be attractive in the context of bicuspid AS, but further clinical research on this topic is needed. Research on captured debris using filter-based embolic protection during TAVR with contemporary THVs identified THV repositioning as the main predictor for more debris and bicuspid phenotype as the main predictor for large debris (>1000 um).

Permanent pacemaker implantation. Presumptive evidence suggests an increased risk of conduction disorders with calcified raphe-type bicuspid valves and fusion of the right and left coronary cusps, as this fusion may cause the radial force of the implanted valve to be translated more toward the membranous septum, thereby generating additional pressure on the conduction system.

12. What features of the newer-generation THVs significantly improved the outcome of TAVR?

In earlier-generation THVs, bicuspid morphology was associated with a higher incidence of PVL, aortic root injury, or second valve implantation. Contemporary THVs are equipped with externally mounted sealing fabric to mitigate PVL. This sealing capacity may allow for less oversizing and arguably less risk for rupture. Repositioning and retrieving features may further optimize results and contribute to improved procedural success.

Bibliography

1 Blackman, D., Gabbieri, D., Del Blanco, B.G. et al. (2021). Expert consensus on sizing and positioning of SAPIEN 3/ultra in bicuspid aortic valves. *Cardiol. Ther.* 10: 277–288.

2 Claessen, B.E., Tang, G.H.L., Kini, A.S., and Sharma, S.K. (2021). Considerations for optimal device selection in transcatheter aortic valve replacement: a review. *JAMA Cardiol.* 6: 102–112.

3 Dowling, C., Firoozi, S., and Brecker, S.J. (2020). First-in-human experience with patient-specific computer simulation of TAVR in bicuspid aortic valve morphology. *JACC Cardiovasc. Interv.* 13: 184–192.

4 Forrest, J.K., Kaple, R.K., Ramlawi, B. et al. (2020). Transcatheter aortic valve replacement in bicuspid versus tricuspid aortic valves from the STS/ACC TVT registry. *JACC Cardiovasc. Interv.* 13: 1749–1759.

5 Hamdan, A., Nassar, M., Schwammenthal, E. et al. (2021). Short membranous septum length in bicuspid aortic valve stenosis increases the risk of conduction disturbances. *J. Cardiovasc. Comput. Tomogr.* 15: 339–347.

6 Jilaihawi, H., Chen, M., Webb, J. et al. (2016). A bicuspid aortic valve imaging classification for the TAVR era. *JACC Cardiovasc. Imaging* 9: 1145–1158.

7 Kroon, H., Von Der Thusen, J.H., Ziviello, F. et al. (2021). Heterogeneity of debris captured by cerebral embolic protection filters during TAVI. *EuroIntervention* 16: 1141–1147.

8 Makkar, R.R., Yoon, S.H., Leon, M.B. et al. (2019). Association between transcatheter aortic valve replacement for bicuspid vs tricuspid aortic stenosis and mortality or stroke. *JAMA* 321: 2193–2202.

9 Ng, A.C., Delgado, V., Van Der Kley, F. et al. (2010). Comparison of aortic root dimensions and geometries before and after transcatheter aortic valve implantation by 2- and 3-dimensional transesophageal echocardiography and multislice computed tomography. *Circ. Cardiovasc. Imaging* 3: 94–102.

10 Rahhab, Z., El Faquir, N., Tchetche, D. et al. (2020). Expanding the indications for transcatheter aortic valve implantation. *Nat. Rev. Cardiol.* 17: 75–84.

11 Roberts, W.C. and Ko, J.M. (2005). Frequency by decades of unicuspid, bicuspid, and tricuspid aortic valves in adults having isolated aortic valve replacement for aortic stenosis, with or without associated aortic regurgitation. *Circulation* 111: 920–925.

12 Schultz, C.J., Van Mieghem, N.M., Van Der Boon, R.M. et al. (2014). Effect of body mass index on the image quality of rotational angiography without rapid pacing for planning of transcatheter aortic valve implantation: a comparison with multislice computed tomography. *Eur. Heart J. Cardiovasc. Imaging* 15: 133–141.

13 Siu, S.C. and Silversides, C.K. (2010). Bicuspid aortic valve disease. *J. Am. Coll. Cardiol.* 55: 2789–2800.

14 Tchetche, D., De Biase, C., Van Gils, L. et al. (2019). Bicuspid aortic valve anatomy and relationship with devices: the BAVARD multicenter registry. *Circ. Cardiovasc. Interv.* 12: e007107.

15 Yoon, S.H., Bleiziffer, S., De Backer, O. et al. (2017). Outcomes in transcatheter aortic valve replacement for bicuspid versus tricuspid aortic valve stenosis. *J. Am. Coll. Cardiol.* 69: 2579–2589.

16 Yoon, S.H., Kim, W.K., Dhoble, A. et al. (2020). Bicuspid aortic valve morphology and outcomes after transcatheter aortic valve replacement. *J. Am. Coll. Cardiol.* 76: 1018–1030.

11

TAVR for Pure Native Valve Aortic Regurgitation

Sergio A. Perez[1] and Antonio Dager[2]

[1] Cardiovascular Service, Baptist Health Medical Center, Montgomery, AL, USA
[2] Angiografia de Occidente SA, Clinica de Occidente, Cali, Colombia

1. How common is aortic regurgitation (AR)?

The prevalence of native aortic valve regurgitation (NAVR) increases with age. In the United States, it is reported to be between 4.9 and 10%. Aortic regurgitation (AR) is more common in males than females, presumably reflecting the 3 : 1 male to female predominance of bicuspid aortic valve (BAV) disease.

2. What are the most common causes of NAVR?

NAVR may result from abnormalities of the valve itself or the aorta, leading to incomplete leaflet coaptation. The development of AR can be acute or chronic. Acute AR is most commonly caused by infective endocarditis, blunt chest trauma, or aortic dissection or as a complication of transcatheter procedures.

Chronic NAVR is most commonly caused by congenital heart disease, particularly BAV, calcified aortic valve disease, and any condition resulting in aortic dilatation. AR can also present in failing bioprosthetic valves. Rheumatic heart disease, rare in industrialized countries, remains a frequent cause in developing countries. An increasing cause of AR is related to continuous-flow left ventricular assist devices (CF-LVADs). The numbers of CF-LVADs have increased exponentially; between 2013 and 2017, approximately 16 000 LVADs were implanted in the US. AR is recognized as a cause of recurrence of symptoms of heart failure in patients with CF-LVADs. It can affect 30% of patients within the first year of implantation and progress with the duration of LVAD support.

3. What are the natural history and prognosis of AR?

Patients with chronic AR have an indolent course and can be asymptomatic for many years. However, with time, there is progressive left ventricular (LV) dilation and dysfunction. Progression of the disease is related to the severity of regurgitation, the etiology of aortic valve disease, the presence of symptoms, and the size and function of the LV. Although patients with mild to moderate AR have an excellent prognosis, patients with severe AR have a rate of progression to symptoms of LV dysfunction of 4.3% per year. The annual mortality in patients with symptomatic severe AR can be as high as 25%.

4. What are the indications and the best timing for intervention of the aortic valve in AR?

According to American College of Cardiology/American Heart Association (ACC/AHA) Valvular Heart Disease Guidelines, aortic valve replacement is indicated in patients with symptomatic severe AR regardless of LV systolic function, in asymptomatic patients with severe AR and LV systolic dysfunction (left ventricular ejection fraction [LVEF] $\leq$ 55%), and in patients with severe AR who are undergoing cardiac surgery for another indication (Class I recommendations). Valve intervention should also be considered in asymptomatic patients with severe AR and normal LV systolic function but severe LV enlargement (left ventricular end-systolic diameter [LVESD] >50 mm or LVESD >25 mm/m^2) and in patients with moderate AR undergoing cardiac surgery for other indications (Class IIa recommendation).

Mastering Structural Heart Disease, First Edition. Edited by Eduardo J. de Marchena and Camilo A. Gomez.
© 2023 John Wiley & Sons Ltd. Published 2023 by John Wiley & Sons Ltd.
Companion website: www.wiley.com/go/deMarchena/Mastering-Structural-Heart-Disease

5. What is the recommended therapy for patients with severe NAVR and indication for intervention?

For patients with severe NAVR who meet guidelines criteria for valve intervention, surgical aortic valve repair or replacement (SAVR) is the conventional treatment. However, the Euro Heart Survey showed that valve intervention was "under-used" in approximately 8% of patients because of an elevated risk of peri-operative mortality due to advanced age or multiple comorbidities. The "under-used" rate was even higher in patients with lower LVEF.

The emergence of transcatheter aortic valve replacement (TAVR) as an established treatment for patients with calcific aortic stenosis (AS) and growing experience and enormous technological improvements have led to an expansion in the scope of transcatheter therapies and their consideration in conditions other than AS. On-label and off-label applications of TAVR are being expanded to patients with failed surgically implanted valves, BAV disease, and pure AR. Pure AR has been considered a contraindication for TAVR due to the technical challenges imposed by the absence of anchoring aortic valve calcification. The 2020 ACC/AHA Valvular Heart Disease Guidelines recommend against TAVR in patients with isolated severe AR who have an indication for valve intervention and are candidates for surgery (Class III). However, as growing experience and evidence with off-label use for pure aortic AR continue to emerge, the door for TAVR in this patient population continues to open.

6. What are the challenges of TAVR in pure NAVR?

TAVR has been discouraged in pure AR because of clinical and anatomical challenges that could compromise procedural success.

From a technical standpoint, the absence of extensive calcification of the aortic annulus and the frequent coexistence of aortic root dilation pose significant difficulties for positioning and anchoring of transcatheter heart valves (THVs), increasing the risk of inadequate sealing, embolization, and residual perivalvular regurgitation. The recommended practice of oversizing up to 25% to facilitate anchoring also comes with an increased risk of annular rupture and conduction abnormalities. Additionally, the excessive stroke volume and the regurgitant flow can increase THV motion, resulting in malposition and embolization.

From a clinical perspective, a significant proportion of patients referred for intervention in chronic AR have advanced cardiac disease with significant LV dysfunction and impaired hemodynamics, adding an incremental risk of procedural complications.

7. What is the available evidence evaluating TAVR for pure NAVR?

Currently, no randomized clinical trials have compared TAVR with SAVR for the treatment of pure AR or compared specific THVs. Existing data comes from single and multicenter series, national registries, and meta-analyses. The available evidence supports the feasibility of TAVR in selected patients; however, despite a trend of improvement in procedural outcomes, the results are not ideal yet.

Roy et al. reported the first multicenter series of 43 patients undergoing TAVR for pure NAVR in 2013. A few more series, mainly using the Medtronic CoreValve system followed, demonstrating technical feasibility with acceptable rates of early adverse events but a significant need for a second valve and overall higher mortality compared to patients treated for AS. In initial studies, the need for valve-in-valve (ViV) ranged from 18 to 20% due to THV malposition and significant residual AR. It is worth mentioning that the first-generation CoreValve system was not repositionable or recapturable. Shortly after, single- and multi-center studies using second-generation THVs such as JenaValve (JenaValve Technology), J-Valve (JC Medical), ACURATE (Boston Scientific), and Direct Flow (Direct Flow Medical) were published. In 2016, a meta-analysis by Franzone et al., including 13 studies using the CoreValve system and second-generation THV, showed a lower need for ViV of 7% and a summary estimated 30-day mortality rate of 7% (range 0–30%).

One of the largest series to date, reported by Yoon et al., included patients treated with first- and second-generation THV and with new-generation devices (Evolut R [Medtronic] and SAPIEN 3 [Edwards Lifesciences]). This study showed that the use of new-generation devices was associated with improved procedural outcomes. The difference was mainly driven by lower rates of need for a second implant and significant residual AR. Similar conclusions were yielded by a meta-analysis published in 2018 by Rawasia et al. The group receiving a new-generation device had lower 30-day mortality (9.1% [6.8–11.7%] vs. 15.3% [10.3–21.1]%) and higher device success rate (92.8% [86.6–97.2%] vs. 75.2% [63.6–85.2%]) compared to the group receiving old-generation devices.

Although the outcomes for patients undergoing TAVR for severe NAVR remain worse when compared with those undergoing TAVR for on-label indications, the difference continues to narrow. In a study using the Society of Thoracic Surgeons/American College of Cardiology (STS/ACC) Transcatheter Valve Therapy (TVT) registry by Hira et al., in-hospital mortality (6.3 vs. 4.7%; p < 0.001) and 30-day mortality (8.5 vs. 6.1%; p < 0.001) were higher in patients receiving TAVR for any off-label indication compared to those for on-label use. However, the subgroup of patients undergoing off-label TAVR for pure NAVR had slightly lower in-hospital (5.6%) and 30-day mortality (7.8%) than the overall off-label group.

With continued refinements of existing TAVR prostheses, development of new technologies, improvement in patient selection, and periprocedural imaging, outcomes of TAVR in pure AR are expected to continue improving and perhaps eventually be established as standard therapy for patients with pure AR.

8. What is the preferred type of THV for TAVR in pure NAVR?

Currently, there is no commercially available AR-specific THV in the United States. Jena Valve (Jena Valve Technology) and J-Valve (JC Medical) are two investigational devices undergoing feasibility studies in the US, designed to treat both stenosis and regurgitation of non-calcified aortic valves. JenaValve is a self-expandable porcine pericardial valve with a low-profile Nitinol stent frame that is individually fixated into the native leaflets using paperclip-like anchors. Similarly, the J-Valve uses U-shaped anchor rings to facilitate self-positioning implantation. An active fixation mechanism and greater size availability to cover an extensive range of annulus sizes are two characteristics that make these valves attractive for use in non-calcified valves with pure or mixed NAVR. At this time, JenaValve and the J-Valve have not received Food and Drug Administration (FDA) approval for commercial use in the United States (US). The JenaValve Trilogy System received CE Mark approval for the treatment of severe, symptomatic AR and aortic stenosis in patients at high surgical risk. The JenaValve ALIGN-AR Pivotal Trial (ALIGN-AR) recently completed enrollment, and its results are awaited.

FDA-approved commercially available platforms have been used for off-label use in pure NAVR in the US. Compared with early-generation devices, new-generation devices are associated with improved procedural outcomes. In the above-mentioned international registry reported by Yoon et al., the use of new-generation devices (Evolut R, SAPIEN 3, JenaValve, Lotus, Direct Flow, ACURATE, and J-Valve) was associated with a higher device success rate of 81.1% compared to 61.3% (p < 0.001) with early-generation devices (CoreValve and SAPIEN XT). There were lower rates of second valve implantation (12.7 vs. 24.4%, p = 0.007), moderate to severe post-procedural AR (4.2% vs. 18.8%, p < 0.001), and cardiovascular mortality (9.6% vs. 23.6%) with new-generation devices. These findings are likely due to technological developments conferring specific features of new-generation devices: longer stent frame and sealing skirt in the SAPIEN 3; and retrievability and repositioning capacity,

external sealing cuff, and redesigned stent frame with better radial force in the Evolut R.

Among early-generation THVs, the self-expanding Medtronic CoreValve was often preferred over the balloon-expandable SAPIEN XT. Currently, both platforms' latest iterations – the self-expanding Evolut R/PRO/PRO + (Medtronic) and the balloon-expandable SAPIEN 3/Ultra (Edwards Lifesciences), are used for off-label procedures in NAVR. Both devices provide adaptive skirting and cover a wide range of annular sizes. The largest Evolut PRO available, 34 mm, can cover annuli with diameters as large as 30 mm and perimeters of 94.2 mm. The 29 mm SAPIEN 3/Ultra can be used in an annulus with an averaged diameter up to 29.5 mm and an area of 680 mm^2, although the balloon can be filled with additional volume for overexpansion. Currently, there is no conclusive data comparing the performance of specific new-generation devices in NAVR. Most operators continue to recommend using a recapturable valve with a sealing skirt for added effectiveness and safety.

9. What are some critical technical considerations?

As mentioned before, proper valve size selection is of paramount importance. In some cases (up to 25%), oversizing may be required to facilitate transcatheter valve anchoring. Therefore, pre-procedural imaging with gated computed tomography and repeated aortograms is critical for a precise definition of annular size and aortic root anatomy. Many patients with pure AR can have large annuli beyond the manufacturer's recommendation. For the balloon-expandable valve SAPIEN 3/Ultra, the balloon can be over-filled to increase the size of the THV.

Fluoroscopic assessment of the spatial relationship of the THV with anatomic landmarks can be challenging due to the absence of calcification. In some cases, two pigtail catheters can be positioned in the non- and right-coronary cusps to facilitate visualization of a coplanar angle.

In general, balloon pre-dilation is not recommended unless there is mixed stenosis or is done to measure the annulus size when pre-procedural imaging was not optimal. Regardless of the type of THV, it is recommended that it be deployed under rapid pacing to decrease stroke and regurgitation volumes and stabilize the valve. Although there is no need for transesophageal echocardiography guidance during the procedure, some operators recommend its use to accurately assess the degree of post-deployment residual AR.

Figures 11.1, 11.2, 11.3, and 11.4 illustrate some technical considerations for a successful TAVR implant in NAVR with a self-expanding valve.

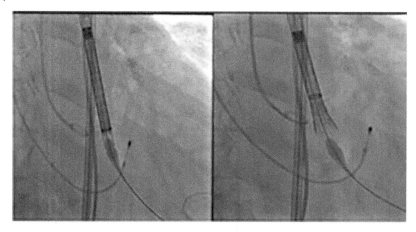

Figure 11.1 (a) Pacing should begin at the initial phase of the deployment (when there is a need to align the device with the aortic annulus to provide a static environment). (b) A static position is reached when we pace above 130 bpm by observing relative motion.

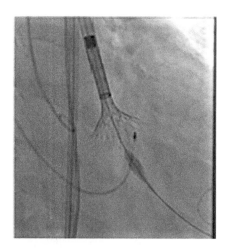

Figure 11.2 To obtain annular contact, the pacing rate should be increased to avoid valve displacement. Device displacement upwards can occur if not a paced at least greater than 130 bpm.

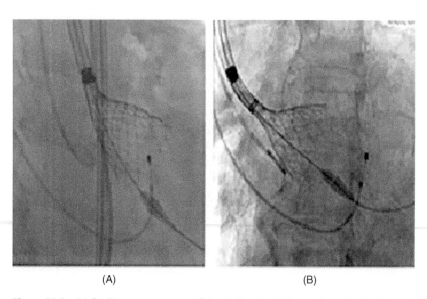

(A)   (B)

Figure 11.3 (a) Oscillatory movement of the device should be confirmed (spinoff) and, if present, must increase the pacemaker rate to achieve adequate tissue contact. (b) After reaching a final and static position, the valve is slowly released under continuous rapid pacing.

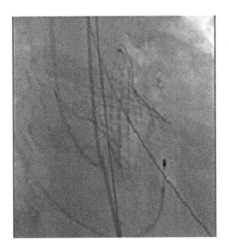

Figure 11.4 Once the valve is deployed, it is recommended not to withdraw the guidewire from the ventricle. Keep it in position for at least 5 to 10 minutes to allow further expansion of the valve.

Bibliography

1 Arias, E.A., Bhan, A., Lim, Z.Y., and Mullen, M. (2019). TAVI for pure native aortic regurgitation: are we there yet? *Interv. Cardiol.* 14: 26–30.

2 Franzone, A., Piccolo, R., Siontis, G.C.M. et al. (2016). Transcatheter aortic valve replacement for the treatment of pure native aortic valve regurgitation: a systematic review. *JACC Cardiovasc. Interv.* 9: 2308–2317.

3 Hira, R.S., Vemulapalli, S., Li, Z. et al. (2017). Trends and outcomes of off-label use of transcatheter aortic valve replacement: insights from the NCDR STS/ACC TVT registry. *JAMA Cardiol.* 2: 846–854.

4 Isogai, T., Saad, A.M., Ahuja, K.R. et al. (2021). Short-term outcomes of transcatheter aortic valve replacement for pure native aortic regurgitation in the United States. *Catheter. Cardiovasc. Interv.* 97: 477–485.

5 Iung, B., Baron, G., Butchart, E.G. et al. (2003). A prospective survey of patients with valvular heart disease in Europe: the euro heart survey on valvular heart disease. *Eur. Heart J.* 24: 1231–1243.

6 Otto, C.M., Nishimura, R.A., Bonow, R.O. et al. (2021). 2020 ACC/AHA guideline for the Management of Patients with Valvular Heart Disease: executive summary: a report of the American College of Cardiology/American Heart Association Joint Committee on Clinical Practice guidelines. *Circulation* 143: e35–e71.

7 Rawasia, W.F., Khan, M.S., Usman, M.S. et al. (2019). Safety and efficacy of transcatheter aortic valve replacement for native aortic valve regurgitation: a systematic review and meta-analysis. *Catheter. Cardiovasc. Interv.* 93: 345–353.

8 Sawaya, F.J., Deutsch, M.A., Seiffert, M. et al. (2017). Safety and efficacy of transcatheter aortic valve replacement in the treatment of pure aortic regurgitation in native valves and failing surgical bioprostheses: results from an international registry study. *JACC Cardiovasc. Interv.* 10: 1048–1056.

9 Yoon, S.H., Schmidt, T., Bleiziffer, S. et al. (2017). Transcatheter aortic valve replacement in pure native aortic valve regurgitation. *J. Am. Coll. Cardiol.* 70: 2752–2763.

12

Aortic Valve-in-Valve Interventions

Guilherme Bratz[1], Pedro F. Gomes Nicz[1,4], Fábio S. de Brito[1,4] and Rogério Sarmento-Leite[2,3]

[1] Structural Heart Disease Intervention, Interventional Cardiology Department at Heart Institute (InCor), University of São Paulo, São Paulo, São Paulo, Brazil
[2] Interventional Cardiology, Heart Institute, Fundação Universitária de Cardiologia (IC – FUC), Porto Alegre, Rio Grande do Sul, Brazil
[3] Interventional Cardiology, Hospital Moinhos de Vento, Porto Alegre, Rio Grande do Sul, Brazil
[4] Interventional Cardiology, Hospital Sírio Libanês, São Paulo, São Paulo, Brazil

1. Why are aortic valve-in-valve procedures needed?

In recent years, surgical aortic valve replacement has been accepted as the standard treatment for aortic stenosis and regurgitation. Both mechanical and bioprosthetic valves are used in this procedure; however, the use of bioprosthetic valves is increasing, even in younger populations, probably because of the bleeding and thromboembolic risks related to the need for anticoagulation therapy and thrombogenicity of mechanical valves. The durability of bioprosthetic valves has increased with newer generations; however, in the best case, it is still around 10–15 years, with the need for reintervention with the failed bioprosthesis. In this context, less invasive alternatives like valve-in-valve (ViV) transcatheter aortic valve replacement (TAVR) have emerged and become good options compared with reoperation, the standard of care, especially in elderly patients with numerous comorbidities and with higher surgical risk.

2. Why are ViV TAVR outcomes better than native valve TAVR?

Large reports are scarce evaluating the ViV approach compared to native valve TAVR. However, according to the analysis of high-risk patients with degenerated bioprosthetic valves (DBVs), in most cases, the ViV approach has been demonstrated to be clinically effective, with excellent hemodynamic performance and improvements in patient functional capacity and quality of life after device implantation and survival benefits and acceptable three-year outcomes. Mortality and stroke rates after VIV procedures are comparable to those in other TAVR cohorts, with fewer procedural complications. Nevertheless, several anatomical, safety, and efficacy concerns emerged in this subgroup of patients. Attention to and prevention of device malposition, ostial coronary obstruction, and high post-procedural gradients should be pursued. Therefore, during patient selection for the procedure, the Heart Team must be familiarized with the characteristics of the previous implanted surgical bioprosthesis: valve anatomy, causes of degeneration, echocardiographic parameters, and risk of coronary compromise.

3. What are the primary limitations of aortic ViV TAVR?

Recent data shows that the rates of serious complications of ViV TAVR are low; however, there are two main limitations related to the procedure: patient-prosthesis mismatch (PPM) and coronary obstruction. Hence correctly identifying the type and size of the bioprosthetic valve is an important step when planning ViV TAR. The interventional cardiologist should be familiar with the valve design and pre-procedure angio-CT interpretation for proper procedure planning. This will prevent and avoid possible complications such as coronary obstruction in externally mounted stented valves or stent-less valves, especially in those with small anatomies, valve malapposition or dislocation in stentless valves, and higher residual gradients leading to mismatch with possible deleterious outcomes.

PPM occurrence is considerably higher after ViV TAVR compared to native valve (NV) TAVR as ViV decreases the minimal outflow area due to the implant of a second valve within a previous one ("Russian doll" effect). The evidence of high gradients in the surgical valve before the ViV procedure may be an obstacle, and the procedure may not be feasible if there's no possibility of balloon valve fracture (BVF). Criteria for high transprosthetic gradients are described in Table 12.1. The severity of the residual gradients is related to three main factors: (i) the size of the surgical valve, (ii) the mode of its failure, and (iii) the size and type of transcatheter heart valve (THV) used. ViV procedure in patients with small bioprosthetic valves are at a higher risk of having elevated residual gradients after the ViV procedure. It can be explained by the non-distensible nature of bioprosthetic valves, resulting in under-expansion of the ViV implants. Larger surgical valve size, supra-annular THV type, and greater THV implantation depth have all been shown to reduce the incidence of mismatch and elevated post-procedural gradients.

Coronary artery obstruction was more frequently seen in the early ViV TAVR series. This severe complication is associated with high mortality rates, and every effort should be made to avoid it. Evaluating the risk of coronary obstruction requires understanding all the mechanisms involved. Usually it is due to the movement of the surgical aortic valve (SAV) leaflets beyond the aortic root above the sinotubular junction after THV deployment. Table 12.2 summarizes the possible risk factors for coronary obstruction.

4. Why does the mechanism of bioprosthetic valve failure matter?

There is a diverse spectrum of surgical valves with different materials, anticalcification treatments, and degeneration modes according to the Valve Academic Research Consortium (VARC)-3 criteria (Table 12.3). Structural valve deterioration (SVD) can be defined as intrinsic permanent changes to the prosthetic valve, such as wear and tear, leaflet disruption, flail leaflet, leaflet fibrosis and/or calcification, or strut fracture. Generally, a valve with bovine pericardial tends to fail due to stenosis, while a porcine valve tends to fail due to regurgitation. Of these two types of valve deterioration, recent data shows that stenosis is more frequent (around 50%), followed by regurgitation (near 30%), and a combinations of both mechanisms (up to 20%). Regardless the mechanism of dysfunction, ViV transcatheter aortic valve implantation (TAVI) is usually considered in SVD and avoided in non-structural valve dysfunction; however, patients with PPM may be suitable for adjunctive procedures (e.g. BVF).

Central regurgitation implies no difference in ViV TAVR compared to stenotic surgical valves. But regurgitation due

Table 12.1 Echocardiographic findings in the presence of high transprosthetic gradients suggestive of PPM.

Normal valve structure and motion
VPeak >3 m/s, MeanG >20 mmHg
EOA >1 cm^2; DVI 0.25–0.34
EOA normal
EOAi ≤0.85 cm^2/m^2
Increase in MeanG <10 mmHg and decrease in EOA <0.3 cm^2 during follow-up

Source: Data from Tarantini, Dvir, and Tang (2021).

Table 12.2 Risk factors for coronary obstruction during ViV procedures.

Anatomic factors
- Low-lying coronary ostia
- Narrow-lying coronary ostia
- Narrow sinotubular junction/low sinus height
- Narrow sinuses of Valsalva
- Previous root repair

Bioprosthetic valve factors
- Supra-annular position
- High leaflet profile
- Internal stent frame
- No stent frame
- Bulky leaflets

Transcatheter valve factors
- Extended sealing cuff
- High implantation

Source: Data from Tarantini, Dvir, and Tang (2021).

Table 12.3 Causes of bioprosthetic valve failure.

Structural valve deterioration (SVD)
Non-structural valve dysfunction
- Paravalvular regurgitation
- Prosthesis-patient mismatch

Valve thrombosis
Endocarditis

Source: Data from Tarantini, Dvir, and Tang (2021).

to paravalvular leaks is an important complication that must be evaluated by echocardiography before the procedure. In this scenario, ViV TAVR itself will not treat the leak since the area of regurgitation is located outside of the surgical valve frame. The use of vascular plugs together with the ViV TAVR may be a good option for patients with severe regurgitation and hemolysis.

5. How do you plan for a ViV procedure?

Planning for ViV TAVI requires special care to evaluate the design of the surgical valve, calcification, coronary level, and relation with the old and the new valve leaflets. However, peripheral vessels also play an important role in choosing the THV and patient selection.

Vascular complications are among the most frequent and serious associated with ViV TAVI, increasing procedure morbidity and mortality. Due to its ability to accurately quantify iliofemoral vessel size, calcification, and tortuosity, computed tomography (CT) allows excellent evaluation of possible vascular complications and can determines whether transfemoral access can be achieved or an alternative access route is required. Risk factors for vascular complications are an external sheath diameter that exceeds the minimal artery diameter, moderate or severe calcification, and vessel tortuosity. Continuous enhancement of delivery systems with smaller devices and expanding sheath designs has substantially decreased the number of vascular complications.

A pre-procedural assessment of the patient is vital for achieving optimal outcomes from the procedure, and as in NV-TAVI, CT is a mainstay for ViV TAVI procedure planning. It allows a complete evaluation of the morphology of the valve, ascending aorta, and coronaries. In cases where surgical heart valve (SHV) information is missing from medical reports, it also allows the identification of the valve type and size. The acquisition protocol in ViV TAVI is the same as in NV-TAVI; however, contrast enhancement is not absolutely necessary for aortic root assessment in patients with stented SHVs. Radiopaque components of the SHV and coronary ostia can easily be identified using non-contrast CT protocols. This technique has limited use for stentless surgical valves.

One of the major determinants of ViV complications is the proximity of the coronary ostia to the final position of the THV. Using pre-procedural CT allows overlapping a virtual ring simulating the size of the THV at maximum expansion, centered in the surgical prosthesis. This makes it possible to calculate the virtual THV-to-coronary distance (VTC).

The ViV Aortic mobile application, developed by Vinayak Bapat, is a helpful tool that can aid operators in planning the procedure. It provides information about surgical valve anatomy, valve size, internal diameter, height, valves with expanding frames, valves that can fracture, and fluoroscopic valve views. Figure 12.1 shows some example images from the app. When the surgical valve and size are selected, it provides THV options for the ViV procedure and fluoroscopic images of both valves in place.

6. How do you avoid PPM in aortic ViV procedures?

The ViV procedure is a strong predictor for PPM, a severe adverse outcome after ViV TAVI. PPM is related to reduced left ventricle mass regression, less improvement in New York Heart Association (NYHA) classification, higher rates of early and late mortality, and increased bleeding complications. Insightful planning may predict and avoid PPM.

Patients with severe PPM with the original SAVR have higher risks for post-procedure gradient ≥20 mmHg and increased 30-day and 1-year mortality. Generally, these patients present sooner with SVD for ViV TAVI than those with moderate PPM. Most of these patients must be considered for redo SAVR instead of ViV procedure.

Following are some techniques used to avoid PPM and increase procedure success.

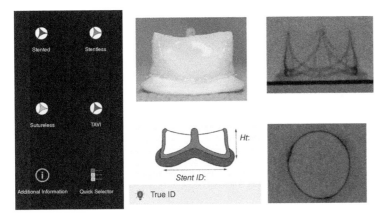

Figure 12.1 Example of ViV app view, surgical valve, and fluoroscopic image. *Source:* Bapat, V., 2014, Europa Group.

Supra-Annular vs. Intra-Annular Design

There are two main mechanisms of THV deployment: self-expandable (SE) and balloon-expandable (BE). Most commercially available SE valves have a supra-annular design with the leaflets sited above the valve annulus, where the frame is least constrained (Figure 12.2). This characteristic makes SE valves indicated for patients with a small annulus and previous PPM. SE valves are associated with a lower post-VIV gradient, primarily in patients with preexisting severe PPM but with higher rates of paravalvular regurgitation (PVR). BE valves have an intra-annular valve design with the leaflets housed within the native annulus (Figure 12.3). These valves are a good choice for patients with intermediate and large surgical valves and low or no PPM.

Implantation Technique (High vs. Low)

Theoretically, the height of the THV implantation may contribute to post-ViV gradients. However, to date, no clinical trial has evaluated the difference in approaches in vivo. Midha et al. evaluated the results of different deployment locations of SE and BE valves in vitro with

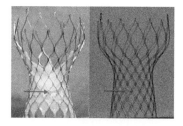

Figure 12.2   Example of supra-annular valve design. *Source:* Bapat, V., 2014, Europa Group.

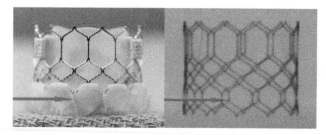

Figure 12.3   Example of intra-annular valve design. *Source:* Bapat, V., 2014, Europa Group.

multiple variables such as hemodynamics, regurgitation fraction (RF), aortic valve area, pinwheeling index, and pullout forces. For SE valves, a range of –3 mm to the normal height was associated with the lowest transvalvular pressure gradient (TVPG). This range was also associated with the least RF. BE valves, however, performed better with increasingly supra-annular deployment, and RF progressively decreased as the deployment height increased (from –6 mm to +6 mm). For both SE and BE valves, pullout forces decreased with supra-annular deployment due to the greater contact area between the THV and the surgical bioprosthesis. As highlighted by the authors, "the results suggest that optimal ViV deployment position exist for both SE and BE valves and must be determined by analysis of benefits (mean gradient, valve area) and risks (PVL, leaflet deformation, and embolization risk)." Figure 12.4 shows the deployment heights used.

High-Pressure Post-Dilation and Balloon Valve Fracture

As already described, high post-ViV gradients significantly affect patient survival. Thus, optimization of transcatheter valve hemodynamics following the ViV procedure is crucial. High-pressure post-dilatation and valve fracture are two techniques that can be used to achieve better hemodynamics results. The ViV Aortic app shows which valves can be fractured and which can be expanded with high-pressure post-dilatation.

High-pressure post-dilatation is intended to optimize post-ViV hemodynamics by overstretching the surgical valve frame (mainly small surgical valve annular frames). It consists of high-pressure post-dilatation with a noncompliant balloon following the ViV procedure. When performed before TAVR, high-pressure pre-dilatation can precipitate acute severe aortic insufficiency and hemodynamic instability. Some trials have shown that high-pressure post-dilatation reduces the valve gradient after the procedure and gives consistent results over 30-day and 1-year follow-up.

Valve fracture is achieved with even higher pressure (16–20 atm) post-dilatation, causing a fracture of the earlier surgical valve frame. Like the previous scenario, a noncompliant balloon should be used, as the compliant balloon can lead to balloon rupture with associated aortic root injury. Valves were often successfully fractured with

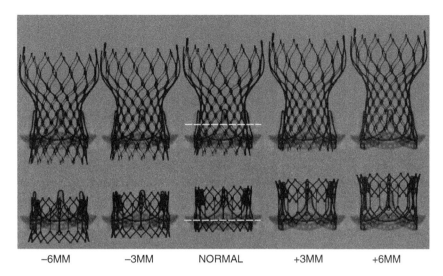

−6MM   −3MM   NORMAL   +3MM   +6MM

Figure 12.4 Schematic representation of deployment heights. The dashed line indicates the base of the leaflets in the transcatheter heart valve. *Source:* Midha, P.A. et al. (2016), Elsevier.

balloons 1 mm larger than the labeled valve size in some trials, while others suggested a balloon at least 3 mm larger than the true ID of the surgical valve. The timing of the BVF involves a balance between the potential for producing catastrophic surgical valve insufficiency versus the unknown influence of high-pressure balloon inflation on the acute structural integrity and long-term durability of the THV leaflets.

7. How do you prevent and treat coronary obstruction?

Coronary obstruction is a rare complication but is associated with high mortality rates after ViV TAVR. The VIV International Data (VIVID) Registry initially reported a coronary obstruction incidence of 3.5%, close to the 2.3% incidence found by Ribeiro et al. in a recent multicenter registry. The coronary obstruction is usually the result of the interaction between a surgical bioprosthesis and the coronary ostium, and the main predisposing factor is the proximity of the coronary ostia to the anticipated final position of the displaced bioprosthetic leaflets after THV implantation. The VTC distance – the distance between this virtual ring and the coronary ostia – may determine an increased hazard of coronary occlusion if the value is small (<4 mm: high risk). Other risk factors are a supra-annular bioprosthetic valve, a narrow and low-lying sino-tubular junction, bulky bioprosthetic leaflets, low-lying

coronaries in the narrow aortic root, and reimplanted coronaries.

Severe hypotension and ST-segment changes are the main presentation of coronary obstruction and occur immediately after valve implantation. This may be explained by the fact that the left main coronary is obstructed in most patients, either alone or associated with the right coronary artery. There are two adjunctive techniques to reduce the coronary obstruction risk: the BASILICA procedure and the chimney technique.

BASILICA Procedure

This is a preventive technique to avoid coronary obstruction during ViV. Both the left and right coronary arteries are suitable for the BASILICA technique to prevent obstruction. It uses an electrified guidewire to transverse the chosen aortic leaflet (right or left) and lacerate and split it to allow blood to blood flow toward the coronary ostia. Figure 12.5 summarizes this approach.

The BASILICA technique may require various sheath accesses, exchange of catheter, and calcified leaflet manipulation; therefore, the risks of vascular complications, stroke, injury of non-target structures, and hemodynamic complications due to aortic regurgitation after the leaflet splitting are high. Due to the complexity of the procedure, associated with its possible complications, physicians must be careful about patient selection.

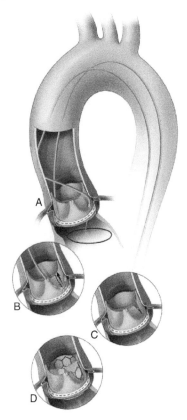

Figure 12.5 BASILICA procedure to prevent coronary obstruction. *Source:* Khan et al. (2018) / With permission of Elsevier.

Chimney Technique

This proposed technique for coronary protection consists of positioning a coronary guidewire, balloon, undeployed stent, or guide extension in the artery at risk before THV deployment. If there is a coronary blood-flow impairment during the procedure, the stent is retracted to extend from the proximal portion of the coronary artery. It's deployed to create a channel for the coronary perfusion like a "chimney." Figure 12.6 shows the steps.

This is a novel technique and needs clinical data to prove its safety. Stent protrusion with residual under-expansion caused by extrinsic compression from the THV and aortic wall associated with a large amount of foreign material inside the aortic root may increase thrombogenicity, jeopardizing the long-term outcome.

8. How important is adjunct pharmacology after ViV-TAVI?

Candidates for ViV are generally patients with multiple comorbidities and higher thromboembolic and bleeding risks. So far, no randomized trial has studied an antithrombotic regimen after the ViV procedure, and the suggested medical treatment is usually based on NV-TAVI trials. The amount of foreign material inside the aortic root (SAV and THV), sinus sequestration, and (sometimes), the presence of residual gradient after the procedure may increase patient thromboembolic risk with a possible benefit of double antithrombotic therapy. The PARTNER 2 (Placement of Aortic Transcatheter Valves) ViV registry recommends aspirin with clopidogrel for up to six months after the procedure. The recent presentation of its three-year follow-up showed a very low rate of thromboembolic risk. Despite the medical treatment used, reassessment of the patient's thromboembolic risk, presence or new onset of atrial fibrillation, or concomitant acute or chronic coronary artery disease should drive tailored antithrombotic or anticoagulant therapy according to current guidelines. Echocardiographic monitoring is also recommended; and when necessary, a CT scan for evaluation of valve thrombosis should be done to prevent or treat possible ViV complications.

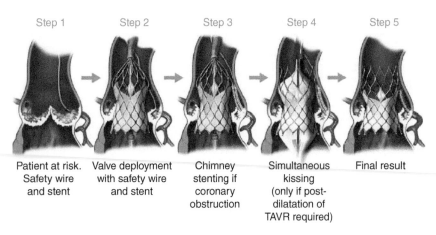

Step 1	Step 2	Step 3	Step 4	Step 5
Patient at risk. Safety wire and stent	Valve deployment with safety wire and stent	Chimney stenting if coronary obstruction	Simultaneous kissing (only if post-dilatation of TAVR required)	Final result

Figure 12.6 Procedural steps for the chimney technique. *Source:* Mercanti et al. (2020) / With permission of Elsevier.

Bibliography

1 Allen, K.B., Chhatriwalla, A.K., Saxon, J.T. et al. (2019). Bioprosthetic valve fracture: technical insights from a multicenter study. *J. Thorac. Cardiovasc. Surg.* 158 (5): 1317–1328.e1.

2 Alperi, A., Garcia, S., and Rodés-Cabau, J. (2021). Transcatheter valve-in-valve implantation in degenerated surgical aortic and mitral bioprosthesis: current state and future perspectives. *Prog. Cardiovasc. Dis.* https://doi.org/10.1016/j.pcad.2021.10.001.

3 Bapat, V. (2014). Valve-in-valve apps: why and how they were developed and how to use them. *EuroIntervention* 10: U44–U51. http://www.pcronline.com/eurointervention/download_pdf.php?issue=U&article=7&art_id=8125%5Cnhttp://ovidsp.ovid.com/ovidweb.cgi?T=JS&PAGE=reference&D=emed12&NEWS=N&AN=2014819857.

4 Blanke, P., Weir-McCall, J.R., Achenbach, S. et al. (2019). Computed tomography imaging in the context of Transcatheter aortic valve implantation (TAVI)/Transcatheter aortic valve replacement (TAVR): an expert consensus document of the Society of Cardiovascular Computed Tomography. *JACC Cardiovasc. Imaging* 12 (1): 1–24.

5 Chakravarty, T., Cox, J., Abramowitz, Y. et al. (2018). High-pressure post-dilation following transcatheter valve-in-valve implantation in small surgical valves. *EuroIntervention* 14 (2): 158–165.

6 Chiocchi, M., Ricci, F., Pasqualetto, M. et al. (2020). Role of computed tomography in transcatheter aortic valve implantation and valve-in-valve implantation: complete review of preprocedural and postprocedural imaging. *J. Cardiovasc. Med.* 21 (3): 182–191.

7 Dahou, A., Mahjoub, H., and Pibarot, P. (2016). Prosthesis-patient mismatch after aortic valve replacement. *Curr. Treat. Options Cardiovasc. Med.* 18 (11).

8 Dunning, J., Gao, H., Chambers, J. et al. (2011). Aortic valve surgery: Marked increases in volume and significant decreases in mechanical valve use – An analysis of 41,227 patients over 5 years from the Society for Cardiothoracic Surgery in Great Britain and Ireland National database. *J. Thorac. Cardiovasc. Surg.* 142 (4): 776.e3–782.e3. http://dx.doi.org/10.1016/j.jtcvs.2011.04.048.

9 Dvir, D., Leipsic, J., Blanke, P. et al. (2015). Coronary obstruction in transcatheter aortic valve-in-valve implantation preprocedural evaluation, device selection, protection, and treatment. *Circ. Cardiovasc. Interv.* 8 (1): 1–10.

10 Dvir, D., Webb, J., Brecker, S. et al. (2012). Transcatheter aortic valve replacement for degenerative bioprosthetic surgical valves: results from the global valve-in-valve registry. *Circulation* 126 (19): 2335–2344.

11 Dvir, D., Webb, J.G., Bleiziffer, S. et al. (2014). Transcatheter aortic valve implantation in failed bioprosthetic surgical valves. *J. Am. Med. Assoc.* 312 (2): 162–170.

12 Hamandi, M., Nwafor, I., Hebeler, K.R. et al. (2020). Bioprosthetic valve fracture during valve-in-valve transcatheter aortic valve replacement. *Baylor Univ. Med. Cent. Proc.* 33 (3): 317–321. https://doi.org/10.1080/08998280.2020.1732267.

13 Khan, J.M., Dvir, D., Greenbaum, A.B. et al. (2018). Transcatheter laceration of aortic leaflets to prevent coronary obstruction during transcatheter aortic valve replacement: concept to first-in-human. *JACC Cardiovasc. Interv.* 11 (7): 677–689.

14 Mercanti, F., Rosseel, L., Neylon, A. et al. (2020). Chimney stenting for coronary occlusion during TAVR: insights from the chimney registry. *JACC Cardiovasc. Interv.* 13 (6): 751–761. https://doi.org/10.1016/j.jcin.2020.01.227.

15 Midha, P.A., Raghav, V., Condado, J.F. et al. (2016). Valve type, size, and deployment location affect hemodynamics in an in vitro valve-in-valve model. *JACC Cardiovasc. Interv.* 9 (15): 1618–1628.

16 Otto, C.M., Nishimura, R.A., Bonow, R.O. et al. (2020, 2021). ACC/AHA guideline for the Management of Patients with Valvular Heart Disease: a report of the American College of Cardiology/American Heart Association Joint Committee on Clinical Practice Guidelines. *J. Am. Coll. Cardiol.* 77 (4): e25–e197. https://doi.org/10.1016/j.jacc.2020.11.018.

17 Paradis, J.M., Del Trigo, M., Puri, R., and Rodés-Cabau, J. (2015). Transcatheter valve-in-valve and valve-in-ring for treating aortic and mitral surgical prosthetic dysfunction. *J. Am. Coll. Cardiol.* 66 (18): 2019–2037.

18 Ribeiro, H.B., Nombela-Franco, L., Allende, R. et al. (2013). Coronary obstruction following transcatheter aortic valve implantation for degenerative bioprosthetic surgical valves: a systematic literature review. *Rev. Bras. Cardiol. Invasiva* 21 (4): 2.

19 Ribeiro, H.B., Webb, J.G., Makkar, R.R. et al. (2013). Predictive factors, management, and clinical outcomes of coronary obstruction following transcatheter aortic valve implantation: insights from a large multicenter registry. *J. Am. Coll. Cardiol.* 62 (17): 1552–1562.

20 Rodés-Cabau, J. and Ribeiro, H.B. (2020). Consolidating the BASILICA technique in TAVI patients at risk of coronary obstruction. *EuroIntervention* 16 (8): 617–619.

21 Romano, V., Buzzatti, N., Latib, A. et al. (2018). Chimney technique for coronary obstruction after aortic valve in valve: pros and cons. *Eur. Heart J. Cardiovasc. Imaging* 19 (10): 1194.

22 Tarantini, G., Dvir, D., and Tang, G.H.L. (2021). Transcatheter aortic valve implantation in degenerated surgical aortic valves. *EuroIntervention* 17 (9): 709–719.

23 Tarantini, G., Nai Fovino, L., and Gersh, B.J. (2018). Transcatheter aortic valve implantation in lower-risk patients: what is the perspective? *Eur. Heart J.* 39 (8): 658–666.

24 Vahanian, A., Beyersdorf, F., Praz, F. et al. (2021). ESC/EACTS guidelines for the management of valvular heart disease. *Eur. Heart J.* 2021: 1–72.

25 Vemulapalli, S., Holmes, D.R., Dai, D. et al. (2018 Jan). Valve hemodynamic deterioration and cardiovascular outcomes in TAVR: a report from the STS/ACC TVT registry. *Am. Heart J.* 1 (195): 1–13.

26 Webb, J.G. and Dvir, D. (2013). Transcatheter aortic valve replacement for bioprosthetic aortic valve failure: the valve-in-valve procedure. *Circulation* 127 (25): 2542–2550.

27 Webb, J.G., Murdoch, D.J., Alu, M.C. et al. (2019). 3-year outcomes after valve-in-valve transcatheter aortic valve replacement for degenerated bioprostheses: the PARTNER 2 registry. *J. Am. Coll. Cardiol.* 73 (21): 2647–2655.

28 Yao, R.J., Simonato, M., and Dvir, D. (2017). Optimising the haemodynamics of aortic valve-in-valve procedures. *Interv. Cardiol. Rev.* 12 (1): 40–43.

13

Prevention and Management of Coronary Artery Obstruction in TAVR

Jonathan D. Wolfe and John M. Lasala

[1] *Cardiovascular Division, Department of Medicine, Washington University School of Medicine, St. Louis, MO, USA*

1. What is the incidence of coronary artery obstruction in transcatheter aortic valve replacement (TAVR)?

Coronary artery obstruction as a consequence of TAVR is uncommon, with an incidence <1% for native aortic valves in multiple case series and registries. In one of the largest multicenter TAVR registries evaluating outcomes in 6688 patients, 0.66% suffered symptomatic coronary obstruction. Coronary obstruction is approximately four times more common when performing TAVR as part of a valve-in-valve (ViV) procedure. The increased risk is likely because most surgical prostheses are in the supra-annular position, resulting in lower coronary heights relative to valve leaflets and because valve suturing draws the coronaries closer, decreasing sinus width. For patients undergoing ViV TAVR, the surgically implanted valves (SIVs) with the highest risk of coronary obstruction are stented bioprostheses with externally mounted leaflets (e.g. Sorin Mitroflow, St. Jude Medical Trifecta) and stentless bioprosthesis (e.g. Sorin Freedom, Medtronic Freestyle, St. Jude Medical Toronto SPV). Stented bioprostheses with internally mounted leaflets (e.g. Edwards Lifesciences PERIMOUNT and Magna, St. Jude Medical Epic, Medtronic Hancock, and Mosaic) have the lowest risk of coronary obstruction.

2. What is the mechanism of coronary artery obstruction in TAVR?

There are five potential mechanisms for coronary artery obstruction in TAVR. The most common mechanism is the displacement of a native or SIV leaflet toward the coronary ostium such that it blankets the ostium. The second is sinus of Valsalva sequestration, which can occur by displacement of native or SIV leaflets and cause obstruction of the entire sinus in an aortic root with a low and narrow sinotubular junction. The third is mass obstruction, typically by a calcium deposit on a native or SIV leaflet that is deflected during TAVR deployment to obstruct the coronary artery. The fourth is valve skirt obstruction, where the valve prosthesis reaches high enough that the skirt covers the coronary ostium. The final mechanism is embolization of thrombus or degenerative material in the aortic root or on the TAVR device to cause coronary obstruction (Figure 13.1).

3. Which coronary artery is most commonly obstructed during TAVR?

The left coronary artery is involved in 80–90% of symptomatic coronary obstruction cases during TAVR. In studies evaluating normal post-mortem hearts or examining the aortic root with multislice computed tomography (CT), the distance from the left coronary artery ostium to the basal attachment point of the aortic valve is typically lower when compared to the right coronary artery ostium. This difference likely explains the increased risk of coronary obstruction on the left.

4. What is delayed coronary obstruction after TAVR?

Coronary artery obstruction typically happens in the seconds or minutes following valve deployment in TAVR. However, delayed coronary obstruction (DCO) has been described, which occurs in the hours and days following the procedure. In a large, international, multicenter registry of 17092 TAVR procedures, the incidence of DCO was 0.22%. Among the patients who experienced DCO, approximately half of cases

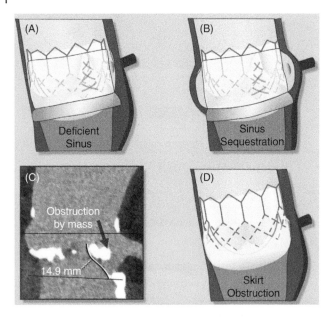

Figure 13.1 Mechanisms of coronary obstruction in transcatheter aortic valve replacement (TAVR). (a) Deficient sinus of Valsalva in which the displaced native or SIV valve leaflets directly obstruct the coronary ostium. (b) In a low sinus of Valsalva with a narrow sinotubular junction, displaced native or SIV leaflets may obstruct the coronary artery by sequestering the sinus. (c) Bulky leaflet mass can be displaced to directly obstruct the coronary ostium during TAVR deployment. (d) In a low-lying coronary ostium, the fabric-covered skirt of a TAVR valve can directly obstruct the coronary artery. *Source:* Lederman et al. (2019) / With permission of Elsevier.

occurred in ≤24 hours. Approximately 15% of patients experienced DCO between 24 hours and ≤7 days, and the remaining 35% of DCO occurred at ≥60 days. Coronary obstruction in cases that occurred in ≤7 days was due to leaflet displacement or minor coronary dissections that later expanded. Coronary obstruction in cases that occurred in ≥60 days was due to endothelization of the TAVR valve with an eventual resultant coronary obstruction or thrombus development on the TAVR valve with subsequent embolization.

5. What are the symptoms of coronary artery obstruction in TAVR?

Coronary artery obstruction after TAVR most commonly presents as severe hypotension after deployment of the valve. Other symptoms include electrocardiographic changes, often ST-segment elevation, and ventricular arrhythmias. Symptoms are due to myocardial ischemia in the distribution of the affected coronary artery.

6. What are the outcomes for patients that have coronary artery obstruction with TAVR?

Although uncommon, coronary artery obstruction after TAVR is a devastating complication with poor outcomes. Registry data suggests that coronary obstruction is associated with approximately a 15–20% rate of procedural death and 40–50% rate of 30-day mortality.

7. What are risk factors for coronary artery obstruction with TAVR?

There are several risk factors for coronary artery obstruction with TAVR in native valves. Coronary height, as measured on CT from the annulus to the base of the coronary ostium, of <12 mm has been associated with coronary obstruction. A narrow sinus of Valsalva of <30 mm is also associated with coronary obstruction. In large-registry data, females have a significantly higher incidence of coronary obstruction than males. Women have a smaller aortic root, which, combined with a lower coronary ostia height, may partially explain this finding. Previous coronary artery bypass surgery (CABG) also appears to have a protective effect against symptomatic coronary obstruction.

For patients undergoing TAVR as part of a ViV procedure, the distance between the annulus and the coronary ostia is less relevant when evaluating the risk of

Table 13.1 Risk factors for coronary obstruction with valve-in-valve transcatheter aortic valve replacement (TAVR) implantation.

Anatomic factors	Bioprosthetic valve factors	Transcatheter valve factors
Low-lying coronary ostia	Supra-annular position	Extended sealing cuff
Narrow sinotubular junction with low sinus height	High leaflet profile	High implantation
Narrow sinuses of Valsalva	Internal stent frame	
Previous aortic root repair	No stent frame	
	Bulky leaflets	

Source: Dvir et al. (2015) / American Heart Association.

coronary obstruction. Instead, the main factor predisposing to coronary obstruction is the proximity of the coronary ostia to the final anticipated position of the displaced SIV leaflets after TAVR implantation. Many factors contribute to the risk of coronary obstruction in this setting, including a supra-annular SIV, low-lying sinotubular junction, and bulky bioprosthetic leaflets (Table 13.1).

8. How do you prevent coronary artery obstruction with TAVR?

The contemporary approach to avoiding coronary obstruction with TAVR is careful patient selection using CT. As described earlier, low coronary ostial height (<12 mm) from the annulus and narrow sinus of Valsalva diameter (<30 mm) are associated with an increased risk of coronary obstruction. However, there is no absolute value for coronary height or sinus of Valsalva diameter at which TAVR should be completely contraindicated, given the low specificity of these measurements to predict coronary obstruction. Instead, these values should be interpreted in the context of annular dimensions, overall aortic root dimensions, and anticipated TAVR valve size. For patients at increased risk of coronary obstruction with TAVR based on their CT findings, surgical valve replacement should be considered. For patients with a high surgical risk precluding surgical valve replacement, the feasibility of "preparatory coronary protection" or the BASILICA procedure should be considered. Both are described in the subsequent sections.

For patients undergoing ViV TAVR implantation, attention to the risk factors described in Table 13.1 is essential. Analogous to assessment before native valve TAVR, relevant anatomic measurements on CT should include the height of the coronary ostia in relation to the sewing ring, the width and height of the sinus of Valsalva, and the width of the sinotubular junction (Table 13.2). For patients undergoing TAVR in stentless SIVs (e.g. Sorin Freedom, Medtronic Freestyle, St. Jude Medical Toronto SPV), implantation is biomechanically similar to TAVR in native valve stenosis due to the absence of the rigid scaffold that is present in stented SIVs. For patients with stented SIVs where the stent post lies above the level of the coronary ostia, the angulation of the SIV can result in significantly higher risk for coronary obstruction than would be predicted by the positioning of the sewing ring. As a result, it

Table 13.2 Computed-tomography assessment for coronary obstruction with valve-in-valve transcatheter aortic valve replacement (TAVR).

Coronary and bypass graft parameters	Aortic root parameters	Bioprosthetic valve parameters	Bioprosthesis-root relationship
Stenosis in coronary ostia	Sinus of Valsalva diameter	Leaflet thickness, calcification, or pannus	Sewing ring to coronary ostial height
Patency of bypass grafts	Sinus height	SIV post height	VTC distance (high risk: <4 mm)

SIV: surgically implanted valve, VTC: virtual transcatheter heart valve to coronary. *Source:* Dvir et al. (2015) / American Heart Association.

is also necessary to evaluate the geometric axis of the SIV at the level of the coronary ostia. This can be accounted for by estimating the anticipated distance of the TAVR valve to the coronary ostia using a virtual transcatheter heart valve to coronary distance (VTC) measurement on CT. A VTC measurement is performed by superimposing a virtual ring simulating the anticipated diameter of the fully expanded TAVR valve along the geometric center of the SIV, followed by a linear measurement from the ring to the coronary ostium. This measurement provides a marker of the capacity of the aortic root to accommodate a TAVR valve while maintaining flow to the coronary arteries and accounts for the frequent eccentric position of the SIV within the aortic root (Figure 13.2). A VTC <4 mm is associated with a high risk of coronary obstruction. If the posts of a stented SIV are below the coronary ostia, the VTC measurement is less relevant. For patients at increased risk of coronary obstruction with ViV TAVR, the decision-making is similar to TAVR in native valves; surgical valve replacement should be considered. If contraindicated, the feasibility of "preparatory coronary protection" or the BASILICA procedure can be evaluated.

9. What is the treatment for coronary artery obstruction with TAVR?

If no preventative strategy is employed, treating coronary obstruction from TAVR is a therapeutic challenge. Treatment strategies include percutaneous coronary intervention,

Patient 1

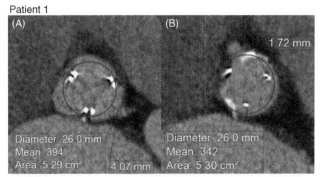

Patient 2

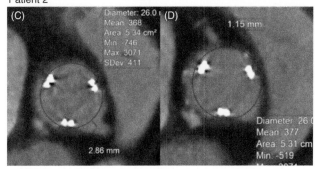

Figure 13.2 Examples of two patients being evaluated for valve-in-valve transcatheter aortic valve replacement (TAVR) with anatomy concerning for high risk of coronary obstruction. (a) Valve to coronary distance (VTC) measurement of 4.07 mm of the left coronary artery in Patient 1; (b) VTC measurement of 1.72 mm of the right coronary artery in Patient 1; (c) VTC measurement of 2.86 mm of the left coronary artery in Patient 2; (d) VTC measurement of 1.15 mm of the right coronary artery of Patient 2. *Source:* Adapted from Blanke, P., Soon, J., Dvir, D. et al. (2016). Computed tomography assessment for transcatheter aortic valve in valve implantation: the Vancouver approach to predict anatomical risk for coronary obstruction and other considerations. *J. Cardiovasc. Comput. Tomogr.* 10 (6): 491–499.

emergency coronary artery bypass surgery, or valve recapture in the case of retrievable TAVR valves (e.g. Medtronic Evolut, Boston Scientific Lotus, Abbott Portico). If the valve is not retrievable, percutaneous coronary intervention is commonly pursued when feasible, given the high mortality associated with emergency bypass surgery in this setting. However, delivery of a wire and subsequent stent to the coronary vasculature in a timely fashion may be challenging due to overlying displaced native or SIV leaflets as well as TAVR struts and because patients are often unstable.

10. What is preparatory coronary protection?

In cases where coronary obstruction is a concern, "preparatory coronary protection" may be used in which a wire and undeployed stent are placed in the coronary vascula-

ture before TAVR implantation. Should coronary obstruction occur, the stent can be pulled back and deployed between the TAVR struts and the aortic root to provide what is variably described as a "snorkel," "chimney," or "periscope" between the aorta and the coronary ostium. While this technique has been employed successfully, cyclic compression and other vascular perturbation around the stent may lead to stent deformation or thrombosis with resultant late ischemic complications.

There are specific technical considerations with regard to coronary intervention in cases where preparatory coronary protection is employed. The optimal guide catheter should approach the coronary ostia from above so as not to interfere with TAVR implantation (e.g. Judkins Left, extra backup). A short-tipped guide catheter should be used when feasible, as it can be more easily pulled out of the left main ostium during TAVR. Large-caliber guide catheters (≥7 Fr) should be used when possible to accommodate the large stent sizes necessary for intervention involving the left main ostium. In many cases, the guide catheter can be used instead of the pigtail that is commonly placed above the aortic valve during TAVR procedures. When the TAVR is deployed, jailing the guiding catheter can be performed because the radial strength of TAVR valves is not high above the annulus, and the guide catheter can be removed later. Finally, using a guide extender (e.g. Vascular Solutions GuideLiner, Boston Scientific GUIDEZILLA, Medtronic Telescope) is prudent because if coronary obstruction occurs, requiring the stent in the coronary artery to be pulled back, the struts of the TAVR can strip off the stent.

11. Explain the BASILICA procedure.

The Bioprosthetic or native Aortic Scallop Intentional Laceration to prevent Coronary Artery obstruction (BASILICA) procedure is used in TAVR implantation where the risk of coronary obstruction is high and entails electrosurgical crossing and laceration of native or SIV valve leaflets to prevent coronary obstruction when the TAVR valve is deployed. The BASILICA technique is performed by first gaining two points of arterial access, usually in the femoral artery. A pair of coaxial catheters are inserted in one access point (e.g. 5 Fr mammary diagnostic catheter inside a 6 Fr extra backup shape-guiding catheter) and positioned over the targeted aortic leaflet scallop. Utilizing a specialized guidewire (e.g. Asahi-Intecc Astato XS 20) sheathed in an insulated polymer jacket (e.g. Vascular Solutions PiggyBack Wire Converter) and electrified to 30 W by clamping the wire to an electrosurgery pencil and generator (e.g. Medtronic Valleylab FX), the target aortic leaflet is punctured with the guidewire at the scallop hinge point using echocardiographic and angiographic guidance. The guidewire is fed into a single-loop snare (e.g. Medtronic Amplatz Goose Neck), which is sized 1 : 1 with the left ventricular outflow tract, and positioned immediately below the leaflet using a separate retrograde catheter that utilizes the second point of arterial access. Once the snare captures the guidewire, the free end of the guidewire is snare-retrieved, allowing externalization of the free end. The guidewire is electrified again to 70 W while maintaining tension on both ends to create a laceration in the leaflet (Figure 13.3). The lacerated leaflet splays after TAVR implantation to allow coronary blood flow.

The first-in-human results using the BASILICA technique were published in 2018, and since then, BASILICA has continued to grow in popularity. In a multicenter inter-national registry of 214 high-risk patients undergoing the BASILICA procedure, leaflet traversal and laceration was successful in 94.4% of patients. The procedure was successful without mortality, coronary obstruction, or reintervention in 86.9% of patients. At 30 days, 2.8% of patients died and 2.8% of patients suffered a stroke. Ten patients (4.7%) had some degree of coronary obstruction despite BASILICA. The technique and appropriate patient selection process for BASILICA continue to be defined.

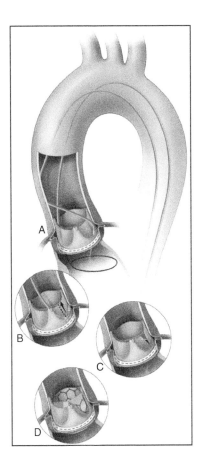

Figure 13.3 Illustration of the BASILICA procedure. (a) A catheter directs an electrified guidewire through the base of the left aortic cusp into a snare in the left ventricular outflow tract. (b) The free end of the guidewire is retrieved using the snare, and the mid-shaft of the guidewire is electrified to lacerate the leaflet. (c) The lacerated aortic valve leaflet. (d) The leaflet splays after transcatheter aortic valve replacement, permitting coronary flow. *Source:* Khan et al. (2018) / With permission of Elsevier.

Bibliography

1 Abramowitz, Y., Chakravarty, T., Jilaihawi, H. et al. (2015). Clinical impact of coronary protection during transcatheter aortic valve implantation: first reported series of patients. *EuroIntervention* 11 (5): 572–581.

2 Blanke, P., Soon, J., Dvir, D. et al. (2016). Computed tomography assessment for transcatheter aortic valve in valve implantation: the Vancouver approach to predict anatomical risk for coronary obstruction and other considerations. *J. Cardiovasc. Comput. Tomogr.* 10 (6): 491–499.

3 Blanke, P., Weir-McCall, J.R., Achenbach, S. et al. (2019). Computed tomography imaging in the context of transcatheter aortic valve implantation (TAVI)/ transcatheter aortic valve replacement (TAVR): an expert consensus document of the Society of Cardiovascular Computed Tomography. *JACC Cardiovasc. Imaging* 12 (1): 1–24.

4 Cavalcanti, J.S., de Melo, N.C., and de Vasconcelos, R.S. (2003). Morphometric and topographic study of coronary ostia. *Arq. Bras. Cardiol.* 81 (4): 359–362, 5–8.

5 Dvir, D., Leipsic, J., Blanke, P. et al. (2015). Coronary obstruction in transcatheter aortic valve-in-valve implantation: preprocedural evaluation, device selection, protection, and treatment. *Circ. Cardiovasc. Interv.* 8 (1): e002079.

6 Jabbour, R.J., Tanaka, A., Finkelstein, A. et al. (2018). Delayed coronary obstruction after transcatheter aortic valve replacement. *J. Am. Coll. Cardiol.* 71 (14): 1513–1524.

7 Khan, J.M., Babaliaros, V.C., Greenbaum, A.B. et al. (2021). Preventing coronary obstruction during transcatheter aortic valve replacement: results from the multicenter international BASILICA registry. *JACC Cardiovasc. Interv.* 14 (9): 941–948.

8 Khan, J.M., Dvir, D., Greenbaum, A.B. et al. (2018). Transcatheter laceration of aortic leaflets to prevent coronary obstruction during transcatheter aortic valve replacement: concept to first-in-human. *JACC Cardiovasc. Interv.* 11 (7): 677–689.

9 Lederman, R.J., Babaliaros, V.C., Rogers, T. et al. (2019). Preventing coronary obstruction during transcatheter aortic valve replacement: from computed tomography to BASILICA. *JACC Cardiovasc. Interv.* 12 (13): 1197–1216.

10 Ribeiro, H.B., Nombela-Franco, L., Urena, M. et al. (2013). Coronary obstruction following transcatheter aortic valve implantation: a systematic review. *JACC Cardiovasc. Interv.* 6 (5): 452–461.

11 Ribeiro, H.B., Rodés-Cabau, J., Blanke, P. et al. (2018). Incidence, predictors, and clinical outcomes of coronary obstruction following transcatheter aortic valve replacement for degenerative bioprosthetic surgical valves: insights from the VIVID registry. *Eur. Heart J.* 39 (8): 687–695.

12 Ribeiro, H.B., Webb, J.G., Makkar, R.R. et al. (2013). Predictive factors, management, and clinical outcomes of coronary obstruction following transcatheter aortic valve implantation: insights from a large multicenter registry. *J. Am. Coll. Cardiol.* 62 (17): 1552–1562.

13 Tops, L.F., Wood, D.A., Delgado, V. et al. (2008). Noninvasive evaluation of the aortic root with multislice computed tomography implications for transcatheter aortic valve replacement. *JACC Cardiovasc. Imaging* 1 (3): 321–330.

14 Vasan, R.S., Larson, M.G., and Levy, D. (1995). Determinants of echocardiographic aortic root size. The Framingham Heart Study. *Circulation* 91 (3): 734–740.

15 Yamamoto, M., Shimura, T., Kano, S. et al. (2016). Impact of preparatory coronary protection in patients at high anatomical risk of acute coronary obstruction during transcatheter aortic valve implantation. *Int. J. Cardiol.* 217: 58–63.

14

Coronary Artery Disease and Transcatheter Aortic Valve Replacement

Timing and Patient Selection for Coronary Intervention in Patients Planned for TAVR

Balaji Shanmugam[1] and Mauricio G. Cohen[2,3]

[1] *University of Miami Miller School of Medicine, Miami, FL, USA*
[2] *Cardiovascular Division, Department of Medicine, University of Miami Miller School of Medicine, Miami, FL, USA*
[3] *Cardiac Catheterization Laboratory, UHealth Tower, University of Miami Hospitals and Clinics, Miami, FL, USA*

1. How common is coronary artery disease (CAD) in patients with severe aortic stenosis (AS)?

The high prevalence of coronary artery disease (CAD) among patients with severe aortic stenosis (AS) may not be surprising given their common risk factors. Despite the variability in the definition of CAD, it has been reported that approximately 15–85% of patients undergoing transcatheter aortic valve replacement (TAVR) had a concomitant presence of CAD, and about half of these have multivessel CAD. The prevalence of CAD is much lower in low-risk patients than in intermediate- or high-risk patients.

2. What is the clinical impact of CAD on TAVR outcomes?

Significant controversy exists regarding the clinical impact of CAD in patients undergoing TAVR. There is significant heterogeneity in published observational data due to variable definitions of CAD, completeness of revascularization, and outcomes. Some studies have been categorized as positive, showing a significant association between CAD and outcomes; as negative, showing no association between CAD and clinical outcomes; or as showing a correlation with CAD severity but not the presence of CAD itself. Therefore, it appears that the presence and extent of CAD may be a surrogate for an increased prevalence of comorbidities rather than an independent risk factor.

3. How do you assess for CAD prior to TAVR?

Since the inception of TAVR, coronary angiography has been the standard method for assessing for the presence of CAD, and the SYNTAX score (SS) is the most commonly utilized tool to quantify the extent of CAD. More recently, with the extension of TAVR indications to lower-risk patients, many operators have proposed an initial screening using coronary computed tomography angiography (CTA). This approach may reduce the need for coronary angiography in 75% of cases. Coronary CTA has an excellent negative predictive value but requires a higher contrast volume. The use of coronary CTA as a "gatekeeper" for invasive coronary angiography is especially well suited for younger patients with a lower probability of CAD and fewer coronary calcifications.

4. Can you use the instantaneous wave-free ratio (iFR) in patients with severe AS?

The use of physiology-guided coronary revascularization has been associated with improved patient outcomes. However, in the setting of AS, functional CAD assessment is problematic due to a combination of microvascular dysfunction, elevated left ventricular end-diastolic pressure, and left ventricular hypertrophy. It has been shown that the hyperemic coronary flow increases significantly post-TAVR compared to baseline. Therefore, the traditional threshold values of fractional flow reserve (FFR) may underestimate stenosis severity. Of note, coronary flow does not change during the diastolic wave-free period before and after TAVR, suggesting that instantaneous free-wave ratio (iFR) may not be affected by AS. In addition, iFR is safer as it does not require the use of adenosine, which can cause hypotension and severe bradycardia – effects not well tolerated by patients with severe AS – even though several studies have shown that the use of intravenous or intracoronary adenosine is safe.

A hybrid approach combining iFR and FFR has been proposed using different cutoff values to determine lesion hemodynamic significance. A cutoff iFR value of 0.93 has been found to have a high negative predictive value (98.4%) to exclude a negative FFR, and a cutoff value of 0.83 has a positive predictive value of 91.3% to identify a positive FFR. In patients with iFR between 0.83 and 0.93, it has been suggested that TAVR can be safely performed with subsequent FFR evaluation of the target lesion (Figure 14.1). FFR and iFR have also been compared with adenosine-stress myocardial perfusion imaging (MPI), showing a good correlation between iFR and FFR and between both physiologic parameters and MPI, demonstrating that iFR can be used as a safe diagnostic tool to evaluate the severity of CAD in patients with severe AS. The results of ongoing trials will provide a definitive answer to the role of coronary physiology testing in guiding revascularization in patients pre-TAVR.

5. What is the role of percutaneous revascularization in TAVR?

In a meta-analysis including 24 observational studies, routine revascularization did not translate into tangible clinical benefit in patients undergoing TAVR. Moreover, revascularization has been associated with increased incidence of vascular complications and 30-day mortality, but not one-year mortality. It is plausible that the impact of CAD and revascularization may be realized after long-term follow-up, especially in younger patients. Most published studies had limited follow-up of up to two years.

PercutAneous Coronary inTervention prIor to transcatheter aortic VAlve implantaTION (ACTIVATION) is the only randomized trial to date assessing the effect of revascularization prior to TAVR. ACTIVATION was a multicenter prospective, randomized, open-label, noninferiority trial designed to assess noninferiority of percutaneous coronary intervention (PCI) prior to TAVR compared with no PCI in patients with mild angina and coexisting significant CAD. The definition of significant CAD included at least one stenosis of >70% in a major epicardial artery that was deemed suitable for PCI (or >50% if protected left main [LM] or vein graft) by the operator. The trial was terminated early due to a low recruitment total of 235 patients, short of the calculated sample size of 310 patients. The distribution and complexity of CAD were similar between groups. Most patients (71.4%) underwent single-vessel PCI with a median of one lesion treated. The most frequently treated vessel was the left anterior descending (LAD;

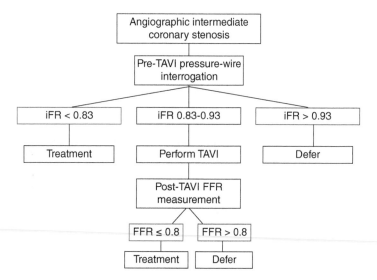

Figure 14.1 Algorithm using a hybrid instantaneous wave-free ratio–fractional flow reserve (iFR-FFR) strategy in patients undergoing transcatheter aortic valve replacement. Using a *deferral iFR* cutoff >0.93 and a *treatment iFR* cutoff <0.83 and measuring FFR only in the gray zone (0.83–0.93) would generate a 97% overall agreement with an FFR classification of lesions while sparing 62.7% of patients from adenosine. *Source:* Scarsini R et al. 2018 / With permission of Elsevier.

61.3%), and there were no target vessel failures. On average, TAVR was performed two weeks post-PCI. The primary endpoint of mortality and rehospitalization at one year was similar in patients who did and did not undergo PCI prior to TAVR, but noninferiority was not met (41.5% vs. 44.0%, absolute difference −2.5%, upper confidence interval [CI] 8.5%, one-sided noninferiority p = 0.0067). The risk of bleeding was higher at 30 days post TAVR among PCI patients (41.2% vs. 26.7%; hazard ratio [HR]: 1.46; 95% CI: 0.93–2.29), driven by the higher use and intensity of antiplatelet therapy. The incidence of acute kidney injury (AKI) was also higher in the PCI arm. Unfortunately, the ACTIVATION trial does not answer all remaining questions regarding revascularization pre-TAVR, as the population comprised highly selected patients with mild angina, mostly with one-vessel disease, and no physiological assessment.

6. What is the recommendation for the management of left main (LM) disease prior to TAVR?

Patients with LM disease are at higher risk for multiple reasons, including fluctuating hemodynamics during TAVR along with potential complications of the prosthesis or native leaflet-induced obstruction of LM during valve implantation due to the anatomical relationship of the annulus to the ostium. The TAVR-LM registry evaluated 204 patients with severe AS and concomitant LM disease who underwent TAVR and PCI. The overall one-year mortality of revascularized patients was similar to a matched control group of patients who did not undergo LM stenting. However, the group of patients who underwent unplanned emergent LM PCI because of TAVR-related complications had greater 30-day and one-year mortality, including the increased incidence of acute renal failure, cardiogenic shock, and CPR. Therefore, in patients at risk for LM occlusion after transcatheter valve deployment (low coronary origin <10 mm, effaced sinuses of Valsalva, long bulky calcified leaflets), it is reasonable to consider protecting the LM ostium during the TAVR procedure by positioning an undeployed stent at the distal LM or its proximal branches.

7. What is the optimal timing for revascularization in patients being evaluated for TAVR?

There are no definite criteria for the optimal timing of PCI in patients undergoing TAVR. In current practice, the timing of PCI is often determined by clinical judgment based on individual patient factors. First and foremost, as with any clinical decisions prior to TAVR, a patient-centered Heart Team approach is of the essence. The advantages and disadvantages of timing PCI before, during, and after TAVR are listed in Table 14.1. Considerations to keep in mind include the risk of an additional vascular access, the need to avoid multiple procedures, contrast media volume, and the need for dual antiplatelet therapy. In pivotal clinical trials, the use of PCI pre-TAVR was approximately 12% (range between 4% and 22%), with the caveat that patients with LM disease or high SS were excluded from clinical trials.

The need for PCI after TAVR is relatively low, with an incidence that ranges from 0.7% to 5.7%. An important technical consideration is the ability to selectively cannulate the coronary ostium through the prosthetic valve struts. In the REVIVAL (Registry Evaluation of Vital Information For VADs in Ambulatory Life) registry (n = 15 325), the need for unplanned PCI post-TAVR was 0.9%. The median time to PCI was 191 days, and acute coronary syndrome was the most common indication, although chronic coronary disease was more frequent beyond two years. PCI success was 100% in patients with balloon-expandable and 96.5% in patients with self-expandable valves. Therefore, maintaining coronary accessibility to selective cannulation is an important consideration in younger patients undergoing TAVR that weighs in the decision of transcatheter prosthetic valve. Young patients who already have moderate CAD may require PCI in the distant future.

8. What about completeness of revascularization in patients undergoing TAVR?

Observational studies have shown that patients with more extensive CAD (SS > 22) experience a higher incidence of adverse cardiovascular outcomes at one year and are less likely to receive complete revascularization. There is discordance among different studies regarding the association between the completeness of revascularization, as assessed by the residual SS, and improved clinical outcomes. In an elderly population with severe AS, Van Mieghem reported similar outcomes in patients with residual SS above and below 8. On the other hand, Witberg found that patients with complete revascularization (residual SS > 8) had outcomes comparable to that of patients without obstructive CAD, whereas those with incomplete revascularization (residual SS > 8) experienced higher event rates of death, myocardial infarction, and stroke at two years (78.6% vs. 16.1%; P < 0.001). A subsequent meta-analysis including six

Table 14.1 Timing of percutaneous coronary intervention (PCI), advantages, and disadvantages.

PCI before TAVR		PCI during TAVR		PCI after TAVR	
Advantages	**Disadvantages**	**Advantages**	**Disadvantages**	**Advantages**	**Disadvantages**
Simplified access to the coronaries before TAVR	Dual antiplatelet therapy after PCI and its impact on bleeding outcomes after subsequent TAVR, especially via non-TF approach	Well-suited for unstable patients	Longer procedure time	Treatment of AS may decrease ischemia, decreasing the need for PCI.	Valve struts may interfere with coronary cannulation.
Less risk of ischemia and hemodynamic instability during rapid pacing and balloon inflation during subsequent TAVR	Safety of performing PCI in the presence of severe AS	No DAPT disruption (non-transfemoral access)	Increased contrast load, risk of CK-AKI	Uncertainty about CAD contribution to symptoms	After recent TAVR, catheter manipulation could dislodge the valve. Small risk of catheter entrapment.
Lower contrast use, minimizing risk of CI-AKI	Patients with complex severe CAD may not tolerate two procedures.	One vascular access; reduces vascular complications and bleeding			
		Preferred for ostial LM or RCA lesions or at risk of coronary occlusion			

Abbreviations: TAVR, transcatheter aortic valve replacement; CI-AKI, contrast-induced acute kidney injury; AS, aortic stenosis; CAD, coronary artery disease; DAPT, dual antiplatelet therapy; LM, left main; RCA, right coronary artery.

observational studies and 3107 patients demonstrated that the degree of pre-TAVR revascularization completeness had important prognostic implications. Compared with patients with non-obstructive CAD, a residual SS > 8 was associated with an increased risk for mortality (OR, 1.85; 95% CI, 1.42–2.40; P < 0.01), whereas a residual SS < 8 was not (OR, 1.11; 95% CI, 0.89–1.39; P = 0.33). Therefore, it appears that among AS patients who have an indication for revascularization prior to TAVR, offering complete revascularization may provide an opportunity to improve long-term prognosis.

9. Are there technical considerations in patients undergoing PCI post-TAVR?

With the expansion of TAVR to low-risk and younger patients, who are likely to need subsequent angiography and revascularization, nonstructural operators need to be familiarized with the nuances of selective coronary cannulation in patients post-TAVR because the alignment of the neo-commissures of the percutaneous prosthetic valves is unpredictable. Sometimes the presence of a TAVR bioprosthesis makes selective cannulation difficult or even impossible.

The technique for cannulation depends on the type of valve. Vascular access in the femoral or radial artery does not make a difference. It is always recommended to perform a nonselective shot to better understand the anatomy and the relation of the coronary ostia to the bioprosthesis. For self-expanding valves, it is recommended to "come from above" using a wire to direct the catheter, crossing the cell coaxial to the coronary ostium. In cases of commissural misalignment, the adjacent cell may be used for subselective cannulation. Six-French catheters with a primary and secondary curve, such as Judkins, are usually preferred. Guide extension catheters may further facilitate the engagement. In patients with balloon-expandable valves, unfavorable access to a coronary ostium located behind the bioprosthesis post is encountered infrequently. A particular challenge occurs when the frame extends above the sinotubular junction. In most cases, the bioprosthesis frame is below the coronary ostia, and Judkins catheters work well in this situation. When the post is in front of the coronary ostium, subselective engagement through the adjacent cell is recommended.

10. What is the current guideline for revascularization in patients undergoing TAVR?

The 2020 American Heart Association/American College of Cardiology (AHA/ACC) Guideline for the Management of Patients with Valvular Heart Disease designates a Class I with level of evidence (LOE) C recommendation for the assessment of CAD, either with coronary CTA or invasive angiography to determine the need for revascularization. Revascularization with PCI in patients undergoing TAVR is reasonable (Class IIa, LOE C) in the presence of significant LM or proximal CAD with or without angina. However, in patients with severe and extensive CAD, with a SS > 33, the guidelines favor surgical aortic valve replacement with coronary artery bypass grafting over TAVR and PCIs with a recommendation Class IIa, LOE C. Figure 14.2 displays the algorithm proposed by the guidelines.

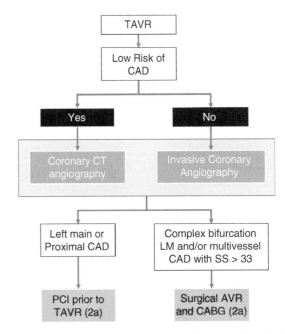

Figure 14.2 Guideline-recommended approach for decision-making in patients undergoing transcatheter aortic valve replacement with concomitant coronary artery disease.

Bibliography

1 Chakravarty, T., Sharma, R., Abramowitz, Y. et al. (2016). Outcomes in patients with transcatheter aortic valve replacement and left main stenting: the TAVR-LM registry. *J. Am. Coll. Cardiol.* 67 (8): 951–960.

2 Chieffo, A., Giustino, G., Spagnolo, P. et al. (2015). Routine screening of coronary artery disease with computed tomographic coronary angiography in place of invasive coronary angiography in patients undergoing transcatheter aortic valve replacement. *Circ. Cardiovasc. Interv.* 8 (7): e002025.

3 Faroux, L., Guimaraes, L., Wintzer-Wehekind, J. et al. (2019). Coronary artery disease and transcatheter aortic valve replacement: JACC state-of-the-art review. *J. Am. Coll. Cardiol.* 74 (3): 362–372.

4 Kotronias, R.A., Kwok, C.S., George, S. et al. (2017). Transcatheter aortic valve implantation with or without percutaneous coronary artery revascularization strategy. A systematic review and meta-analysis. *J. Am. Heart Assoc.* 6 (6): e005960.

5 Otto, C.M., Nishimura, R.A., Bonow, R.O. et al. (2021). 2020 ACC/AHA guideline for the management of patients with valvular heart disease: a report of the American College of Cardiology/American Heart Association joint committee on clinical practice guidelines. *Circulation* 143 (5): e72–e227.

6 Patterson, T., Clayton, T., Dodd, M. et al. (2021). ACTIVATION (PercutAneous Coronary inTervention prIor to transcatheter aortic VAlve implantaTION): a randomized clinical trial. *JACC Cardiovasc. Interv.* 14 (18): 1965–1974.

7 Scarsini, R., Pesarini, G., Lunardi, M. et al. (2018). Observations from a real-time, iFR-FFR "hybrid approach" in patients with severe aortic stenosis and coronary artery disease undergoing TAVI. *Cardiovasc. Revasc. Med.* 19 (3 Pt B): 355–359.

8 Stefanini, G.G., Cerrato, E., Pivato, C.A. et al. (2021). Unplanned percutaneous coronary revascularization after TAVR: a multicenter international registry. *JACC Cardiovasc. Interv.* 14 (2): 198–207.

9 Stefanini, G.G., Stortecky, S., Cao, D. et al. (2014). Coronary artery disease severity and aortic stenosis: clinical outcomes according to SYNTAX score in patients undergoing transcatheter aortic valve implantation. *Eur. Heart J.* 35 (37): 2530–2540.

10 Van Mieghem, N.M., van der Boon, R.M., Faqiri, E. et al. (2013). Complete revascularization is not a prerequisite for success in current transcatheter aortic valve implantation practice. *JACC Cardiovasc. Interv.* 6 (8): 867–875.

11 Witberg, G., Lavi, I., Harari, E. et al. (2015). Effect of coronary artery disease severity and revascularization

completeness on 2-year clinical outcomes in patients undergoing transcatether aortic valve replacement. *Coron. Artery Dis.* 26 (7): 573–582.

12 Witberg, G., Zusman, O., Codner, P. et al. (2018). Impact of coronary artery revascularization completeness on outcomes of patients with coronary artery disease undergoing transcatheter aortic valve replacement: a meta-analysis of studies using the residual SYNTAX score (synergy between PCI with Taxus and cardiac surgery). *Circ. Cardiovasc. Interv.* 11 (3): e006000.

13 Yamanaka, F., Shishido, K., Ochiai, T. et al. (2018). Instantaneous wave-free ratio for the assessment of intermediate coronary artery stenosis in patients with severe aortic valve stenosis: comparison with myocardial perfusion scintigraphy. *JACC Cardiovasc. Interv.* 11 (20): 2032–2040.

15

Conduction Disturbances Associated with TAVR

Clinical Impact and Techniques to Minimize

Camilo A. Gomez[1], Alexandre C. Ferreira[1] and Eduardo J. de Marchena[2]

[1] *Department of Cardiology, Jackson Memorial Health System, Miami, FL, USA*
[2] *Cardiovascular Division, University of Miami Miller School of Medicine, Miami, FL, USA*

1. What is the relationship between the aortic valve structures and the conduction system?

There is a close anatomical relationship between the aortic valve, the aortic annulus, and the conduction system. The bundle of His is located just below the aortic leaflets, just below the level of the membranous septum, 2–3 mm downstream from the space between the right and non-coronary cusps. The bundle of His continues beneath the membranous septum and becomes more superficial at the crest of the interventricular septum, giving rise to the left bundle. The left bundle is more superficial at the basal attachment of the right and non-coronary commissures, which makes it more vulnerable to contact and mechanical interaction during transcatheter aortic valve replacement (TAVR). Mechanical interactions may cause trauma and potential damage during TAVR, leading to tissue injury such as hematoma, edema, necrosis, or compression. These injuries can be transient or permanent, subject to the severity of the trauma. Mechanical injury can occur at different stages of the procedure: during guidewire insertion, balloon pre-dilation, valve deployment, or post-dilatation.

Aside from the mechanical interaction between the transcatheter valve and the conduction system, there is an association between aortic stenosis and baseline conduction abnormalities, mainly due to calcium deposits in the conduction system and the development of cardiomyopathy that is associated with a vulnerable conduction system. This close relationship is the key to understanding the conduction disturbances associated with TAVR (Figure 15.1).

2. What is the incidence of conduction disturbances associated with TAVR?

Despite the improvement in the incidence of periprocedural complications and death associated with TAVR, which have progressively decreased over time, conduction disturbances (new-onset persistent left bundle branch block [NOP-LBBB]) and high-degree atrioventricular block [AVB] requiring permanent pacemaker implantation [PPI]) remain the most frequent complication of TAVR procedures. These occur because of a complex interplay of patient, device, and procedural factors. The high incidence of conduction disturbances is explained by a high frequency of conduction system disease and the close anatomic proximity of the aortic valve with the conduction system. It is well described that there is a higher rate of conduction abnormalities with the self-expanding platforms in comparison to balloon-expandable valves. However, the incidence has decreased since the first-generation devices. This is the result of the improvement in transcatheter heart valve (THV) technology and engineering, in addition to better implantation techniques, in particular the depth of THV implantation.

Studies have shown a wide range of NOP-LBBB post-TAVR, ranging from 4 to 65% depending on the valve type. The incidence is higher with the self-expanding Medtronic CoreValve series, with an average of 27% (range 9–65%) and a reported incidence of 11% (range 4–18%) for the balloon-expandable Edwards Lifesciences SAPIEN valve.

Recent systematic reviews showed that the rate of PPI after TAVR with the new-generation platforms ranges from 2.3 to 36.1%. A higher incidence is reported using the

Mastering Structural Heart Disease, First Edition. Edited by Eduardo J. de Marchena and Camilo A. Gomez.
© 2023 John Wiley & Sons Ltd. Published 2023 by John Wiley & Sons Ltd.
Companion website: www.wiley.com/go/deMarchena/Mastering-Structural-Heart-Disease

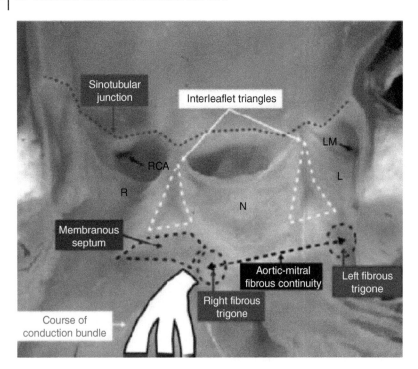

Figure 15.1 Relationship between the aortic valve structures and annulus with the conduction system. The conduction system runs below the membranous septum at the base of a triangle formed by the separation of the non-coronary and the right coronary leaflets. *Source:* Ferreira et al. (2010).

self-expanding Medtronic CoreValve/Evolut valve (14.7–26.7%) compared to the balloon-expandable Edwards SAPIEN 3 valve (4 to 24%). There is a reported incidence of 17.4% in the Evolut Low Risk Trial and 6.6% in the PARTNER 3 (Placement of Aortic Transcatheter Valves) trial. More recent smaller observations suggest a reduction in PPI after TAVR to less than 10% with self-expanding valves with expert operators and the introduction of newer implantation techniques. Other new-generation valves have demonstrated relatively low rates of PPI: 15% with the Portico valve with the FlexNav system (Abbott Vascular) and 10% with the ACURATE *neo* valve (Boston Scientific).

3. What is the clinical impact of conduction disturbances after TAVR?

The clinical impact of NOP-LBBB and complete heart block (CHB) requiring PPI remains controversial, with conflicting and limited evidence of the impact on prognosis. Compelling evidence establishes the detrimental effects of NOP-LBBB in morbidity and mortality. NOP-LBBB causes ventricular desynchrony that can negatively impact left ventricular function and also predisposes to ventricular arrhythmias. On top of that, LBBB with a very wide QRS interval (more than 160 ms) is associated with sudden cardiac death. In addition, NOP-LBBB impacts left ventricular ejection fraction (LVEF) recovery post-procedure in those with systolic dysfunction.

The clinical impact of PPI is more controversial, with some signals of a protective effect on cardiac mortality, likely explained by the prevention of high-degree aortic valve (AV) block. However, the association of PPI with late hazards such as tricuspid regurgitation, infection, pocket complications, and lead dislodgement is well described in the electrophysiology (EP) literature. Additionally, chronic right ventricular pacing has direct consequences on the myocardium because it produces ventricular desynchrony that can result in adverse LV remodeling and reduced ejection fraction.

A recent meta-analysis showed an increased risk of all-cause death and heart failure hospitalization at one year in both NOP-LBBB and PPI groups after TAVR. NOP-LBBB was associated with an increased risk of cardiac death, heart failure hospitalization, and need for a permanent pacemaker at one year following the procedure. In contrast, PPI was not associated with an increase in cardiac death but was associated with an increase in heart failure hospitalizations (Figure 15.2). Longer-term follow-up data recently published by the SWEDEHEART registry at 5–10 years showed no clear association of PPI with mortality.

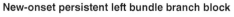

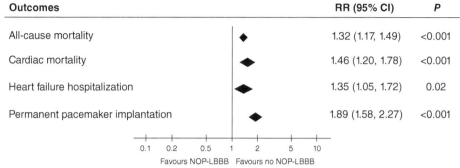

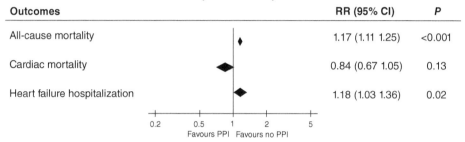

Figure 15.2 Meta-analysis assessing the risk of all-cause mortality, cardiac mortality, and heart failure hospitalization in patients with new-onset persistent left bundle branch block and patients with permanent pacemaker implantation following transcatheter aortic valve replacement. *Source:* Faroux et al. (2020) / Oxford University Press.

In terms of economic implications, conduction disturbances, and, in particular, PPI are associated with an increase in length of hospitalization and periprocedural and long-term costs.

4. What are the predictors of conduction disturbances and PPI associated with TAVR?

The predictors of conduction disturbances associated with TAVR can be divided into clinical, electrocardiographic, anatomic, or procedural factors (Figure 15.3). Operators should be aware of the conditions that increase these risks. The most important predictors are baseline conduction disturbances, use of a self-expanding valve, depth of implantation, and percentage of oversizing.

Pre-procedural conduction abnormalities – such as pre-existing right bundle branch block (RBBB), seen in 10–14% of patients and pre-existing LBBB, seen in 9–12% – increase the risk of PPI after TAVR. Other pre-existing conduction abnormalities such as baseline first-degree atrioventricular block increase the risk but with less impact on the incidence of PPI. RBBB is one of the most consistent and strong predictors of PPI; this is explained by the anatomic location of the left bundle, which makes it vulnerable to mechanical injury during the procedure. Valve platform selection is important for patients with baseline conduction abnormalities. As discussed, self-expandable valves have a higher incidence of conduction disturbances compared to balloon-expandable valves. In recent years, special attention has been paid to implantation depth in relation to the annulus, as it is strongly associated with an increased risk of PPI after TAVR regardless of the prosthesis used.

Another independent predictor is left ventricular outflow tract (LVOT) calcium location and burden: a strong association has been identified between dense calcification in the LVOT – particularly under the left and right coronary cusp, resulting in an oblique asymmetric expansion of the THV – and uneven distribution of the mechanical stress on the conduction system. More recently, with the widespread use of cardiac computed tomography (CT), the membranous septum length was identified as a predictor of PPI.

5. What strategies can be implemented to prevent or minimize conduction disturbances associated with TAVR?

Careful and meticulous planning is important, including a patient-specific risk assessment. Cardiac CT is mandatory

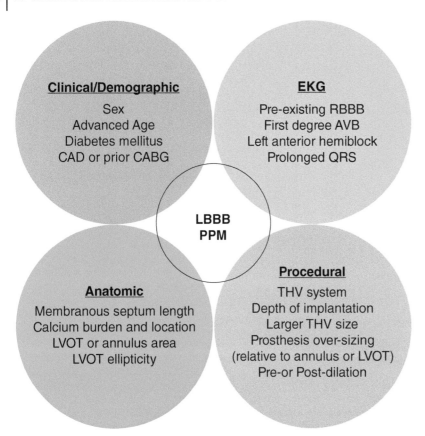

Figure 15.3 Predictors of PPI and NO-LBBB after transcatheter aortic valve replacement. *Source:* Adapted from Chen et al. (2020) / AME Publishing Company.

to evaluate the anatomy and identify predictors of conduction disturbances. Particular attention should be given to potentially modifiable risk factors. Valve selection is remarkably important for high-risk patients. A valve should be selected that best accommodates the anatomy and provides the safest profile for each individual case. Precise sizing of the valve is another important aspect to prevent overstretching and mechanical injury to the conduction system or other structures at risk of mechanical complications. Moreover, conscious pre or post balloon dilation in high-risk patients should be part of the procedure strategy. Importantly, in recent years, newer and refined implantation techniques have been introduced to prevent the impact of TAVR in the conduction system.

MIDAS Approach

As discussed, the conduction system runs below the membranous septum (MS). In 2015, the concept of the inverse relationship between MS length and the risk of AV block was first introduced by Hamdan et al. More recently,

Jilaihawi et al. described the MIDAS approach (Minimizing Depth According to the Membranous Septum), which attempts to have an implantation depth less than the MS length. This approach achieved a decreased incidence in the rate of PPI from 9.3 to 3%, and new LBBB decreased from 25.8 to 9% with the use of self-expanding valves.

Cusp Overlap Technique

The cusp overlap technique is an implantation technique introduced in recent years with the objective of lowering the potential risk of interaction of the THV and the conduction system by providing a more accurate assessment of THV depth during deployment. Observational studies have shown a decrease in the rate of conduction disturbances during TAVR using this technique. The reasoning is based on the fact that the virtual annulus or implanting plane is an imaginary structure created from the lowest points of the aortic cusps. During valve deployment, a 3D structure is created and seen as a 2D structure on fluoroscopy; this results in a perceptual change in the configuration of some structures, with the potential for foreshortening. The traditional view for implantation is the coplanar view, with the virtual annulus projected with the non-coronary cusp (NCC) on the right, the right coronary cusp (RCC) in the middle, and the left coronary cusp (LCC) on the left. The coplanar view works well for balloon-expandable valves because the valve is centered and deployed in a perpendicular view to the annulus, with the RCC projected in the center. In contrast, self-expanding valves engage the aortic valve from the outer aortic curvature and expand from the NCC toward the LCC. During the procedure, multiple adjustments to the C-arm views are frequently required to eliminate the fore-shortening of the delivery catheter. The cusp overlap view displays the LCC and RCC overlapping and isolates the NCC inferiorly. The non-right commissure is displayed in the center of the image, allowing implantation of the valve in relation to the conduction system (Figure 15.4).

Advantages of the Cusp Overlap Technique

Observational studies have demonstrated a reduction in the incidence of advanced atrioventricular block and the need for PPI using the cusp overlap technique for deploy-ment of self-expandable valves, decreasing the rates of PPI to single digits. The relationship between the cusps is better perceived during THV deployment. This approach creates a good anatomical reference for deployment depth; with this view, the LVOT and aortic root are elongated (the heart is imaged in a three-chamber view), providing an accurate perception of the THV implant depth (the opposite of the traditional three-cusp left anterior oblique (LAO)-cranial

view, where the heart is imaged in a four-chamber view with the LVOT foreshortened). This eliminates the parallax of the delivery catheter and obviates C-arm adjustments. The delivery catheter is more centered across the aortic valve. There is a perceived shorter visual distance to engage the RCC and LCC. This position results in an enface view of the NCC that facilitates higher valve implantation with-out device "pop-out" upon release (Figure 15.5).

Disadvantages of the Cusp Overlap View

In a right anterior oblique/caudal (RAO/CAU) view, the ten-sion of the delivery system and the position of the delivery catheter in relation to the inner or outer aortic curvature can-not be assessed. Once the implant depth is assessed prior to valve deployment, it is recommended to use an LAO projec-tion to check the delivery catheter position and depth in rela-tion to the LCC before the final release. Occasionally an extreme RAO/CAU angulation is required, affecting the ergonomic comfort of the operator; this is the case with verti-cal aortic annulus and obese patients. In these cases, a modi-fied projection is recommended with less extreme angulation.

High-implantation Technique for the Balloon-Expandable SAPIEN 3 Valve

Similar to the cusp overlap technique for self-expandable valves, this technique was introduced for the balloon-expandable SAPIEN 3. It is a modification of the cusp

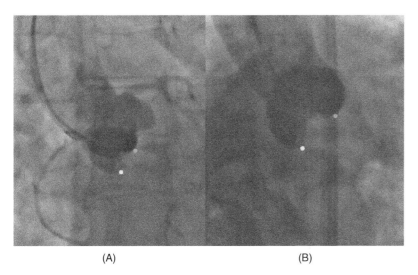

(A)   (B)

Figure 15.4 Comparison of the (a) coplanar view and (b) cusp overlap view in the same patient. In the coplanar view, the virtual annulus is projected with the non-coronary cusp (NNC) on the right, the right coronary cusp (RCC) in the middle, and the left coronary cusp (LCC) on the left. The cusp overlap view displays the LCC and RCC overlapping and isolates the NCC.

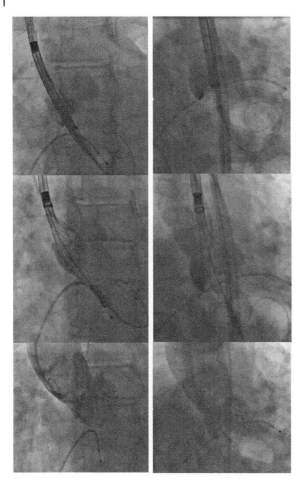

Figure 15.5 Comparison of the coplanar view (right column) and cusp overlap view (left column) in the same patient during a self-expanding transcatheter heart valve (THV) implantation. With the cusp overlap view, the relationship of all the cusps is better perceived during deployment, the delivery catheter is more centered across the aortic valve, and parallax of the delivery catheter is eliminated. There is a shorter perceived visual distance to engage the right coronary cusp (RCC) and left coronary cusp (LCC) from the non-coronary cusp (NCC). An enface view of the NCC with elongation of the left ventricular outflow tract and aortic root provides a good anatomical reference of the virtual annulus and a better assessment of the implant depth, facilitating a higher THV implantation.

overlap view: after the THV is advanced into the aortic valve and the parallax is removed, the valve is deployed in an RAO/CAU projection. The distal radiolucent line close

to the distal portion of the struts is aligned with the NCC; this permits positioning the catheter in reference to the lowest portion of the annulus, which is the NCC. A retrospective single-center analysis using this technique found that the need for PPI was reduced to 5.5% in the high implantation technique vs. 13.1% in the conventional deployment group.

6. Describe post-procedural monitoring and electrophysiological assessment after TAVR.

In patients with normal sinus rhythm and no new conduction disturbances on immediate post-procedure electrocardiogram (ECG), the risk of developing delayed AV block is less than 1%. The temporary pacemaker (TPM) can be removed immediately after the procedure. Telemetry monitoring should be continued for at least 24 hours.

Rapid atrial pacing immediately post-implant has recently been used to assess the risk of developing high-degree AV block post-TAVR. The TPM electrode can be used for rapid atrial pacing up to 120 beats per minute to predict the need for permanent pacing: patients who developed second-degree Mobitz I AV block had pacemaker rates of 13.1% vs. 1.3% (p < 0.001) at 30 days post-implant. The negative predictive value for PPM implantation in the group without Mobitz I AV block was 98.7%.

For patients with new LBBB, new PR interval prolongation or increase in QRS duration of >20 ms, or transient CHB during implant, it is reasonable to keep the TPM for 24 hours and continue telemetry monitoring for 48 hours. Patients with underlying RBBB have an incidence of CHB as high as 25%, and maintaining the ability to pace and prolonged monitoring are also advised.

The role of electrophysiological study after TAVR to guide PPM has not been studied in a randomized prospective clinical trial. Patients with RBBB, old or new LBBB with an increase in PR duration >20 ms, an isolated increase in PR duration >40 ms, and atrial fibrillation with a ventricular response <100 bpm, particularly when post-procedure LBBB is noted, are reasonable candidates for EPS.

Bibliography

1 Abdel-Wahab, M., Mehilli, J., Frerker, C. et al. (2014). Comparison of balloon-expandable vs self-expandable valves in patients undergoing transcatheter aortic valve replacement: the CHOICE randomized clinical trial. *JAMA* 311: 1503–1514. https://doi.org/10.1001/jama.2014.3316.

2 Ander Regueiro, M.D., Altisent, O.A.-J., Del Trigo, M. et al. (2016). Impact of new-onset left bundle branch block and Periprocedural permanent pacemaker implantation on clinical outcomes in patients undergoing Transcatheter aortic valve replacement. *Circ. Cardiovasc. Interv.* 9 (5): e003635. https://doi.org/10.1161/CIRCINTE RVENTIONS.115.003635.

3 Andreas Rück, A., Nawzad Saleh, A., and Glaser, N. (2021). Outcomes following permanent pacemaker implantation after Transcatheter aortic valve replacement: SWEDEHEART observational study. *J. Am. Coll. Cardiol. Intv.* 14 (19): 2173–2181. https://doi.org/10.1016/j.jcin.2021.07.043.

4 Armario, X., Rosseel, L., and Mylotte, D. Cusp overlap technique in TAVR. TAVR implantation optimization- CT analysis and practical aspects of the cusp overlap technique. *Cardiac Interv. Today* https://citoday.com/articles/2021-jan-feb-supplement/cusp-overlap-technique-in-tavr.

5 Auffret, V., Puri, R., Urena, M. et al. (2017). Conduction disturbances after Transcatheter aortic valve replacement. Current status and future perspectives. *Circulation* 136: 1049–1069. https://doi.org/10.1161/CIRCULATIONAHA.117.028352.

6 Chen, S., Chau, K., and Nazif, T. (2020). The incidence and impact of cardiac conduction disturbances after Transcatheter aortic valve replacement. *Ann. Cardiothorac. Surg.* 9 (6): 452–467. https://doi.org/10.21037/acs-2020-av-23.

7 Faroux, L., Chen, S., Muntané-Carol, G. et al. (2020). Clinical impact of conduction disturbances in transcatheter aortic valve replacement recipients: a systematic review and meta-analysis. *Eur. Heart J.* 41 (29): 2771–2781. https://doi.org/10.1093/eurheartj/ehz924.

8 Ferreira, N.D., Caeiro, D., Adão, L. et al. (2010). Incidence and predictors of permanent pacemaker requirement after transcatheter aortic valve implantation with a self-expanding bioprosthesis. *Pacing Clin. Electrophysiol.* 33: 1364–1372. https://doi.org/10.1111/j.1540-8159.2010.02870.x.

9 Hamdan, A., Guetta, V., Klempfner, R. et al. (2015). Inverse relationship between membranous septal length and the risk of atrioventricular block in patients undergoing transcatheter aortic valve implantation. *JACC Cardiovasc. Interv* 8: 1218–1228.

10 Jilaihawi, H., Zhao, Z., Du, R. et al. (2019). Minimizing permanent pacemaker following repositionable self-expanding transcatheter aortic valve replacement. *J. Am. Coll. Cardiovasc. Interv.* 12: 1796–1807. https://doi.org/10.1016/j.jcin.2019.05.056.

11 Krishnaswamy, A., Sammour, Y., Mangieri, A. et al. (2020). The utility of rapid atrial pacing immediately post-TAVR to predict the need for pacemaker implantation. *J. Am. Coll. Cardiol. Intv.* 13: 1046–1054.

12 Mack, M.J., Leon, M.B., Thourani, V.H. et al. (2019). Transcatheter aortic-valve replacement with balloon expandable valve in low-risk patients. *N. Engl. J. Med.* 380: 1695–1705.

13 Pisaniello, A.D., Makki, H.B.E., Jahangeer, S. et al. (2021). Low rates of permanent pacing are observed following self-expandingtranscatheter aortic valve replacement using an annular plane projection forDeployment. *Circ. Cardiovasc. Interv.* 14: e009258.

14 Popma, J.J., Deeb, G.M., Yakubov, S.J. et al. (2019). Transcatheter aortic-valve replacement with a self-expanding valve in low-risk patients. *N. Engl. J. Med.* 380: 1706–1715.

15 Regueiro, A., Abdul-Jawad Altisent, O., Del Trigo, M. et al. (2016). Impact of new-onset left bundle branch block and periprocedural permanent pacemaker implantation on clinical outcomes in patients undergoing transcatheter aortic valve replacement: a systematic review and meta-analysis. *Circ. Cardiovasc. Interv.* 9: e003635.

16 Sammour, Y., Banerjee, K., Kumar, A. et al. (2021). Systematic approach to high implantation of SAPIEN-3 valve achieves a lower rate of conduction abnormalities including pacemaker implantation. *Circ. Cardiovasc. Interv.* 14: e009407.

17 Tang, G.H.L., Zaid, S., Michev, I. et al. (2018). "Cusp-overlap" view simplifies fluoroscopy-guided implantation of self-expanding valve in transcatheter aortic valve replacement. *JACC Cardiovasc. Interv.* 11: 1663–1665. https://doi.org/10.1016/j.jcin.2018.03.018.

18 Tovia-Brodie, O., Ben-Haim, Y., Joffe, E. et al. (2017). The value of electrophysiologic study in decision-making regarding the need for pacemaker implantation after TAVI. *J. Interv. Card. Electrophysiol.* 48: 121–130.

16

Management of Conduction Disturbances Post-TAVR

Alex H. Velasquez and Raul Mitrani

Division of Cardiology, University of Miami, Miami, FL, USA

1. What are the components of normal conduction from sinus node to ventricular tissue?

Impulses generated from the sinus node propagate through atrial tissue, the atrioventricular node, the atrioventricular (AV) bundle (bundle of His), the right and left bundle branches (RBB and LBB) (the LBB bifurcates into the left anterior and left posterior fascicles); and Purkinje fibers that terminate at the myocardial cells.

2. Match the components of the conduction system to the following intervals

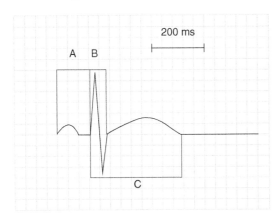

a. PR
b. QRS
c. QT

1. Depolarization of atrium
2. Depolarization of AV node
3. Depolarization of AV bundle (bundle of His)
4. Depolarization of bundle branches
5. Depolarization of fascicles
6. Depolarization of myocardium
7. Depolarization and repolarization of the myocardium

The PR segment includes several components of cardiac conduction. It includes the intra-atrial conduction time, AV node conduction time, and the AV bundle (bundle of His) conduction time. Differences in conduction time or conduction block between the bundles and fascicles can lead to bundle branch block or fascicular block. The QRS duration results from myocardial depolarization. Delay or block in either of the bundle branches results in propagation of action potentials from one cell to adjacent cells through low resistance intercellular gap junctions, which occurs at a slower rate for the portion of myocardium not depolarized rapidly through the His-Purkinje system. Thus, a longer time is required to complete ventricular depolarization. The QT includes both the time required to depolarize the ventricle and the time required to re-polarize the ventricle.

3. What components of the conduction system are susceptible to injury during transcatheter aortic valve replacement (TAVR) implantation?

The AV node resides within the triangle of Koch defined by the tendon of Todaro, the attachment of the tricuspid valve, and the ostium of the coronary sinus.

The AV bundle (Bundle of His) resides in the inferior-anterior border of the membranous septum (MS). This is in proximity to the aortic root complex adjacent to the commissure between the right and non-coronary cusps.

The LBB is a continuation of the branching portion of the AV bundle, which resides in the anterior one-half to two-thirds of the infra-anterior border of MS. The LBB penetrates the deep ventricular septum at various levels. It can enter the superficial portion of the left ventricular septum close to the MS (Figure 16.1).

4. At what operative stage can AV conduction abnormalities be encountered?

AV conduction abnormalities can be encountered pre-operatively, during the procedure prior to valve deployment, during valve deployment, and after. A significant portion of patients can be observed to have high-degree AV conduction abnormalities or severe bradycardia with 24 hours of continuous ECG monitoring prior to TAVR. Transient Injury to the AV bundle can be seen with manipulation of wires and catheters during the pre-deployment phase of TAVR implantation. Although a majority of patients will develop high-degree AV block/complete heart block (HAVB/CHB) within 48 hours after TAVR implantation, up to 10% of patients will develop HAVB/CHB beyond 48 hours when observed with ambulatory 30 day real-time mobile cardiac telemetry device.

5. What changes to the EKG can be anticipated after TAVR?

Bradycardia can manifest as sinus node dysfunction or AV conduction disturbance. AV conduction abnormalities include a new left bundle branch block (LBBB), prolongation of PR interval, second-degree AV block, and CHB. Sinus node dysfunction is often pre-existing and discovered during continuous EKG monitoring in the pre- and post-TAVR phase. PR prolongation can manifest from slow conduction through the AV node or impaired conduction through the AV bundle because of injury to these structures.

6. What pre-operative EKG finding is the strongest predictor of post-TAVR conduction disturbances and pacemaker requirement? Why?

Pre-operative right bundle branch block (RBBB) is recognized as the strongest predictor of post-operative HAVB/CHB necessitating permanent pacemaker implantation. Although injury to the AV bundle proximal to the diverging AV bundle can result in CHB, injury to the proximal LBB is common, persisting at discharge or 30 days after TAVR in ~55% of cases. Combined with RBBB, LBBB results in CHB.

7. What procedural factors have been associated with higher risk of post-TAVR conduction disturbances?

Several procedural factors affect the likelihood that post-TAVR pacemaker implantation will be required, including valve pre-dilation with balloon valvuloplasty, prosthetic valve type, final prosthetic valve position (including depth and proximity to the AV bundle), and valve oversizing.

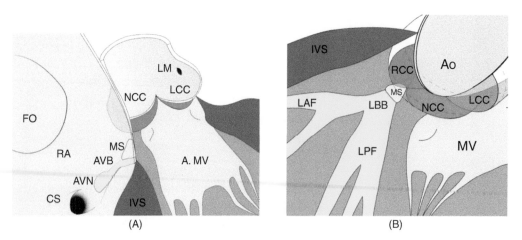

Figure 16.1 Atrioventricular junction. AMV, anterior mitral valve; Ao, aorta; AVB, atrioventricular bundle; AVN, atrioventricular node; CS, coronary sinus; FO, fossa ovalis; IVS, interventricular septum; LAF, left anterior fascicle; LBB, left bundle branch; LCC, left coronary cusp; LM, left main; LPF, left posterior fascicle; MS, membranous septum; MV, mitral valve; NCC, non-coronary cusp; RA, right atrium.

8.   At what point should a 12-lead EKG be performed to determine the duration of temporary pacing wire and post-operative telemetry?

A 12-lead EKG should be performed prior to the case and at the end of the case before removal of the trans-venous catheter to assess PR interval and QRS duration. CHB during the case if not present at the end of the case should be noted.

9.   A patient with the pre-operative EKG shown here undergoes TAVR. No change in EKG is seen at the end of the procedure. What is recommended for the duration of temporary pacing and telemetry monitoring?

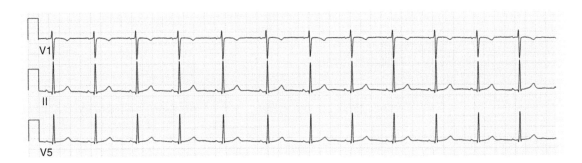

The patient's temporary pacemaker may be discontinued at the end of the procedure since no change to the PR or QRS was noted. The patient should still be observed for 24 hours (or at least overnight) by telemetry for bradyarrhythmia or new conduction disturbances. Without any further changes, the patient may be discharged on the first post-operative day.

10.   What is the likelihood that a patient with this EKG will require a pacemaker implant after TAVR?

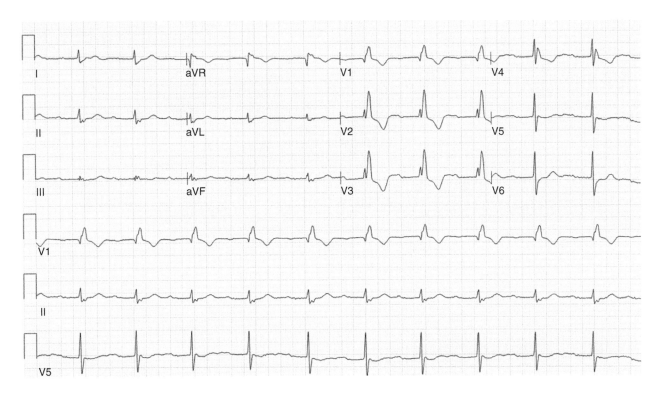

More than 25% of patients with pre-existing RBBB will develop HAVB/CHB that requires pacemaker implantation. Using a valve prosthesis that is not self-expanding and has a higher valve position reduces the risk of AV block.

11. The patient in question 10 has no change in the 12-lead EKG at the end of the procedure. How long after the TAVR procedure is temporary pacing recommended?

Temporary transvenous pacing is recommended for 24 hours or at least overnight. Abrupt loss of conduction in the left bundle can result in CHB. Without a reliable ventricular escape rhythm, asystole can occur.

12. A patient who undergoes TAVR has the pre-operative EKG shown in (a) and the post-procedure EKG shown in (b). What management decisions are recommended for this scenario?

A transvenous RV lead should be continued for 24 hours or at least overnight for new-onset LBBB (Figure 16.2). An EKG should be repeated at 24 hours to determine if the PR interval and QRS are stable. If PR is seen to lengthen or QRS widens further, a temporary pacemaker should be left in place for another 24 hours. Progression to CHB requires pacemaker implantation. Resolution of PR lengthening

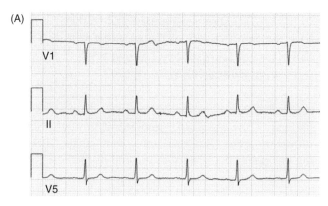

(A)

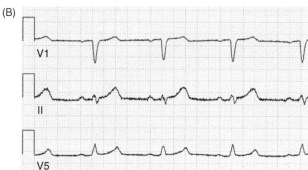

(B)

and LBBB allow removal of temporary pacemaker and observation of EKG for 24 hours.

13. The patient from question 12 develops the following EKG 10 hours after LBBB was noticed after TAVR. What pacemaker configuration will maintain atrioventricular synchrony?

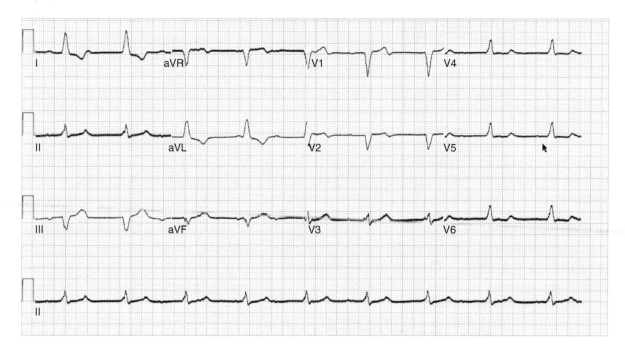

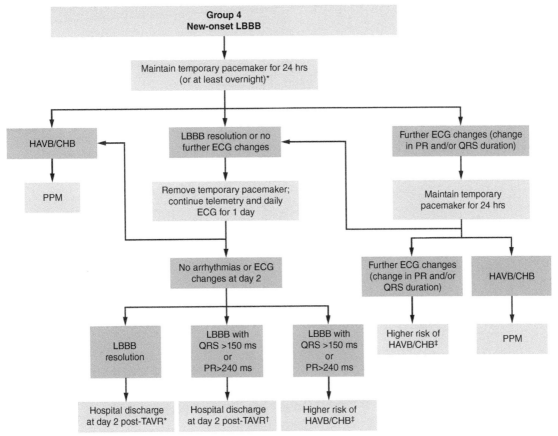

* Consider earlier discontinuation of temporary pacing along with hospital discharge at day 1 if partial/complete resolution of LBBB in <24h.

† Consider continuous ECG monitoring at hospital discharge.

‡ Consider: 1) invasive EPS to guide the decision about PPM; 2) continuous ECG monitoring at hospital discharge; 3) PPM.

Figure 16.2 Strategy algorithm proposal for the management of patients with new-onset left bundle branch block post-TAVR.

AV synchrony is best maintained by a dual-chamber pacemaker with an atrial and ventricular lead. Alternatively, a leadless pacemaker with an atrial sensing accelerometer algorithm can provide up to 89% AV synchrony. However, this configuration may not be optimal if atrial tracking is expected to be above 105 bpm.

14. A patient with severe aortic stenosis and moderately reduced systolic function receives TAVR and develops the rhythm shown here, associated with dizziness, post-TAVR. What kind of pacing configuration is less likely to result in persistent systolic dysfunction?

The EKG shows second-degree AV block with a 2 : 1 pattern. With a 2 : 1 pattern, Mobitz I or Mobitz II second-degree AV block is possible. Two characteristics of this tracing indicate that the level of AV block is lower than the AV node. First, the PR segment is short, suggesting that the AV node conduction time is preserved and unlikely to block abruptly. Second, the QRS is wide, with a right bundle branch pattern indicating a diseased His-Purkinje system. These findings associated with dizziness are sufficient to justify pacemaker implantation. This patient is likely to require high-degree or right ventricular pacing. Up to 20% of patients with high right ventricular pacing burden develop systolic dysfunction. For those with mild systolic dysfunction at the time of pacing indication, cardiac resynchronization or physiologic pacing has been shown to reduce re-hospitalization. Biventricular pacing or His-bundle pacing is recommended (IIa) for patients with systolic dysfunction (left ventricular ejection fraction [LVEF] <50%) and right ventricular pacing requirement anticipated to be >40%

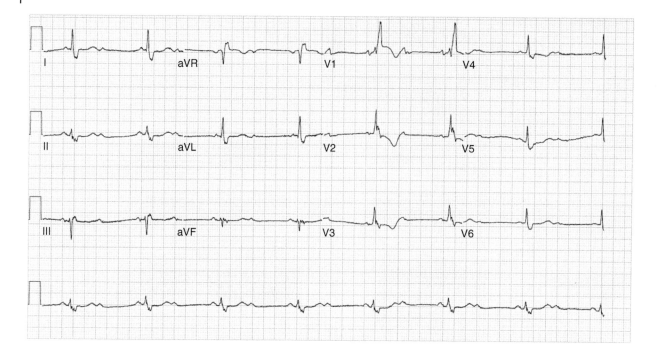

15. Pre-operatively, an 88-year-old man has the EKG shown in (a); 48 hours after TAVR, he has the EKG shown in (b). An electrophysiology study is performed. The intra-cardiac electrocardiograms are shown in (c). Does this patient require a pacemaker?

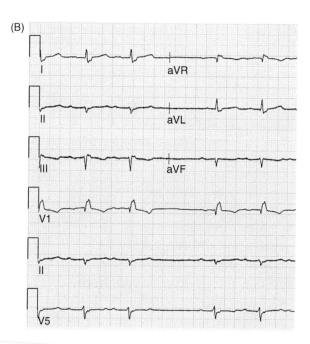

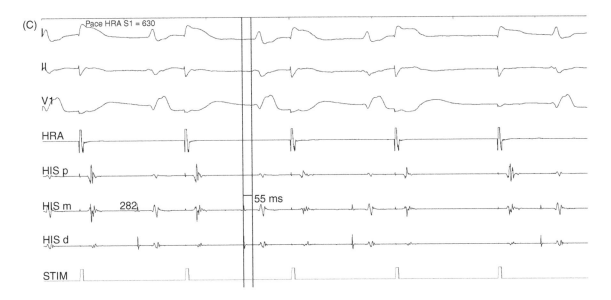

The patient's pre-operative EKG shows sinus rhythm with first-degree AV block, RBBB, and left anterior fascicular block. The baseline PR interval and QRS duration were 270 ms and 156 ms, respectively. The likelihood of developing CHB post-TAVR due to infra-His block in this setting is high. At 48 hours post-TAVR, the EKG shows prolongation of the PR interval (304 ms), QRS duration of 154 ms, and blocked premature atrial complexes. The intra-cardiac EGM shows a normal His-ventricular (HV) conduction time of 55 ms. The PR interval comprises the intra-atrial conduction time, Atrial–His conduction time (A–H interval), and HV conduction. The PR interval was prolonged due to prolonged AH conduction time. HV conduction time >100 ms is an indication for pacemaker implantation due to the high risk of CHB. Increased HV time >65 has been associated with a need for pacemaker implantation. 30-day real-time mobile cardiac telemetry monitoring can be employed to detect worsening of AV block. Delayed HAVB necessitating permanent pacemaker implantation can occur in patients beyond 48 hours. In patients with RBBB, the incidence of delayed HAVB is higher.

Bibliography

1 Auffret, V., Puri, R., Urena, M. et al. (2017). Conduction disturbances after transcatheter aortic valve replacement. *Circulation* 136 (11): 1049–1069. https://doi.org/10.1161/circulationaha.117.028352.

2 Auffret, V., Webb, J.G., Eltchaninoff, H. et al. (2017). Clinical impact of baseline right bundle branch block in patients undergoing transcatheter aortic valve replacement. *JACC Cardiovasc. Interv.* 10 (15): 1564–1574. https://doi.org/10.1016/j.jcin.2017.05.030.

3 Ferreira, T., Da Costa, A., Cerisier, A. et al. (2021). Predictors of high-degree conduction disturbances and pacemaker implantation after transcatheter aortic valve replacement: prognostic role of the electrophysiological study. *Pacing Clin. Electrophysiol.* 44 (5): 843–855. https://doi.org/10.1111/pace.14225.

4 Kawashima, T. and Sato, F. (2014). Visualizing anatomical evidences on atrioventricular conduction system for TAVI. *Int. J. Cardiol.* 174 (1): 1–6. https://doi.org/10.1016/j.ijcard.2014.04.003.

5 Kusumoto, F.M., Schoenfeld, M.H., Barrett, C. et al. (2019). 2018 ACC/AHA/HRS guideline on the evaluation and management of patients with bradycardia and cardiac conduction delay: a report of the American College of Cardiology/American Heart Association task force on clinical practice guidelines and the heart rhyth. *Circulation* 140 (8): https://doi.org/10.1161/cir.0000000000000628.

6 Niu, H.X., Liu, X., Gu, M. et al. (2021). Conduction system pacing for post transcatheter aortic valve replacement patients: comparison with right ventricular pacing. *Front. Cardiovasc. Med.* 8: 772548. (In eng). https://doi.org/10.3389/fcvm.2021.772548.

7 Ream, K., Sandhu, A., Valle, J. et al. (2019). Ambulatory rhythm monitoring to detect late high-grade atrioventricular block following transcatheter aortic valve replacement. *J. Am. Coll. Cardiol.* 73 (20): 2538–2547. https://doi.org/10.1016/j.jacc.2019.02.068.

8 Rodés-Cabau, J., Ellenbogen, K.A., Krahn, A.D. et al. (2019). Management of conduction disturbances associated with transcatheter aortic valve replacement. *J. Am. Coll. Cardiol.* 74 (8): 1086–1106. https://doi.org/10.1016/j.jacc.2019.07.014.

9 Steinwender, C., Khelae, S.K., Garweg, C. et al. (2020). Atrioventricular synchronous pacing using a leadless ventricular pacemaker. *JACC Clin. Electrophysiol.* 6 (1): 94–106. https://doi.org/10.1016/j.jacep.2019.10.017.

10 Urena, M., Hayek, S., Cheema, A.N. et al. (2015). Arrhythmia burden in elderly patients with severe aortic stenosis as determined by continuous electrocardiographic recording. *Circulation* 131 (5): 469–477. https://doi.org/10.1161/circulationaha.114.011929.

11 Vijayaraman, P., Cano, Ó., Koruth, J.S. et al. (2020). His-Purkinje conduction system pacing following transcatheter aortic valve replacement. *JACC Clin. Electrophysiol.* 6 (6): 649–657. https://doi.org/10.1016/j.jacep.2020.02.010.

17

TAVR Mechanical Complications Prevention and Management

Christian McNeely and John M. Lasala

Cardiovascular Division, Department of Medicine, Washington University School of Medicine, St. Louis, MO, USA

Annular Rupture

1. What constitutes annular rupture in TAVR?

Annular rupture is a term that encompasses a spectrum of procedural-related injuries in the region of the aortic root and left ventricular outflow tract during transcatheter aortic valve replacement (TAVR). Annular rupture can be uncontained, with frank extravasation, or contained, as manifested by new periaortic hematoma.

2. How do you classify annular rupture after TAVR?

We can classify annular rupture by whether it is contained or uncontained and also by the region of injury. The region of injuries can be intra-annular; sub-annular, such as the intraventricular septum; supra-annular, such as the sinus of Valsalva or sinotubular juncture; or a combined rupture that involves multiple anatomic areas.

3. How often does annular rupture occur?

Annular rupture occurs in about 1% of all TAVR procedures. In the largest cohort studying annular rupture, root rupture accounted for approximately two-thirds of these cases and periaortic hematoma one-third. The prevalence of undetected annular rupture remains unknown, particularly contained ruptures, especially with increasing use of transthoracic in place of transesophageal echo.

4. Why does annular rupture happen with TAVR?

Annular injury and rupture may occur during multiple phases of the procedure, including balloon pre-dilatation of the native aortic valve, prosthetic valve deployment, or valve post-dilatation for paravalvular leakage (PVL). Annular rupture is largely seen with balloon-expandable valves, although there are case reports of rupture with self-expandable valves during post-dilatation of the prosthesis to treat residual PVL.

5. What are the risk factors for annular rupture with TAVR?

In a large cohort of TAVR patients, moderate to severe left ventricular outflow tract (LVOT)/sub-annular calcifications and aggressive annular oversizing ($\geq$20%) were shown to be the strongest risk factors for annular rupture. Moderate to severe LVOT calcifications were defined by two or more nodules of calcium or one extending >5mm or covering >10% of the LVOT. Ruptures tend to occur in patients with both of these risk factors; however, they can occur in patients with one or none of these established risk factors. A number of other risk factors have been reported, including post-dilatation, small annuli, narrow root, annulus eccentricity, chronic immunosuppressive therapy, and heavy leaflet/annular calcification/sinus of Valsalva calcification.

Mastering Structural Heart Disease, First Edition. Edited by Eduardo J. de Marchena and Camilo A. Gomez.
© 2023 John Wiley & Sons Ltd. Published 2023 by John Wiley & Sons Ltd.
Companion website: www.wiley.com/go/deMarchena/Mastering-Structural-Heart-Disease

6. What are the outcomes of annular rupture?

Overall, in-hospital mortality is high, reported at around 50%. The mortality rate varies considerably depending on whether the rupture is contained. In one of the largest series studying annular ruptures, all of the deaths occurred in patients with uncontained ruptures, with an overall mortality rate of 75%. However, of patients who are able to undergo emergent surgery, likely at least 50% will survive. The long-term complications and prognosis, particularly of contained ruptures managed conservatively, remain unknown.

7. How do you diagnose annular rupture?

The presentation of annular rupture can range from asymptomatic to immediate hemodynamic collapse, depending on the location and severity of the injury. Rupture should be suspected in the case of new-onset pericardial effusion, hemodynamic changes, aortic wall thickening or dissection, hematoma between the aorta and pulmonary artery, or a new intracardiac shunt such as a ventricular septal defect (VSD). Intraprocedurally, transesophageal echocardiography (TEE) is typically able to identify annular rupture as well as characterize any associated paravalvular regurgitation. Angiography can also be helpful but is of less value in the case of intra-annular injury, particularly if there is no relevant paravalvular or valvular regurgitation. Post-procedurally, cardiac computed tomography (CT) and/or TEE can be used for surveillance, depending on the location of the rupture and whether there is any relevant regurgitation.

8. How do you treat annular rupture?

The treatment for rupture depends on the location, type of rupture, and sequelae of the injury (Figure 17.1). In the typical case where the diagnosis is made intraprocedurally,

Surgical Treatment According to the Type of Annular Rupture	
Type of Rupture	**Treatment**
1. Intra-annular	Repair* of the lesion + AVR
2. Subannular	
a. Injury of the free myocardial wall	Reconstruction of the LVOT from inside the LVOT with a pericardial patch using transaortic approach† + AVR
b. Injury of the anterior mitral leaflet	Repair with a pericardial patch ± MVR‡ + AVR
c. Injury of the interventricular septum	Repair* + AVR
3. Supra-annular	
a. Injury of the wall of sinus of Valsalva	Repair* of the lesion + AVR or composite valved graft
b. Injury of a coronary ostium	Composite valved graft or repair of the lesion + AVR ± stenting of a coronary ostium/CABG
c. Injury of the sinotubular junction	Repair* of the lesion ± AVR or supracoronary aortic tube graft replacement ± AVR
4. Combined	
a. Intra- and supra-annular	Repair* of the lesion + AVR or composite valved graft
b. Intra-annular and subannular	Repair* of the lesion + AVR ± MVR
c. Intra-annular, supra-annular, and subannular	Composite valved graft ± MVR or repair* of the lesion + AVR ± MVR

*Using pericardial patch or pledgeted sutures. †No attempts should be made to close the rupture from outside the left ventricle by using U-stitches because bleeding stops when the LVOT is reconstructed. The danger of damaging the coronary arteries by myocardial sutures from the outside is very high; this would lead to myocardial infarction and unsuccessful weaning from cardiopulmonary bypass. ‡Performed via a transaortic approach with additional incision of the left atrial roof and reconstruction of the intervalvular fibrous body using 2 pericardial patches.

AVR = aortic valve replacement; CABG = coronary artery bypass grafting; LVOT = left ventricular outflow tract; MVR = mitral valve replacement.

Figure 17.1 Surgical treatment according to the type of annular rupture. *Source:* Pasic et al. (2015) / With permission of Elsevier.

the immediate goal is to restore or maintain hemodynamics, with initiation of cardiopulmonary bypass, usually via the femoral route. At this point, the exact nature of the injury can be explored via TEE, angiography if needed, and direct visualization through sternotomy. Typically, for uncontained ruptures, surgical repair of the lesion and aortic valve replacement is the preferred strategy. If there is supra-annular injury, repair of the aorta will need to be done; and in the case of sub-annular injury, LVOT repair with patching will frequently be necessary. For small lesions, such as a periaortic hematoma, conservative therapy may be considered, with reversal of anticoagulation and close surveillance, particularly if the patient is of high surgical risk. Percutaneous coil embolization or use of vascular plugs has also been reported in select cases, although this is not the default treatment for the large majority of patients. The long-term outcomes of patients treated conservatively remain in question, but it has been observed that some of these patients die during the post-operative period.

9. How do you prevent annular rupture?

Identifying and characterizing the risk for rupture pre-procedurally is the most crucial component of preventing this complication. These risk factors were previously described, but severe LVOT calcification, large (4–5 mm) calcific nodules and heavily calcified bicuspid valves should raise concern. Once a patient is considered to be at high anatomic risk for rupture, the Heart Team should discuss whether conventional surgical AVR, TAVR, or even conservative therapy is the best treatment option. If not already being treated at a high-volume TAVR center, referral to one should be made. If TAVR is decided on, procedural modifications should be employed to reduce the risk for this complication. One should avoid significantly ($\geq$20%) oversizing the valve, consider high valve deployment in the case of LVOT calcium, avoid valve post-dilatation for residual leak, and consider the use of a self-expandable valve.

Perforation and Tamponade

10. How does cardiac tamponade occur in TAVR?

Typically, tamponade is the result of perforation of one of three different structures: the right ventricle (RV), left ventricle (LV), or aortic root. We addressed aortic root rupture earlier.

11. Why does ventricular perforation occur?

RV perforation is usually secondary to improper placement or manipulation of the temporary pacing wire. LV perforation typically is secondary to trauma from the stiff delivery wire. LV perforation from the delivery wire is likely more common with the use of pre-shaped stiff wires.

12. How common is ventricular perforation in TAVR?

Ventricular perforation has been reported at around 1% of most series. Overall, RV perforation accounts for the majority of ventricular perforations.

13. How do you diagnose and manage perforation?

The diagnosis of perforation should always be suspected in the case of new pericardial effusion or hemodynamic deterioration of the patient. Typically, TEE is able to characterize the size and hemodynamic consequences of perforation. RV perforations can almost always be managed conservatively or with pericardiocentesis, rarely requiring surgical repair. However, in the case of a posterior effusion, these may be difficult to access from a percutaneous approach.

For LV perforations, management depends on the type and extent of injury, clinical status, and operative candidacy. In free LV perforations, there is typically rapid hemodynamic instability requiring immediate initiation of cardiopulmonary bypass, sternotomy, and open repair. If there is a small LV perforation, percutaneous drainage may be possible, but vigilant monitoring is required. In cases of LV pseudoaneurysm, percutaneous plug placement and open repair are treatment options, depending on the size of the defect and overall operative candidacy.

14. What are the outcomes after perforation?

If recognized early and managed with drainage, RV perforations usually have a favorable outcome and rarely need surgical repair. LV perforations with subsequent tamponade carry a very high mortality, with the majority of patients dying in-hospital.

15. How can you prevent cardiac perforations in TAVR?

RV perforation is likely more frequent with the use of screw-in leads rather than passive balloon-tipped pacing catheters, so screw-in leads should be avoided whenever possible. With balloon-tipped catheters, overly aggressive wire manipulation in an attempt to achieve optimal thresholds should also be discouraged. This is particularly relevant in elderly patients and patients on chronic steroids due to the thinner and more fragile RV. LV perforations are typically secondary to the improper use of self-shaped, stiff support wires. The use of a dedicated TAVR wire (e.g. Safari or Confida) is likely safer than self-shaped wires. If the operator chooses to - shape stiff wires, one should be diligent in ensuring an appropriate curve has been made. One should closely monitor the transition point in the LV from the soft tip to the stiff wire as monitor wire position during manipulations and balloon inflation. Direct LV pacing via the standard delivery wire is also a strategy used by some centers that avoids an additional vascular access and replaces the need for a temporary RV pacemaker. However, inconsistent capture is a frequent criticism of pacing via the standard LV delivery wire.

There is likely to be continued device innovation in this space. A dedicated bipolar pacing wire that supports TAVR valve deployment (Wattson wire) is currently being tested; it would obviate the need for a temporary RV pacemaker and potentially provide more stable pacing.

Bioprosthetic Valve Infolding

16. What is prosthetic valve infolding?

Prosthetic valve infolding is an uncommon complication seen with the use of self-expanding valves (SEVs) for TAVR. It occurs when the valve frame is infolded during deployment with secondary distortion and malfunction of the prosthesis. This was initially described in the first-generation CoreValve, but it has also been reported in the Evolut R and Evolut Pro.

17. What are the consequences of prosthetic valve infolding?

Infolding can lead to severe paravalvular and intravalvular leakage with hemodynamic collapse owing to valve dysfunction. Infolding is also associated with an increased rate of peri-procedural stroke, likely secondary to the need for further manipulation of the valve.

18. Why does valve infolding occur?

The mechanism for infolding is unclear but is likely related to the low radial force of the Nitinol frame. This is particularly relevant with larger valves because they have lower radial force by nature of their design.

19. What are risk factors for valve infolding?

Risk factors include valve- and patient-related characteristics. Valve-related characteristics that predispose to infolding of SEVs include re-sheathing and larger valves (≥29 mm). Patient-related risk factors include bicuspid valves and heavy calcification.

20. How common is valve infolding?

The largest available case series, which included patients from 2015 to 2020 and included first- and second-generation SEVs, reported a valve infolding rate of 3.15%. More contemporary case series with only Evolut R reported a lower rate: 0.7% (3/420).

21. How can you diagnose valve infolding?

If there is severe paravalvular leak and/or hemodynamic instability after valve SEV deployment, valve infolding should be suspected. Signs of valve infolding can be seen on fluoroscopy, including a narrower than expected valve prosthesis and a vertical line along the valve frame. Meticulous attention should be paid to evaluating the valve frame with multiple fluoroscopic angles or the cusp-overlap technique prior to release. In addition, a right anterior oblique (RAO) – cranial view looking down the valve on the short axis can confirm this diagnosis. On echocardiography, the infolded valve is easily recognized, particularly on the short axis (Figure 17.2).

22. How do you treat valve infolding?

If valve infolding is recognized prior to release, recapture and replacement with a new transcatheter heart valve (THV) is preferred, given the severe potential consequences of

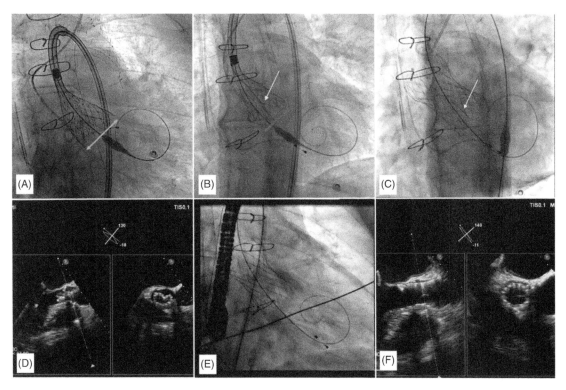

Figure 17.2 Fluoroscopic and echocardiographic diagnosis of a 34 mm Evolut R stent frame that infolded and required repositioning after complete valve release. (a) Fluoroscopy shows a normal transverse diameter (green arrow) after the first deployment. (b, c) After resheathing and redeployment, the transverse diameter of the prosthesis is narrower than expected (red arrow), and the string sign (yellow arrow) is visible as a vertical line after complete valve release. (d) Transesophageal echocardiography shows the Pac-Man sign confirming prosthesis infolding. (e, f) Infolding is resolved after balloon post-dilatation of the prosthesis: the string sign is no longer visible at fluoroscopy, and the prosthesis appears circular at transesophageal echocardiography Color figure can be viewed at http://wileyonlinelibrary.com. *Source:* Ancona et al. (2020).

infolding. If this complication is not noticed until after valve deployment, immediate post-dilatation is required to restore the valve function and avoid hemodynamic collapse. Typically, post-dilatation can eliminate the infolding. If this is unsuccessful, retrieval and deployment of a new valve will be necessary. Whether there are long-term consequences to the valve after post-dilatation for infolding is unknown.

Valve Embolization

23. What is transcatheter valve embolization?

The term *valve embolization* implies permanent loss of contact of the valve prosthesis with the native valve structure. The valve most commonly embolizes to the ascending aorta but can also be in the LV or descending aorta. Migration of the THV can also occur, where there can be varying degrees of displacement within minutes or even days after implantation.

24. How common is valve embolization?

With increasing experience, the incidence of valve embolization has become quite uncommon. In the low-risk PARTNER (Placement of Aortic Transcatheter Valves) trial, there were no reported cases of valve embolization. However, in real-world experience, valve embolization occurs more frequently than in trials with carefully selected patients and highly experienced centers. In a large TAVR registry, transcatheter valve embolization or migration (TVEM) occurred in 273 patients (0.92%) of 29 636 procedures. Of these cases, 20% THVs embolized to the LV, while the majority migrated or embolized to the ascending aorta.

25. What is the cause of TVEM?

There are multiple potential causes for TVEM, most technical in nature. Malpositioning is the most common cause, accounting for around 50% of cases. Other technical causes were improper valve manipulation and use of the delivery catheter, significant valve undersizing, and failure of rapid pacing. The main patient-related factor that is a risk factor for TVEM is a bicuspid valve with slightly higher rates of implantation of a second valve or conversion to open surgery.

26. How do you treat TVEM?

The treatment strategy largely depends on the embolized location (Figure 17.3). If the valve has embolized to the LV, open surgery typically is performed for removal; however, there have been reports of balloon-assisted retrieval with a second attempt at reimplantation after identifying the cause. If the valve embolizes to the aorta, it can typically be managed with percutaneous techniques. A balloon-expandable valve can typically be maneuvered with a balloon in place, while SEVs usually require snares (Medtronic Amplatz Goose Neck or Merit Medical EN Snare).

The THV is typically pulled to an area of the lumen that is sized appropriately for the valve and does not compromise flow to important branches. Pulling the THV back across the arch should be avoided whenever possible due to the risk of arch dissection and stroke. There have been reports of implanting a covered stent across this maldeployed valve, but this is not typically required as the second prosthesis in the aorta does not appear to cause hemodynamic consequences. After the embolized valve is deployed in a stable position, a second THV is implanted by traversing through the first valve and realigning with the annulus.

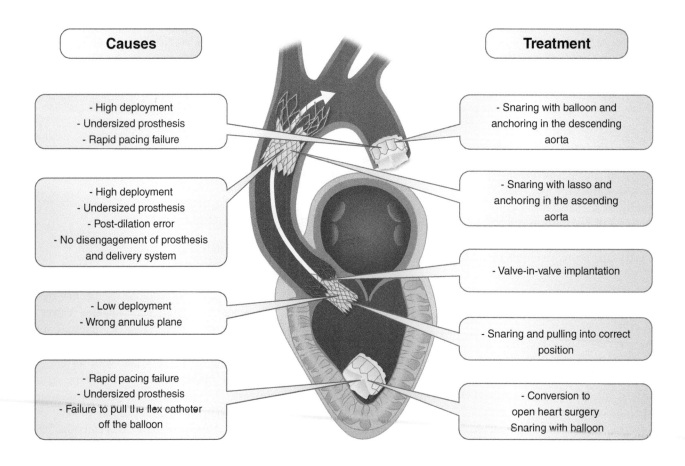

Figure 17.3 Causes and treatments for transcatheter heart valve malpositioning, migration, and embolization. *Source:* Binder and Webb (2019) / Oxford University Press.

This assumes the operator has reasonably identified/addressed the cause of the embolization.

27. How can you prevent TVEM?

Given that the majority of causes are technical, TVEM can typically be avoided. Ensuring stable pacing capture and position is crucial to avoid loss of capture during valve deployment. Significant valve undersizing can be avoided by careful pre-procedural planning with annulus sizing by multidetector CT. Good communication between operators and technicians and adequate training can avoid most issues with improper delivery catheter manipulation and technique.

Bibliography

1 Ancona, M.B., Beneduce, A., Romano, V. et al. (2020). Self-expanding transcatheter aortic valve infolding: current evidence, diagnosis, and management. *Catheter. Cardiovasc. Interv.* https://doi.org/10.1002/ccd.29432. Epub ahead of print, PMID: 33315300.

2 Barbanti, M., Yang, T.H., Rodès Cabau, J. et al. (2013). Anatomical and procedural features associated with aortic root rupture during balloon-expandable transcatheter aortic valve replacement. *Circulation* 128 (3): 244–253. https://doi.org/10.1161/CIRCULATIONAHA.113.002947. Epub 2013 Jun 7. PMID: 23748467.

3 Binder, R.K. and Webb, J.G. (2019). Transcatheter heart valve migration and embolization: rare and preventable? *Eur. Heart J.* 40 (38): 3166–3168. https://doi.org/10.1093/eurheartj/ehz562. PMID: 31377802.

4 Hodson, R.W., Jin, R., Ring, M.E. et al. (2020). Intrathoracic complications associated with trans-femoral transcatheter aortic valve replacement: implications for emergency surgical preparedness. *Catheter. Cardiovasc. Interv.* 96 (3): E369–E376. https://doi.org/10.1002/ccd.28620. Epub 2019 Dec 3. PMID: 31794142.

5 Karrowni, W., Fakih, S., and Nassar, P. (2020). Infolding of self-expandable transcatheter heart valve: case report and review of literature. *Cureus* 12 (8): e10093. https://doi.org/10.7759/cureus.10093. Published 2020 Aug 28.

6 Langer, N.B., Hamid, N.B., Nazif, T.M. et al. (2017). Injuries to the aorta, aortic annulus, and left ventricle during transcatheter aortic valve replacement: management and outcomes. *Circ. Cardiovasc. Interv.* 10 (1): e004735. https://doi.org/10.1161/CIRCINTERVENTIONS.116.004735. PMID: 28039322.

7 Musallam, A., Rogers, T., Ben-Dor, I. et al. (2020). Self-expanding transcatheter aortic valve-frame infolding: a case series with a warning message. *JACC Cardiovasc. Interv.* 13 (6): 789–790. https://doi.org/10.1016/j.jcin.2019.11.035. PMID: 32192702.

8 Pasic, M., Unbehaun, A., Buz, S. et al. (2015). Annular rupture during transcatheter aortic valve replacement: classification, pathophysiology, diagnostics, treatment approaches, and prevention. *JACC Cardiovasc. Interv.* 8 (1 Pt A): 1–9. https://doi.org/10.1016/j.jcin.2014.07.020. PMID: 25616813.

9 Rezq, A., Basavarajaiah, S., Latib, A. et al. (2012). Incidence, management, and outcomes of cardiac tamponade during transcatheter aortic valve implantation: a single-center study. *JACC Cardiovasc. Interv.* 5 (12): 1264–1272. https://doi.org/10.1016/j.jcin.2012.08.012. PMID: 23257375.

18

Pathological Insights of TAVR Degeneration and Thrombosis

Yu Sato and Renu Virmani

[1] *CVPath Institute, Gaithersburg, MD, USA*

Introduction

Transcatheter aortic valve replacement (TAVR) or implantation (TAVI) has become the standard of care for elderly patients and for patients with severe symptomatic aortic stenosis regardless of age. Randomized controlled clinical trials (RCTs) between TAVR and surgical aortic valve replacement (SAVR) have demonstrated similar or superior clinical outcomes in prohibited-, high-, intermediate-, and low-risk patients with aortic stenosis (AS). Surgical bioprosthetic valve studies have shown excellent but limited durability beyond 10 years, especially in younger patients. On the other hand, recent clinical trials also demonstrated a lower rate of structural valve deterioration (SVD) in TAVR compared to SAVR, but data is limited to eight years of follow-up. However, these results are diluted by a high mortality rate during follow-up because TAVR was limited to older age patients with high- or prohibited surgical risk patients when it was introduced in the clinic. The lack of this evidence can be covered by pathological studies with detailed observation of explanted valves. In this chapter, we review the causes of transcatheter aortic bioprosthesis valve failure from a pathological point of view.

Bioprosthetic Valve Failure (BVF)

1. What types of valve failure modes are observed in TAVR bioprostheses?

Despite the clinical success of TAVR, transcatheter bioprosthetic valve failure (BVF) is still observed, including valve thrombosis, infective endocarditis (IE), and SVD. Mylotte et al. reported a systematic review exploring transcatheter BVF following TAVR. A total of 87 cases of transcatheter aortic valve failure were identified from 70 publications between 2002 and 2014; 34 cases were IE, 15 cases were valve thrombosis, and 13 cases were SVD. In SVD cases, severe calcification of the leaflets was observed in 3 cases after 3.5 years of follow-up. All three cases were treated with surgical valve replacement or transcatheter valve-in-valve placement.

IE and surgical damage to the valve are the most common cause of early bioprosthetic heart valve (BHV) failure. Other causes of early valve failure are the development of extensive tissue overgrowth (pannus) and leaflet thrombosis. The main reason for late-phase valve failure is SVD, which is a slow and gradual process mainly caused by leaflet calcification.

Infective Endocarditis

2. What are the incidence and causative microorganisms of IE after TAVR?

IE following the TAVR procedure is reported to occur in the first year in 1.5% of patients (range 0.5–3.1%), which is similar to the incidence of IE following SAVR. Butt et al. conducted a nationwide observational cohort study that compared the incidence of IE among patients who underwent TAVR and SAVR. During a median follow-up of 3.6 years, the cumulative 1-year and 5-year risk of IE was 2.3 and 5.8% in TAVR, and 1.8 and 5.1% in SAVR, respectively; these differences were not statistically significant. Stortecky et al. also reported the incidence of IE from the Swiss TAVI registry, which includes 7203 patients. The incidence of IE for the peri-procedural phase (<100 days), delayed early phase (100–365 days), and late phase (>365 days) after TAVR was 2.59, 0.71, and 0.40 events per 100 person-years. These studies suggest that the risk of IE during the first year following TAVR is not trivial. The three most common causative organisms were *Enterococcus* species, *Staphylococcus, and Streptococcus* species; these account for 60–70% of all organisms. Among patients with early IE, *Enterococcus* species were the commonest isolated microorganisms.

3. What are the pathological findings of IE?

In our CVPath TAVR registry (N = 43), IE was observed in three patients: two occurred in SAPIEN (Edwards Lifesciences) and one in CoreValve (Medtronic) bioprostheses. In the cases of SAPIEN, IE occurred 65 and 60 days after the implantation with *Aspergillus* species and gram-positive cocci, respectively. In the former case, large vegetations were seen, involving all three leaflets and the stent frame, consisting of chronic organizing granulation tissue

with chronic inflammation and fungal organisms. In this case, gram-positive cocci platelet-fibrin thrombi were seen in all three leaflets, along with acute and chronic inflammation interspersed with bacterial colonies. In the case of CoreValve, endocarditis occurred eight months after the implantation with *Staphylococcus aureus,* involving two of three leaflets with small fibrin-rich vegetations, frame thrombus, and bacterial colonies with inflammatory cell infiltrates around the pericardial skirt (Figure 18.1).

Leaflet Thrombosis

4. What are the clinical relevancies of leaflet thrombosis?

Leaflet thrombosis after TAVR in the clinical setting is one of the most important causes of BVF because it can lead to

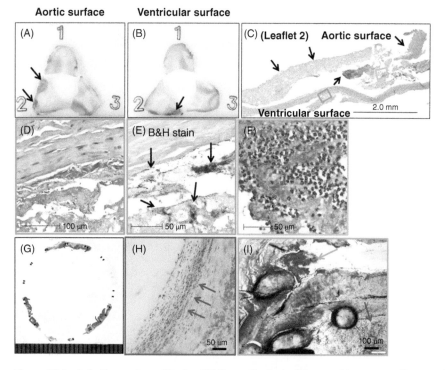

Figure 18.1 Infective endocarditis in a TAVR prosthesis. An 83-year-old man was diagnosed with infective endocarditis eight months following implantation of a TAVR prosthesis. The patient was febrile with an increased white blood cell count; blood cultures were positive for *Staphylococcus aureus,* and the patient was started on intravenous antibiotics. An echocardiogram showed vegetation on the prosthetic valve. The valve was explanted and replaced surgically. Photographs of the (a) ventricular surface and (b) aortic surface of excised leaflets are shown. Note the small thrombotic vegetation on leaflet 2 (black arrows). (c–f) Histologic images of leaflet 2 show platelet-fibrin thrombus intermingled with acute inflammation and bacterial organisms. (d) Leaflet 2 section stained with hematoxylin and eosin (H&E) shows a small platelet-fibrin thrombus with organisms seen clearly with Brown & Hopps (B&H) stain: (e) clumps of cocci (black arrows) and (f) a dense neutrophilic infiltrate. (g–i) Histologic images of valve stent flame. (h) A high-power image of the red boxed area in (g) shows acute inflammation in the neointimal lesion of the valve flame. (i) A high-power image of the blue boxed area in (g) shows a thrombus with bacterial colonies (i.e. vegetation) (blue arrow) and inflammatory cells (difficult to see in this magnification) around the pericardial skirt (red arrows). (c, d, f–i) are stained with H&E; (e) is stained with B&H.
Source: Modified and reproduced with permission from Torii, S. et al. (2021). The Pathologist Perspective. In *Aortic Valve Transcatheter Intervention* (eds. M. Zimarino, R. Waksman, I.J. Amat-Santos and C. Tamburino).

valve stenosis, leaflet degeneration, and embolic events. However, symptomatic valve thrombosis following TAVR is rare (<1%) and occurs at a frequency similar to that with surgical bioprosthetic valves.

In 2015, Boourgugnon et al. reported not a single case of clinical valve thrombosis among 2659 Carpentier-Edwards Perimount valves with long-term follow-up at their institution from 1984 to 2008 (median follow-up of 6.7 years). Similarly, no clinical valve cases of thrombosis were observed in the NOTION (Nordic Aortic Valve Intervention) lower-risk trial in the TAVR or SAVR group with up to six years of follow-up. Two retrospective analyses have shown the prevalence of clinical valve thrombosis to be between 0.6 and 2.8% after TAVR. However, until Makker et al. reported in 2015 using four-dimensional, volume-rendered computed tomography (4DCT) scans, the presence of subclinical leaflet thrombosis and associated restricted leaflet motion had not been described. The presence of subclinical leaflet thrombosis in bioprosthetic valves is an incidental finding on 4DCT or trans-esophageal echocardiography (TEE) imaging and does not cause symptoms or hemodynamic changes. In CT imaging, leaflet thrombus is characterized by hypoattenuating leaflet thickening (HALT). The prevalence of HALT has been reported to vary from 7 to 16.5% at one month and 24–30.9% at one year. However, the clinical significance of HALT remains unknown. Some studies have shown that the presence of HALT is clinically relevant and associated with death, thromboembolic events (i.e. stroke, or transient ischemic attack [TIA], and changes in hemodynamics), but the majority of studies have shown no association of HALT with such events. Anticoagulants seem to be an effective treatment for bioprosthetic valve thrombosis, whereas antiplatelet therapies are not effective for its prevention.

5. What are the pathological findings of valve thrombosis?

We have examined valve thrombosis in our two registries (CoreValve and SAPIEN) involving 43 patients. Of these, moderate or severe leaflet thrombosis was observed in 21% of the cases (9 of 43 patients) following TAVR (83 ± 160 days) (Figures 18.2 and 18.3). The valve thrombi at the early time point (≤30 days) were mainly platelet-rich. At a later time point (>30 days), the predominant type of thrombus was fibrin-rich with or without organization (beyond 30 days); this type was observed in 44% of cases, including the formation of granulation tissue, smooth muscle cells infiltration, and proteoglycan-collagen matrix. Although minimal thrombus attachment on the leaflet surface was common even in cases >90 days after TAVR, it was rarely associated

with BVF. Thrombus on the leaflet can calcify and causes extrinsic calcification and lead to BVF (Figure 18.4).

Del Trigo et al. demonstrated that the absence of anticoagulation therapy was one of the predictors of hemodynamic valve deterioration post-TAVR. Thus, anticoagulants have the potential to extend the durability of the valve leaflets and may be a good strategy for young patients who are likely to have fewer bleeding complications. Further randomized controlled studies are needed to determine the efficacy of anticoagulants after TAVR.

Neointimal Coverage and Pannus Formation

6. Is pannus formation seen in the TAVR valve?

Neointima is formed as a result of the healing process and is accompanied by an organizing thrombus and inflammation attached to the valve frame that extends onto the leaflets. Intimal growth is predominantly observed on the aortic surface, especially at the base of the leaflets. Host tissue growth after SAVR is expected around the suture ring and is considered part of the healing process. However, its extension onto the leaflets with an exuberant growth is associated with restricted leaflet motion and BV and is defined as pannus. Generally, foreign materials after implantation acquire a host protein layer at first, which primarily includes fibrin and platelets (thrombus) with inflammatory cell infiltration. Leaflet neointimal growth increases over time; however, complete neointimal coverage is rare even in valves implanted for >90 days.

A pannus formation tissue consists of smooth muscle cells within a rich collagen matrix, retracts as it matures, and results in harmful shortening and stiffness of the valve that either obstructs the bioprosthetic valve opening (stenosis) or may lead to regurgitation. Koo et al. evaluated patients who underwent TAVI and follow-up cardiac CT scans and revealed that the prevalence of pannus formation occurred in 1% (2/138) of the patients.

7. What are the pathological findings of pannus formation and leaflet endothelialization in TAVR bioprostheses?

We have observed two cases with pannus formation from our TAVR bioprosthesis registries and other institutions.

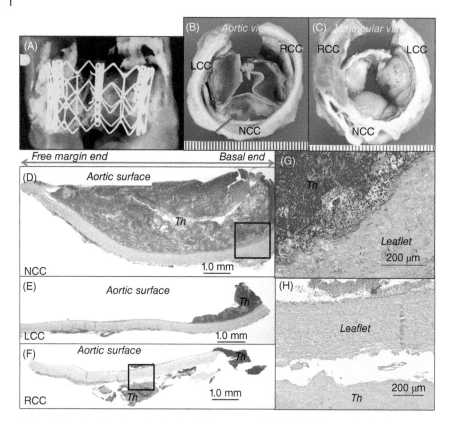

Figure 18.2 Leaflet thrombosis in a balloon-expandable TAVR bioprosthesis. (a) Radiograph of an Edwards SAPIEN prosthesis following removal of the valve along with the aorta and outflow tract and cutting open the transcatheter valve at autopsy. (b, c) Gross images show the stented valve excised with the aortic root (aortic surface at left; ventricular surface at right). Note the presence of a tan-white thrombus (Th, red arrow) on the aortic surface of the NCC. (d) A large platelet fibrin thrombus on the aortic surface of the NCC involves the entire cusp. (e) The LCC shows a valve thrombus on the aortic surface near the basal attachment site. (f) Focal fibrin thrombus attachved to the ventricular surface of RCC. (g, h) High-power images show the interface between the thrombus and the pericardial valve. (d–g) are stained with Movat pentachrome; (h) is stained with hematoxylin and eosin. NCC, non-coronary cusp; LCC, left coronary cusp; RCC, right coronary cusp. *Source:* Reproduced with permission from de Marchena, E. et al., *JACC Cardiovasc Interv* 2015; 8: 728–39.

One case was an Edwards SAPIEN valve implanted 1826 days before death; this case also showed severe leaflet calcification (Figure 18.5). The other was a CoreValve implanted 350 days prior to death. The pannus consisted of smooth muscle cells in a proteoglycan-collagen matrix on the leaflet and was seen near the leaflet attachment site and predominantly on the aortic surface of the leaflet. Within a few days after implantation, the leaflets become covered with a layer of fibrin, platelets, and a few erythrocytes consisting of macrophages and giant cells.

The endothelialization of bioprosthetic valve leaflets occurs gradually from the basal regions of the cusps. The endothelium is usually absent in the acute phase (<30 days), and it may take from several months to several years. It is predominantly seen on the basal regions of the leaflet and usually as a single layer, overlying a substrate of neointima (Figure 18.6).

Leaflet Calcification

8. What is the cause of leaflet calcification?

Leaflet calcification in surgical BHV is the most common contributor to SVD and has been comprehensively studied. It is reported that the presence of calcification in surgical bioprosthetic valve leaflets detected by CT is strongly and independently associated with hemodynamic valve deterioration as well as clinical outcomes. It is thought that glutaraldehyde is one of the leading causes of SVD and interacts with phospholipids and circulating calcium ions, although glutaraldehyde fixation is necessary to reduce allograft immunogenicity and promote collagen linkage to establish a solid tissue structure. Various types of anti-calcific treatments have been developed, such as alcohol

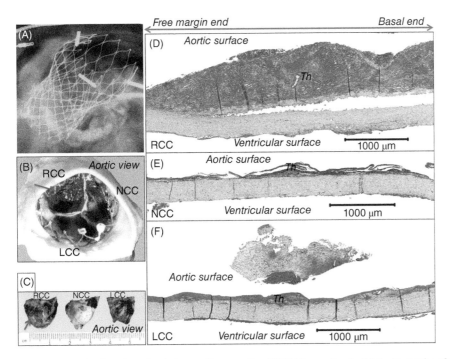

Figure 18.3 Leaflet thrombosis in a self-expanding TAVR bioprosthesis. (a) Radiographs of the CoreValve prosthesis and surgical clips from the previous bypass graft procedure. (b) Gross image of the aortic surface of the CoreValve. Note that the thrombus on the aortic surface of the valve cusps is greater on the RCC (red arrow) than on the LCC and NCC. (c) Excised valve cusps, aortic views. Red arrow indicates an adherent mural thrombus on the surfaces of the RCC. (d) RCC with organizing fibrin thrombus on the aortic surface. (e) NCC with a mild fibrin thrombus on the aortic surface. (f) LCC with an organizing fibrin thrombus on the aortic surface. (d–f) are stained with Movat pentachrome. NCC, non-coronary cusp; LCC, left coronary cusp; RCC, right coronary cusp. *Source:* Reproduced with permission from de Marchena, E. et al., *JACC Cardiovasc Interv* 2015; 8: 728–39.

tissue pretreatment, thermal treatment, and application of specific surfactants, but none of them convincingly reduced the incidence of SVD *in vivo*.

9. When is leaflet calcification seen after implantation?

Although valve dysfunction due to calcification does not begin before five years, histologic evidence of calcification can be seen within three years (usually focal mild calcification); it does not lead to untoward effects except for cases with IE or patients on hemodialysis, which can show severe calcification regardless of the duration of the implant. Moderate to severe calcification leads to stiffening of the leaflets that often results in aortic stenosis or regurgitation or both and is usually accompanied by tears.

Because the main cause of SVD is leaflet calcification and the process is slow, early valve failure from SVD is quite rare (<1% after 5 years, and 10% after 10 years) from long-term SAVR experience. Although the prevalence of leaflet calcification depends on the patient's age, the younger the

patient at the time of bioprosthetic valve implantation, the higher the risk of SVD because younger patients have a higher metabolic rate and a stronger immune system. Also, any conditions that influence calcium metabolism (e.g. chronic kidney disease) accelerate SVD related to calcification. Based on our experience with SAVR, patients who received TAVR at a young age may demonstrate a high rate of SVD compared to elderly patients.

10. What are the pathological findings of leaflet calcification?

From our pathological registry of 43 cases of TAVR from the PARTNER trial and the CoreValve U.S. Pivotal High-Risk Trial, valve calcification was observed in only two Edwards SAPIEN valves with bovine pericardial leaflets. The first case showed a mild intrinsic leaflet calcification at 1293 days (3.5 years) following the procedure; the subject was asymptomatic without valve dysfunction (Figure 18.5). The second case showed severe leaflet calcification with pannus formation 1739 days (4.8 years) after implantation (Figure 18.5). The patient showed symptoms of heart

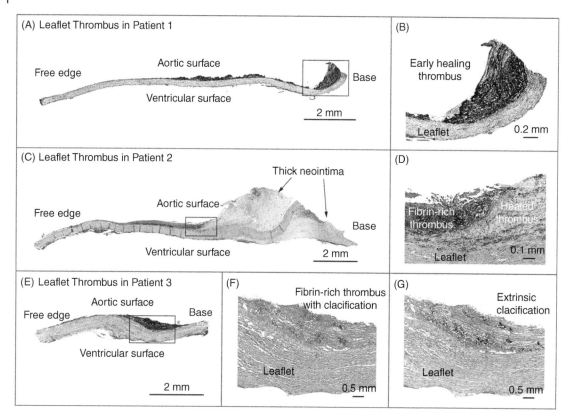

Figure 18.4 Histologic images of leaflet thrombi from three patients after TAVR. (a) Low-power image of a leaflet with a fibrin-rich thrombus on the aortic surface at 38 days after implantation. (b) An inset of the boxed area shows a high-power image revealing that the thrombus is attached to the base of the leaflet; the early organization of the thrombus is indicated by visible proteoglycan (green areas interspersed in the magenta-colored thrombus). (c) A low-power image of a leaflet with fibrin-rich thrombus in the mid portion and thick neointima from a healed thrombus at the base of both the aortic and ventricular surfaces at 105 days after implantation. (d) An inset of the boxed area shows a high-power image of the organizing thrombus. The fibrin-rich thrombus is healing with replacement by smooth-muscle cells in a proteoglycan matrix (green). (e) A low-power image of a leaflet with a fibrin-rich thrombus on the aortic surface at 517 days after implantation. (f) The first inset of the boxed area shows a high-power image of the leaflet thrombus, with purple areas indicating calcification (hematoxylin and eosin stain). (g) The second inset shows early spotty extrinsic calcification of the thrombus (von Kossa stain). (a–e) are stained with Movat pentachrome. TAVR: transcatheter aortic valve replacement. *Source:* Reproduced with permission from Yahagi, K. et al. *N Engl J Med* 2020; 383 (2): e8.

failure with significant hemodynamic changes (mean aortic valve pressure gradient was 51 mmHg).

Sellers et al. also reported five cases of leaflet calcification. One case had IE and showed severe calcification at 145 days after the procedure; the other 4 cases showed calcification at 1598 days (4.4 years), 1611 days (4.4 years), 2496 days (6.8 years), and 2583 days (7.1 years) after TAVR. In this study, calcification was seen in the attached thrombus and fibrosis (extrinsic calcification) and the leaflets themselves (intrinsic calcification).

Mylotte et al. confirmed three cases of SVD attributed to severe leaflet calcification, including two CoreValve and one Edwards SAPIEN bioprostheses. The duration of the implants ranged from 3.5 to 5.5 years following the procedure.

The 10 cases mentioned had histologically validated leaflet calcification. From these reports, leaflet calcification in TAVR valves is likely to occur three or more years after implantation in a few cases.

Leaflet calcification is observed at the commissure of the leaflets and the base of the cusps. The calcification initiates in areas with collagen fiber disruption, proteoglycan deposition, or phospholipid deposition. Leaflet calcification is typically observed in the center with surrounding collagen (intrinsic calcification) and is composed of calcium phosphate, with a crystal structure related to bone mineralization (hydroxyapatite). The thrombus attached to the leaflets is also prone to calcification (extrinsic calcification), and similarly, vegetations in IE tend to calcify.

Severe leaflet calcification/Pannus

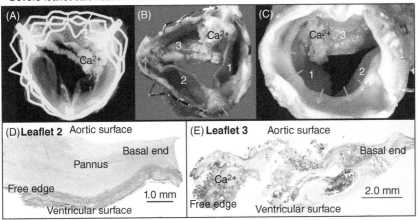

Early (mild) leaflet calcification

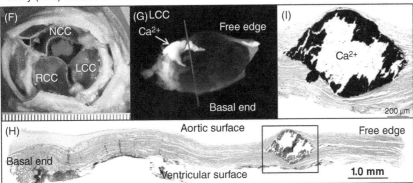

Figure 18.5 Edwards SAPIEN TAVR leaflet calcification and pannus formation. (a–e) Severe leaflet calcification with pannus formation in a surgically removed TAVR valve five years following implantation. (a) Radiograph of the valve. Note the presence of severe leaflet calcification (Ca^{2+}). Calcification involving the commissure sites was predominantly seen between leaflets 1 and 3. (b, c) Gross images from the aortic and ventricular surfaces, respectively. Green arrows show pannus formation, which was also predominantly present on the ventricular surface. (d) Histologic section with a thick pannus consisting of smooth muscle cells in a proteoglycan (green) collagenous matrix on leaflet 2. (e) Severe calcification with neointima growth in leaflet 3. (f–i) Early (mild) leaflet calcifications four years after implantation. (f) Gross image from the aortic surface with commissural fusion (green arrows). (g) Radiograph with focal calcification (Ca^{2+}) at the commissure site. (h) Histologic section with focal intrinsic calcification of the valve leaflet (Movat stain). (i) High-power image of the black boxed area in (h) is a calcium stained section. (d, e, and h) are stained with Movat pentachrome. (i) is stained with von Kossa. TAVR: transcatheter aortic valve replacement. *Source:* Modified and reproduced with permission from Yahagi, K. et al. Pathology of balloon-expandable transcatheter aortic valves. *Catheter Cardiovasc Interv* 2017; 90: 1048–1057.

Structural Changes (Non-calcific Structural Valve Deterioration)

11. What are the other causes of SVD besides calcification?

SVD is mostly characterized by leaflet calcification; however, non- or minimal calcific SVD is attributed to reoperations, such as leaflet tears and perforations, which account for 25% of cases. Leaflet tears in surgical bioprosthetic valves are seen more than 10 years post-implantation, resulting in aortic regurgitation. Ishihara et al. classified them into four groups: type I, linear tears involving the free edge of the cusp; type II, linear tears running parallel to the sewing ring, along the basal regions of the cusp; type III, large round or oval perforations occupying the central regions of the cup; and type IV, small and multiple pinholes like fenestrations in the cusp. Butany et al. reported that type I and type II were more common in the bovine pericardial Carpentier-Edwards Perimount valve in an autopsy study. Our autopsy studies of TAVR bioprostheses evaluated the degree of structural changes in bioprosthetic TAVR valve leaflets. The leaflet structural changes increased over time, and overall changes were mild even beyond one year of implantation.

Leaflet tears and perforations have been observed following TAVR at the sewing ring, usually occurring early within

Day 17

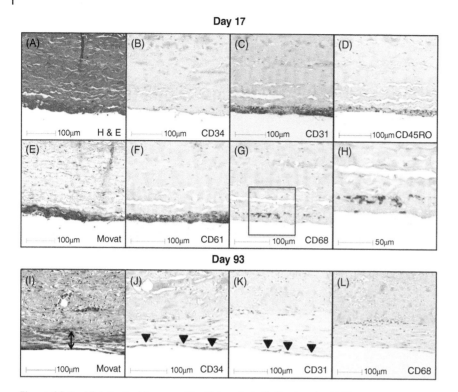

Figure 18.6 Histological images of leaflet endothelialization. (a–h) Platelet-rich surface thrombus on the ventricular surface from a 90-year-old male who died of pneumonia 17 days post-implantation. Note the positive staining in (c) CD31 and (f) CD61 with (d, g, h) inflammatory cell infiltration. (b) CD34 was negative. (i–l) Neointimal coverage (arrow) on the ventricular surface from a 90-year-old female who died of multiple organ failure 93 days after implant. Note endothelialization on the top of smooth muscle cells in a proteoglycan matrix with (j) CD34 and (k) CD31 positive cells (arrowheads). (l) There is minimal inflammation at the pericardial neointimal junction but no inflammation on the luminal surface. TAVR, transcatheter aortic valve replacement; CD34, endothelial cell marker; CD68, macrophage marker; CD45RO, common leukocyte antigen marker; CD31, non-specific stain marker for endothelial cell and platelet; CD61, platelet marker. *Source:* Modified and reproduced with permission from Torii, S., et al. *JACC Cardiovasc Imaging* 2019; 12: 566–567.

one year. The histological findings of structural changes are characterized by fluid insudation, fraying, and separation of collagen bundles (Figure 18.7). These changes are similar to those observed in SAVR bioprosthetic valve leaflets. Longer follow-up studies are needed to confirm structural changes in TAVR leaflets.

Durability of Bioprosthetic Valves

12. Is the durability of TAVR bioprostheses similar to that of SAVR bioprostheses?

Clinical trials with five to eight years of follow-up have demonstrated that the rate of moderate/severe SVD or BVF based on European Association of Percutaneous Cardiovascular Interventions / European Society of Cardiology / European Association for Cardio-Thoracic Surgery (EAPCI/

ESC/EACTS) definitions in TAVR bioprostheses ranges from 3.0 to 14.9% or 2.6 to 7.5%, respectively. However, a competing risk of mortality is related to very elderly and/or high surgical risk patients having received TAVR, which could result in bias. For example, Tesla et al. reported long-term clinical data including 990 inoperable or high-risk patients (mean age 82 ± 6 years and Society for Thoracic Surgery Predictor of Mortality [STS PROM] score 9 ± 10). The rates of moderate SVD, severe SVD, and BVF at eight years were 3.0, 1.6, and 2.5%, respectively. However, the mortality rate at eight years was 78.3% (728 patients had died during follow-up), which may have affected the results.

Unlike TAVR bioprostheses, the long-term durability of surgical bioprostheses has been comprehensively studied. From a recent systematic review of long-term follow-up data of surgical bioprosthetic valves, the actual freedom from SVD rate of the Carpentier-Edwards Perimount valve (Edwards Life Sciences) ranged from 86 to 98.1% at 10 years and 78.6 to 87.7% at 15 years and was 85% at 20 years.

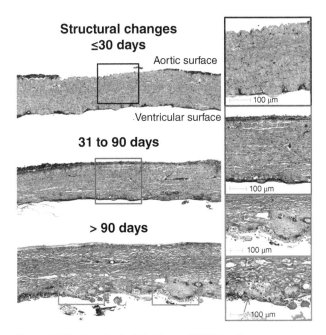

Structural changes ≤30 days

Aortic surface

Ventricular surface

⊢——⊣ 100 µm

31 to 90 days

⊢——⊣ 100 µm

> 90 days

⊢——⊣ 100 µm

⊢——⊣ 100 µm

Figure 18.7 Histological findings of TAVR leaflet structural changes. Structural degenerative changes were mostly absent or minimal before 90 days, whereas mild structural changes, including separation of collagen bundles near the leaflet surface with fluid insudation (red arrows), were seen beyond 90 days, especially after one year. All histologic images are stained with Movat pentachrome. TAVR: transcatheter aortic valve replacement. *Source:* Yahagi, K. et al. (2017). Reproduced with permission from John Wiley & Sons.

However, most studies used reoperation as the definition of SVD instead of valve hemodynamic performance, which may have led to underdiagnosis of the real incidence of SVD. Long-term, controlled comparison data between surgical and transcatheter aortic bioprosthesis with the uniform definition of SVD and BVF is warranted.

13. Is the long-term durability the same in both TAVR and SAVR bioprostheses?

Although both bioprostheses are made from porcine or bovine pericardium and consist of three leaflets, the durability of TAVR bioprostheses may theoretically be different from that of SAVR bioprostheses. Valve manufacturing/preparation processes, stent crimping processes, and ballooning during the procedure may damage the leaflets; however, none of these have been definitely proven. The non-circular opening of the stent and leaving native cusp calcifications in situ in TAVR may affect valve hemodynamics. These factors may contribute to varying leaflet durability. In an *in vitro* soft tissue fatigue simulation study, the TAVR valve durability is expected to be about 7–8 years, whereas the durability of the SAVR valve was assumed as 20 years. Given the concerns highlighted here, initial comprehensive 10-year follow-up data is warranted.

Conclusion

The majority of explanted TAVR bioprostheses up to five years following implantation demonstrated intact leaflets with mild changes, including thrombus, calcification, neointimal formation, and structural deterioration. Clinical trials also showed a low rate of SVD in TAVR valves for up to eight years of follow-up. However, these results are biased by a high mortality rate, as TAVR was initially introduced for inoperable or high-risk older patients. Further studies with a longer duration of implants are needed to confirm the significance of these findings and the durability of TAVR valves.

Bibliography

1 Adams, D.H., Popma, J.J., and Reardon, M.J. (2014). Transcatheter aortic-valve replacement with a self-expanding prosthesis. *N. Engl. J. Med.* 371: 967–968.

2 Agnihotri, A.K., Mcgiffin, D.C., Galbraith, A.J., and O'Brien, M.F. (1995). The prevalence of infective endocarditis after aortic valve replacement. *J. Thorac. Cardiovasc. Surg.* 110: 1708–1720. discussion 1720–1724.

3 Arsalan, M. and Walther, T. (2016). Durability of prostheses for transcatheter aortic valve implantation. *Nat. Rev. Cardiol.* 13: 360–367.

4 Blanke, P., Leipsic, J.A., Popma, J.J. et al. (2020). Bioprosthetic aortic valve leaflet thickening in the Evolut low risk sub-study. *J. Am. Coll. Cardiol.* 75: 2430–2442.

5 Bourguignon, T., Bouquiaux-Stablo, A.L., Candolfi, P. et al. (2015). Very long-term outcomes of the Carpentier-Edwards Perimount valve in aortic position. *Ann. Thorac. Surg.* 99: 831–837.

6 Brown, M.L., Park, S.J., Sundt, T.M., and Schaff, H.V. (2012). Early thrombosis risk in patients with biologic valves in the aortic position. *J. Thorac. Cardiovasc. Surg.* 144: 108–111.

7 Butany, J., Nair, V., Leong, S.W. et al. (2007). Carpentier-Edwards Perimount valves--morphological findings in surgical explants. *J. Card. Surg.* 22: 7–12.

8 Butt, J.H., Ihlemann, N., De Backer, O. et al. (2019). Long-term risk of infective endocarditis after transcatheter aortic valve replacement. *J. Am. Coll. Cardiol.* 73: 1646–1655.

9 Chakravarty, T., Søndergaard, L., Friedman, J. et al. (2017). Subclinical leaflet thrombosis in surgical and transcatheter bioprosthetic aortic valves: an observational study. *Lancet* 389: 2383–2392.

10 Cohn, L.H., Collins, J.J. Jr., Rizzo, R.J. et al. (1998). Twenty-year follow-up of the Hancock modified orifice porcine aortic valve. *Ann. Thorac. Surg.* 66: S30–S34.

11 Côté, N., Pibarot, P., and Clavel, M.A. (2017). Incidence, risk factors, clinical impact, and management of bioprosthesis structural valve degeneration. *Curr. Opin. Cardiol.* 32: 123–129.

12 David, T.E., Ivanov, J., Armstrong, S. et al. (2001). Late results of heart valve replacement with the Hancock ii bioprosthesis. *J. Thorac. Cardiovasc. Surg.* 121: 268–277.

13 De La Fuente, A.B., Wright, G.A., Olin, J.M. et al. (2015). Advanced integrity preservation technology reduces bioprosthesis calcification while preserving performance and safety. *J. Heart Valve Dis.* 24: 101–109.

14 De Marchena, E., Mesa, J., Pomenti, S. et al. (2015). Thrombus formation following transcatheter aortic valve replacement. *JACC Cardiovasc. Interv.* 8: 728–739.

15 Del Trigo, M., Muñoz-García, A.J., Latib, A. et al. (2018). Impact of anticoagulation therapy on valve haemodynamic deterioration following transcatheter aortic valve replacement. *Heart* 104: 814–820.

16 Del Trigo, M., Muñoz-Garcia, A.J., Wijeysundera, H.C. et al. (2016). Incidence, timing, and predictors of valve hemodynamic deterioration after transcatheter aortic valve replacement: multicenter registry. *J. Am. Coll. Cardiol.* 67: 644–655.

17 Fatima, B., Mohananey, D., Khan, F.W. et al. (2019). Durability data for bioprosthetic surgical aortic valve: a systematic review. *JAMA Cardiol.* 4: 71–80.

18 Ferrans, V.J., Tomita, Y., Hilbert, S.L. et al. (1987). Pathology of bioprosthetic cardiac valves. *Hum. Pathol.* 18: 586–595.

19 Généreux, P., Webb, J.G., Svensson, L.G. et al. (2012). Vascular complications after transcatheter aortic valve replacement: insights from the PARTNER (Placement of Aortic TraNscatheter Valve) trial. *J. Am. Coll. Cardiol.* 60: 1043–1052.

20 Gleason, T.G., Reardon, M.J., Popma, J.J. et al. (2018). 5-year outcomes of self-expanding transcatheter versus surgical aortic valve replacement in high-risk patients. *J. Am. Coll. Cardiol.* 72: 2687–2696.

21 Hammerstingl, C., Nickenig, G., and Grube, E. (2012). Treatment of a degenerative stenosed CoreValve(®) aortic bioprosthesis by transcatheter valve-in-valve insertion. *Catheter. Cardiovasc. Interv.* 79: 748–755.

22 Hansson, N.C., Grove, E.L., Andersen, H.R. et al. (2016). Transcatheter aortic valve thrombosis: incidence, predisposing factors, and clinical implications. *J. Am. Coll. Cardiol.* 68: 2059–2069.

23 Hoffmann, R., Möllmann, H., and Lotfi, S. (2013). Transcatheter aortic valve-in-valve implantation of a CoreValve in a degenerated stenotic Sapien heart valve prosthesis. *Catheter. Cardiovasc. Interv.* 82: E922–E925.

24 Ishihara, T., Ferrans, V.J., Boyce, S.W. et al. (1981a). Structure and classification of cuspal tears and perforations in porcine bioprosthetic cardiac valves implanted in patients. *Am. J. Cardiol.* 48: 665–678.

25 Ishihara, T., Ferrans, V.J., Jones, M. et al. (1981b). Occurrence and significance of endothelial cells in implanted porcine bioprosthetic valves. *Am. J. Cardiol.* 48: 443–454.

26 Jose, J., Sulimov, D.S., El-Mawardy, M. et al. (2017). Clinical bioprosthetic heart valve thrombosis after transcatheter aortic valve replacement: incidence, characteristics, and treatment outcomes. *JACC Cardiovasc. Interv.* 10: 686–697.

27 Kapadia, S.R., Leon, M.B., Makkar, R.R. et al. (2015). 5-year outcomes of transcatheter aortic valve replacement compared with standard treatment for patients with inoperable aortic stenosis (PARTNER 1): a randomised controlled trial. *Lancet* 385: 2485–2491.

28 Koo, H.J., Choe, J., Kang, D.Y. et al. (2020). Computed tomography features of Cuspal thrombosis and subvalvular tissue ingrowth after transcatheter aortic valve implantation. *Am. J. Cardiol.* 125: 597–606.

29 Latib, A., Naganuma, T., Abdel-Wahab, M. et al. (2015). Treatment and clinical outcomes of transcatheter heart valve thrombosis. *Circ. Cardiovasc. Interv.* 8.

30 Leon, M.B., Smith, C.R., Mack, M. et al. (2010). Transcatheter aortic-valve implantation for aortic stenosis in patients who cannot undergo surgery. *N. Engl. J. Med.* 363: 1597–1607.

31 Leon, M.B., Smith, C.R., Mack, M.J. et al. (2016). Transcatheter or surgical aortic-valve replacement in intermediate-risk patients. *N. Engl. J. Med.* 374: 1609–1620.

32 Mack, M.J., Leon, M.B., Thourani, V.H. et al. (2019). Transcatheter aortic-valve replacement with a balloon-expandable valve in low-risk patients. *N. Engl. J. Med.* 380: 1695–1705.

33 Makkar, R.R., Blanke, P., Leipsic, J. et al. (2020a). Subclinical leaflet thrombosis in transcatheter and surgical bioprosthetic valves: PARTNER 3 cardiac computed tomography substudy. *J. Am. Coll. Cardiol.* 75: 3003–3015.

34 Makkar, R.R., Fontana, G., Jilaihawi, H. et al. (2015). Possible subclinical leaflet thrombosis in bioprosthetic aortic valves. *N. Engl. J. Med.* 373: 2015–2024.

35 Makkar, R.R., Thourani, V.H., Mack, M.J. et al. (2020b). Five-year outcomes of transcatheter or surgical aortic-valve replacement. *N. Engl. J. Med.* 382: 799–809.

36 Martin, C. and Sun, W. (2015). Comparison of transcatheter aortic valve and surgical bioprosthetic valve durability: a fatigue simulation study. *J. Biomech.* 48: 3026–3034.

37 Mylotte, D., Andalib, A., Theriault-Lauzier, P. et al. (2015). Transcatheter heart valve failure: a systematic review. *Eur. Heart J.* 36: 1306–1327.

38 Noble, S., Asgar, A., Cartier, R. et al. (2009). Anatomo-pathological analysis after CoreValve Revalving system implantation. *EuroIntervention* 5: 78–85.

39 Ong, S.H., Mueller, R., and Iversen, S. (2012). Early calcific degeneration of a CoreValve transcatheter aortic bioprosthesis. *Eur. Heart J.* 33: 586.

40 Otto, C.M., Nishimura, R.A., Bonow, R.O. et al. (2021). 2020 ACC/AHA guideline for the Management of Patients with Valvular Heart Disease: a report of the American College of Cardiology/American Heart Association Joint Committee on Clinical Practice Guidelines. *Circulation* 143: e72–e227.

41 Pache, G., Schoechlin, S., Blanke, P. et al. (2016). Early hypo-attenuated leaflet thickening in balloon-expandable transcatheter aortic heart valves. *Eur. Heart J.* 37: 2263–2271.

42 Popma, J.J., Deeb, G.M., Yakubov, S.J. et al. (2019). Transcatheter aortic-valve replacement with a self-expanding valve in low-risk patients. *N. Engl. J. Med.* 380: 1706–1715.

43 Reardon, M.J., Van Mieghem, N.M., Popma, J.J. et al. (2017). Surgical or transcatheter aortic-valve replacement in intermediate-risk patients. *N. Engl. J. Med.* 376: 1321–1331.

44 Regueiro, A., Linke, A., Latib, A. et al. (2016). Association between transcatheter aortic valve replacement and subsequent infective endocarditis and in-hospital death. *JAMA* 316: 1083–1092.

45 Ruel, M., Rubens, F.D., Masters, R.G. et al. (2004). Late incidence and predictors of persistent or recurrent heart failure in patients with aortic prosthetic valves. *J. Thorac. Cardiovasc. Surg.* 127: 149–159.

46 Ruile, P., Minners, J., Breitbart, P. et al. (2018). Medium-term follow-up of early leaflet thrombosis after transcatheter aortic valve replacement. *JACC Cardiovasc. Interv.* 11: 1164–1171.

47 Saleeb, S.F., Newburger, J.W., Geva, T. et al. (2014). Accelerated degeneration of a bovine pericardial bioprosthetic aortic valve in children and young adults. *Circulation* 130: 51–60.

48 Schoen, F.J. and Levy, R.J. (1999). Founder's Award, 25th Annual Meeting of the Society for Biomaterials, perspectives. Providence, Ri, April 28 May 2, 1999. Tissue heart valves: current challenges and future research perspectives. *J. Biomed. Mater. Res.* 47: 439–465.

49 Sellers, S.L., Turner, C.T., Sathananthan, J. et al. (2018). Transcatheter aortic heart valves: histological analysis providing insight to leaflet thickening and structural valve degeneration. *JACC Cardiovascular imaging* 12 (1): 135–145.

50 Sellers, S.L., Turner, C.T., Sathananthan, J. et al. (2019). Transcatheter aortic heart valves: histological analysis providing insight to leaflet thickening and structural valve degeneration. *JACC Cardiovasc. Imaging* 12: 135–145.

51 Smith, C.R., Leon, M.B., Mack, M.J. et al. (2011). Transcatheter versus surgical aortic-valve replacement in high-risk patients. *N. Engl. J. Med.* 364: 2187–2198.

52 Søndergaard, L., Ihlemann, N., Capodanno, D. et al. (2019). Durability of transcatheter and surgical bioprosthetic aortic valves in patients at lower surgical risk. *J. Am. Coll. Cardiol.* 73: 546–553.

53 Stortecky, S., Heg, D., Tueller, D. et al. (2020). Infective endocarditis after transcatheter aortic valve replacement. *J. Am. Coll. Cardiol.* 75: 3020–3030.

54 Testa, L., Latib, A., Brambilla, N. et al. (2020). Long-term clinical outcome and performance of transcatheter aortic valve replacement with a self-expandable bioprosthesis. *Eur. Heart J.* 41: 1876–1886.

55 Tomazic, B.B., Brown, W.E., and Schoen, F.J. (1994). Physicochemical properties of calcific deposits isolated from porcine bioprosthetic heart valves removed from patients following 2–13 years function. *J. Biomed. Mater. Res.* 28: 35–47.

56 Torii, S., Romero, M.E., Kolodgie, F.D. et al. (2019). Endothelial cell coverage on the leaflet after transcatheter aortic valve replacement. *JACC Cardiovasc. Imaging* 12: 566–567.

57 Vollema, E.M., Kong, W.K.F., Katsanos, S. et al. (2017). Transcatheter aortic valve thrombosis: the relation between hypo-attenuated leaflet thickening, abnormal valve haemodynamics, and stroke. *Eur. Heart J.* 38: 1207–1217.

58 Yahagi, K., Ladich, E., Kutys, R. et al. (2017). Pathology of balloon-expandable transcatheter aortic valves. *Catheter. Cardiovasc. Interv.* 90: 1048–1057.

59 Yahagi, K., Sato, Y., and Virmani, R. (2020). A controlled trial of rivaroxaban after transcatheter aortic-valve replacement. *N. Engl. J. Med.* 383: e8.

60 Yahagi, K., Torii, S., Ladich, E. et al. (2018). Pathology of self-expanding transcatheter aortic valves: findings from the CoreValve us pivotal trials. *Catheter. Cardiovasc. Interv.* 91: 947–955.

61 Zhang, B., Salaun, E., Côté, N. et al. (2020). Association of bioprosthetic aortic valve leaflet calcification on hemodynamic and clinical outcomes. *J. Am. Coll. Cardiol.* 76: 1737–1748.

19

Clinical Implications of Valve Thrombosis and Early Thickening

Management of Antiplatelets and Anticoagulation Post TAVI

David "Chip" Sosa, Shazib Sagheer and Nestor F. Mercado

[1] *University of New Mexico Health Sciences Center, Albuquerque, NM, USA*

1. What are the risk factors for transcatheter heart valve (THV) thrombosis?

Some of the predictors of bioprosthetic valve thrombosis include (i) >50% increase in mean transvalvular gradient, (ii) increased leaflet thickness, (iii) abnormal leaflet mobility, (iv) presence of atrial fibrillation, (v) small valve size and under-expansion, (vi) aggressive post-dilation, (vii) geometric deformation of THV, and (viii) the underlying thrombophilia.

2. What is the role of the routine use of anticoagulation post-transcatheter aortic valve implantation (TAVI) in the absence and a concurrent anticoagulation indication (such as atrial fibrillation)?

The 2020 American College of Cardiology/American Heart Association (ACC/AHA) guidelines for the management of patients with valvular heart disease recommend aspirin 75–100 mg once daily as a reasonable antiplatelet therapy for patients with a bioprosthetic TAVI (Class IIa indication). There is a class IIb indication for Aspirin 75–100 mg and Clopidogrel 75 mg for three to six months post-TAVI. Currently, patients deemed to be low bleeding risk carry a Class IIb indication for anticoagulation with a vitamin K antagonist (VKA) for at least three months after implantation. However, the efficacy and safety of empiric anticoagulation in the absence of an alternative indication remains unclear and is currently under investigation.

3. For bioprosthetic TAVI patients who do not have other indications for anticoagulation, is it appropriate to use a single antiplatelet agent, or is dual antiplatelet always necessary?

Current guidelines indicate that for bioprosthetic TAVI, a regimen of aspirin 75–100 mg daily is reasonable in the absence of other indications for oral anticoagulation. This recommendation is based on a recent meta-analysis as well as the ARTE (Aspirin vs. Aspirin + Clopidogrel Following Transcatheter Aortic Valve Implant) trial, a small study that showed that aspirin monotherapy seemed to reduce the risk of major or life-threatening events without increasing the risk for myocardial infarction or stroke.

4. In the setting of bioprosthetic TAVI, for whom would dual antiplatelet therapy be indicated?

Current guidelines support the use of dual antiplatelet therapy using aspirin 75–100 mg daily and Clopidogrel 75 mg daily post-implant, stating it "may be reasonable" for three to six months after implantation (Class IIb indication). However, as mentioned in question 3, recent data does seem to show that aspirin alone appears to reduce events without increasing thromboembolic risk compared to dual antiplatelet therapy.

Mastering Structural Heart Disease, First Edition. Edited by Eduardo J. de Marchena and Camilo A. Gomez.
© 2023 John Wiley & Sons Ltd. Published 2023 by John Wiley & Sons Ltd.
Companion website: www.wiley.com/go/deMarchena/Mastering-Structural-Heart-Disease

5. For bioprosthetic TAVI patients who have a stroke while on antiplatelet therapy, would it be reasonable to start on oral anticoagulation in place of antiplatelet therapy?

Yes. Based on previous reviews and observational data on valve thrombosis, there is a Class IIb indication for patients with TAVI who experience a stroke or systemic embolic event while on antiplatelet therapy to consider VKA anticoagulation instead of antiplatelet therapy after consideration of bleeding risk.

6. For bioprosthetic TAVI patients who have suspected valve thrombosis and are clinically stable, what would be the initial anticoagulation choice?

Based on current data, anticoagulation with a VKA is considered reasonable in patients with suspected or confirmed bioprosthetic valve thrombosis (Class IIa indication).

7. In the setting of bioprosthetic TAVI, what regimen would be indicated for a patient with concurrent atrial fibrillation and a CHA$_2$DS$_2$-Vasc Score of 4, but no other indication for antiplatelet therapy?

For patients with an indication for anticoagulation but not antiplatelet therapy (i.e. atrial fibrillation), direct-acting oral anticoagulant (DOAC), or VKA agents, anticoagulation only is recommended with no need for additional antithrombotic therapy.

8. In the setting of bioprosthetic TAVI, what regimen would be indicated for a patient with concurrent atrial fibrillation and a CHA$_2$DS$_2$-Vasc Score of 4, as well as a recent coronary artery stent?

In TAVI patients with an indication for anticoagulation and antiplatelet therapy, it is generally recommended that anticoagulation plus a single antiplatelet agent be used. However, consensus guidelines on which antiplatelet agent

to use and for what duration are lacking and currently undergoing clinical investigation. The POPular TAVI trial (Antiplatelet Therapy for Patients Undergoing Transcatheter Aortic Valve Implantation) compared anticoagulation only to anticoagulation plus Clopidogrel and found similar rates of stroke and mortality among the two groups but a higher rate of bleeding among those treated with Clopidogrel. However, an adjusted analysis of the PARTNER 2 (Placement of Aortic Transcatheter Valves) trial showed reduced rates of death and stroke in patients treated with anticoagulation and antiplatelet therapy.

9. Which bioprosthetic TAVI patients should be on concurrent dual antiplatelet therapy as well as anticoagulation (i.e. triple therapy)?

It is recommended that "triple therapy" (anticoagulation plus dual antiplatelet therapy) be avoided after TAVI. A large meta-analysis has clearly shown a higher mortality rate in triple therapy than anticoagulation plus antiplatelet or anticoagulation alone.

10. For bioprosthetic TAVI patients with a concurrent indication for anticoagulation, are DOACs a reasonable alternative to VKAs?

DOAC and VKA agents are both reasonable post-TAVI. However, there is growing evidence that DOAC would be preferred to VKA if feasible. For example, the ENVISAGE-TAVI AF (Edoxaban Compared to Standard Care After Heart Valve Replacement Using a Catheter in Patients With Atrial Fibrillation) trial compared Edoxaban to VKA agents in TAVI patients with atrial fibrillation and found Edoxaban to be non-inferior to VKA but to have higher rates of major bleeding. Another large observational analysis of French TAVI registry data showed higher mortality and bleeding complications in these patients treated with VKA than DOAC.

11. What are the clinical implications of subclinical valve thrombosis, also called hypoattenuating leaflet thrombosis (HALT)?

Subclinical valve thrombosis, also called hypo-attenuating leaflet thickening (HALT), is described as a hypoattenuating lesion on the aortic side of the leaflets as seen on multidetector CT (MDCT). This can impair the valve function, in which case it is called hypo-attenuation affecting motion (HAM). Based on the current literature, HALT has been associated with transient ischemic attacks. There is insufficient evidence to recommend routine post-TAVI surveillance CT scan. Based on expert opinion and observational data, it is perhaps reasonable to obtain MDCT at 30 days post-TAVI in patients who have risk factors of THV thrombosis. If HALT is present, then a short course (three months) of anticoagulation should be considered, followed by repeat serial imaging to document resolution of HALT.

Bibliography

1 Brouwer, J., Nijenhuis, V., Rodés-CAbau, J. et al. (2021). Aspirin alone versus dual antiplatelet therapy after transcatheter aortic valve implantation: a systematic review and patient-level meta-analysis. *J. Am. Heart Assoc.* 10 (8): e019604.

2 Chakravarty, T., Sondergaard, L., Friedman, J. et al. (2017). Subclinical leaflet thrombosis in surgical and transcatheter bioprosthetic aortic valves: an observational study. *Lancet* 389 (10087): 2383–2392.

3 Dangas, G.D., Weitz, J.I., Giustino, G., et al., Prosthetic heart valve thrombosis. *J. Am. Coll. Cardiol.*, 2016. 68(24) 2670–2689.

4 De Marchena, E., Mesa, J., Pomenti, S. et al. (2015). Thrombus formation following transcatheter aortic valve replacement. *JACC Cardiovasc. Interv.* 8 (5): 728–739.

5 Didier, R., Lhermusier, T., Auffret, V. et al. (2021). TAVR patients requiring anticoagulation: direct oral anticoagulant or vitamin K antagonist? *JACC Cardiovasc. Interv.* 14 (15): 1704–1713.

6 Egbe, A.C., Pislaru, S.V., Pellikka, P.A. et al. (2015). Bioprosthetic valve thrombosis versus structural failure: clinical and echocardiographic predictors. *J. Am. Coll. Cardiol.* 66 (21): 2285–2294.

7 Jochheim, D., Barbanti, M., Capretti, G. et al. (2019). Oral anticoagulant type and outcomes after transcatheter aortic valve replacement. *JACC Cardiovasc. Interv.* 12 (16): 1566–1576.

8 Jose, J., Sulimov, D.S., El-Mawardy, M. et al. (2017). Clinical bioprosthetic heart valve thrombosis after transcatheter aortic valve replacement: incidence, characteristics, and treatment outcomes. *JACC Cardiovasc. Interv.* 10 (7): 686–697.

9 Kosmidou, I., Liu, Y., Alu, M.C. et al. (2019). Antithrombotic therapy and cardiovascular outcomes after transcatheter aortic valve replacement in patients with atrial fibrillation. *JACC Cardiovasc. Interv.* 12 (16): 1580–1589.

10 Kuneman, J.H., Singh, G.K., Hansson, N.C. et al. (2021). Subclinical leaflet thrombosis after transcatheter aortic valve implantation: no association with left ventricular reverse remodeling at 1-year follow-up. *Int. J. Cardiovasc. Imaging* .

11 Martín, M., Cuevas, J., Cigarran, H. et al. (2021). Transcatheter aortic valve implantation and subclinical and clinical leaflet thrombosis: multimodality imaging for diagnosis and risk stratification. *Eur. Cardiol.* 16: e35–e35.

12 Nijenhuis, V.J., Brouwer, J., Delewi, R. et al. (2020). Anticoagulation with or without Clopidogrel after transcatheter aortic-valve implantation. *N. Engl. J. Med.* 382 (18): 1696–1707.

13 Otto, C.M., Nishimura, R.A., Bonow, R.O. et al. (2021). 2020 ACC/AHA guideline for the management of patients with valvular heart disease: a report of the American College of Cardiology/American Heart Association joint committee on clinical practice guidelines. *J. Thorac. Cardiovasc. Surg.* 162 (2): e183–e353.

14 Rodés-Cabau, J., Masson, J.-B., Welsh, R.C. et al. (2017). Aspirin versus aspirin plus Clopidogrel as antithrombotic treatment following transcatheter aortic valve replacement with a balloon-expandable valve: the ARTE (aspirin versus aspirin + Clopidogrel following transcatheter aortic valve implantation) randomized clinical trial. *JACC Cardiovasc. Interv.* 10 (13): 1357–1365.

15 Van Mieghem, N.M., Underdorben, M., Hengstenberg, C. et al. (2021). Edoxaban versus vitamin K antagonist for atrial fibrillation after TAVR. *N. Engl. J. Med.* 385 (23): 2150–2160.

16 Zuo, W., Yang, M., He, Y. et al. (2019). Single or dual antiplatelet therapy after transcatheter aortic valve replacement: an updated systemic review and meta-analysis. *J. Thorac. Dis.* 11 (3): 959–968.

20

TAVR and Stroke

Shashvat M. Desai[1], Adam A. Dmytriw[2], Tannavi Prakash[3], Abhishek Sharma[4], Priyank Khandelwal[3] and Dileep R. Yavagal[5]

[1] Department of Neuroscience, HonorHealth Research Institute, Scottsdale, AZ, USA
[2] Harvard Medical School, Neuroradiology and Neurointervention Service, Brigham & Women's Hospital, Boston, MA, USA
[3] Department of Neurological Surgery, New Jersey Medical School, Rutgers, University Hospital Newark, Newark, NJ, USA
[4] Department of Cardiology, New Jersey Medical School, Rutgers, University Hospital Newark, Newark, NJ, USA
[5] Department of Neurology and Neurological Surgery, University of Miami Miller School of Medicine and Jackson Health System, Miami, FL, USA

Introduction

Transcatheter aortic valve replacement (TAVR) is a minimally invasive percutaneous procedure in which an aortic valve is replaced through an endovascular technique that wedges a replacement valve into an old valve to treat severe aortic stenosis (AS). It is sometimes also called transcatheter aortic valve implantation (TAVI). It uses chemically fixed xenografts for leaflets. It was initially indicated for inoperable high-risk patients with AS and recently has been approved for intermediate and low-risk patients. It is the new standard of care for symptomatic severe AS patients at risk of surgical valve replacement. Some advantages of TAVR include shorter hospital stays and lower mortality compared to surgical aortic valve replacement (SAVR). In this chapter, we discuss the incidence of ischemic stroke, the risk and benefit of the TAVR procedure, and future directions.

1. Describe the evidence for TAVR.

The Placement of Aortic Transcatheter Valves (PARTNER) trial was the first multicenter, randomized clinical trial comparing TAVR with standard therapy in high-risk patients with severe AS. PARTNER 1B reported the outcomes with TAVR compared with standard therapy among 358 patients in the PARTNER trial who were not suitable candidates for SAVR [30]. Patients who underwent TAVR had significantly reduced all-cause mortality, repeat hospitalization, and cardiac symptoms, despite the higher incidence of major strokes and major vascular events compared to the control arm. PARTNER 1A reported similar rates of survival at one year among 699 high-risk patients with severe AS who were randomly assigned to undergo either TAVR or SAVR. At 30 days, rates of stroke were higher with TAVR compared to SAVR (8.3% vs. 4.3%, $P < 0.05$). In high-risk patient populations, the mortality rates were similar even on two-year follow up (33.9% for TAVR vs. 35.0% for SAVR [$P = 0.78$]). In the PARTNER 2A randomized trial, TAVR was compared with SAVR in intermediate-risk patients. The primary endpoint of all-cause mortality or disabling stroke at two years was similar among 2032 patients who were randomly assigned to either TAVR or SAVR ($N_{on-inferiority} = 0.001$).

Another multicenter randomized clinical trial, Surgical Replacement and Transcatheter Aortic Valve Implantation (SURTAVI), enrolled 1746 patients at intermediate surgical risk. Of these patients, 1660 underwent either TAVR or SAVR. TAVR was reported to be non-inferior to SAVR, with an incidence of the primary endpoint (a composite of death from any cause or disabling stroke) of 12.6 and 14% at 24 months in the two groups, respectively.

Given promising results in high- and intermediate-risk patients, PARTNER 3 compared the TAVR and SAVR in 1000 low-risk patients. The rate of the primary composite endpoint (composite of death, stroke, or rehospitalization) at one year was significantly lower in the TAVR arm compared to the surgical arm (8.5 vs. 15.1%; absolute difference, −6.6% points; 95% confidence interval [CI], −10.8 to −2.5; P < 0.001 for noninferiority; hazard ratio [HR], 0.54; 95% CI, 0.37–0.79; P = 0.001 for superiority).

Furthermore, at 30 days, TAVR resulted in a lower rate of stroke (P = 0.02) and a shorter index hospitalization (P < 0.001) than surgery.

In another randomized multicenter clinical trial involving a self-expanding supranuclear bioprosthesis, TAVR was found to be non-inferior to surgery with respect to the composite end point of death or disabling stroke at 24 months among low surgical risk patients. Taking into account these high-quality randomized data, the latest American College of Cardiology/American Heart Association (ACC/AHA) valvular heart disease guidelines provide a new roadmap and direction for the assessment and management of patients with AS and support TAVR as the preferred therapeutic management tool among elderly (>80 years) patients with symptomatic severe AS.

Stroke Following TAVR

2. What is the incidence of stroke following TAVR?

TAVR serves as an alternative to SAVR in eligible AS patients. While the surgical technique involves the precise removal of calcium deposits from the stenosed valve followed by valve replacement, TAVR is associated with lateral compression and exclusion of calcifications by the new prosthetic valve. Such technical variations, along with other hemodynamic factors, lead to a twofold higher incidence of stroke following TAVR as compared to SAVR. Stroke following TAVR is a dreaded complication that principally occurs in the peri-procedural period or within the 30 days following. Strokes that occur immediately (early) or in the first few days are commonly attributed to the embolization of procedural debris. In patients who receive timely neuroimaging following TAVR, it is felt that some degree of post-implantation ischemia is close to guaranteed. Much akin to post-neuro-interventional ischemic lesions, the ultimate morbidity related to silent strokes (which may occur in 84–94% of patients) is unknown but is surmised to have long-term neurocognitive implications. Delayed strokes are considered those which are not detected immediately but occur more than 24 hours later, and there is debate as to whether they occur due to slow thrombus formation or simply delays in neuroimaging. From 7 to 30 days later is considered delayed and is typically felt to be related to patient factors.

Table 20.1 provides a comprehensive review of high-quality data (randomized trials, meta-analyses, and real-world registries) on the 30-day and one-year incidence of stroke following TAVR across an important period of evolving experience with TAVR. As experience and technology progress, the incidence of stroke following TAVR appears to be declining from approximately 11% to 3% at one year and from approximately 7% to 2% at 30 days. This data needs to be appreciated with respect to the period of the study, the definition of stroke used, and the patient population included in the trials.

Table 20.1 Various studies showing rate of stroke in transcatheter aortic valve replacement patients.

Study name	Type of study	Publication year	N in TAVR arm	Incidence of any stroke	
				30 d	1 yr
PARTNER-B	RCT	2010	179	6.7%	10.6%
PARTNER-A	RCT	2011	348	5.5%	8.3%
Eggebrecht et al.	Meta-analysis	2012	10 037	3.3%	5.2%
CoreValve	RCT	2014	390	4.9%	8.8%
Homes et al.	Pooled analysis	2015	12 182	2.5%	4.1%
PARTNER meta-analysis	Meta-analysis	2016	2621	3.3%	5.2%
Muralidharan et al.	Meta-analysis	2016	29 043	NA	3.1%
Krasopoulos et al.	Meta-analysis	2016	9786	NA	3%
Huded et al.	Registry	2019	101 430	2.3%	NA
SWENTRY	Registry	2021	4205	NA	2%

RCT, randomized controlled trial.

3. What are the predictors and impact of stroke associated with TAVR?

Stroke after TAVR is associated with a more than fivefold increase in mortality and significantly worse long-term outcomes as compared to TAVR without a stroke. One-year mortality following an early or late stroke in the CoreValve study was 46.2% and 44.6%, respectively, and of course was greatest in patients with major stroke. Moreover, 7% of patients with a peri-procedural stroke had a recurrent stroke at one-year follow-up. TIA and stroke had a major impact compared to expected one-year survival rates in the PARTNER trial at 64% and 47% compared to 83% and 82%. A large Swedish nationwide study of TAVR from 2008 to 2018 identified reduced renal function, diabetes, history of stroke, age, and male sex as risk factors for developing stroke after TAVR. This investigation found a one-year mortality rate of 44%, which was similar to that of CoreValve. Another study identified the following elements as predictors of stroke following TAVR: new-onset atrial fibrillation (HR 2.27–4.40), smaller aortic valve area (HR 11.8), balloon post-dilatation (HR 1.94), valve dislodgment (HR 4.36), and severe aortic calcification (HR 2.26). In contrast, late stroke is felt to be predicted by chronic AF (HR 1.44–2.84), prior stroke within 6–12 months (HR 1.93), non-transfemoral candidacy (HR 2.30), peripheral vascular disease (2.02), and cerebrovascular disease (2.04) [36]. Appropriate management of stroke, primary and secondary, after TAVR is necessary to avoid increased disability and increased mortality.

Management of TAVR-Related Stroke

4. How can you prevent stroke related to TAVR?

Given the substantial negative impact of stroke after TAVR, primary prevention of stroke after TAVR is important. The etiology of stroke after TAVR is variable and dependent on the timing of the stroke. It may be grouped into three phases: early (0–24 hours), delayed (2–30 days), and late (>30 days).

Early stroke after TAVR is due to procedural factors and immediate post-procedural risk of thromboembolism. Careful imaging-based characterization of the stenotic valve (size, calcification), aortic arch anatomy (type, disease burden), and prosthetic valve deployment technique (balloon expansion vs. self-expanding valves, smaller lumen caliber catheters) has the potential to limit embolic strokes during TAVR. The use of embolic protection devices (EPDs) has been shown to limit the degree of diffusion-weighted imaging (DWI) lesions during the procedure. Choosing and deploying the appropriate embolic protection device may be a promising method of reducing early stroke risk. The EPDs have been designed to protect supra-aortic vessels by capturing emboli during the TAVR procedure. Currently, there are different devices three devices are available for this purpose: Embrella, Sentinel, and TriGUARD.

Despite studies that have demonstrated the technical feasibility and safety of these devices, no clear data exists to support their clinical efficacy in stroke prevention. A meta-analysis that included 16 studies (a total of 1170 patients) showed no benefit of EPDs in terms of rates of clinically evident stroke, number of brain lesions, and 30-day mortality. This meta-analysis looked at a cumulative effect across all EPDs for stroke prevention. These results are also supported by recent data from the Transcatheter Aortic Valve Registry showing no benefit of EPDs for stroke prevention. In contrast, another meta-analysis has investigated only studies using the Sentinel device (four studies with a total of 1330 patients), suggesting its benefit in terms of lower rates of 30-day symptomatic stroke (3.5% vs. 6.1%) and 30-day mortality (0.8% vs. 2.7%). To this end, the PROTECTED-TAVR (Stroke PROTECTion With SEntinel During Transcatheter Aortic Valve Replacement) trial randomizing 3000 patients to TAVR with or without a Sentinel device is ongoing and will hopefully provide us with the answer to the current equipoise in their efficacy in the prevention of TAVR-related strokes.

Intra-procedural manipulation of the aorta, valve, and surrounding structures coupled with prolonged exposure to thrombogenic devices increases the risk of thromboembolism. Additionally, pre-existing atrial fibrillation in the setting of AS and new-onset atrial fibrillation due to cardiac surgery contribute to higher early stroke risk. Hence, the cornerstone of stroke prevention in TAVR patients remains antithrombotic treatment. The American College of Cardiology Foundation & Society for Cardiovascular Angiography and Intervention/Society of Thoracic Surgeons guideline recommends intra-procedural use of heparin (aim to achieve activated clotting time of >300 seconds). Unfractionated heparin (UFH) is a standard therapy during the TAVR procedure with up to 17% risk of peri-procedural bleeding. For this reason, the BRAVO (Effect of Bivalirudin on Aortic Valve Intervention Outcomes) 3 study compared the use of direct thrombin inhibitor bivalirudin to UFH but failed to show its superiority in terms of risk reduction both of thromboembolic events and periop-erative bleeding. Clinically, antiplatelet medication for post-TAVR-related risk of thrombosis is routine. However, the debate over mono therapy versus dual agent therapy is ongoing. In patients with atrial fibrillation anticoagulation is recommended. Stroke prevention after TAVR in the time window beyond one year is similar to prevention strategies employed for the larger at-risk population and includes optimal vascular risk factor control and better cardiovascu-lar health.

5. What is the best way to treat stroke related to TAVR?

A novel challenge with respect to peri-TVAR strokes is the timely recognition of signs and symptoms of acute stroke due to sedation/anesthesia. Intra-operative neurophysio-logical monitoring (electroencephalogram [EEG], tran-scranial Doppler) is an emerging tool for recognizing TAVR-related strokes. Acute reperfusion therapy, includ-ing systemic thrombolysis and mechanical thrombec-tomy, is the mainstay of acute ischemic stroke treatment. As such, American Heart Association and American Stroke Association (AHA/ASA) guidelines offer Class 1A recommendations for thrombolysis of acute ischemic strokes in the 0–3-hour time window and for mechanical thrombectomy for selected patients in the 0–24-hour time window. The guidelines do not provide any specific rec-ommendations concerning TAVR patients. Neuroimaging plays a central role in the diagnosis and triage of post-TAVR stroke patients. Two primary objectives of neuro-imaging include exclusion of intracranial hemorrhage for potential thrombolysis therapy and vascular imaging to identify a targetable large vessel occlusion for mechanical thrombectomy.

Data on acute reperfusion therapy for strokes after TAVR is limited. Alkhouli et al. utilized the Vizient Clinical Database of >400 US hospitals and studied management patterns and outcomes of acute ischemic strokes after TAVR. Between 2016 and 2020, over 72 000 TAVR proce-dures were identified, and acute ischemic strokes occurred in 1.6% of patients (1135). Overall utilization of acute reperfusion therapy was low: 4.8% of patients received thrombolysis, and 4.4% of patients received mechanical thrombectomy. Low thrombolysis utilization is likely attributed to ineligibility arising out of delayed recognition (>4.5 hours since last known well), pre- or peri-procedural use of anticoagulants, or other thrombolysis-specific exclu-sion criteria. Among patients treated with thrombolysis

(when compared to patients who do not receive thromboly-sis), Alkhouli et al. demonstrate higher rates of in-hospital deaths (13% vs. 8%) and intracerebral hemorrhage (11% vs. 3%), and similar rates of acute kidney injury (33% vs. 26%) and discharge to a skilled nursing facility (SNF) or long-term acute care facility (LTAC) (26% vs. 29%). These results do suffer from selection bias but provide an insight into the overall performance of thrombolysis in post-TAVR stroke patients.

Cline et al. report on an eight-year experience of the safety and efficacy of IV-tPA for stroke after TAVR. Of 779 patients undergoing TAVR, 22 had acute ischemic stroke and 8 received IV-tPA. There was no difference between adverse neurological or cardiac outcomes at discharge and 90 days in the tPA group vs. non-tPA group. More tPA patients had groin bleeding, which did not cause any long-term functional impairment. There was a trend toward tPA patients having a lower discharge NIHSS. Overall, tPA appears to be a safe intervention for stroke after TAVR. A case series by Warner et al. reports the use of protamine reversal of heparin for acute ischemic stroke caused after cardiac catheterization. Six similar cases have been reported in the literature and suggest that tPA may be safe even in patients with reversal of heparin (no case reporting intracranial hemorrhage after tPA administration).

In the presence of a large vessel occlusion after TAVR, mechanical thrombectomy (MT) may be a potential man-agement option. It can be offered up to 24 hours from stroke onset and can also be performed without thromboly-sis. Alkhouli et al. report that 4.4% of patients in the Vizient database received MT after TAVR-related stroke, suggest-ing low utilization. The most likely reasons would be lack of large vessel occlusion and delayed recognition of stroke. D'Anna et al. report two cases of thrombolysis and thrombectomy after TAVR: thrombolysis infusion had to be halted in the first case due to groin bleeding, but the patient received a successful thrombectomy with a 24-hour NIH Stroke Scale (NIHSS) score of 3. In the second case, a 98-year-old man received thrombectomy (with TICI 3 rep-erfusion) and an NIHSS score of 5 at 24 hours. Hamandi et al. report two more successful cases of thrombolysis and thrombectomy after TAVR-related stroke. Ramirez-Moreno et al. report a case of thrombectomy post-TAVR stroke involving retrieval of a calcified embolus in the first pass of thrombectomy. The patient went on to be functionally independent at three months.

Figure 20.1 highlights a patient who underwent TAVR at a large academic center in Miami and experienced severe stroke symptoms during the procedure.

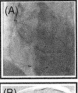
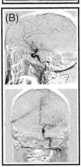
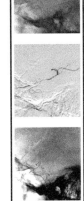
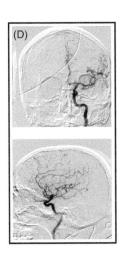

Figure 20.1 A patient underwent (a) transcatheter aortic valve replacement and experienced severe stroke symptoms during the procedure. The patient was taken directly to the neuro-angiography suite for emergent angiography. (b) Digital subtraction angiography confirmed a left MCA M1 occlusion. (c) The patient received stent-retriever-based mechanical thrombectomy, and (d) high-grade reperfusion was established (mTICI 2C).

Conclusions

Stroke in the setting of TAVR is not uncommon and leads to severe disability and mortality. Appropriate management is complex but necessary to realize the benefit of the procedure. Acute reperfusion therapy must be considered, and the utilization of thrombolysis and thrombectomy should be tailored to the specific patients after consultation with an interdisciplinary team of neurologists and cardiologists along with patients' families. More studies are needed to optimize prevention and treatment strategies for acute stroke after TAVR.

Bibliography

1 Adams, D.H., Popma, J.J., and Reardon, M.J. (2014). Transcatheter aortic-valve replacement with a self-expanding prosthesis. *N. Engl. J. Med.* 371: 967–968.

2 Alkhouli, M., Alqahtani, F., Hartsell Harris, A. et al. (2021). Management patterns and outcomes of acute ischemic stroke complicating transcatheter aortic valve replacement. *Stroke* 52: e94–e96.

3 Amat-Santos, I.J., Rodes-Cabau, J., Urena, M. et al. (2012). Incidence, predictive factors, and prognostic value of new-onset atrial fibrillation following transcatheter aortic valve implantation. *J. Am. Coll. Cardiol.* 59: 178–188.

4 Anetakis, K.M., Dolia, J.N., Desai, S.M. et al. (2020). Last electrically well: intraoperative neurophysiological monitoring for identification and triage of large vessel occlusions. *J. Stroke Cerebrovasc. Dis. Official J. Natl. Stroke Assoc.* 29 (10): 105158.

5 Astarci, P., Glineur, D., Kefer, J. et al. (2011). Magnetic resonance imaging evaluation of cerebral embolization during percutaneous aortic valve implantation: comparison of transfemoral and trans-apical approaches using Edwards sapiens valve. *Eur. J. Cardio-thorac. Surg. Official J. Eur. Assoc. Cardio-thorac. Surg.* 40: 475–479.

6 Bagur, R., Solo, K., Alghofaili, S. et al. (2017). Cerebral embolic protection devices during transcatheter aortic valve implantation: systematic review and meta-analysis. *Stroke* 48: 1306–1315.

7 Bjursten, H., Norrving, B., and Ragnarsson, S. (2021). Late stroke after transcatheter aortic valve replacement: a nationwide study. *Sci. Rep.* 11: 9593.

8 Butala, N.M., Makkar, R., Secemsky, E.A. et al. (2021). Cerebral embolic protection and outcomes of transcatheter aortic valve replacement: results from the transcatheter valve therapy registry. *Circulation* 143: 2229–2240.

9 Cline, T.E., Burchette, R., Cheng, P. et al. (2021). Abstract MP1: safety and efficacy of IV-tPA for acute ischemic stroke after transcatheter aortic valve replacement. *Stroke* 52 (**Suppl_1**): AMP1–AMP1.

10 Cribier, A. (2016). The development of transcatheter aortic valve replacement (TAVR). *Glob. Cardiol. Sci. Pract.* (4): e201632.

11 Dangas, G.D., Lefevre, T., Kupatt, C. et al. (2015). Bivalirudin versus heparin anticoagulation in transcatheter aortic valve replacement: the randomized BRAVO-3 trial. *J. Am. Coll. Cardiol.* 66: 2860–2868.

12 D'Anna, L., Demir, O., Banerjee, S., and Malik, I. (2019). Intravenous thrombolysis and mechanical thrombectomy in patients with stroke after TAVI: a report of two cases. *J. Stroke Cerebrovasc. Dis. Official J. Natl. Stroke Assoc.* 28: 104277.

13 Davlouros, P.A., Mplani, V.C., Koniari, I. et al. (2018). Transcatheter aortic valve replacement and stroke: a comprehensive review. *J. Geriatr. Cardiol* 15: 95–104.

14 Eggebrecht, H., Schmermund, A., Voigtländer, T. et al. (2012). Risk of stroke after transcatheter aortic valve implantation (TAVI): a meta-analysis of 10,037 published patients. *EuroIntervention, J. Eur. Collab. Work. Group Interv. Cardiol. Eur. Soc. Cardiol.* 8: 129–138.

15 European Heart Rhythm Association (2006). ACC/AHA/ESC 2006 guidelines for the management of patients with atrial fibrillation--executive summary: a report of the American College of Cardiology/American Heart Association task force on practice guidelines and the European Society of Cardiology Committee for practice guidelines (Writing Committee to revise the 2001 guidelines for the management of patients with atrial fibrillation). *J. Am. Coll. Cardiol.* 48: 854–906.

16 Fanning, J.P., Walters, D.L., Platts, D.G. et al. (2014). Characterization of neurological injury in transcatheter aortic valve implantation: how clear is the picture? *Circulation* 129: 504–515.

17 Fontaine, G.V. and Smith, S.M. (2017). Alteplase for acute ischemic stroke after heparin reversal with protamine: a case report and review. *Pharmacotherapy* 37: e103–e106.

18 Ghanem, A., Muller, A., Nahle, C.P. et al. (2010). Risk and fate of cerebral embolism after transfemoral aortic valve implantation: a prospective pilot study with diffusion-weighted magnetic resonance imaging. *J. Am. Coll. Cardiol.* 55: 1427–1432.

19 Guevara, C., Quijada, A., Rosas, C. et al. (2017). Acute ischemic stroke after cardiac catheterization: the protamine low-dose recombinant tissue plasminogen activator pathway. *Blood Coagul. Fibrinolysis Int. J. Haemost. Thromb.* 28: 261–263.

20 Hamandi, M., Farber, A.J., Tatum, J.K. et al. (2018). Acute stroke intervention after transcatheter aortic valve replacement. *Proc. Bayl. Univ. Med. Cent.* 31: 490–492.

21 Haussig, S., Manger, N., Dwyer, M.G. et al. (2016). Effect of a cerebral protection device on brain lesions following transcatheter aortic valve implantation in patients with severe aortic stenosis: the CLEAN-TAVI randomized clinical trial. *J. Am. Med. Assoc.* 316: 592–601.

22 Hecker, F., Arsalan, M., and Walther, T. (2017). Managing stroke during transcatheter aortic valve replacement. *Interv. Cardiol. Lond. Engl.* 12: 25–30.

23 Holmes, D.R., Brennan, J.M., Rumsfeld, J.S, et al. (2015). Clinical outcomes at 1 year following transcatheter aortic valve replacement. *J. Am. Med. Assoc.* 313: 1019–1028.

24 Holmes, D.R., Mack, M.M., Kaul, S. et al. (2012). 2012 ACCF/AATS/SCAI/STS expert consensus document on transcatheter aortic valve replacement. *J. Am. Coll. Cardiol.* 59: 1200–1254.

25 Huded, C.P., Tuzcu, E.M., Krishnaswamy, A. et al. (2019). Association between transcatheter aortic valve replacement and early postprocedural stroke. *J. Am. Med. Assoc.* 321: 2306–2315.

26 Kapadia, S.R., Kodali, S., Makkar, R. et al. (2017). Protection against cerebral embolism during transcatheter aortic valve replacement. *J. Am. Coll. Cardiol.* 69: 367–377.

27 Kapadia, S., Agarwal, S., Miller, D.C. et al. (2016). Insights into timing, risk factors, and outcomes of stroke and transient ischemic attack after transcatheter aortic valve replacement in the PARTNER trial (placement of aortic transcatheter valves). *Circ. Cardiovasc. Interv.* 9: e002981.

28 Krasopoulos, G., Falconieri, F., Benedetto, U. et al. (2016). European real world trans-catheter aortic valve implantation: systematic review and meta-analysis of European national registries. *J. Cardiothorac. Surg.* 11: 159.

29 Lansky, A.J., Schofer, J., Tchetche, D. et al. (2015). A prospective randomized evaluation of the TriGuard™ HDH embolic DEFLECTion device during transcatheter aortic valve implantation: results from the DEFLECT III trial. *Eur. Heart J.* 36: 2070–2078.

30 Leon, M.B., Smith, C.R., Mack, M.J. et al. (2010). Transcatheter aortic-valve implantation for aortic stenosis in patients who cannot undergo surgery. *N. Engl. J. Med.* 363: 1597–1607.

31 Leon, M.B., Smith, M.D., Mack, M.J. et al. (2016). Transcatheter or surgical aortic-valve replacement in intermediate-risk patients. *N. Engl. J. Med.* 374: 1609–1620.

32 Linke, A., Hollriegel, R., Walther, T. et al. (2008). Ingrowths of a percutaneously implanted aortic valve prosthesis (corevalve) in a patient with severe aortic stenosis. *Circ. Cardiovasc. Interv.* 1: 155–158.

33 Mack, M.J., Leon, M.D., Thourani, V.H. et al. (2019). Transcatheter aortic-valve replacement with a balloon-expandable valve in low-risk patients. *N. Engl. J. Med.* 380: 1695–1705.

34 Macle, L., Cairns, J.A., Andrade, J.A. et al. (2015). The 2014 atrial fibrillation guidelines companion: a practical approach to the use of the Canadian cardiovascular society guidelines. *Can. J. Cardiol.* 31: 1207–1218.

35 Maisel, W.H., Rawn, J.D., and Stevenson, W.G. (2001). Atrial fibrillation after cardiac surgery. *Ann. Intern. Med.* 135: 1061–1073.

36 Mastoris, I., Schoos, M.M., Dangas, G.D., and Mehran, R. (2014). Stroke after transcatheter aortic valve replacement: incidence, risk factors, prognosis, and preventive strategies. *Clin. Cardiol.* 37: 756–764.

37 Miller, D.C., Blackstone, E.H., Mack, M.J. et al. (2012). Transcatheter (TAVR) versus surgical (AVR) aortic valve replacement: occurrence, hazard, risk factors, and consequences of neurologic events in the PARTNER trial. *J. Thorac. Cardiovasc. Surg.* 143: 832–843.e13.

38 Möllmann, H., Kim, W.-K., Kempfert, J. et al. (2015). Complications of transcatheter aortic valve implantation (TAVI): how to avoid and treat them. *Heart Br. Card. Soc.* 101: 900–908.

39 Muralidharan, A., Thiagarajan, K., Van Ham, R. et al. (2016). Meta-analysis of perioperative stroke and mortality in transcatheter aortic valve implantation. *Am. J. Cardiol.* 118: 1031–1045.

40 Naber, C.K., Ghanem, A., Abizaid, A.A. et al. (2012). First-in-man use of a novel embolic protection device for patients undergoing transcatheter aortic valve implantation. *EuroIntervention, J. Eur. Collab. Work. Group Interv. Cardiol. Eur. Soc. Cardiol.* 8: 43–50.

41 Nuis, R.-J., Van Mieghem, N.M., Schultz, C.J. et al. (2012). Frequency and causes of stroke during or after transcatheter aortic valve implantation. *Am. J. Cardiol.* 109: 1637–1643.

42 Otto, C.O., Nishimura, R.A., Bonow, R.O. et al. (2021). 2020 ACC/AHA guideline for the management of patients with valvular heart disease: executive summary: a report of the American College of Cardiology/American Heart Association joint committee on clinical practice guidelines. *J. Am. Coll. Cardiol.* 77: 450–500.

43 Popma, J.J., Deeb, M., Yakubov, S.J. et al. (2019). Transcatheter aortic-valve replacement with a self-expanding valve in low-risk patients. *N. Engl. J. Med.* 380: 1706–1715.

44 Powers, W.J., Rabinstein, A.A., Ackerson, T. et al. (2019). Guidelines for the early management of patients with acute ischemic stroke: 2019 update to the 2018 guidelines for the early management of acute ischemic stroke: a guideline for healthcare professionals from the American Heart Association/American Stroke Association. *Stroke* 50: e344–e418.

45 Ramírez-Moreno, J.M., Trinidad-Ruiz, M., Ceberino, D., and Fernández de Alarcón, L. (2017). Mechanical thrombectomy during ischaemic stroke due to a calcified cerebral embolism. *Neurol. Engl. Ed.* 32: 270–273.

46 Ranasinghe, T., Mays, T., Quedado, J., and Adcock, A. (2019). Thrombolysis following heparin reversal with protamine sulfate in acute ischemic stroke: case series and literature review. *J. Stroke Cerebrovasc. Dis. Official J. Natl. Stroke Assoc.* 28: 104283.

47 Reardon, M.J., Van Mieghem, N.M., Popma, J.J. et al. (2017). Surgical or transcatheter aortic-valve replacement in intermediate-risk patients. *N. Engl. J. Med.* 376: 1321–1331.

48 Rodés-Cabau, J., Dumont, E., Boone, R.H. et al. (2011). Cerebral embolism following transcatheter aortic valve implantation: comparison of transfemoral and transapical approaches. *J. Am. Coll. Cardiol.* 57: 18–28.

49 Schoenhagen, P., Tuzcu, E.M., Kapadia, S.R. et al. (2009). Three-dimensional imaging of the aortic valve and aortic root with computed tomography: new standards in an era of transcatheter valve repair/implantation. *Eur. Heart J.* 30: 2079–2086.

50 Smith, C.R., Leon, M.D., Mack, M.J. et al. (2011). Transcatheter versus surgical aortic-valve replacement in high-risk patients. *N. Engl. J. Med.* 364: 2187–2198.

51 Sundt, T.M. and Jneid, H. (2021). Guideline update on indications for transcatheter aortic valve implantation based on the 2020 American College of Cardiology/American Heart Association guidelines for management of valvular heart disease. *JAMA Cardiol.* 6: 1088–1089.

52 Van Mieghem, N.M., Schipper, M.E.I., Lasich, E. et al. (2013). Histopathology of embolic debris captured during transcatheter aortic valve replacement. *Circulation* 127: 2194–2201.

53 Warner, D.S., Schwartz, B.G., Babygirija, R. et al. (2018). Thrombolysis after protamine reversal of heparin for acute ischemic stroke after cardiac catheterization: case report and literature review. *Neurologist* 23: 194–196.

54 Werner, N., Zeymer, U., Schneider, S. et al. (2016). Incidence and clinical impact of stroke complicating transcatheter aortic valve implantation: results from the German TAVI registry. *Catheter. Cardiovasc. Interv. Official J. Soc. Card. Angiogr. Interv.* 88: 644–653.

21

Current Evidence of Neuroprotection in TAVR

Herbert G. Kroon and Nicolas M. Van Mieghem

Department of Interventional Cardiology, Thoraxcenter, Erasmus University Medical Center, Rotterdam, The Netherlands

Peri-Procedural Stroke

1. Is the occurrence of peri-procedural strokes still the Achilles' heel of TAVR?

Approximately 5% of patients suffered from stroke in the early transcatheter aortic valve replacement (TAVR) era. TAVR-related stroke incidence appeared twice as high as the stroke rate after surgical aortic valve replacement (SAVR). Stroke negatively impacts quality of life and is associated with higher mortality rates at one year. Increasing operator experience, evolution to lower-profile devices, and expanding to younger and lower-risk patients have diminished the stroke rate after TAVR. Nowadays, up to 3% of TAVR patients experience a stroke within 30 days after the procedure, which is in line with the SAVR benchmark. Still, stroke continues to have a tremendous effect on patients' lives, including prolonged hospital admissions, greater morbidity, increased healthcare costs, and curtailed survival.

2. What is the underlying mechanism of stroke in TAVR patients?

Stroke up to 48 hours post-TAVR is considered to be related to particle dislodgement and embolization to the brain. A transcranial Doppler study demonstrated an excess of high-intensity signals as a surrogate for debris embolization during valve positioning and subsequent implantation. Particles may completely or partially obstruct blood flow in focal brain areas and may result in an immediate or delayed neurological event. Beyond 48 hours after the index procedure, atrial fibrillation seems to be the dominant cause of stroke. Up to 30% of patients may experience new-onset atrial fibrillation after TAVR. Other risk factors for stroke include a history of stroke, peripheral artery disease, chronic kidney disease, atherosclerotic disease (especially in the aortic arch) and excessive aortic root calcifications.

3. What are the consequences of debris embolizing to the brain?

So far, the overall clinical implications of debris that embolizes to the brain during TAVR are unresolved. Magnetic resonance imaging (MRI) studies performed before and after TAVR reveal new (ischemic) brain lesions in the vast majority of patients. Most of these new brain lesions appear transient and do not seem to have an immediate clinical impact. However, silent lesions have been associated with frank neurocognitive decline and early dementia. Systematic clinical examination by a trained neurologist before and after TAVR has also led to enhanced awareness of neurological events and higher reported stroke rates. This was demonstrated in the randomized SENTINEL Cerebral Protection in Transcatheter Aortic Valve Replacement (trial), as it reported a 9.1% stroke rate in patients with no brain protection vs. 5.6% in patients with brain protection.

The Rationale for Cerebral Embolic Protection Devices

4. How many TAVR patients are affected by embolized debris?

The conceptual framework of cerebral embolic protection (CEP) is sound: devices should prevent debris that is dislodged during a TAVR procedure from reaching the brain. Histopathological studies demonstrated captured debris in up to 98% of patients who underwent TAVR with filter-based embolic protection devices (EPDs). Cerebral EPDs can be roughly divided into filter-based and deflector-based devices or hybrid technologies. Deflector devices redirect particles away from the brain downstream toward the descending aorta. Filter-based devices capture debris and allow debris removal from the bloodstream.

5.   What kind of EPDs are currently available for TAVR?

Currently, the only CE marked and FDA approved EPD is the filter-based Sentinel device (Boston Scientific). The Sentinel is inserted through the right radial or brachial artery (6 French [F] delivery system) and consists of two poly-urethane mesh filters with a current pore size of 140 μm. The proximal filter is deployed in the brachiocephalic trunk and the distal filter in the left common carotid artery, leaving the left vertebral artery unprotected. Difficulty deploying the device has been occasionally reported due to radial artery spasm, excessive tortuosity, atherosclerotic disease at landing zones, or anatomical variation of the cerebral vasculature. Pre-procedural planning includes computed tomography (CT) to evaluate the device landing zones (Figure 21.1); the instructions for use propose diameters of 9.0–15.0 mm and 6.5–10.0 mm for the brachiocephalic trunk and left common carotid artery, respectively. The TriGUARD 3 (Keystone Heart) is a CE-marked deflector device that incorporates a mesh with pores sized 115–145 μm. This device requires an 8F sheath and a common femoral artery approach.

6.   Are other technologies in the pipeline?

Several devices are currently under investigation. The ProtEmbo system (Protembis) is a deflector device with 60 μm pores that delivers full cerebral coverage and is deployed through a 6F sheath and a left radial artery approach (unique for deflector devices). POINT-GUARD (Transverse Medical) is a deflector with 105 μm pores and requires a 10F sheath through a common femoral artery access.

The 9F Emboliner (Emboline) features a sock-like circumferential design with 150 μm pores and contains an expandable port for passage of the TAVR catheter. It captures and removes emboli from the body. The Emblok system (Innovative Cardiovascular Solutions) is an 11F conic-shaped filter system with an integrated 4F pigtail catheter for anatomical landmarking that is deployed just proximal to the brachiocephalic trunk in the ascending aorta for complete protection. A TAVR delivery catheter can be advanced next to the Emblok system, which is deployed while essential TAVR procedural steps are performed (balloon dilatation, valve deployment, post-dilatation, etc.). The device needs to be resheathed between steps but can be reopened for additional valve manipulation. Thus the device offers complete protection while fully opened but does not protect against debris that is dislodged during catheter passage in the aortic arch. The CAPTIS device (Filterlex Medical) is a hybrid system that includes a deflector section that is deployed in the aortic arch to protect all extracranial arteries and a filter section that is deployed in the descending aorta and collects all deflected debris. This device leverages the large bore arterial access used for the TAVR delivery system and thus precludes additional (large-bore) arterial access for embolic protection. Table 21.1 summarizes contemporary EPDs.

Characteristics of Dislodged Debris

7.   What kind of debris may embolize toward the brain?

Microscopic debris is captured in almost all patients. The majority of captured debris is thrombotic and can be found in approximately 90% of patients. Calcified particles stemming from the aortic valve or wall are also common (approximately 60–80% of patients).

Furthermore, foreign body material coming from catheters/delivery systems is present in 30–60% of patients.

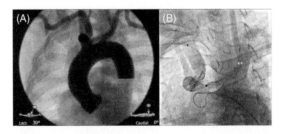

Figure 21.1   Pre-procedural computed tomography planning for the Sentinel embolic protection device (EPD). (a) Angiographic reconstruction of the aortic arch, brachiocephalic trunk, and carotid arteries in the left anterior oblique projection using 3mensio software (Pie Medical Imaging BV). (b) The EPD in situ with the proximal and distal filter deployed in the brachiocephalic trunk (*) and left common carotid artery (**), respectively, in a TAVR patient with a bovine arch. In general, this pre-procedural reconstruction allows the operator to deploy the EPD without using extra contrast.

Table 21.1 Overview of embolic protection devices currently being evaluated.

Device	Sheath size (F)	Type	Cerebral coverage	Pore size (µm)	Access site	Clinical state	Current trial
Sentinel	6	Filter	Partial	140	Right radial	CE mark/FDA approved	PROTECTED TAVR/ BHF PROTECT TAVI
TriGuard 3	8	Deflector	Full	115–145	Femoral	CE mark	REFLECT II
Emblok	11	Filter	Full	125	Femoral	Investigational	EMBLOK in TAVR
Emboliner	9	Filter	Full	150	Femoral	Investigational	SafePass 2
Captis	Unknown	Filter	Full	Unknown	Femoral	Investigational	Unknown
ProtEmbo	6	Deflector	Full	60	Left radial	Investigational	PROTEMBO SF
Point-Guard	10	Deflector	Full	105	Femoral	Investigational	CENTER

Source: Haussig et al. (2020) / Springer Nature.

Endothelium, myocardial tissue, and collagen can also be identified in the filters after TAVR but seems to be less common (<30%).

8. What is the captured debris size?

Histopathological analysis has been performed with the 140 µm pore-size Sentinel EPD after TAVR. Most particles measure <1000 µm. Still, particles >1000 µm (and in some cases even larger than 2000 µm or 2 mm and therefore macroscopically visible) are not uncommon and are reported in 20–50% of filters after TAVR (10–15% for particles >2 mm) (Figure 21.2).

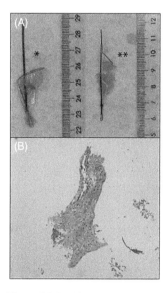

Figure 21.2 Macroscopy and histopathology of filters with captured debris following the transcatheter aortic valve replacement (TAVR) procedure. (a) Proximal (*) and distal (**) filter as received at the pathology department. (b) Aortic valve material, hematoxylin–eosin stain, 10× magnification.

9. Are there any predicting factors for the dislodgement of debris?

Currently, there is no compelling evidence that one particular transcatheter heart valve is more prone to debris embolization than others. However, repositioning the valve may increase the amount of debris released for embolization, according to some observational filter-based cerebral embolic protection studies. TAVR in calcified (functional) bicuspid valves may result in the capture of larger particles.

10. Who might benefit most from protected TAVR?

Currently, no strong predictors for clinically relevant debris embolization have been identified to justify the selective use of EPDs. Debris has been identified across the age and operative risk spectrum and all commercially available TAVR platforms.

Clinical Evidence of Neuroprotection In TAVR

11. Is there a proven clinical benefit from randomized controlled trials (RCTs) to underpin the systematic use of cerebral embolic protection in TAVR?

Three RCTs have been performed with the Sentinel device with MRI-based primary endpoints. The CLEAN-TAVI

(CLaret Embolic Protection ANd TAVI) trial found fewer lesions and smaller lesion volume in protected patients, but the other two did not observe significant differences. These studies suffered from patient drop-out and had incomplete follow-up MRI data. Furthermore, because the primary endpoints were imaging-based, these studies were not sufficiently powered for clinical endpoints like stroke or death. The TriGUARD deflector device has been studied in three RCTs but failed to demonstrate clinically relevant benefits. In aggregate, there is no compelling clinical evidence from RCTs that EPDs would reduce the incidence of neurological events with TAVR. A large interrogation of the Transcatheter Valve Therapy database suggested a modest reduction in new strokes with filter-based embolic protection in a propensity weighted analysis. Table 21.2 provides an overview of RCTs with EPDs.

Various observational studies with the Sentinel device reported a relative risk reduction of up to 80% for any stroke

Table 21.2 Overview of clinical randomized controlled trials studying embolic protection.

Study/Device	EPD (N)	No EPD (N)	Stroke	MRI lesion volume (mm^3)	MRI number of lesions	AKI	Major VC
CLEAN-TAVI Sentinel	50	50	5 (10%) vs. 5 (10%)	466 (349–711) vs. 800 (594–1407), **P = 0.02**	8.0 [5.0–12.0] vs. 16.0 [9.8–24.3], **P = 0.002**	1 (2%) vs. 5 (10%)	5 (10%) vs. 6 (12%)
MISTRAL-C[4] Sentinel	32	33	0 (0%) vs. 2 (7%)	95 [10–257] vs. 197 [95–525], NS	No lesions 27% vs. 13%, NS 1–9 lesions 73% vs. 67%, NS 10 or more 0% vs. 20%, **P = 0.03**	0 (0%) vs. 1 (3%)	0 (0%) vs. 6 (19%)
SENTINEL Sentinel	244	119	13 (6%) vs. 10 (9%), NS	294.0 [69.2–786.4] vs. 309.8 [105.5–859.6], NS	3 [2–10] vs. 5 [2–10], NS	Stage III 1 (<1%) vs. 0 (0%), NS	21 (9%) vs. 7 (6%), NS
DEFLECT III TriGuard	46	39	2 (4%) vs. 2 (6%), NS	Maximum lesion volume 58.5 vs. 68.3, NS	Freedom from lesions 21.2% vs. 11.5%	Stage II/III 1 (2%) vs. 0 (0%), NS	8 (17%) vs. 8 (21%), NS
REFLECT I TriGuard	141	63	14 (11%) vs. 4 (7%), NS	229 [46–631] vs. 235 [81–484], NS	5.5 ± 6.4 vs. 5.0 ± 5.9, NS	Stage II/III 0 (0%) vs. 0 (0%), NS	16 (12%) vs. 1 (2%), **P = 0.02**
REFLECT II TriGuard 3	116	57	13 (8%)[a] vs. 3 (5%), NS	215.4 [68.1–619.7] vs. 188.1 [52.1–453.1], NS	6.0 ± 8.3 vs. 4.6 ± 5.9, NS	Stage II/III 4 (3%)[a] vs. 0 (0%), NS	11 (7%)[a] vs. 0 (0%), **P = 0.039**
PROTECTED TAVR Sentinel	Overall 3.000 patients	–	–	–	–	–	–
BHF PROTECT TAVI Sentinel	Overall 7.730 patients	–	–	–	–	–	–

Clinical outcomes at 30 days after the index procedure according to Valvular Academic Research Consortium (VARC)-2 criteria. Magnetic Resonance Imaging was normally performed between 2 and 7 days after TAVR. Treatment arm with EPD vs. Control arm without EPD. Some studies did not report p-values for specific data. Data presented as number N (percentage), mean $\pm$ SD, median [Interquartile Range], or median (95% Confidence Interval).

Abbreviations: EPD = Embolic Protection Device; MRI = Magnetic Resonance Imaging; AKI = Acute Kidney Injury; VC = Vascular complication; NS = Not Significant.

[a] Indicates numbers including the 41 roll-in patients.

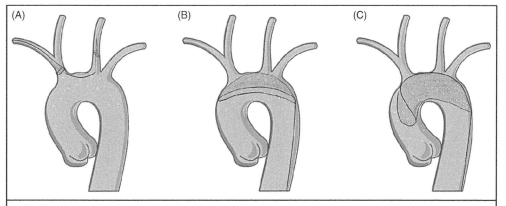

Figure 21.3 Key points of neuroprotection in TAVR. *Source:* Haussig et al. (2020) / Springer Nature.

after TAVR with cerebral protection. Despite inherent selection bias with observational studies, the mechanistic concept of embolic protection seems sound and could justify its use to prevent debris from entering the brain in practically all patients undergoing TAVR. Imaging studies also confirmed (silent) cerebral injury in the vast majority of TAVR patients, which may be associated with early dementia and neurocognitive decline. EPDs may reduce new brain lesion volume and number and thus hypothetically protect against premature neurocognitive decline.

12. What will the future bring?

Currently, two properly powered RCTs are evaluating filter-based embolic protection with the Sentinel device. The

PROTECTED TAVR (Stroke PROTECTion With SEntinel During Transcatheter Aortic Valve Replacement) study plans to enroll 3000 patients, while the British Heart Foundation PROTECT TAVI (Randomised Trial of Routine Cerebral Embolic Protection in TAVI) trial will include 7730 patients. The primary endpoint for both studies is all-cause stroke at 72 hours or discharge, adjudicated by an independent clinical event committee. These studies are expected to provide a more definite answer about whether embolic protection during TAVR reduces neurological events and makes TAVR safer.

In conclusion, this chapter discussed the mechanism and clinical impact of stroke after TAVR, current available embolic protection devices, histopathological characteristics of captured debris, and available evidence of neuroprotection in TAVR (Figure 21.3)

Bibliography

1 Butala, N.M., Makkar, R., Secemsky, E.A. et al. (2021). Cerebral embolic protection and outcomes of transcatheter aortic valve replacement: results from the transcatheter valve therapy registry. *Circulation* 143: 2229–2240.

2 Davlouros, P.A., Mplani, V.C., Koniari, I. et al. (2018). Transcatheter aortic valve replacement and stroke: a comprehensive review. *J. Geriatric Cardiol. JGC* 15: 95–104.

3 Eggebrecht, H., Schmermund, A., Voigtlander, T. et al. (2012). Risk of stroke after transcatheter aortic valve implantation (TAVI): a meta-analysis of 10,037 published patients. *EuroIntervention* 8: 129–138.

4 Haussig, S., Linke, A., and Mangner, N. (2020). Cerebral protection devices during transcatheter interventions: indications, benefits, and limitations. *Curr. Cardiol. Rep.* 22: 96.

5 Haussig, S., Mangner, N., Dwyer, M.G. et al. (2016). Effect of a cerebral protection device on brain lesions following

transcatheter aortic valve implantation in patients with severe aortic stenosis: the CLEAN-TAVI randomized clinical trial. *JAMA* 316: 592–601.

6 Kahlert, P., Al-Rashid, F., Dottger, P. et al. (2012). Cerebral embolization during transcatheter aortic valve implantation: a transcranial Doppler study. *Circulation* 126: 1245–1255.

7 Kapadia, S.R., Kodali, S., Makkar, R. et al. (2017). Protection against cerebral embolism during transcatheter aortic valve replacement. *J. Am. Coll. Cardiol.* 69: 367–377.

8 Kroon, H., von der Thusen, J.H., Ziviello, F. et al. (2021). Heterogeneity of debris captured by cerebral embolic protection filters during TAVI. *EuroIntervention* 16: 1141–1147.

9 Kroon, H.G., van der Werf, H.W., Hoeks, S.E. et al. (2019). Early clinical impact of cerebral embolic protection in patients undergoing transcatheter aortic valve replacement. *Circ. Cardiovasc. Interv.* 12: e007605.

10 Lansky, A.J., Makkar, R., Nazif, T. et al. (2021). A randomized evaluation of the TriGuard HDH cerebral embolic protection device to reduce the impact of cerebral embolic LEsions after TransCatheter aortic valve ImplanTation: the REFLECT I trial. *Eur. Heart J.* 42: 2670–2679.

11 Lansky, A.J., Schofer, J., Tchetche, D. et al. (2015). A prospective randomized evaluation of the TriGuard HDH embolic DEFLECTion device during transcatheter aortic valve implantation: results from the DEFLECT III trial. *Eur. Heart J.* 36: 2070–2078.

12 Nazif, T.M., Moses, J., Sharma, R. et al. (2021). Randomized evaluation of TriGuard 3 cerebral embolic protection after transcatheter aortic valve replacement: REFLECT II. *JACC Cardiovasc. Interv.* 14: 515–527.

13 Schmidt, T., Leon, M.B., Mehran, R. et al. (2018). Debris heterogeneity across different valve types captured by a cerebral protection system during transcatheter aortic valve replacement. *JACC Cardiovasc. Interv.* 11: 1262–1273.

14 Seeger, J., Gonska, B., Otto, M. et al. (2017). Cerebral embolic protection during transcatheter aortic valve replacement significantly reduces death and stroke compared with unprotected procedures. *JACC Cardiovasc. Interv.* 10: 2297–2303.

15 Seeger, J., Romero, M., Schuh, C. et al. (2019). Impact of repositioning during transcatheter aortic valve replacement on embolized debris. *J. Invasive Cardiol.* 31: 282–288.

16 Seeger, J., Virmani, R., Romero, M. et al. (2018). Significant differences in debris captured by the sentinel dual-filter cerebral embolic protection during transcatheter aortic valve replacement among different valve types. *JACC Cardiovasc. Interv.* 11: 1683–1693.

17 Van Mieghem, N.M., van Gils, L., Ahmad, H. et al. (2016). Filter-based cerebral embolic protection with transcatheter aortic valve implantation: the randomised MISTRAL-C trial. *EuroIntervention* 12: 499–507.

18 Vermeer, S.E., Prins, N.D., den Heijer, T. et al. (2003). Silent brain infarcts and the risk of dementia and cognitive decline. *N. Engl. J. Med.* 348: 1215–1222.

22

Difficult Transfemoral Access for TAVR and Bailout Techniques

Camilo A. Gomez[1] and Eduardo J. de Marchena[2]

Department of Cardiology,, Jackson Memorial Health System, Miami, FL, USA
Division of Cardiovascular Medicine, University of Miami Miller School of Medicine, University of Miami Hospital, Miami, FL, USA

1. What are the benefits of transfemoral access?

Transfemoral (TF) is the preferred approach for TAVR. It has been shown to have better outcomes than alternative accesses for TAVR. Some of the benefits are shorter length of stay, lower cost, less use of sedation or general anesthesia, and, in some centers, performance with only local anesthesia. Additionally, it provides an ergonomic advantage for the implanter. Unfortunately, not all patients have favorable TF anatomy; many patients have complex anatomic features that have led to the development of sophisticated techniques and advancements in the technology of TAVR platforms and delivery systems. The transfemoral approach has evolved and now has increased safety and procedural success. With these advancements, femoral access is increasingly available and is the approach in more than 94% of TAVR procedures; only a small percentage of cases need to be performed via an alternative access. Alternative access significantly increases the rate of complications and mortality compared to the TF approach and therefore should be avoided if possible.

2. What is considered "high-risk" vascular anatomy for transfemoral TAVR?

High-risk vascular anatomy for TAVR includes anatomical features or advanced disease of the peripheral vasculature that threatens the success of the TF approach. High-risk anatomy means a greater risk of vascular complications and, in many instances, requires an alternative access approach to perform the TAVR procedure. Some of the most common challenging anatomies are small size vessels, extensive obstructive peripheral artery disease, significant calcification, and severe tortuosity. In a single-center retrospective study, Staniloae et al. identified patients with "hostile access" over 12 months, 7.4% of the patients met the definition.

According to Staniloae et al., hostile (high-risk) vascular access is defined as follows:

- Arterial diameter < 5.0 mm
- Arterial diameter < 5.5 mm with severe calcification or severe tortuosity
  - Severe calcification = 270–360° circumferential calcium
  - Severe tortuosity = any iliofemoral angle of <90°
- Severe tortuosity with severe calcification irrespective of arterial diameter

3. How common is severe peripheral arterial disease in severe aortic stenosis patients?

Peripheral artery disease (PAD) is frequently found in aortic stenosis (AS) patients, especially because both are more frequent in the same age groups and have common cardiovascular risk factors. In older high-risk AS patients, significant PAD has been reported in at least 25% of the patients. Significant obstruction and calcified lesions obstruct and compromise the advancement of TAVR delivery sheaths and catheters, increasing the risks of vascular complications secondary to the trauma caused by the mechanical interaction with the rigid structures, thereby increasing the

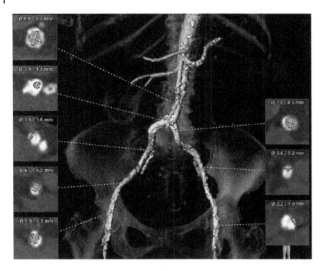

Figure 22.1 Patient with significant peripheral vascular disease and multiple features of a hostile (high-risk) vascular access.

risk of perforation, dissection, plaque disruption, and vessel occlusion (Figure 22.1).

4. How do you plan for a successful transfemoral TAVR procedure?

TF TAVR carries an inherent risk of vascular access complications. Meticulous pre-procedural planning is the key to a successful procedure; thus it is important to evaluate the vascular anatomy and anticipate potential obstacles. It is mandatory to perform pre-procedural computed tomography (CT) with extension to the abdomen and pelvis. Ideally, there should be a three-dimensional reconstruction to correctly delineate the anatomy and aid procedural planning. Some of the important CT features to assess are as follows:

- Height of femoral artery bifurcation
- Size of the femoral and iliac arteries
- Location and extent of calcifications
- Stenosis characteristics of the obstructive plaques
- Iliofemoral and aorta tortuosity, aneurysms, and ectasias
- Inguinal and abdominal soft tissue, and depth to the femoral puncture site

The Heart Team's discussion of individual cases is extremely important, especially with an experienced surgeon's input in cases where a surgical alternative is contemplated. When the procedure strategy is decided, be sure to have all the tools and equipment in the catheterization laboratory to overcome potential difficulties and guarantee a successful TF procedure.

5. What are the most important technology developments for TF access success?

Size and Design of TAVR Delivery Systems

The most important technological improvement is the evolution in the size and design of the delivery systems, which have evolved to lower-profile systems. The first-generation devices were bulky and used catheters and sheaths that were rigid and had a large diameter. The systems have evolved to have a lower profile and more flexibility to adapt to different vascular anatomies (Figure 22.2).

In the case of the self-expanding Medtronic CoreValve system, the delivery system has evolved. The first-generation system was 18 Fr to 24 Fr in size. With improvements in design and engineering, the most recent Medtronic system, the Evolut PRO+, provides a lower delivery profile that makes it possible to access 5 mm vessels with the 23–29 mm valves and 6 mm vessels with the 34 mm valve. The most recent delivery catheter system with the InLine sheath is 14 Fr equivalent for the 23, 26, and 29 mm valves and 18 Fr equivalent for the 34 mm valve (Figure 22.2a). For the SAPIEN S3 (Edwards Lifesciences) balloon-expandable system, the Axela Sheath (commonly called the eSheath) is an expandable and self-collapsible device with a hydrophilic coating that has numerous advantages favoring a smooth transit through the arterial vasculature into the aorta. For the latest S3 Ultra delivery system, the 14 Fr sheath is compatible with all valve sizes (20, 23, 26, and 29 mm). For the SAPIEN S3, the 29 mm valve requires a 16 Fr Axela sheath (Figure 22.2b). The ACURATE *neo* self-expanding valve uses a 14 Fr introducer set, the iSLEEVE. It is a hydrophilic-coated introducer that dynamically expands and contracts with all the ACURATE *neo* valve sizes (S, M, and L) (Figure 22.2c). The Portico valve is delivered using the FlexNav delivery system; it is hydrophilic coated to reduce friction through the vasculature, has an atraumatic nosecone to reduce vascular complications and prevent calcium dislodgement, and has a flexible shaft to adapt to the anatomy. The system uses an integrated sheath that comes in two sizes: 14 Fr for 5 mm vessels and 15 Fr for 5.5 mm vessels (Figure 22.2d).

Ultrasound-Guided Vascular Access

Ultrasound guidance helps to identify the optimal puncture site of the femoral artery above the femoral bifurcation and, usually, below the inguinal ligament. It helps to identify and avoid anterior, posterior, and circumferential calcifications within the artery. It is recommended that it be used in all cases to increase the safety and success of the TF procedure.

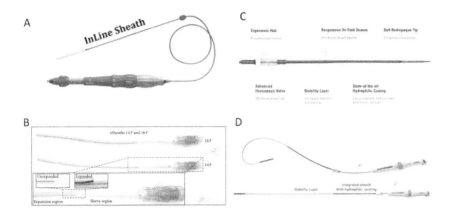

Figure 22.2 TAVR delivery systems. (a) Medtronic CoreValve system delivery catheter with the InLine sheath. *Source:* Medtronic, Inc. (b) Edwards SAPIEN S3 balloon-expandable system with the Axela sheath (eSheath). *Source:* Adapted from Koehler et al., Changes of the eSheath Outer Dimensions Used for Transfemoral Transcatheter Aortic Valve Replacement, *BioMed Research International*, vol. 2015, Article ID 572681, 6 pages, 2015, https://doi.org/10.1155/2015/572681, Figure 1. (c) The ACURATE *neo* self-expanding valve uses an introducer set, the iSLEEVE. *Source:* Adapted from Boston Scientific, https://www.bostonscientific.com/en-EU/products/transcatheter-heart-valve/acurateneo2-tavi-valve-system.html. (d) The Portico valve is delivered using the FlexNav delivery system. *Source:* Adapted from Fontana, G.P. et al. *J Am Coll Cardiol Intv.* 2020; 13 (21):2467–78 https://www.jacc.org/doi/abs/10.1016/j.jcin.2020.06.041.

Shockwave Intravascular Lithotripsy

The Shockwave intravascular lithotripsy (IVL) system (Shockwave Medical) is a relatively new technology designed to treat calcified stenosis of the peripheral arteries by lithotripsy. IVL uses sonic pressure waves that disrupt the intima and media calcification, modify vessel compliance, and permit vessel expansion and the passage of large bore equipment. The IVL balloon catheter is composed of an array of lithotripters that are incorporated into a semi-compliant balloon. The catheter is advanced to the calcified lesion over a wire (0.014″ guide wire), the balloon is inflated with a mixture of contrast and saline and inflated to a subnominal pressure of around 4 atm, sufficient to be opposed to the vessel wall. These sealing provides an effective fluid-tissue interface that facilitates the acoustic transmission of energy waves to the vessel wall. Balloon catheters range from 3.5 to 7.0 mm in diameter and require a 6 Fr or 7 Fr sheath, depending on the balloon size. Data have shown Shockwave's effectiveness and safety. Even concentrically calcified and stenotic vessels can be enlarged and have their bio-elasticity improved by pretreatment with Shockwave (Figure 22.3).

Presently there is little observational data on the use of Shockwave to facilitate TF TAVR, but this technology is revolutionizing the TF approach and leaving a negligible number of cases that must be performed by an alternative access.

How to Approach High-Risk Vascular Anatomies

6. How do you approach small vessels?

The minimal vessel dimension depends on the platform to be used and the size of the selected valve. Currently,

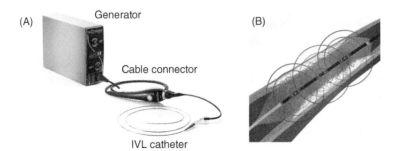

Figure 22.3 (a) Shockwave portable generator with the IVL catheter and peripheral IVL balloon. *Source:* Adapted from Galougahi et al. (2020). (b) Shockwave IVL catheter positioned and inflated. Integrated emitters discharge compressive shockwaves that affect superficial and deep calcium. *Source:* Dean et al. (2021) / With permission of Elsevier.

low-profile sheaths and delivery systems make it possible to access vessels as small as 5.0 mm vessels. For borderline diameter and rigid vessel walls, hydrophilic dilators facilitate the passage of large-bore sheaths.

7. Can endovascular pretreatment of iliofemoral atherosclerotic disease be performed?

Endovascular pretreatment for high-risk anatomy can be performed in most cases with plain balloon angioplasty without stent placement. Usually it is performed at the same time as the TAVR procedure and can be performed from the same access or the contralateral access site. If iliac stents are implanted, it is recommended to do so using a stage approach if the patient's condition permits. If stents are placed, the TAVR procedure can be performed via the TF approach safely six to eight weeks after, as the stents are expected to be endothelialized, decreasing the risk of friction and mechanical interaction. If stenting is performed at the same time as the TAVR procedure, it is preferred to implant the stents after delivering the valve and removing the large-bore equipment at the end of the procedure prior to vessel closure.

8. How do you approach significant calcific peripheral disease?

Significant calcific peripheral disease should be identified with pre-procedural CT. In the case of femoral arterial calcific disease, the location of calcium within the artery is important for the puncture site; anterior, circumferential, and bulky posterior calcium can prevent a successful TF puncture and large-bore access placement. Additionally, successful closure with suture-based devices at the end of the procedure can be impaired. Surgical femoral cut-down is a safe, controlled approach in heavily calcified vessels. It permits direct visualization and tactile palpation of the wall to identify a less calcified segment for the access site, enables surgical endarterectomy if needed, and provides direct control of hemostasis and vessel repair at the end of the procedure. For significant circumferential iliofemoral disease, Shockwave IVL is a safe, successful approach that allows the modification of the calcified vessel compliance and dilation of dense calcified lesions so the TAVR sheath and delivery system can be advanced in a safe and effective manner. If Shockwave IVL technology is not available, when the stenotic calcified lesion is not completely circumferential, and it is considered that that the vessel is large

enough to permit vessel expansion, advancement of large-bore TAVR equipment can be attempted with the following techniques:

1. Use stiffer wires (Lunderquist or Amplatz Super Stiff). Provides more support for the force of the push that is transmitted while the equipment is advanced.
2. In the case of Iliac lesions and stiff vessels, an ipsilateral or contralateral stiff wire can be used as a "buddy wire" to provide support and railing to the system at the level of the bifurcation. This also helps to modify the angulation of the iliac bifurcation, assisting the passage of the equipment into the aorta, especially in the presence of eccentric lesions that may be obstructing and causing resistance. The same principle applies to rigid, stiff vessels: a contralateral stiff wire provides support and external anchorage to allow advancement and delivery of the equipment.

9. How do you approach severe vascular tortuosity?

Significant vascular tortuosity predisposes the vessel wall to mechanical injury and adds extrinsic resistance when the sheaths and delivery system are advanced through the vasculature (Figure 22.4). There are no pre-specified

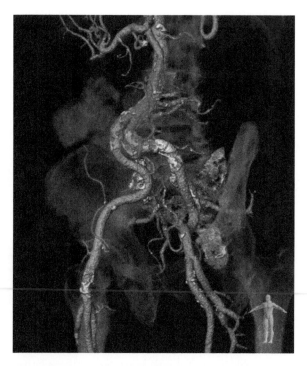

Figure 22.4 Significant tortuosity of the bilateral iliac arteries and abdominal aorta.

cutoffs for severe tortuosity that may prohibit a TF access; it should be evaluated independently in each case. The same principles apply for iliofemoral tortuosity and abdominal aorta tortuosity. Using guide wires with a stiff shaft helps to straighten the vessels and the entire aorto-iliofemoral axis, providing support for the delivery of the equipment. Some of the stiffer wires on the market are Lunderquist Extra-Stiff (Cook Medical), Amplatz Super Stiff (Boston Scientific), Back-Up Meier (Boston Scientific), and Amplatz Extra-Stiff (Cook Medical). In more challenging scenarios, especially when the vessels have rigid walls, the operator may need to use more than one wire to provide extra support and help to straighten the vasculature. The use of long sheaths is recommended to protect the vessel wall and retain the support necessary to accomplish the TF TAVR procedure.

10. Can TF TAVR be performed in patients with abdominal aortic aneurysms?

A successful TAVR can be performed in patients with abdominal aortic aneurysms (Figure 22.5). Extra caution should be used in all procedure steps, especially when wires and equipment are advanced. We recommend using soft-tip wires; always direct them under fluoroscopy guidance through the aneurysm before exchanging them for more rigid wires over a 5 or 6 Fr catheter. This permits safe delivery of a large sheath through the aneurysm. Long delivery sheaths, such as the Gore DrySeal sheath or the Edwards eSheath, can be delivered past the upper extent of the aneurysm, providing extra safety.

Bibliography

1 Cruz-Gonzalez, I., Gonzalez Ferreiro, R., Moreiras, J. et al. (2019). Facilitated transfemoral access by shockwave lithoplasty for transcatheter aortic valve replacement. *JACC Cardiovasc. Interv.* 12 (5): e35–e38. https://doi.org/10.1016/j.jcin.2018.11.041.

2 Di Mario, C., Goodwin, M., Ristalli, F. et al. (2019). A prospective registry of intravascular lithotripsy-enabled vascular access for transfemoral transcatheter aortic valve replacement. *JACC Cardiovasc. Interv.* 12: 502–504. https://doi.org/10.1016/j.jcin.2019.01.211.

3 Galougahi, K.K., Petrossian, G., Hill, J., and Ali, Z.. (2020). Intravacular lithotripsy in cardiovascular interventions. Expert analysis. JACC. https://www.acc.org/Latest-in-Cardiology/Articles/2020/07/17/08/00/Intravascular-Lithotripsy-in-Cardiovascular-Interventions.

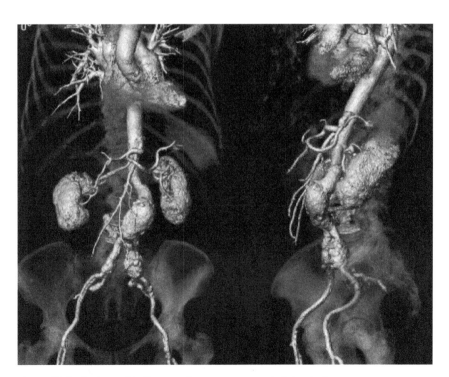

Figure 22.5 Patient with iliac arteries aneurysms and abdominal aorta aneurysm.

4 Grossman, Y., Silverberg, D., Berkovitch, A. et al. (2018). Long-term outcomes of Iliofemoral artery stents after transfemoral aortic valve replacement. *J. Vasc. Interv. Radiol.* 29 (12): 1733–1740, ISSN 1051-0443. https://doi.org/10.1016/j.jvir.2018.06.003.

5 Kereiakes, D.J., Virmani, R., Hokama, J.Y. et al. (2021). Principles of intravascular lithotripsy for calcific plaque modification. *J. Am. Coll. Cardiol. Intv.* 14 (12): 1275–1292. https://doi.org/10.1016/j.jcin.2021.03.036.

6 Ruge, H., Burri, M., Erlebach, M., and Lange, R. (2020). Access site related vascular complications with third generation transcatheter heart valve systems. *Catheter. Cardiovasc. Interv.* 97: 325–332. https://doi.org/10.1002/ccd.29095.

7 Saad, M., Seoudy, H., and Frank, D. (2021). Challenging anatomies for TAVR—bicuspid and beyond. *Front.* Cardiovasc. Med. 8: 654554. https://doi.org/10.3389/fcvm.2021.654554.

8 Sardar, M.R., Goldsweig, A.M., Abbott, J.D. et al. (2017). Vascular complications associated with transcatheter aortic valve replacement. *Vasc. Med.* 22: 234–244. https://doi.org/10.1177/1358863X17697832.

9 Singh, G. and Southard, J. (2019). Hostile territory: navigating complex Iliofemoral access for a transfermoral first strategy in patients undergoing transcatheter aortic valve replacement. *Struct. Heart* 3 (1): 41–43. https://doi.org/10.1080/24748706.2018.1556829.

10 Staniloae, C., Jilaihawi, H., Amoroso, N. et al. (2019). Systematic Transfemoral Transarterial Transcatheter aortic valve replacement in hostile vascular access. *Struct. Heart* 3 (1): 34–40. https://doi.org/10.1080/24748706.2018.1556828.

23

Alternative Access for TAVR

Pedro Engel Gonzalez, Tiberio Frisoli, Brian P. O'Neill, Dee Dee Wang, James C. Lee, William W. O'Neill and Pedro Villablanca

[1] *Division of Cardiology, Center for Structural Heart Disease, Henry Ford Hospital, Detroit, MI, USA*

1. Why is TF access the gold standard for TAVR?

Percutaneous transfemoral (TF) access for retrograde transarterial transcatheter aortic valve replacement (TAVR) with percutaneous access and closure has become the most common approach and is used in 95% of cases in contemporary practice. Due to the improvement in technology with small-caliber access catheters and delivery systems, as well as a decrease in patient risk profile and increase in operator experience, the rate of vascular access complications with TAVR has decreased dramatically using TF access. Vascular complication rates have decreased to 1–3% from 12–16%. TF access has been associated with better outcomes, including lower bleeding rates and reduced length of stay in the hospital.

2. How are transapical and direct aortic access performed?

Transapical TAVR begins with a limited thoracotomy and apical exposure of the heart. It is followed by a horizontal mattress pledgeted suture placement surrounding the intended access area, usually lateral to the true apex. Puncture is performed with an 18-gauge needle, and the apex is cannulated with a small sheath and then exchanged for a stiff wire in the descending aorta. After a large delivery sheath is placed over the stiff wire, the next step is the transcatheter heart valve (THV) implantation. Hemostasis is achieved by lowering the blood pressure using rapid pacing, sheath withdrawal, and pledget tightening of the sutures. A chest tube is typically left in place, and the thoracotomy is closed. Apical tissue integrity is somewhat unpredictable, and cases have been aborted because of degeneration of apical tissue architecture or large amounts of apical adiposity, making it difficult for pledget suture placement. Currently, the SAPIEN 3 Ultra balloon-expandable THV (Edwards Lifesciences) uses the Certitude delivery system with an internal diameter of 18 to 21 F, depending on the valve size used. Even though the technology has improved, thoracic access is still associated with increased death, stroke, vascular complications, myocardial injury, and new atrial fibrillation.

More recently, given the concerns for complications with transapical access and increased comfort with limited sternotomy for aortic cannulation, transaortic access (TAo) was developed. TAo access is feasible as long as the aorta is not excessively calcified and there is at least 6.5–7 cm of length between the proposed entry side and aortic annulus to allow valve preparation. Aortic access is achieved using a J-sternotomy or right lateral thoracotomy, depending on the position of the aorta. After placing pledgeted sutures at the access site, a direct puncture is performed with an 18-gauge needle. A small sheath is inserted to facilitate crossing the aortic valve and then exchanged for a stiff wire that enables large-sheath delivery. Following THV implantation, the pledgeted sutures are tightened, and the thorax is closed in the usual fashion. TAo is often preferred over transapical access because of less surgical site pain and minimal myocardial injury; in addition, apical tissue integrity is not a limitation. Rare complications include dissections or intramural hematomas. TAo is associated with 8% in-hospital mortality, a 40% rate of renal failure, a minority of patients able to be discharged home, and prolonged convalescence. Transapical and TAo access account for less than 2.8% of all SAPIEN TAVR cases in the STS/ACC Transcatheter Valve Therapy (TVT) registry between 2015 and 2018. These transthoracic alternatives were more

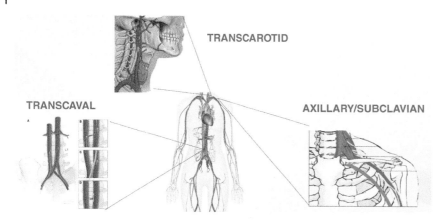

Figure 23.1 Peripheral options for alternative access.

common in the first-generation SAPIEN valve delivery systems, which usually required 22–24 F sheaths for transfemoral access. Peripheral alternative access strategies (Figure 23.1) have become increasingly more common and have been shown to have less morbidity and mortality (Table 23.1).

3. What are the important considerations when selecting transaxillary (TAx) access for TAVR?

This access route was initially performed as an alternative access for Medtronic CoreValve implantation with surgical exposure for sheath insertion, and it has evolved to complete percutaneous access and closure. It has become the most frequently used alternative access in the United States. Advantages of axillary access are the relative lack of atherosclerosis relative to iliofemoral vessels, accessibility, and extra-thoracic locations. Disadvantages are the proximity of the brachial plexus and the potential of compromising the upper extremity via peripheral nerve injury or distal

embolism. Observational studies suggest high rates of technical success and similar procedure outcomes between TF and TAx routes. The axillary artery is divided into three segments, with the most proximal section between the lateral margin of the first rib and the medial border of the pectoralis minor muscle; the second segment is deep to the pectoralis minor muscle, and the third segment is between the lateral border of the pectoralis minor and inferior border of the teres major muscle (Figure 23.2). The axillary artery is, on average, 1.5 mm smaller than the lower-extremity vessels. It is not uncommon for elderly patients undergoing TAVR to have a permanent pacemaker or implantable cardioverter defibrillator crowding the spaces in the deltopectoral groove. Another consideration is that large-bore axillary access should be avoided in the presence of an ipsilateral patent mammary graft to prevent ischemia.

4. How is TAx TAVR performed?

Operators should aim to access the distal end of the first segment or proximal second segment at a shallow angle to

Table 23.1 Summary of published outcomes for each alternative access used for transcatheter aortic valve replacement.

	Antegrade	Transaortic	Transapical	Surgical axillary	Percutaneous axillary	Transcarotid	Transcaval
In-hospital mortality, %	0	8.1	7.4	4.3	3.4	2.5	4
Longer-Term mortality	22% 6 mo	19% 1 y	9% 30 d	2.9% 30 d; 20% 1 y	5.4% 30 d	4.3% 30 d	8% 30 d
Major bleeding, %	44.4	5	7.2	NA	0.5	0.1	12
Acute kidney injury, %	22.2	39.6	NA	NA	NA	NA	12
Stroke, %	0	2.5	2.8	3	6.1	4.2	5
Vascular complications, %	33.3	0.5	3.8	2	2.5	1.5	13

N/A, not available or not applicable.

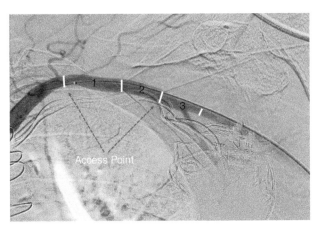

Figure 23.2 Digital subtraction angiography of the axillary artery, its three divisions, and side branches. Transaxillary access target site for puncture is shown.

avoid sheath kinking. The left axillary artery is more commonly used, given that it has a more favorable angle into the ascending aorta to achieve coaxial alignment. Right axillary access is feasible, but additional technical challenges are encountered in regard to achieving coaxial alignment. For recommendations on setting up the catheterization laboratory for TAx and other peripheral alternative access options, see Figure 23.3. In preparation for large-bore TAVR access, the ipsilateral radial artery is frequently accessed with a 7 Fr sheath and a 0.014–0.18″ wire for endovascular management and bailout if needed. Using a combination of fluoroscopy and ultrasound, the axillary artery is punctured and dilated, and ProGlide

sutures are implanted in a typical fashion before large-sheath insertion. Balloon tamponade between sheath exchanges is recommended to minimize blood loss: compression against a bony structure is difficult but can be done against the second rib to maintain hemostasis. The large-bore sheath should be inserted over a stiff wire. Following THV implantation in a typical fashion, a "dry closure" technique with short-duration balloon tamponade while tightening the Perclose sutures can be helpful to minimize blood loss and facilitate hemostasis. In case of closure failure, a flexible self-expanding or balloon-expandable covered stent (i.e. VBX; Gore Medical) is recommended. The latter option is preferable because of its large range and ability to fit through a 7 F sheath.

5. What are the advantages and important considerations of transcarotid (TC) access?

There is deep surgical experience with accessing the carotid artery, and its superficial location and sturdy constitution make it a good target. Carotid exposure is achieved surgically, and proximal and distal control of the vessels is established with tourniquets (Figure 23.4). The vessel is accessed near the level of the thyroid cartilage. After a small sheath insertion using a Seldinger technique, the aortic valve is crossed and exchanged for a stiff wire, allowing for the introduction of a large-bore sheath. Following THV implantation, the sheath is withdrawn, and hemostatic

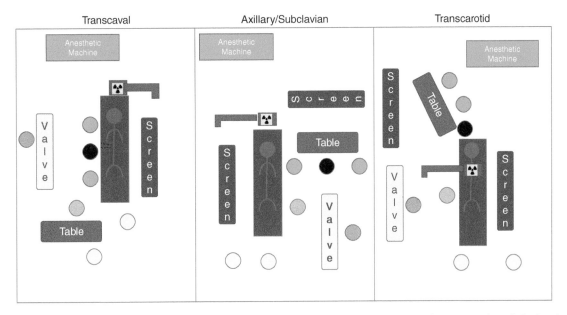

Figure 23.3 Catheterization lab setup for alternative access. The green dots represent the structural cardiologist, the black dots represent the cardiac surgeon, the blue dots represent the valve representative, the orange dot represents the scrub technician, and the yellow dots represent the circulating nurses.

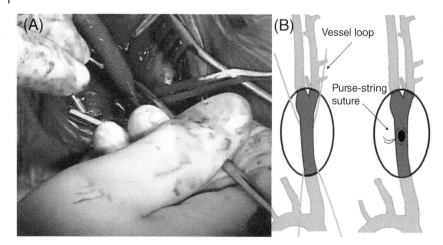

Figure 23.4 Transcarotid access for transcatheter aortic valve replacement. (a) Surgical exposure of the carotid artery. (b) Proximal and distal control of the carotid artery is established surgically using tourniquets, and closure is performed with surgical repair.

control is established by tightening the tourniquets. Surgical repair of the arteriotomy can be performed in a standard fashion. Some valve centers with expertise with this access route screen for advanced atherosclerosis in the contralateral carotid and circle of Willis prior to selecting this route. TC access is usually performed under general anesthesia; however, some data from France suggests the feasibility of TC TAVR using local and conscious sedation and noted that this was associated with lower stroke rates and shorter hospitalization. Retrospective data shows that TC access is associated with better outcomes than thoracic access. Compared with TAx TAVR, TC TAVR has similar mortality, less fluoroscopy, shorter procedure time, and numerically lower stroke rates (not a statistically significant difference), making it a favorable alternative access.

6. What is the physiology that allows for transcaval (TCV) access and prevents a life-threatening retroperitoneal bleed?

At first glance, creating a vascular track into the retroperitoneal space from the inferior vena cava (IVC) into the abdominal aorta would be expected to result in exsanguination. However, because the hydrostatic pressure of the abdomen exceeds the IVC pressure, arterial blood preferentially shunts into the IVC. The normal mean arterial pressure in the aorta is usually between 70 and 100 mm hg, the normal IVC pressure is usually ~5 mmHg, and the normal retroperitoneal interstitial pace pressure is 15 mmHg (Figure 23.5). Successful TCV hinges on these pressure gradients, and the IVC essentially serves as a sink for arterial blood from the abdominal aorta. The technique of

harnessing electrosurgical power to create a track between the abdominal aorta, the retroperitoneal space, and the IVC was first validated in animal models, and its safety and feasibility were subsequently demonstrated in humans.

TCV access planning requires detailed anatomical analysis of the IVC/abdominal aorta to determine the crossing level, extension of calcification, aortic size, distance from renal arteries (accessory renal arteries), distance from the iliacs, coplanar crossing angle, presence of interposed structures, and distance from the femoral vein. Many of these considerations are beyond the scope of this chapter, but some important concepts involve finding a crossing window that is free of calcium and interposed structures (i.e. bowel, major veins, arterial branches); identifying vascular structures at risk during the closure if endograft rescue is required (crossing site should be at least 15 mm away from aortoiliac bifurcation and renal arteries); and avoiding crossing sites with high-risk anatomy such as pedunculated atheroma, abdominal aneurysms, dissections, leftward aorta, or prior device implants. Multidetector CT is the preferred modality for planning prior to TCV access. The coplanar angle for crossing is also pre-identified using CT analysis.

7. How is TCV access for TAVR performed?

After the appropriate assembly of all the necessary equipment, the procedure can be started (Figure 23.6). The largest magnification on fluoroscopy using the predetermined coplanar angle is selected. Scout angiogram using digital subtraction angiogram (DSA) of the abdominal aorta in the coplanar view is performed. A 6 Fr internal mammary or

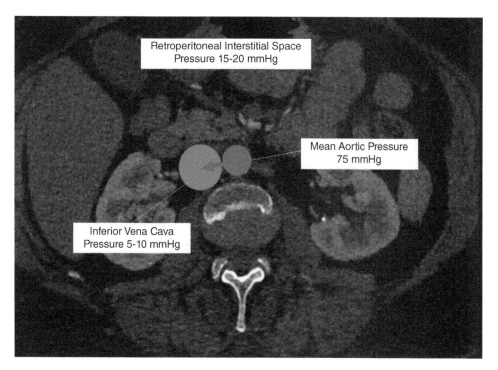

Figure 23.5 Physiology of an iatrogenic aortic-caval fistula. A tunnel is created between the aorta and vena cava, and because the interstitial pressure of the retroperitoneal space exceeds the venous pressure, blood preferentially shunts from the aorta to the vena cava (straight red arrow).

renal double curve guide catheter is oriented in the IVC, pointed toward the abdominal aorta aimed at the snare at the corresponding lumbar spine level. A 6 Fr JR4 guide catheter with a single-loop snare (i.e. Amplatz Goose Neck; Medtronic) is positioned in the abdominal aorta at the proposed crossing point oriented orthogonally to the coplanar angle in preparation for wire crossing. A 0.014" Astato 20 wire, a 0.014" microcatheter, and a 0.035" braided catheter are assembled in a serial telescoping configuration. The back of the 0.014" wire is clamped with a hemostat to the electrosurgical pencil. Then the coaxial trajectory of the wire is confirmed using coaxial projections by rotating the image intensifier 90° to the coplanar angle. Once confirmed, the 0.014" wire is advanced while applying a short burst of 50 W of electrosurgical cutting, halting the advancement of the wire when it approaches the snare in the aorta. The snare is closed around the wire, and then the wire is dragged cephalad to the thoracic descending aorta. The 0.014" catheter and the 0.035" catheter are then advanced in a telescoping fashion into the descending aorta. The aortic wall may sometimes be resistant to catheter crossing despite wire traversal, in which case a 2.5 to 3.0 mm noncompliant coronary balloon can be used to dilate the track. Once in the descending aorta, the snare is released, and then the 0.014" wire is exchanged for a 0.035" stiff wire such as the Lunderquist. Finally, the large-bore

sheath is advanced over the stiff 0.035" wire into the aorta using high-resolution fluoroscopy to ensure smooth passage. The THC can now be implanted in a typical fashion.

8. How is TCV access closure performed?

After THC deployment, protamine can be administered to normalize the activated clotting time. A 0.014" 300-cm safety wire (i.e. Balanced Middle Weight) is advanced to the aorta and left across the tract. A small curl deflectable catheter is advanced through the delivery sheath. A Nitinol closure device, preferably an Amplatzer Duct Occluder I (ADO 1; Abbott), is usually used to close the aortic puncture site. The large-bore sheath is pulled back to the crossing site, and the ADO 1 is passively exposed, forming a "ball." Next, the large-bore sheath is briskly retracted to the IVC with care to ensure the venous side is not obstructed to allow venous decompression. Finally, a retention disc is formed on the aortic side; the deflectable catheter is flexed to 90° and retracts the system with sufficient tension to appose to the aortic wall but avoid pulling through. Once apposed, the remainder of the device can be passively exposed. DSA angiography is repeated at this point to recognize any bleeding.

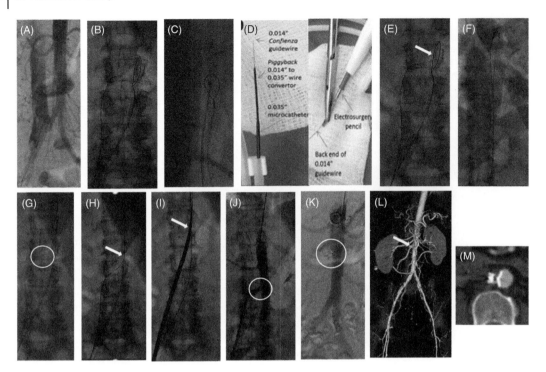

Figure 23.6 Transcaval access and closure transcatheter aortic valve replacement. (a) Scout angiogram using a digital subtraction angiogram (DSA) of the abdominal aorta and vena cava in the coplanar view. (b) A 7F RDC-1 guide catheter is oriented in the inferior vena cava and pointed toward the abdominal aorta. A 25-mm Gooseneck snare advanced via a 6F JR4 guide catheter is in the abdominal aorta in preparation for wire crossing. (c) The image intensifier is oriented 90° to the coplanar angle to confirm adequate RDC-1 catheter trajectory into the open snare in the abdominal aorta. (d) Assembly of a serial telescoping system composed of a 0.014″ Confianza Pro 12 within a 2.0 mm over-the-wire (OTW) balloon inside a 0.035″ microcatheter. (e) An electrified 0.014″ wire (applying 50 W of "cut" electrosurgical energy) crosses from the IVC into the abdominal aorta at the level of the snare. (f) The 0.014″ wire is captured with the snare, and the whole unit is advanced to the thoracic aorta. (g) The OTW balloon is advanced over the 0.014″ wire and used to dilate the arteriotomy in the abdominal aorta. (h) The 0.035″ microcatheter is advanced into the aorta, which facilitates the delivery of a 0.035″ stiff wire into the aorta. (i) With the support of a stiff 0.035″ wire, the Edwards Lifesciences eSheath is advanced into the abdominal aorta. (j) Abdominal aortogram performed from above arteriotomy site, demonstrating how a small curl Agilis catheter is used to deploy an Amplatzer Duct Occluder 10/8 against the abdominal aortic wall. (k) DSA abdominal aortogram demonstrates complete occlusion with no bleeding after closure (type 0). (l) Post-procedural computer tomography-based 3D reconstruction, showing the Amplatzer Duct Occluder positioned in the wall of the abdominal aortic wall. (m) Cross-sectional computed tomography image again showing the Amplatzer Duct Occluder apposed to the aortic wall occluding the transcaval fistula.

Generally, there are four patterns of results after closure: complete occlusion with no bleeding (type 0), patent funnel-shaped fistula flow (type 1), patent fistula with a cruciform pattern of flow (type 2), and frank extravasation (type 3). Types 0 to 2 can be observed without intervention, but type 3 requires intervention. Transient blood pressure drops of 10–15 mmHg are typical with shunting. In the event of extravasation, rapidly exchange for an aortic occlusion balloon (i.e. Reliant Aortic Occlusion Balloon [Medtronic] or Coda Aortic Occlusion Balloon [Cook Medical]) and tamponade the TCV tract. Occlusion of the tract for three- to five-minute cycles can be done several times, but if there is no improvement, it is important to proceed with covered stent implantation. A self-expanding covered stent 10–20% larger than the aortic lumen is recommended, and the stent of choice is an Ovation iX aortic limb extender (Endologix); however, a balloon-expandable stent (VBX) has also been used successfully.

Conclusion

Although THV delivery systems, ancillary equipment, and operator expertise have evolved and TF access is performed successfully in the vast majority of cases, a significant number of cases are better suited for alternative access. Given the prevalence of elderly patients, morbid obesity, peripheral vascular disease, and earlier onset diabetes, the need for familiarity and expertise with nonfemoral access is imperative for a high-quality valve center. The infrequent use of alternative access requires that operators focus on developing expertise with at least one or two techniques or refer patients to experienced tertiary centers. The access route decision should be individualized to each patient, and the best access should be pursued for each individual. This is why alternative access remains central to building a high-quality TAVR program and obtaining the best outcomes for most patients with symptomatic severe AS.

Bibliography

1 Adams, D.H., Popma, M.D., Reardon, M.J. et al. (2014). Transcatheter aortic-valve replacement with a self-expanding prosthesis. *N. Engl. J. Med.* 370: 1790–1798.

2 Allen, K., Chhatriwalla, A.K., Cohen, D. et al. (2019). Transcarotid versus transapical and transaortic access for transcatheter aortic valve replacement. *Ann. Thorac. Surg.* 108: 715–722.

3 Bapat, V., Frank, D., Cocchieri, R. et al. (2016). Transcatheter aortic valve replacement using transaortic access: experience from the multicenter, multinational, prospective ROUTE registry. *JACC Cardiovasc. Interv.* 9: 1815–1822.

4 Blackstone, E.H., Suri, R.M., Rajeswaran, J. et al. (2015). Propensity-matched comparisons of clinical outcomes after transapical or transfemoral transcatheter aortic valve replacement: a placement of aortic transcatheter valves (PARTNER)-I trial substudy. *Circulation* 131: 1989–2000.

5 Carroll, J.D., Mack, M.J., Vemulapalli, S. et al. (2020). STS-ACC TVT registry of transcatheter aortic valve replacement. *J. Am. Coll. Cardiol.* 76: 2492–2516.

6 Chamandi, C., Abi-Akar, R., Roses-Cabau, J. et al. (2018). Transcarotid compared with other alternative access routes for transcatheter aortic valve replacement. *Circ. Cardiovasc. Interv.* 11: e006388. https://doi.org/10.1161/CIRCINTERVENTIONS.118.006388.

7 Dahle, T.G., Kaneko, T., McCabe, J. et al. (2019). Outcomes following subclavian and axillary artery access for transcatheter aortic valve replacement: Society of the Thoracic Surgeons/American College of Cardiology TVT registry report. *JACC Cardiovasc. Interv.* 12: 662–669.

8 Eng, M.H., Qintar, M., Apstolou, D. et al. (2021). Alternative access for transcatheter aortic valve replacement: a comprehensive review. *Interv. Cardiol. Clin.* 10: 505–517.

9 Eng, M.H., Villablanca, P., Frisoli, T. et al. (2019). Transcaval access for large bore devices. *Curr. Cardiol. Rep.* 21: 134.

10 Fanaroff, A.C., Manandhar, P., Holmes, D.R. et al. (2017). Peripheral artery disease and transcatheter aortic valve replacement outcomes: a report from the Society of Thoracic Surgeons/American College of Cardiology Transcatheter Therapy Registry. *Circ. Cardiovasc. Interv.* http://dx.doi.org/10.1161/CIRCINTERVENTIONS.117.005456.

11 Kundi, H., Strom, J.B., Valsdottir, L.R. et al. (2018). Trends in isolated surgical aortic valve replacement according to hospital-based transcatheter aortic valve replacement volumes. *JACC Cardiovasc. Interv.* 11: 2148–2156.

12 Lederman, R.J., Babaliaros, V., Rogers, T. et al. (2019). The fate of transcaval access tracts: 12-month results of the prospective NHLBI transcaval transcatheter aortic valve replacement study. *JACC Cardiovasc. Interv.* 12: 448–456.

13 Leon, M.B., Smith, C.R., Mack, M.J. et al. (2016). Transcatheter or surgical aortic-valve replacement in intermediate-risk patients. *N. Engl. J. Med.* 374: 1609–1620.

14 Reardon, M.J., Van Mieghem, N.M., Popma, J.J. et al. (2017). Surgical or transcatheter aortic-valve replacement in intermediate-risk patients. *N. Engl. J. Med.* 376: 1321–1331.

15 Smith, C.R., Leon, M.B., Mack, M.J. et al. (2011). Transcatheter versus surgical aortic-valve replacement in high-risk patients. *N. Engl. J. Med.* 364: 2187–2198.

24

Vascular Access and Closure Options for TAVR

Diego Celli, Joao Braghiroli, Michael Dangl, Jelani K. Grant, Alexandre C. Ferreira and Cesar E. Mendoza

Department of Cardiology, Jackson Memorial Health System, Miami, FL, USA

1. What constitutes pre-procedural vascular access evaluation?

A comprehensive evaluation of the patient and the access site is paramount during the pre-procedural assessment of the vascular access. This evaluation includes detailed clinical and imaging reviews.

A thorough history must be obtained to determine the suitable vascular access and recognize features that increase the risk of complications. This must include the patient's functional status, pertinent comorbidities, the feasibility of procedural tolerance (ability to lie prone), and accurate documentation of peripheral vascular (arterial, venous, lymphatic) disease, prior radiation therapy, and previous percutaneous or surgical vascular procedures.

Physical examination should be focused on inspection for signs of skin infection and palpation at the desired insertion site and distal extremity pulses.

It is mandatory to obtain pre-procedural imaging of the vascular access site(s) for most left-sided structural heart disease interventions. This strategy provides valuable information for planning and executing the procedure and is central to avoiding or minimizing the risk of vascular complications.

2. What is the gold standard imaging technique for the anatomic evaluation of arterial access sites before TAVR?

While femoral access is commonly used and technically easy for a variety of procedures requiring small sheath sizes such as coronary angiography, percutaneous coronary interventions, and hemodynamic monitoring; structural heart procedures and mechanical circulatory support devices require large-bore vascular sheaths that demand careful anatomical assessment. Adventitious access should be avoided, given the potential risk of life-threatening complications.

When planning for an elective large-bore vascular access procedure, it is of the utmost importance to delineate and evaluate the patient's vascular anatomy. Computed tomography (CT)-angiography is a fundamental and standard protocol used in multidisciplinary Heart Team discussions to assess the feasibility of transcutaneous access and enable clinical outcome optimization. It is usually accompanied by 3D reconstruction, extending from the aortic annulus to the superficial femoral artery. It is an essential tool to delineate the vessel's caliber, trajectory, calcification, and relationship with surrounding structures.

3. What is the optimal arterial puncture technique for common femoral artery access?

The common femoral artery (CFA) continues from the external iliac artery immediately after the take-off of the inferior epigastric artery when crossing the inguinal ligament, forming an anatomical landmark. Importantly, CFA puncture sites (not skin puncture) close to this proximal region are usually noncompressible, as there is a lack of bony structures and a puncture at this level is frequently associated with retroperitoneal bleeding. The CFA continues its vertical descent, passing in front of the femoral head and becoming more accessible for manual compression in cases of bleeding just before its bifurcation. Punctures below the femoral bifurcation are associated with higher rates of pseudoaneurysms and arteriovenous fistulas and, given their smaller caliber, might be unsuitable for large-sized sheaths.

Mastering Structural Heart Disease, First Edition. Edited by Eduardo J. de Marchena and Camilo A. Gomez.
© 2023 John Wiley & Sons Ltd. Published 2023 by John Wiley & Sons Ltd.
Companion website: www.wiley.com/go/deMarchena/Mastering-Structural-Heart-Disease

Although anatomical landmarks have been traditionally used for femoral access, is associated with suboptimal access location, which increases the risk for vascular complications in a significant proportion of patients. Therefore, the use of ultrasound (US) supported by fluoroscopy monitoring is generally the preferred approach. Using a linear US probe, the operator can get a real-time, cross-sectional image of the femoral artery above its bifurcation, in addition to differentiating it from the compressible and non-pulsating femoral vein, evaluating calcium, and monitoring needle entry into the vessel. Moreover, the use of US to gain femoral access has been associated with improved CFA cannulation in patients with high CFA bifurcations along with reduced number of attempts, time to access, risk of venipuncture, and vascular complications compared to fluoroscopic-guided methods.

The choice of access needle is also essential in reducing vascular complications. Traditionally, 18-gauge needles have been used for femoral access. However, 21-gauge micropuncture needles are 56% smaller and have been shown to reduce rates of vascular access complications compared to standard 18-gauge needles (2.5 vs. 3.6%).

4. What is the best technique for fluoroscopic confirmation of vascular sheath insertion in the common femoral artery?

Regardless of the technique used for CFA access, it is good practice to confirm the position of the initial small vascular sheath with a limited angiographic view. Although one could use the US probe to demonstrate the insertion site and track it up or down, it becomes challenging to ascertain its position once the artery deepens. For this purpose, fluoroscopy and angiography play a significant role, especially before advancing large-bore devices or systems. Femoral angiograms should be recorded in the 30° to 50° ipsilateral anterior oblique view without cranial or caudal angulation. The goal is to open the CFA bifurcation and define the take-off of the inferior epigastric artery.

5. What are the technical considerations to obtain optimal carotid and axillary artery access?

Arterial access through the percutaneous transfemoral approach for transcatheter aortic valve replacement (TAVR) has been associated with less morbidity and mortality compared to transthoracic accesses (transapical or transaortic).

As such, it remains the default route for procedures requiring extensive bore access, including mechanical circulatory support devices. Nevertheless, some patients remain ineligible for transfemoral access due to unsuitable anatomy with peripheral artery disease (i.e. tortuosity, circumferential calcification, and small caliber). In such cases, alternative approaches are considered. They can be categorized as transthoracic (transapical and transaortic, which are more invasive due to opening the chest), transcaval, transcarotid, or transaxillary/subclavian. Given their accessibility, transcarotid and transaxillary/subclavian access have recently emerged as favorable substitutes for fully percutaneous TAVR in transfemoral-ineligible patients.

Similar to the transfemoral approach, pre-procedural planning with CT-angiography is paramount to delineate the vessel's caliber, trajectory, calcification, and relationship with surrounding structures. It is worth noting that the required protocol for proper assessment differs from the typical TAVR CT protocol, as the window needs to be wide enough to capture both arteries and high enough to screen for the ostial and proximal segments of the left vertebral artery.

The desired target for axillary artery cannulation lies in the first segment distal to the clavicle and proximal to the superior border of the pectoralis minor muscle, significantly distanced from vascular and nerve branches with surrounding bony structures for compression. The procedure can be done percutaneously or using a limited size cut-down.

Theoretically, the left axillary artery is preferred due to a lower chance of carotid compromise relative to the innominate artery and better coaxial orientation of the TAVR prosthesis in the aortic annulus; however, there is no convincing data to support choosing between the right or left axillary arteries. Therefore, it is generally recommended to be cautious in patients who previously underwent myocardial revascularization using a mammary artery graft or patients with only one functional arm. In these cases, we should as much as possible avoid using the axillary artery corresponding to the patent internal mammary artery or supplying the functional limb.

In the case of the transcarotid approach, pre-procedural planning is geared toward understanding the carotid, vertebral and intracerebral arterial anatomy (including assessment of the patency of the circle of Willis). When accessed for TAVR, the left carotid artery is preferred given its superior coaxial alignment of the prosthesis with the aortic annulus; however, both sides can be used.

The procedure is typically done using a cut-down, because this provides clean access to the vessel under direct visualization.

Vascular access closure for the transradial/subclavian approach is done either surgically or percutaneously. For the latter approach, most of the current experience includes suture-based closure devices, especially the Perclose ProGlide (Abbott Vascular). Nevertheless, manual pressure is also plausible. Transcarotid vascular access is usually closed by direct surgical closure.

6. What are the technical considerations to obtain optimal transcaval access, and what techniques are helpful to achieve hemostasis after removal of large-caliber sheaths following transcaval approach?

Transcaval access is a fully percutaneous procedure that facilitates the passage of TAVR or percutaneous left ventricular mechanical circulatory support in patients who are unsuitable candidates for transfemoral, transaxillary/transsubclavian or transthoracic approaches. The procedure involves bypassing the iliofemoral arteries employing a retroperitoneal channel between the inferior vena cava and the abdominal aorta. This procedure has proven to be feasible and is associated with acceptable higher rates of bleeding complications (compared to traditional transfemoral approaches) in this high-risk cohort. But there were no late bleeding or vascular complication events related to the access point or closure device at one-year CT analysis follow-up.

CT angiography is indispensable to determine if the abdominal aorta considered for traverse is calcium-free and, as such, conducive for transcaval access. Therefore, the desired target for this approach is situated in an area that is neither so low as to be close to the aortic bifurcation nor so high as to be adjacent to the renal arteries.

The closure technique includes the use of a slightly oversized Amplatzer Ductal Occluder 1 (Abbott Vascular) across the aortotomy with no other devices needed for venotomy closure as the entire retroperitoneal space has a resting pressure that supersedes the IVC.

7. What vascular closure devices are currently recommended after transfemoral interventions with large-caliber vascular sheaths?

Large-bore vascular interventions have created challenges in closure management; fortunately, multiple percutaneous devices have been designed, moving from the traditional manual compression to achieve hemostasis and closure of arteriotomy sites. These arteriotomy closure devices (ACDs) can be broadly classified as suture- or plug-based (Table 24.1). Although all available devices have been shown to shorten the time to hemostasis and ambulation (compared to manual compression), none of them has been proven superior to the others.

Suture-based closure devices are the most frequently used method for percutaneous closure. Two devices are currently employed: the Prostar XL and the Perclose ProGlide (Abbott Vascular) are percutaneous devices that work by approximating the intravascular structures with the use of pretied absorbable sutures with no re-access restriction. However, there is conflicting data regarding the superiority of any suture-base closure device; as such, a general recommendation is that each center master one suture-based technique.

Collagen-based closure devices include the ANGIO-SEAL (Terumo) and the new MANTA (Teleflex). They are designed explicitly for large-bore femoral arterial access site closure but have proven successful in complete percutaneous closure of axillary arteriotomies after TAVR. Both devices create a mechanical seal by sandwiching the arteriotomy between a bioabsorbable anchor and collagen sponge/plug, which dissolves in three to six months.

Other dedicated large-bore closure devices have been designed and tested, including InSeal (InSeal Medical) and PerQseal (Vivasure Medical).

Despite technological advancements, vascular complications resulting from vascular closure device failure remain common and are associated with increased morbidity and length of stay (Figure 24.1). A recent pilot randomized controlled trial compared the plug-based large-bore arteriotomy closure MANTA to suture-based vascular closure with two ProGlides. The incidence of the primary endpoint of access site-related vascular complications between MANTA and ProGlide was 10 vs. 4%, respectively, but not considered statistically superior. Patient-specific factors should be considered to decide on the most appropriate device.

8. What accounts for vascular access-site and access-related complications?

The most frequent access-related vascular injuries are related to either ischemic or bleeding events, and both have been associated with higher morbidity and mortality. Ischemic complications include dissection, stenosis, and

Table 24.1 Femoral arteriotomy closure devices and device-specific complications.

Device/manufacturer	Frequent major complications	
ANGIO-SEAL (Terumo)	Groin bleeding Vessel occlusion due to the intraluminal deployment of a collagen plug	*Source:* Terumo Medical Corporation.
Perclose ProGlide (Abbott Vascular)	Groin bleeding Vessel occlusion due to laceration or dissection of the arterial wall by the foot pedals	*Source:* Abbott.
MANTA (Teleflex)	Persistent bleeding Vessel occlusion Access site infection	*Source:* Teleflex Inc.

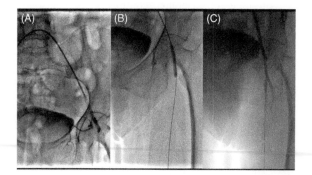

Figure 24.1 (a) Subtotal occlusion of the left common femoral artery after tightening the sutures of a pair of Perclose ProGlide vascular closure devices (arrow). (b) Balloon angioplasty using a dedicated peripheral balloon advanced through contralateral vascular access. (c) Successful revascularization of the subtotal occlusion of the left common femoral artery.

distal embolization, potentially leading to distal limb ischemia. Hematoma, aneurysm, pseudoaneurysm, and retroperitoneal hemorrhage are the most frequent bleeding complications. The Valve Academic Research Consortium (VARC) formulated clear endpoints for vascular complications, which allow for comparison and meta-analysis using independent studies.

Major vascular complications include:

- Any thoracic aortic dissection
- Access site or access-related vascular injury leading to death, need for significant blood transfusions (≥4 U), unplanned percutaneous or surgical intervention, or irreversible end-organ damage
- Distal embolization (noncerebral) from a vascular source requiring surgery or resulting in amputation or irreversible end-organ damage

Minor vascular complications include:

- Access site or access-related vascular injury not requiring unplanned percutaneous or surgical intervention and not resulting in irreversible end-organ damage
- Distal embolization treated with embolectomy and thrombectomy and not resulting in amputation or irreversible end-organ damage failure of percutaneous access site closure resulting in interventional or surgical correction and not associated with death, need for significant blood transfusions, or irreversible end-organ damage

9.   What is the incidence of vascular access complications?

Vascular access complications in TAVR randomized controlled trials and registries vary between 4 and 30%, most frequently associated with bleeding events. The significant bleeding rates at 30 days after TAVR have ranged from 17–24% in extreme-risk cohorts to 7–10% in international registries. In the TVT registry, the significant bleeding rates were 4.2% in 2014. This wide range can be explained by an initial lack of clear definitions and graduations of vascular complications, continuous improvements in both technical skills and technology of the delivery system designs, and the different degrees of comorbidities among population cohorts.

10.   What is the most appropriate management of an arterial dissection?

Treatment will depend on the presence of hemodynamic compromise; if present, a balloon can be quickly introduced, inserted, and inflated to obtain apposition of the intima and underlying media. If this strategy fails, stent deployment or a surgical graft might be considered.

11.   What is the most appropriate management of an arterial perforation?

For small perforations, crossover balloon insertion from the ipsilateral or contralateral location and inflation for 5–10 minutes is generally sufficient to achieve hemostasis; nevertheless, a covered stent is sometimes required to control an ongoing bleed fully. In addition, when a significant vascular injury occurs, temporizing maneuvers such as rapid insertion of dilators or sheaths with a quick introduction of other highly compliant occlusion balloons are needed to control hemostasis before definitive surgical therapies can be implemented.

12.   What is the most appropriate management of retroperitoneal bleeding?

Retroperitoneal bleeding is a rare but potentially serious complication of transfemoral vascular access. The vasculature in the retroperitoneum is noncompressible, and large volumes of blood may accumulate without any signs or symptoms. Once identified, initial management of retroperitoneal bleeding consists of ensuring large-bore intravenous access, reversing coagulopathies, measuring hemoglobin, and preparing blood products. Further management depends on the degree of hemodynamic instability: (i) stable patients can be managed conservatively with close monitoring, serial blood counts, and imaging, whereas (ii) unstable patients may require fluid resuscitation and transfusion of blood products. Patients should be taken to the catheterization lab, where angiography should be performed to identify the source of bleeding. Tamponade with balloon angioplasty can be utilized as a temporizing measure. Large-vessel bleeding can be treated with the placement of a covered stent, and small-vessel bleeding can be treated with coiling. If these measures fail to achieve hemostasis, surgical consultation is required.

13.   What is the most appropriate management of acute limb ischemia?

Defined as a sudden decrease in limb perfusion that threatens limb viability, this is an emergency that should be promptly recognized in the cardiac laboratory, the recovery area, or the critical care unit due to high amputation and mortality rates. Treatment relies on immediate initiation of unfractionated heparin accompanied by a revascularization strategy that will vary by location, duration, and comorbidities. Blood-flow restoration might be achieved through endovascular procedures such as percutaneous mechanical thrombectomy, thromboaspiration, or catheter-directed thrombolysis.

14. What methods can be used to prevent ischemic limbs when large bore access is occlusive?

The large-bore access sheaths required for TAVR can occlude the femoral artery and prevent blood flow distally. Ipsilateral femoral external bypass, contralateral femoral external bypass, and contralateral femoral internal bypass are several different methods for antegrade access that allow for distal perfusion and prevention of limb ischemia. Ipsilateral femoral external bypass occurs when the occlusive sheath is connected to an antegrade sheath in the ipsilateral femoral artery. Contralateral femoral external bypass consists of a contralateral femoral artery sheath connected to an ipsilateral femoral artery sheath antegrade to the occlusion. Contralateral femoral internal bypass is obtained by accessing the contralateral femoral artery with a 7 Fr sheath and advancing a 4 Fr sheath retrograde to the ipsilateral CFA and then continuing to advance it until antegrade to the site of occlusion. Additionally, a radial-to-femoral bypass method has been described where a sheath from the radial artery is connected to an ipsilateral femoral sheath that is antegrade to the site of occlusion.

Bibliography

1 Arnett, D.M., Lee, J.C., Harms, M.A. et al. (2018). Caliber and fitness of the axillary artery as a conduit for large-bore cardiovascular procedures. *Catheter. Cardiovasc. Interv.* 91: 150–156. https://doi.org/10.1002/ccd.27416.

2 Barbanti, M., Capranzano, P., Ohno, Y. et al. (2015). Comparison of suture-based vascular closure devices in transfemoral transcatheter aortic valve implantation. *EuroIntervention* 11: 690–697. https://doi.org/10.4244/EIJV11I6A137.

3 Barbash, I.M., Barbanti, M., Webb, J. et al. (2015). Comparison of vascular closure devices for access site closure after transfemoral aortic valve implantation. *Eur. Heart J.* 36: 3370–3379. https://doi.org/10.1093/eurheartj/ehv417.

4 Ben-Dor, I., Sharma, A., Rogers, T. et al. (2021). Micropuncture technique for femoral access is associated with lower vascular complications compared to standard needle. *Catheter. Cardiovasc. Interv.* 97: 1379–1385. https://doi.org/10.1002/ccd.29330.

5 Blackstone, E.H., Suri, R.M., Rajeswaran, J. et al. (2015). Propensity-matched comparisons of clinical outcomes after transapical or transfemoral transcatheter aortic valve replacement: a placement of aortic transcatheter valves (PARTNER)-I trial substudy. *Circulation* 131: 1989–2000. https://doi.org/10.1161/CIRCULATIONAHA.114.012525.

6 Cheney, A.E. and McCabe, J.M. (2019). Alternative percutaneous access for large bore devices. *Circ. Cardiovasc. Interv.* 12: e007707. https://doi.org/10.1161/CIRCINTERVENTIONS.118.007707.

7 De Palma, R., Rück, A., Settergren, M., and Saleh, N. (2018). Percutaneous axillary arteriotomy closure during transcatheter aortic valve replacement using the MANTA device. *Catheter. Cardiovasc. Interv.* 92: 998–1001. https://doi.org/10.1002/ccd.27383.

8 Greenbaum, A.B., Babaliaros, V.C., Chen, M.Y. et al. (2017). Transcaval access and closure for transcatheter aortic valve replacement: a prospective investigation. *J. Am. Coll. Cardiol.* 69: 511–521. https://doi.org/10.1016/j.jacc.2016.10.024.

9 Kaki, A., Alraies, M.C., Kajy, M. et al. (2019). Large bore occlusive sheath management. *Catheter. Cardiovasc. Interv.* 93: 678–684. https://doi.org/10.1002/ccd.28101.

10 Lederman, R.J., Babaliaros, V.C., Rogers, T. et al. (2019). The fate of transcaval access tracts: twelve month results of the prospective NHLBI transcaval TAVR study. *JACC Cardiovasc. Interv.* 12: 448–456. https://doi.org/10.1016/j.jcin.2018.11.035.

11 Leon, M.B., Piazza, N., Nikolsky, E. et al. (2011). Standardized endpoint definitions for transcatheter aortic valve implantation clinical trials: a consensus report from the valve academic research consortium. *J. Am. Coll. Cardiol.* 57: 253–269. https://doi.org/10.1016/j.jacc.2010.12.005.

12 Leon, M.B., Smith, C.R., Mack, M.J. et al. (2016). Transcatheter or surgical aortic-valve replacement in intermediate-risk patients. *N. Engl. J. Med.* 374: 1609–1620. https://doi.org/10.1056/NEJMoa1514616.

13 Lichaa, H. (2020). The "lend a hand" external bypass technique: external radial to femoral bypass for antegrade perfusion of an ischemic limb with occlusive large bore sheath – a novel and favorable approach. *Catheter. Cardiovasc. Interv.* 96: E614–E620. https://doi.org/10.1002/ccd.29187.

14 Mak, G.Y., Daly, B., Chan, W. et al. (1993). Percutaneous treatment of post catheterization massive retroperitoneal hemorrhage. *Cathet. Cardiovasc. Diagn.* 29: 40–43. https://doi.org/10.1002/ccd.1810290109.

15 Mathur, M., Hira, R.S., Smith, B.M. et al. (2016). Fully percutaneous technique for transaxillary implantation of the impella CP. *JACC Cardiovasc. Interv.* 9: 1196–1198. https://doi.org/10.1016/j.jcin.2016.03.028.

16 Nuis, R.-J., Wood, D., Kroon, H. et al. (2021). Frequency, impact and predictors of access complications with plug-based large-bore arteriotomy closure – a patient level meta-analysis. *Cardiovasc. Revasc. Med.* https://doi.org/10.1016/j.carrev.2021.02.017.

17 Pitta, S.R., Prasad, A., Kumar, G. et al. (2011). Location of femoral artery access and correlation with vascular complications. *Catheter. Cardiovasc. Interv.* 78: 294–299. https://doi.org/10.1002/ccd.22827.

18 Seto, A.H., Abu-Fadel, M.S., Sparling, J.M. et al. (2010). Real-time ultrasound guidance facilitates femoral arterial access and reduces vascular complications: FAUST (Femoral Arterial Access With Ultrasound Trial). *JACC Cardiovasc. Interv.* 3: 751–758. https://doi.org/10.1016/j.jcin.2010.04.015.

19 Toggweiler, S., Leipsic, J., Binder, R.K. et al. (2013). Management of vascular access in transcatheter aortic valve replacement: part 2: vascular complications. *J. Am. Coll. Cardiol. Intv.* 6: 767–776. https://doi.org/10.1016/j.jcin.2013.05.004.

20 van Wiechen, M.P., Tchétché, D., Ooms, J.F. et al. (2021). Suture- or plug-based large-bore arteriotomy closure: a pilot randomized controlled trial. *J. Am. Coll. Cardiol. Intv.* 14: 149–157. https://doi.org/10.1016/j.jcin.2020.09.052.

Part II

Structural Interventions for the Mitral Valve

25

The Natural History of Mitral Valve Disease

Blase A. Carabello

[1] *East Carolina Heart Institute, Brody School of Medicine, and Vidant Medical Center, East Carolina University, Greenville, NC, USA*

Mitral Stenosis

1. What are the causes of mitral stenosis (MS)?

Worldwide, the most common cause of mitral stenosis (MS) is rheumatic fever. While the attack rate of rheumatic fever is roughly equal between men and women, women develop MS three to four times more often than men. Rheumatic MS is an inflammatory disease caused by an immunologic reaction to streptococcal infection. It is characterized by mitral leaflet thickening and calcification that may also involve the subvalvular mitral apparatus. In developed countries, the prevalence of rheumatic fever has declined so that rheumatic MS has now become a rare disease. Most often, it is seen in patients who have emigrated from countries where rheumatic fever is still endemic. However, because patients often live longer in the developed world, mitral annular calcification (MAC), a non-rheumatic inflammatory involvement of the annulus, causes encroachment on the mitral orifice, reducing its aperture and causing MS.

2. What are the hemodynamic consequences of MS?

In normal subjects, the open mitral valve forms a near-common chamber between the left atrium (LA) and left ventricle (LV). As such, the pressures in those chambers rapidly equalize early in diastole. As MS worsens, the narrowed orifice leads to a pressure gradient between the LA and LV (Figure 25.1). Higher pressure in the LA is transmitted to the lungs, potentially causing pulmonary congestion. At the same time, MS limits LV filling, reducing LV stroke volume and cardiac output. Because the right ventricle (RV) supplies some of the impetus for LV filling, increased LA pressure places a pressure overload upon the RV. This pressure overload is often compounded by reflexive pulmonary vasoconstriction, leading to potentially severe pulmonary hypertension and RV failure.

3. How are the hemodynamics of MS translated into symptoms?

Increased LV filling pressure and reduced cardiac output cause the patient to experience dyspnea on exertion. During exercise, the heart rate increases, reducing the diastolic filling time and thereby exacerbating already increased LA pressure and pulmonary congestion. Elevated LA pressure at rest also usually causes orthopnea and, sometimes, paroxysmal nocturnal dyspnea. If pulmonary hypertension has ensued, RV failure may lead to ascites and peripheral edema. Hemoptysis during or immediately after exercise is rare in other heart diseases but more common in MS. This occurs when the sudden increase in LA pressure noted previously causes rupture of anastomoses between bronchial and pulmonary veins. In extreme cases, LA enlargement may compress the left recurrent laryngeal nerve, leading to hoarseness (Ortner's Syndrome). Left atrial enlargement and inflammation frequently cause atrial fibrillation, especially in older patients.

4. How are the hemodynamics of MS translated into physical exam findings?

The physical exam of MS is unique and, when performed by an experienced practitioner, should be diagnostic. However, the findings are subtle and often are only

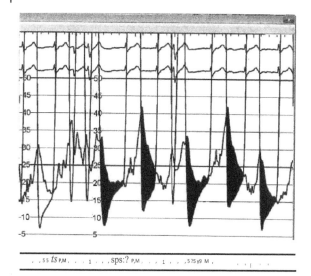

Figure 25.1 The gradient between the left atrium (pulmonary capillary wedge pressure) and left ventricle in a patient with mitral stenosisis demonstrated by the areas shaded in black.

observed when the patient is examined in a very quiet room and placed in the left lateral decubitus position. Palpation of the LV apex may reveal a diastolic thrill, while palpation of the sternum may demonstrate an RV lift if pulmonary hypertension has ensued. The transmitral gradient holds the mitral valve open during diastole instead of allowing it to partially close, in turn increasing the intensity of S1, although in severe cases, S1 becomes soft as mitral valve movement is reduced. The pulmonic component of S2 is increased when pulmonary hypertension is present. S2 is followed by an opening snap (OS) as the stenotic valve opens, and the OS is followed by a diastolic rumble. If the patient has remained in sinus rhythm, there may be presystolic accentuation of the rumble due to

LA contraction. The interval between S2 and OS is key to estimating MS severity. The more severe the MS is, the higher the LA pressure will be, causing the mitral valve to open earlier in diastole than if LA pressure is lower. Thus an S2-OS interval of 60 msec (just slightly longer than the interval between A2 and P2 during inspiration) indicates severe MS. An S2-OS interval of 120 msec (more like the S2, S3 cadence) suggests lower LA pressure and thus milder disease.

5. How is MS diagnosed (imaging and invasive hemodynamics)?

Echocardiography is the mainstay for diagnosing MS. Nonetheless, the standard chest x-ray is often diagnostic. Characteristic findings include a double density at the right heart border as the enlarged LA is projected outside of the normal right atrial contour. There is also enlargement of the pulmonary artery segment and the presence of Kerley B lines (hypertrophied septae) in the lung fields.

In rheumatic MS, echocardiography demonstrates that the mitral leaflets are thickened and often calcified, presenting a "hockey stick" appearance. In the en fosse 3D view, the open valve has a "fish mouth" appearance (Figure 25.2). MS severity is estimated echocardiographically in three ways: (i) calculations of the transmitral flow velocity and gradient from Doppler interrogation of the valve, (ii) direct planimetry of the open valve, and (iii) using an empiric formula: 220/pressure half time. Because the development of symptoms dramatically worsens the MS patient's prognosis, symptom onset is a crucial demarcation point in the natural history of the disease. Symptoms often arise when the mitral valve area (MVA) is reduced to </=1.5 cm^2, about

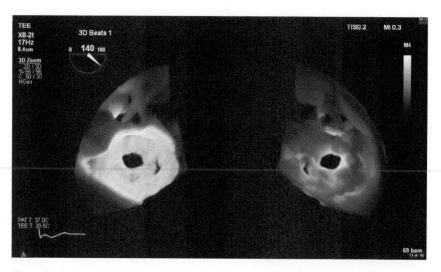

Figure 25.2 An echocardiographic 3D view of rheumatic mitral stenosis. The restricted opening presents a "fish mouth" appearance.

one-third of its normal orifice area. Thus *severe* MS is defined when the valve area is narrowed to this degree. Severe MS is almost always accompanied by an enlarged left atrium, another diagnostic criterion.

When MS is due to MAC, the leaflet anatomy is usually normal, but there is reduced orifice area due to encroachment by the calcified annulus producing a gradient across the valve.

In most cases, echocardiography is the prime tool for diagnosing and quantifying MS severity. However, in some cases, severity may be in doubt after non-invasive imaging. Here, invasive hemodynamics are used to measure the transmitral gradient directly and then relate the gradient to cardiac output through the Gorlin formula to calculate $MVA = flow/\sqrt{}$ gradient. Measurement of hemodynamics during exercise may be very helpful, uncovering severe abnormalities not present at rest.

6. What are the indications for medical therapy of MS, and what do those therapies consist of?

MS is a mechanical obstruction of LV inflow requiring mechanical correction. However, medical therapy is appropriate in some cases. The risk of stroke in MS patients who also have a history of atrial fibrillation is high, up to 20% per year. Thus anticoagulation is necessary in these patients. Because of this high risk and because there is little experience with non-vitamin K antagonists, warfarin is the appropriate anticoagulant therapy.

Because tachycardia shortens the LV filling period, tachycardia increases LA pressure. Thus heart rate control may be beneficial in lowering LA pressure and improving symptoms. In patients in atrial fibrillation, beta-blockers, rate-affective calcium channel blockers, digoxin, and ivabradine may be effective in slowing heart rate and improving symptoms. In patients in sinus rhythm, digoxin is unlikely to be effective, while the other agents listed may be helpful. If mechanical therapy is not anticipated, diuretics may be useful in lowering LA pressure and improving symptoms

7. What are the indications for mechanical therapy of MS, and what do those therapies consist of?

Mechanical relief of rheumatic MS is indicated for symptomatic patients with severe stenosis, indicated by a MVA of $\leq 1.5 \, cm^2$. For appropriate valve anatomy, relief is provided by balloon mitral valvotomy, wherein a large balloon is percutaneously maneuvered into the mitral orifice and inflated, breaking the rheumatic adhesions in the commissures and thereby increasing the MVA. Balloon valvotomy is appropriate when there is no more than mild mitral regurgitation (MR), as the procedure may worsen MR. Valve anatomy is assessed according to valve calcification, leaflet mobility, leaflet thickening, and pliability of the sub-valvular apparatus, each of which is given a score of 1–4. Valves with a total score of ≤ 8 are predicted to have a good result with balloon valvotomy, while valves with a higher score are more likely to require surgical valve replacement.

MS due to MAC is much more problematic; both balloon valvotomy and simple surgical valve replacement are usually ineffective. While debridement of the calcium from the annulus followed by mitral valve replacement (MVR) is possible, the procedure may cause catastrophic annular rupture and or disruption of LA-LV continuity. MVR in MAC patients is reserved for surgical teams with substantial experience in this area.

8. What is the prognosis of MS?

For symptomatic patients who do not undergo mechanical therapy, prognosis is poor, with a <50% five-year survival. Prognosis for patients undergoing mechanical therapy varies according to age, the presence of atrial fibrillation and/or pulmonary hypertension, and the success of balloon valvotomy. Overall, for a 50-year-old undergoing balloon valvotomy, the 10-year event-free survival is about 60%.

Mitral Regurgitation

9. What are the two major classes of MR? How do they differ in prognosis and therapy?

Mitral regurgitation is classified as primary or secondary MR. Despite the similarity in name, these two diseases are remarkably separate from one another, differing in patho-anatomy, pathophysiology, therapy, and prognosis.

The mitral valve is composed of its leaflets, the chordae tendineae, the papillary muscles, and the mitral annulus. Disease in any one or all of these components can cause the valve to leak. Thus the valve itself causes MR, defining primary MR (PMR). When PMR is severe, the volume overload placed on the LV causes LV eccentric hypertrophy, dilatation, and myocardial damage, leading to heart failure and eventually, if uncorrected, death. The MR **is** the disease, and proper timing of its therapy is consistent with a normal lifespan.

In secondary MR (SMR), the valve itself is often normal. Rather, disease of the LV leads to LV dilatation, wall motion abnormalities, and papillary muscle displacement that cause failure of the mitral leaflets to coapt. Thus there are at least two diseases present: intrinsic LV disease and MR. Correcting MR addresses only one of them, and accordingly, prognosis is much worse for SMR than for PMR.

Primary Mitral Regurgitation

10. What are the major etiologies of PMR?

The major causes of PMR are myxomatous valve degeneration, infective endocarditis, collagen vascular disease, rheumatic heart disease, and MAC.

11. What are the hemodynamics of PMR?

In PMR, a portion of the LV stroke volume is ejected into the LA during systole. With chronic severe MR, the heart compensates with LV enlargement, allowing it to increase its total stroke volume and compensate for that lost to regurgitation. In concert, the LA enlarges to accommodate the extra volume at normal filling pressure. However, when PMR is severe and acute, the fall in forward stroke volume is also severe, while the volume overload on both the LA and LV causes a dangerous increase in pulmonary venous pressure, potentially leading to both cardiogenic shock and pulmonary edema (Figure 25.3). Invasive hemodynamics find elevated LV diastolic pressure and elevated LA pressure, usually with a large v wave, together with a widened A-V O_2 difference, indicating reduced cardiac output. Because LA pressure is elevated, right ventricular and pulmonary artery pressure are also increased, eventually leading to pulmonary hypertension and RV failure.

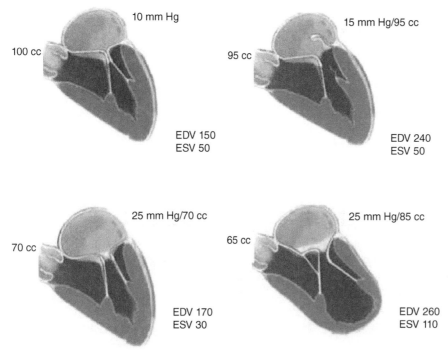

Figure 25.3 The stages of primary MR. Normal physiology (control) is compared to that of acute MR (chordal rupture), compensated MR, and decompensated chronic MR. The sudden opening of a new pathway for regurgitant flow into the left atrium increases left atrial pressure and preload (SL), in turn mildly increasing EDV because resting SL is still 90% of maximum length. Afterload (ESS) is decreased, allowing more complete left ventricular EF and reducing ESV. These changes in loading increase EF and total stroke volume, but because 50% of the total stroke volume is lost to regurgitation (regurgitant fraction), forward stroke volume is decreased. Therefore, despite normal contractile fraction and increased EF, the patient presents with the hemodynamics of congestive heart failure. In the presence of decompensated chronic MR, muscle damage caused by prolonged severe volume overload reduces the effectiveness of ventricular ejection, and ESV increases. There is a further increase in diastolic volume, which is not compensatory, resulting in a decrease in total and forward stroke volumes. EDV, end-diastolic volume; EF, ejection fraction; ESS, end-systolic stress; ESV, end-systolic volume; MR, mitral regurgitation; SL, sarcomere length. *Source:* Modified from O'Gara et al. (2008) and Costillo et al. (2017).

12. How are PMR hemodynamics translated into symptoms?

In compensated severe PMR, the patient may be asymptomatic and remain so for months to years. But eventually, symptoms of dyspnea on exertion, orthopnea, and paroxysmal nocturnal dyspnea become manifest. Low output leads to fatigue. If pulmonary hypertension has intervened, the patients may complain of edema and ascites.

13. How are PMR hemodynamics translated into physical signs?

The typical physical finding of PMR is a holosystolic, sometimes honking murmur heard best at the LV apex, sometimes radiating to the shoulder or elbow. Murmur intensity does not vary with RR interval. In diastole, there may be an s3 representing the large volume of blood filling the LV but not necessarily indicating heart failure. The LV apical beat is shifted downward and to the left. If pulmonary hypertension has developed a loud P2, jugular venous distension and ascites may be present. It should be noted that in acute severe MR, the large v wave reduces the systolic gradient between LV and LA, causing the murmur to be short and often unimpressive.

14. How is PMR diagnosed (imaging and invasive hemodynamics)?

Imaging with transthoracic echocardiography (TTE) is the mainstay of PMR diagnosis. It is usually adequate to define the mitral pathoanatomy responsible for the regurgitation. It allows for assessment of LA and LV enlargement, which occurs to accommodate the regurgitant volume as noted earlier. Doppler interrogation of the valve allows for quantification of MR severity by visualizing the regurgitant jet of flow from LV to LA during systole and estimating regurgitant volume using the proximal isovelocity surface area (PISA) method. (Figure 25.4). If tricuspid regurgitation is present, RV systolic pressure can be accurately estimated. The criteria for diagnosing severe MR are given in Table 25.1.

If transthoracic images are inadequate for diagnosis, TEE provides excellent mitral valve images that help further define valve abnormalities and can provide a 3D reconstruction that is similar to that seen by the surgeon during mitral repair. In acute MR, TTE often underestimates PMR severity. In the patient with unexplained pulmonary congestion in the face of a hyperdynamic LV but only mild MR during TTE, TEE should be considered to re-evaluate MR severity.

Because cardiac MRI can provide precise cardiac volumes, it also can be used to calculate an accurate regurgitant fraction to further quantify MR severity.

While in most cases, resting non-invasive imaging is adequate to diagnose the cause and severity of PMR, exercise imaging and/or exercise invasive hemodynamics may help clarify the clinical picture in cases when symptoms and imaging are discordant with one another. In some cases, MR may worsen with exercise causing exercise-related symptoms not explained by apparently less-than-severe MR at rest. Imaging during exercise may reveal worsening MR, or invasive hemodynamics may reveal elevated LA and PA pressures that were normal at rest.

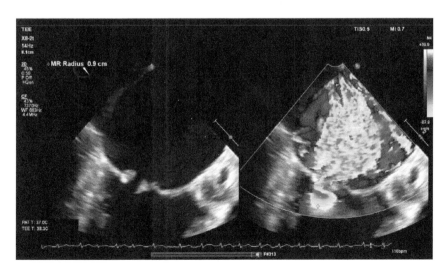

Figure 25.4 Doppler interrogation of a patient with mitral regurgitation reveals the mitral regurgitation jet and the proximal convergence zone used to help estimated regurgitant flow.

Table 25.1 Decision-making for intervention in primary mitral regurgitation.

Class I indications for mitral valve repair or replacement (repair favored over replacement whenever possible)

1) Severe symptomatic MR, with "severe" defined as integration of the following parameters (some or all may be present):

    A. Holosystolic apical murmur
    B. Regurgitant fraction >/=50% by echo or CMR
    C. Central MR jet >40% of LA
    D. Vena contracta >/= 0.7 cm
    E. Regurgitant volume >/= 60 cc
    F. Effective regurgitant orifice area >/=0.4 cm^2

2) Severe asymptomatic MR with LV dysfunction defined as LV EF < 0.60 or LV end-systolic dimension >40 mm

Class IIa indications:

    A. Surgical mitral repair but not replacement for asymptomatic MR patients with normal LV function, especially if LV function is declining but still within "normal" as noted in the text.

    B. Transcatheter repair for inoperable patients with severe symptomatic MR

Additional evidence of decompensation that may be incorporated into decision-making regarding intervention:

1. Brain natriuretic peptide levels >3× normal for patient age and sex
2. Abnormal global longitudinal strain
3. Exercise capacity <75% of predicted for age

CMR, cardiac magnetic resonance imaging; EF, ejection fraction; LA, left atrium; LV, left ventricular; MR, mitral regurgitation.

15. What are the indications for medical therapy in PMR, and what do those therapies consist of?

PMR is a mechanical problem that normally requires a mechanical solution (mitral repair or replacement) for adequate therapy. However, in PMR patients who develop atrial fibrillation, proper anticoagulation with either vitamin K antagonists or nonvitamin antagonists is indicated.

16. What are the indications for mechanical therapy of PMR, and what do those therapies consist of? What is the prognosis following treatment?

As noted previously, severe PMR is a potentially fatal disease leading to myocardial damage, heart failure, and death. However, timely mechanical correction (Table 25.1) of PMR is consistent with a normal lifespan and lifestyle.

No medical therapy has been proven effective. The onset of symptoms, usually dyspnea on exertion, marks a turning point in the illness with a marked decline in survival if PMR is left untreated. Some consider the onset of atrial fibrillation equivalent to symptom onset. Likewise, the development of LV dysfunction also has a major negative impact on survival even if symptoms are absent. Because MR enhances LV ejection and survival worsens for patients with ejection fraction (EF) < 60%, an EF decreasing toward 60% is an indication for mitral intervention. Likewise, if the LV is unable to contract to an end-systolic dimension of </=40 mm, there is likely myocardial dysfunction, and prognosis is worsened. Increasing levels of natriuretic peptides, especially to >3× times normal, and/or worsening of LV global longitudinal strain are worrisome and may help in the decision for MR correction. Patients with severe PMR should be followed with examination and echocardiography every 6–12 months until definitive therapy is instituted.

Mitral valve repair is superior to MVR when valve anatomy and surgical expertise permit repair. Operative mortality is about half that of MVR, and the very long-term outcome is also superior. These results are thought to be due to better LV function with repair and the absence of prosthetic valve complications. For this reason, many would consider early repair before either symptoms or LV dysfunction develop. When valve anatomy does not permit repair, MVR is performed. In patients at prohibitive surgical risk, transcatheter repair wherein the valve leaflets are clipped together with a percutaneously inserted device is a satisfactory option.

Secondary Mitral Regurgitation

17. What are the major etiologies of SMR?

The term *secondary MR* indicates that the valve leak is secondary to another process rather than due to abnormalities of the mitral valve itself. SMR is almost always due to LV dysfunction created by previous myocardial infarction or primary myocardial disease. Both lead to LV dilatation, papillary muscle displacement, mitral annular dilatation, and reduced valve closing force, all acting in concert to restrict leaflet motion and prevent leaflet coaptation. Myocardial infarction may also cause regional wall motion abnormalities, further interfering with coordinated valve closing. In some cases of SMR, atrial fibrillation leads to LA and annular dilatation, preventing leaflet closure.

18. What are the hemodynamics of SMR?

In most cases of SMR, the LV dysfunction that led to valvular insufficiency will also cause heart failure. As such, reduced cardiac output and elevated left-sided pressures are likely to present even before SMR develops. The superimposition of SMR worsens these hemodynamics because more LV stroke volume is diverted into the LA, further reducing forward output while simultaneously increasing LA pressure and pulmonary congestion.

19. What are common myths about the hemodynamics of SMR?

Some believe that SMR acts as a "pop-off" valve, reducing LV afterload such that correction of SMR increases load and reduces ejection. In fact, this is usually not true. The regurgitant orifice area in severe SMR is on the order of $0.4\,cm^2$, a small hole considering the normal MVA is about $4.0\,cm^2$. Thus while LA pressure is low compared to aortic pressure, actual impedance to flow is usually higher, not lower, than impedance to aortic flow. EF may fall after mitral surgery, but this is usually due to a reduction in end-diastolic volume as the volume overload of SMR had been removed by the procedure. However, in some cases of very severe SMR or if the mitral apparatus is damaged by repair, end-systolic volume may increase, thereby lowering EF.

20. How are SMR hemodynamics translated into symptoms?

Because SMR is a manifestation of heart failure, the patient with SMR usually has symptoms typical of heart failure, including dyspnea, orthopnea, paroxysmal nocturnal dyspnea, and – if there is also right-sided failure – ascites and edema. However, small changes in LV volume may cause changes in the mitral regurgitant orifice, leading to sudden increases in SMR. Thus evidence of worsened SMR should be sought when a heart failure patient develops sudden symptomatic decline. The presence of angina helps point to an ischemic cause of SMR.

21. How are SMR hemodynamics translated into physical signs?

Because SMR often exists in a hemodynamic milieu of high LA pressure and reduced LV systolic pressure, the transmitral gradient driving SMR may be relatively reduced compared to that of PMR. As such, the murmur of SMR may be unimpressive or even absent.

22. How is SMR diagnosed (imaging and invasive hemodynamics)?

Because the murmur of SMR may be unimpressive, the severity of SMR may not be suspected until TTE is performed. As with PMR, TEE may be warranted to further investigate SMR if signs and symptoms suggest worse MR than is appreciated by TTE. Either method helps assess the mechanisms causing SMR, degree of LV dysfunction, and presence of wall motion abnormalities that may suggest an ischemic etiology for the patient's SMR. As the issue of whether the SMR is of ischemic or non-ischemic origin usually arises, assessment of the coronary anatomy by either coronary computed tomography (CT) or left heart catheterization is usually warranted. If an invasive strategy is planned, both right and left heart catheterization are indicated. The criteria for severe SMR are similar to those of PMR (Table 25.1), although the regurgitant volume is usually <60 cc/beat

23. What are the indications for medical therapy in SMR, and what do those therapies consist of?

Because heart failure is usually co-existent with SMR, intensive guideline-directed therapy for heart failure is indicated. Beta-blockers, angiotensin-converting enzyme (ACE) inhibitors, angiotensin receptor blockers, spironolactone, and the addition of neprilysin inhibitors are indicated. In many cases, SMR greatly improves or even resolves with these therapies. If a left bundle branch block is present, cardiac resynchronization may also greatly reduce SMR.

24. What are the indications for mechanical therapy of SMR, and what do those therapies consist of?

By definition, SMR is due to another condition, usually ischemic heart disease, primary cardiomyopathy, or atrial fibrillation. Thus, correction of the MR by itself does not "cure" the patient as it does in PMR. Mechanical treatment of SMR is reserved for patients with severe MR and advanced symptoms despite aggressive therapy for heart failure. Surgical repair of SMR is usually problematic because the valve itself is anatomically normal, leaving little for the surgeon to repair. There is often a successful surgical reduction in MR, only to have it reappear shortly after the operation. Currently, no large randomized trials demonstrate that surgical treatment of SMR prolongs life, and surgery may increase the risk of stroke. Therefore mitral surgery is usually employed as an additional procedure when coronary revascularization is performed.

Several non-surgical approaches to SMR have been attempted. The most successful of these is the Abbott MitraClip, a device that clips the two bellies of the mitral leaflets together at their midsections. This catheter-based technique is successful in reducing SMR and, in at least one trial, reduced the incidence of hospital admission for heart failure and improved survival.

25. What is the prognosis of SMR?

Because SMR is a product of LV dysfunction and heart failure, those conditions drive prognosis. Unlike in PMR, where life span may be normal after timely surgery, Mortality in SMR is about 10–15% per year.

Bibliography

1 Bargiggia, G.S., Tronconi, L., Sahn, D.J. et al. (1991). A new method for quantitation of mitral regurgitation based on color flow Doppler imaging of flow convergence proximal to regurgitant orifice. *Circulation* 84: 1481–1489.

2 Bertrand, P.B., Mihos, C.G., and Yucel, E. (2019). Mitral annular calcification and calcific mitral stenosis: therapeutic challenges and considerations. *Curr. Treat. Options Cardiovasc. Med.* 21: 19.

3 Bouleti, C., Iung, B., Laouénan, C. et al. (2012). Late results of percutaneous mitral commissurotomy up to 20 years: development and validation of a risk score predicting late functional results from a series of 912 patients. *Circulation* 125: 2119–2127.

4 Costillo, J.G., Adams, D.H., Carabello, B.A., and Sangupta, P.P. (2017). Degenerative mitral valve disease. In: *Hurst's the Heart*, 14e (ed. V. Fuster, R.A. Harrington, J. Narula and Z.J. Eapen), 1215–1238. New York: McGraw Hill.

5 David, T.E., David, C.M., Tsang, W. et al. (2019). Long-term results of mitral valve repair for regurgitation due to leaflet prolapse. *J. Am. Coll. Cardiol.* 74: 1044–1053.

6 Enriquez-Sarano, M., Tajik, A.J., Schaff, H.V. et al. (1994). Echocardiographic prediction of survival after surgical correction of organic mitral regurgitation. *Circulation* 90: 830–837.

7 Feldman, T., Kar, S., Elmariah, S. et al. (2015). Randomized comparison of percutaneous repair and surgery for mitral regurgitation: 5-year results of EVEREST II. *J. Am. Coll. Cardiol.* 66: 2844–2854.

8 Goldstein, D., Moskowitz, A.J., Gelijns, A.C. et al. (2016). Two-year outcomes of surgical treatment of severe ischemic mitral regurgitation. *N. Engl. J. Med.* 374: 344–353.

9 Gorlin, R. and Gorlin, S.G. (1951). Hydraulic formula for calculation of the area of the stenotic mitral valve, other cardiac valves, and central circulatory shunts. *Am. Heart J.* 41 (1): 1–29.

10 Hiemstra, Y.L., Tomsic, A., van Wijngaarden, S.E. et al. (2020). Prognostic value of global longitudinal strain and etiology after surgery for primary mitral regurgitation. *JACC Cardiovasc. Imaging* 13: 577–585.

11 Meneguz-Moreno, R.A., Costa, J.R. Jr., Gomes, N.L. et al. (2018). Very long term follow-up after percutaneous balloon mitral valvuloplasty. *JACC Cardiovasc. Interv.* 11: 1945–1952.

12 Mentias, A., Patel, K., Patel, H. et al. (2016). Prognostic utility of brain natriuretic peptide in asymptomatic patients with significant mitral regurgitation and preserved left ventricular ejection fraction. *Am. J. Cardiol.* 117: 258–263.

13 O'Gara, P., Sugeng, L., Lang, R. et al. (2008). The role of imaging in chronic degenerative mitral regurgitation. *JACC Cardiovosc Imaging* l (2): 221–237.

14 Olesen, K.H. (1962). The natural history of 271 patients with mitral stenosis under medical treatment. *Br. Heart J.* 24: 349–357.

15 Rajesh, G.N., Sajeer, K., Sajeev, C.G. et al. (2016). A comparative study of ivabradine and atenolol in patients with moderate mitral stenosis in sinus rhythm. *Indian Heart J.* 68: 311–315.

16 Stone, G.W., Lindenfeld, J., Abraham, W.T. et al. (2018). Transcatheter mitral-valve repair in patients with heart failure. *N. Engl. J. Med.* 379: 2307–2318.

17 Tribouilloy, C., Grigioni, F., Avicrinos, J.F. et al. (2009). Survival implication of left ventricular end-systolic diameter in mitral regurgitation due to flail leaflets a long-term follow-up multicenter study. *J. Am. Coll. Cardiol.* 54: 1961–1968.

18 Tribouilloy, C.M., Enriquez-Sarano, M., Schaff, H.V. et al. (1999). Impact of preoperative symptoms on survival

after surgical correction of organic mitral regurgitation: rationale for optimizing surgical indications. *Circulation* 99: 400–405.

19 Watkins, D.A., Johnson, C.O., Colquhoun, S.M. et al. (2017). Global, regional, and National Burden of rheumatic heart disease, 1990–2015. *N. Engl. J. Med.* 377 (8): 713–722.

20 Writing Committee Members, Otto, C.M., Nishimura, R.A. et al. (2021). 2020 ACC/AHA guideline for the Management of Patients with Valvular Heart Disease: executive summary: a report of the American College of Cardiology/American Heart Association Joint Committee on Clinical Practice Guidelines. *J. Am. Coll. Cardiol.* 77 (4): 450–500.

26

Hemodynamic Assessment of the Mitral Valve

Calvin C. Sheng, Samir R. Kapadia and Serge Harb

[1] *Department of Cardiovascular Medicine, Cleveland Clinic, Cleveland, OH, USA*

Mitral Stenosis

1. Why is it important to distinguish between rheumatic and nonrheumatic calcific mitral stenosis?

Rheumatic mitral stenosis (MS) remains the most common cause of MS globally in developing countries as a late complication of rheumatic fever and typically presents in young adults with commissural fusion of otherwise pliable noncalcified valve leaflets. Conversely, nonrheumatic calcific MS is much more commonly seen in developed countries in older patients due to mitral annular calcification (MAC) and/or leaflet calcification (Figure 26.1). These differences in underlying pathology and risk factors lead to differences in intervention. In rheumatic MS, patients with favorable anatomy (Wilkins' score ≤ 8 on echocardiography, pre-procedural mitral regurgitation (MR) <2+, and absence of left atrial thrombus) or some with unfavorable anatomy but no significant MR may benefit from percutaneous mitral balloon valvuloplasty (PMBV). Otherwise, mitral valve surgery can be considered.

2. What is the pathophysiology leading to the hemodynamic consequences of MS?

As the MV orifice area decreases, the obstruction impedes left ventricular diastolic filling, thus leading to decreased cardiac output and increased pressure gradient between the left atrium (LA) and left ventricle (LV) generated by rising LA pressure and subsequent enlargement of the LA chamber. This is then transmitted to the pulmonary circulation with increases in pulmonary artery pressures and pulmonary vascular resistance (PVR). With chronicity and remodeling, the resulting pulmonary hypertension may become irreversible without early intervention and may also lead to right ventricular (RV) dilatation and right-sided heart failure.

3. When is it reasonable to consider intervention for MS?

Stages of MS are defined by patient symptoms, valve anatomy, and hemodynamics. Severe MS is defined by a mitral valve area (MVA) $\leq 1.5\,cm^2$ in the 2020 American College of Cardiology/American Heart Association (ACC/AHA) valvular heart disease guidelines. This typically corresponds to a transmitral mean gradient >5 mmHg. If clinical symptoms are discordant with resting echo findings, exercise testing with echo Doppler or invasive hemodynamic assessment can be used to assess physiologic changes in mean mitral gradient and pulmonary artery (PA) pressures.

4. What are the findings on invasive hemodynamic assessment to suggest severe MS?

- Hallmark: elevated LA or pulmonary capillary wedge pressure (PCWP) relative to LV end-diastolic pressure (LVEDP), leading to an elevated diastolic transmitral gradient ranging from 5 to 25 mmHg
- Reduced cardiac output (3.5–4.5 l/min) due to obstruction in flow across MV
- Calculated valve area $\leq 1.5\,cm^2$ based on a simplified Gorlin formula

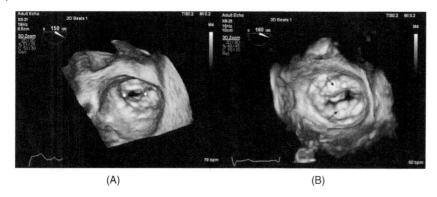

(A)   (B)

Figure 26.1   3D transesophageal echocardiography illustrations from an atrial or "surgeon's" view of (a) rheumatic mitral stenosis (MS) vs. (b) calcific MS. Asterisks (*) show the anterolateral and posteromedial commissural fusion. Arrows point to the severe anterior and posterior mitral annular calcification.

- Abnormalities in LA pressure tracing affecting both *a* and *v* waves
- Shallow slope of y descent due to the delayed emptying of LA
- Pulmonary hypertension with elevated PA pressures and increased PVR

5.   What are the pitfalls of using PCWP as surrogate for LA pressure?

There is a good correlation between mean PCWP and LA pressure when the PCWP is low (<25 mmHg), but it becomes more variable above that (Figure 26.2). Due to the intrinsic nature of PCWP as transmitted pressure from the LA across the pulmonary bed, there may be a considerable time delay, leading to the *v* wave partially appearing in diastole and dampening of the waveform. The former can be adjusted for by phase-shifting the peak of the *v* wave to the downslope of the LV waveform. Furthermore, in the presence of severe pulmonary hypertension, obtaining

true PCWP may be technically challenging, and a hybrid PCWP-PA pressure may be sampled. All of these factors can result in inaccurate estimations of the transmitral gradient. True PCWP position can be confirmed by obtaining an oximetry saturation >90%. Alternatively, a transseptal puncture across the fossa ovalis or retrograde crossing of the mitral valve can be considered for direct LA pressure monitoring.

6.   What can cause an elevated transmitral gradient?

Aside from rheumatic MS and nonrheumatic calcific MS with MAC, other causes of the differential include:

- Severe MR leading to an increase in flow across the valve, although typically this only contributes to early diastole
- Obstruction of flow from mass effect (e.g. atrial myxoma, infective endocarditis)

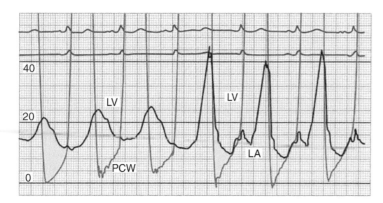

Figure 26.2   Pulmonary capillary wedge pressure (PCWP) as a surrogate for left atrium (LA) pressure can lead to overestimation of the transmitral gradient. *Source:* Figure adapted from Ragosta, M. (2017). *Textbook of Clinical Hemodynamics E-Book.* Elsevier Health Sciences.

- Bioprosthetic MV degeneration
- High cardiac output (CO) states (and some have described this for acute ventricular septal defect [VSD]; a large *v* wave is classic)

7. What are the expected hemodynamics before and after PMBV?

In select patients with severe symptomatic MS and favorable anatomy, as outlined in question 1, PMBV can be performed with results comparable to surgical commissurotomy. Both double-balloon and Inoue PMBV techniques are done (Figure 26.3). After each balloon inflation, carefully reassess the transmitral gradient and interval development of worsening MR.

A successful valvuloplasty will show an immediate reduction in LA pressure with a decrease in transmitral gradient of ≥50% and a post-procedural MV area ≥1.5 cm². Depending on the chronicity of pulmonary hypertension, PA pressures may improve but may not revert to normal due to remodeling of the pulmonary vasculature.

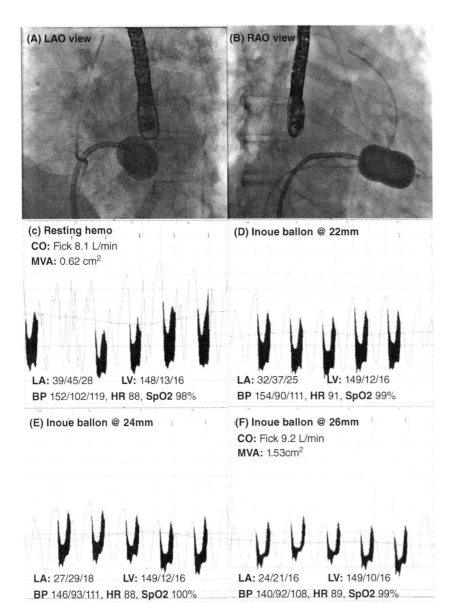

Figure 26.3 (a, b) Fluoroscopic left anterior oblique and right anterior oblique views of the Inoue technique. (c–f) Resting hemodynamics followed by serial incremental balloon dilatations to achieve improvement in mitral valve area and mean gradient without worsening mitral regurgitation or pulmonary artery pressures.

8. What is a dreaded immediate complication to monitor for during PMBV?

While rare, the incidence of developing severe MR after PMBV occurred with a frequency ranging from 1.4 to 9.4%. This can result from excessive tearing of the commissures or leaflets or chordal/subvalvular apparatus rupture. The post-valvuloplasty hemodynamics will show an increase rather than an expected decrease in LA pressure with a large prominent *v* wave with steep *y* descent. Depending on the severity and clinical stability, this may require urgent surgical or percutaneous MV intervention.

Mitral Regurgitation

9. What are the common causes of primary and secondary MR?

Primary MR (degenerative):

- Myxomatous degeneration
- Spontaneous chordal rupture
- Fibroelastic deficiency
- Valvulitis (rheumatic, radiation)
- Infectious endocarditis
- Mitral annular calcification related MR
- Prosthetic MV dysfunction and/or prosthetic paravalvular leak

Secondary MR (functional):

- Annular dilatation due to LA and/or LV dysfunction
- Ischemic MR due to tethering of leaflets

10. What is the difference in pathophysiology leading to the hemodynamic consequences of acute vs. chronic MR?

Severe acute MR, most commonly from spontaneous chordal rupture or infarction-related papillary muscle rupture, is usually diagnosed based on acute clinical presentation and confirmed by a transthoracic or transesophageal echo. Acute MR leads to a rapid increase in regurgitant volume in an otherwise unadapted LA and subsequent increases in LA and pulmonary venous pressures, which clinically manifest as pulmonary edema. The diminished forward stroke volume (SV) results in compensatory tachycardia and peripheral vasoconstriction and may ultimately progress to shock and death if urgent surgical intervention is not performed.

In chronic MR, there is an inevitable progression in severity over time as the body tries to adapt. There is an interval increase in total LV volume to maintain forward SV and enlargement of LA to accommodate the regurgitant volume. As the compensatory mechanisms fail, patients clinically become more symptomatic. A corresponding increase in PCWP and decrease in cardiac output are observed hemodynamically.

Classically, severe MR is associated with a prominent *v* wave on PCWP or LA pressure tracing, which has been previously described as (i) peak *v* wave >40 mmHg, (ii) difference between peak *v* wave and mean PCWP ≥10 mmHg, and (iii) ratio of peak *v* wave to mean PCWP >2. However, studies have shown that this is insensitive and that its absence or presence does not always correlate to the severity of MR.

11. What are mimickers that lead to a prominent *v* wave on PCWP or LA pressure tracings?

Normally, the *v* wave represents atrial filling at the end of ventricular systole and reflects the compliance of the LA. Even a small change in volume can produce a large pressure response in a stiff LA, whereas in a compliant LA, a larger change in volume would be needed to generate the same pressure response. In addition to severe MR, any process that leads to increased volume and pressure inside the LA can also generate this:

- Ventricular septal defect
- Mitral stenosis
- Left-sided heart failure
- Tachycardia leading to incomplete atrial emptying
- Processes that result in decreased LA compliance (i.e. infiltrative disease, tumor, constriction, etc.)

12. When is it reasonable to consider percutaneous intervention for MR?

Detailed indications are outlined in the 2020 ACC/AHA valvular heart disease guidelines. In general, patients with severe primary MR in the presence of symptoms and/or LV systolic dysfunction (ejection fraction [EF] ≤60% or left ventricular end-systolic diameter [LVESD] ≥40mm) should be evaluated for percutaneous or surgical options. For primary MR, the percutaneous approach is generally only considered when surgery is high risk and the procedure is technically feasible with patient anatomy (Class 2a recommendation). Similarly, in patients with severe secondary MR, a subset with reduced EF <50% who are symptomatic despite maximally tolerated guideline-directed medical therapy (GDMT) and favorable MV anatomy may be considered for percutaneous options.

13. What is the concept of *proportionately* and *disproportionately* severe secondary MR?

Traditionally, MR is categorized as primary versus secondary MR depending on whether the underlying pathology is due to the leaflets or in the LV, respectively. The latter is a heterogeneous group that can be conceptualized as either (i) *proportionately* or (ii) *disproportionately* severe MR relative to the degree of LV dilatation (Figure 26.4). Quantitatively, severe MR is defined by effective regurgitant orifice area (EROA) ≥0.4cm^2, although it may be limited by interobserver variability and regurgitant fraction ≥50%. However, it is important not to neglect the LV's contributions to MV hemodynamics in terms of volume (measured by LV end-diastolic volume [LVEDV]) and function (measured by left ventricular ejection fraction [LVEF]). The ratio of EROA to LVEDV can be a useful index for predicting a favorable response to transcatheter mitral valve repair (TMVr). For example, in a patient without significant adversely remodeled LV (i.e. LVEDV 160–200 ml), the presence of severe MR by EROA means a *disproportionate*

degree of MR relative to LV size and is more likely to confer mortality benefits, as demonstrated in the COAPT (Cardiovascular Outcomes Assessment of the MitraClip Percutaneous Therapy for Heart Failure Patients With Functional Mitral Regurgitation) trial. Conversely, in a patient with significantly remodeled LV (i.e. LVEDV >200ml), the presence of severe MR by EROA (may be <0.40cm^2 due to elliptical ROA) may be *proportionate* to the degree of LV dilatation, and TMVr may not provide mortality benefit as concluded by the MITRA-FR (Multicentre Study of Percutaneous Mitral Valve Repair MitraClip Device in Patients With Severe Secondary Mitral Regurgitation) trial. In an otherwise normotensive patient with reduced LVEF, an EROA ≤0.2cm^2 is unlikely to contribute a hemodynamically or clinically relevant degree of MR requiring intervention.

14. Alternatively, what is the difference between atrial and ventricular functional MR (AFMR vs. VFMR)?

Ventricular functional MR (VFMR) is the classic secondary MR due to LV dilatation and systolic dysfunction from leaflet tethering-tenting in the setting of ischemic or dilated cardiomyopathy. More recently, atrial functional MR (AFMR) has gained traction as a distinct entity highlighting the role of LA and mitral annulus (MA) dynamics in LA enlargement and MA dilatation despite preserved EF, as seen in atrial fibrillation and heart failure with preserved ejection fraction. While these changes lead to leaflet malcoaptation, contributions from other mechanisms, including atriogenic leaflet tethering, inadequate compensatory

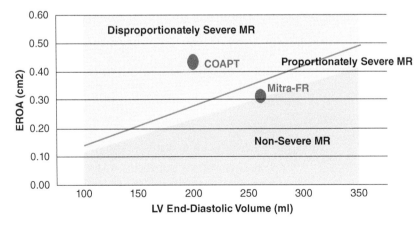

Figure 26.4 Relationship of effective regurgitant orifice area to left ventricle end-diastolic volume in discerning *proportionate* and *disproportionate* mitral regurgitation (MR) versus non-severe MR. Patients with *disproportionately* severe MR would likely benefit the most from percutaneous intervention. *Source:* Grayburn et al. (2019) / With permission of Elsevier.

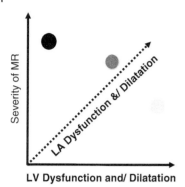

Figure 26.5 Relationship of mitral regurgitation (MR) severity to degree of left atrium and left ventricle (LV) dysfunction and/or dilatation. Patients with severe atrial functional MR and severe ventricular functional MR without severe LV dilatation (black and gray circles) would likely benefit the most from percutaneous intervention.

leaflet remodeling, and MA dysfunction, remain to be fully elucidated. During systole, the MA has a threefold motion that can be affected: (i) anteroposterior "sphincter-like" contraction, (ii) annular height and saddle-shaped increase leading to "folding," and (iii) downward "translational" motion. A recent study also demonstrated the association between MA dysfunction and both LA- and LV-dilatation and dysfunction. Maintaining sinus rhythm and euvolemia may be key in preventing progression of AFMR, while in severe cases, treatment should target MA dilatation with annuloplasty devices or reduction of the anterior–posterior MA diameter with TMVr (Figure 26.5). Often, AFMR and VFMR co-exist but with varying degrees of atrial versus ventricular contributions, further illustrating the fine balance in defining MV hemodynamics.

15. What are the percutaneous MV interventions currently available and under investigation?

Compared to the aortic valve, the MV has an added level of complexity due to the subvalvular apparatus (chordae tendineae and papillary muscle displacement) and the non-planar saddle-shaped geometry of the annulus, where the peaks are the anterior and posterior landmarks of the leaflets and the troughs are the anterolateral and posteromedial commissures. The devices and technologies can be broadly categorized as edge-to-edge repair, annuloplasty, mitral valve replacement, and miscellaneous. Currently, the only percutaneous device approved by the US Food and Drug Administration (FDA) for either primary or secondary MR is edge-to-edge repair with the MitraClip device (Abbott Vascular).

16. What are the expected hemodynamic changes after the most common percutaneous edge-to-edge repair with MitraClip?

Real-time hemodynamic response can be observed after successful MitraClip repair. With a reduction in regurgitant volume, there is increased forward SV and cardiac output with a decrease in systemic vascular resistance. If the peak *v* wave and LA pressure are elevated pre-procedurally, then post-procedurally, there should be expected improvements along with a reduction in LV end-diastolic pressure. In fact, the improvements in hemodynamics with MitraClip have also been shown to reverse LA and LV remodeling. Chronic pulmonary hypertension may not improve significantly since the improvement seen in MR may be partly offset by a mild increase in MS caused by the creation of a double MV orifice from the nature of the edge-to-edge repair design. Several studies have demonstrated the feasibility and efficacy of continuous LA pressure monitor to help guide placement of the MitraClip. Ultimately, there is a tradeoff with every additional clip between minimal incremental improvements in the degree of MR on Doppler and invasive hemodynamics with *v* wave and LA pressure at the cost of potentially causing worsening MS (Figure 26.6).

Bibliography

1 Chen, C.-R., Cheng, T.O., and Group, M.S. (1995). Percutaneous balloon mitral valvuloplasty by the Inoue technique: a multicenter study of 4832 patients in China. *Am. Heart J.* 129: 1197–1203.

2 Deferm, S., Bertrand, P.B., Verbrugge, F.H. et al. (2019). Atrial functional mitral regurgitation: JACC review topic of the week. *J. Am. Coll. Cardiol.* 73: 2465–2476.

3 Fuchs, R.M., Heuser, R.R., Yin, F.C., and Brinker, J.A. (1982). Limitations of pulmonary wedge V waves in diagnosing mitral regurgitation. *Am. J. Cardiol.* 49: 849–854.

4 Gajjar, M., Yadlapati, A., Van Assche, L.M. et al. (2017). Real-time continuous left atrial pressure monitoring during mitral valve repair using the MitraClip NT system:

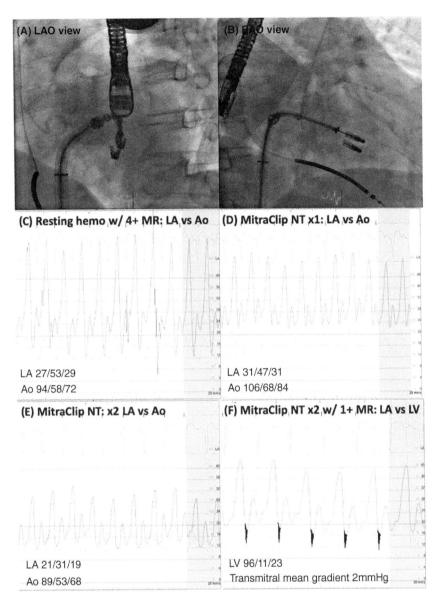

Figure 26.6 (a, b) Fluoroscopic left anterior oblique and right anterior oblique views of MitraClips. (c–e) Resting hemodynamics followed by sequential deployment of MitraClip NT #1 and #2, monitoring left atrium and aortic pressures. (f) Closing pressures with residual mild 1+ mitral regurgitation and a transmitral mean gradient of 2 mmHg.

a feasibility study. *J. Am. Coll. Cardiol. Intv.* 10: 1466–1467.

5 Grayburn, P.A., Foster, E., Sangli, C. et al. (2013). Relationship between the magnitude of reduction in mitral regurgitation severity and left ventricular and left atrial reverse remodeling after MitraClip therapy. *Circulation* 128: 1667–1674.

6 Grayburn, P.A., Sannino, A., and Packer, M. (2019). Proportionate and disproportionate functional mitral regurgitation: a new conceptual framework that reconciles the results of the MITRA-FR and COAPT trials. *JACC Cardiovasc. Imaging* 12: 353–362.

7 Kuwata, S., Taramasso, M., Czopak, A. et al. (2019). Continuous direct left atrial pressure: intraprocedural measurement predicts clinical response following MitraClip therapy. *J. Am. Coll. Cardiol. Intv.* 12: 127–136.

8 Meneguz-Moreno, R., Costa, J., and Gomes, N. (2018). Very long-term follow-up after percutaneous mitral balloon valvuloplasty. *J. Am. Coll. Cardiol. Intv.* 11: 1945–1952.

9 Mihaila Baldea, S., Muraru, D., Miglioranza, M.H. et al. (2020). Relation of mitral annulus and left atrial dysfunction to the severity of functional mitral regurgitation in patients with dilated cardiomyopathy. *Cardiol. Res. Pract.* 2020.

10 Obadia, J.-F., Messika-Zeitoun, D., Leurent, G. et al. (2018). Percutaneous repair or medical treatment for secondary mitral regurgitation. *N. Engl. J. Med.* 379: 2297–2306.

11 Otto, C.M., Nishimura, R.A., Bonow, R.O. et al. (2021). 2020 ACC/AHA guideline for the management of patients with valvular heart disease: executive summary: a report of the American College of Cardiology/ American Heart Association Joint Committee on Clinical Practice Guidelines. *J. Am. Coll. Cardiol.* 77: 450–500.

12 Palacios, I.F., Sanchez, P.L., Harrell, L.C. et al. (2002). Which patients benefit from percutaneous mitral balloon valvuloplasty? Prevalvuloplasty and postvalvuloplasty variables that predict long-term outcome. *Circulation* 105: 1465–1471.

13 Ragosta, M. (2017). *Textbook of Clinical Hemodynamics E-Book*. Elsevier Health Sciences.

14 Reyes, V.P., Raju, B.S., Wynne, J. et al. (1994). Percutaneous balloon valvuloplasty compared with open surgical commissurotomy for mitral stenosis. *N. Engl. J. Med.* 331: 961–967.

15 Silbiger, J.J. (2014). Does left atrial enlargement contribute to mitral leaflet tethering in patients with functional mitral regurgitation? Proposed role of atriogenic leaflet tethering. *Echocardiography* 31: 1310–1311.

16 Snyder, R.W. II, Glamann, D.B., Lange, R.A. et al. (1994). Predictive value of prominent pulmonary arterial wedge V waves in assessing the presence and severity of mitral regurgitation. *Am. J. Cardiol.* 73: 568–570.

17 Stone, G.W., Lindenfeld, J., Abraham, W.T. et al. (2018). Transcatheter mitral-valve repair in patients with heart failure. *N. Engl. J. Med.* 379: 2307–2318.

18 Zoghbi, W.A., Adams, D., Bonow, R.O. et al. (2017). Recommendations for noninvasive evaluation of native valvular regurgitation: a report from the American Society of Echocardiography developed in collaboration with the Society for Cardiovascular Magnetic Resonance. *J. Am. Soc. Echocardiogr.* 30: 303–371.

27

Echocardiographic Assessment Prior to Mitral Valve Edge-to-Edge Repair

Jonatan D. Nunez and Martin Bilsker

Division of Cardiology, University of Miami, Miami, FL, USA

1. What is edge-to-edge mitral valve repair?

Edge-to-edge mitral valve repair Is a minimally invasive percutaneous procedure for patients with significant mitral regurgitation (MR) and increased surgical risk. It consists in using a MitraClip (Abbot) to attach both the anterior and posterior leaflets of the mitral valve, thus creating a double orifice. This procedure is derived from the surgical Alfieri stitch.

2. What is the role of pre-procedural transthoracic echocardiography (TTE) prior to edge-to-edge mitral valve repair?

Pre-procedural TTE is the initial and arguably the most important diagnostic tool. It is a fundamental part of screening and classifying the severity of MR, as well as clarifying the etiology of MR and the initial anatomic suitability for percutaneous intervention.

3. How is MR classified?

According to the Carpentier classification, the mechanism of MR is described as follows:

Type I: Normal leaflet motion	Type II: Excessive leaflet motion	Type III: Restricted leaflet motion
Annular dilation or perforation	Prolapse or flail leaflet	a) Thickening/ Fusion
		b) LV/LA dilation

For simplification, MR is also described as primary or secondary. Primary MR is mostly caused by myxomatous or calcific leaflet degeneration. Secondary MR is further divided into regional left ventricle (LV) dysfunction (due to inferior myocardial infarction) and global LV dysfunction (in cases of nonischemic cardiomyopathy, large anterior, or multiple myocardial infarctions).

4. Which patients with primary MR would benefit the most from percutaneous edge-to-edge repair?

According to the most recent American College of Cardiology (ACC) guidelines, the transcatheter edge-to-edge mitral valve repair in primary MR has 2a recommendations in the following circumstances:

- Severe MR (vena contracta (VC) ≥ 0.7 cm, regurgitant volume ≥ 60 ml, regurgitant fraction $\geq 50\%$, effective regurgitant orifice area (EROA) ≥ 0.40 cm^2); symptoms due to MR; high or prohibitive risk of mitral valve surgery; favorable anatomy, and life expectancy >1 year
- Severe MR, high or prohibitive risk of mitral valve surgery, favorable anatomy, life expectancy >1 year, and no symptoms due to MR but evidence of LV dysfunction such as left ventricular ejection fraction (LVEF) $\leq 60\%$ or end-systolic diameter (ESD) ≥ 40 mm

5. Which patients with secondary MR would benefit the most from percutaneous edge-to-edge repair?

According to the most recent ACC guidelines, edge-to-edge mitral valve repair has a 2a indication in patients with

Mastering Structural Heart Disease, First Edition. Edited by Eduardo J. de Marchena and Camilo A. Gomez.
© 2023 John Wiley & Sons Ltd. Published 2023 by John Wiley & Sons Ltd.
Companion website: www.wiley.com/go/deMarchena/Mastering-Structural-Heart-Disease

guideline-directed medical therapy (GDMT) supervised by a heart failure specialist, with LVEF <50%, persistent symptoms on GDMT, favorable mitral anatomy, EF 20–50%, ESD ≤ 70 mm, and pulmonary artery systolic pressure ≤ 70 mmHg.

As explained in the guideline, a key factor for success in selecting patients with secondary MR is the degree of MR and the severity of LV dilation. This component played an important role in the discordant results between the COAPT (Cardiovascular Outcomes Assessment of the MitraClip Percutaneous Therapy for Heart Failure Patients With Functional Mitral Regurgitation) and MITRA-FR (Multicentre Study of Percutaneous Mitral Valve Repair MitraClip Device in Patients With Severe Secondary Mitral Regurgitation) trials.

In the COAPT trial, there was a statistically significant decrease in hospitalization for heart failure within 24 months in the device group (35.8 vs. 67.9%) and decreased mortality (29.1 vs. 46.1%); this was in contrast to the MITRA-FR trial, where no difference was found between the device and medical therapy groups. In the COAPT trial, the EROA was about 30% higher, and LV volumes were about 30% smaller, indicating disproportionally severe MR (see Figure 27.1).

6.   Which are the most important views in the pre-procedural TTE?

- *Parasternal long-axis view:* Excellent to visualize middle scallops (A2/P2), sub-valvular apparatus, thickening or calcifications of the leaflets, LV/annular dimension, and etiology of the MR and estimate severity.
- *Apical four-chamber view:* Can reveal primary valve abnormalities such as thickening, restriction, prolapse, and flailing. This view is also instrumental for the quantitative assessment of MR by obtaining the proximal isovelocity surface area (PISA), EROA, and transvalvular gradient and calculating the mitral valve area (MVA). Pulmonary veins can sometimes be adequately assessed for systolic flow reversal in this view.
- *Two-chamber view:* The plane should be parallel to the zone of coaptation; usually, the entire width of the regurgitant jet from the medial to the lateral commissure is observed. If the jet is broad, more than one mitral clip might be needed.
- *Parasternal short-axis view:* With this view, MVA can be measured directly and the origin of the jet can often be clarified. With the help of 3D or bi-plane echocardiography, an accurate MVA (independently from loading conditions, pressure, and compliance) can be measured; MVA is particularly important to determine suitability for edge-to-edge repair. 3D imaging is often challenging in TTE; therefore, it is not done routinely.

7.   Why is pre-procedure transesophageal echocardiography (TEE) important?

It allows a superior visualization of the mitral valve apparatus to clarify the etiology, location, and mechanism of regurgitation, assess the suitability of edge-to-edge repair, and rule out left atrial appendage thrombus. It also provides a better assessment of the interatrial septum, quantifies the MR severity, and most accurately measures MVA by planimetry. This test is exceptionally important in patients with poor windows for TTE. The superior resolution and image quality often allow good 3D views.

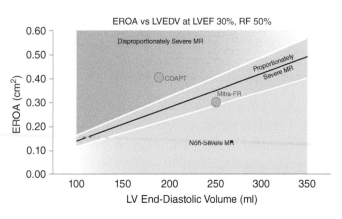

Figure 27.1 Graphic comparing the differences between the COAPT and MITRA-FR trials. *Source:* Grayburn et al. (2019) / With permission of Elsevier.

8. Which are the most important pre-procedural TEE views to assess for edge-to-edge mitral valve repair?

- *Mid-esophageal view 0°:* Depending on the level of the probe, the lateral (A1/P1) scallops can be seen; but by advancing the probe deeper, the medial (A2/P3) scallops are observed (see Figure 27.2a).
- *Intercommissural view:* In the mid-esophageal position at 45°–60°, P1/A2/P3 are usually seen. The anterior and posterior leaflets can be assessed with clockwise and counterclockwise rotation of the probe, respectively (see Figure 27.2b).
- *Long-axis view:* Usually, in the mid esophageal position at 135°–150° – similarly to the transthoracic long parasternal axis view – the A2/P2 scallops and the long axis of the aortic valve are pictured. Rotating the probe clockwise will move the plane medially to the interatrial septum, and counterclockwise will move the plane laterally to the left atrial appendage (see Figure 27.2c).

9. What are the applications of 3D pre-procedural TEE for edge-to-edge repair?

Accurate anatomical views of the entire mitral valve can be obtained using 3D TEE for better spatial orientation (see Figure 27.3). 3D images can unambiguously identify the location of the regurgitant jet and identify multiple jets in relation to the anterior and posterior scallops. Another key benefit of 3D TEE is the measurement of MVA by planimetry. Any 2D echocardiographic plane that includes the entire valve can be used, but there is an inverse relationship between temporal resolution (frame rate) and the size of the sample. Furthermore, the spatial resolution depends on the number of 2D sectors in the 3D volume; therefore, the greater the number of sectors and lines, the higher the spatial resolution and the lower the temporal resolution. In conclusion, the narrower the pyramidal data, the higher the spatial and temporal resolution.

10. What are the differences between real-time 3D and multi-beat 3D acquisition, and how does this affect edge-to-edge mitral valve repair?

Real-time 3D is acquired in a single beat, avoiding "stitch artifacts" caused by breathing, movement, or arrhythmia; but since the whole volume is acquired in a single beat, both the temporal and spatial resolution are affected. On the other hand, multi-beat acquisition using electrocardiogram (ECG) gating captures sub-volumes from two to six cardiac cycles, maintaining both high temporal and high spatial resolution. 3D color Doppler can be obtained with both modalities; this is especially useful in pinpointing the location of the jet (see Figure 27.4). Despite multi-beat acquisition having higher temporal and spatial resolution, real-time is superior to guide percutaneous interventions and in the setting of irregular heart rate.

11. Does 3D TEE add any information to the quantification of MR?

In 2D color echocardiography, both VC and EROA derived from PISA have been widely used to quantify and classify the severity of MR based on these assumption: (i) the VC is circular (in fact, in most cases it is not) and (ii) PISA is a perfect hemisphere (when it is hemi-ellipsoidal). 3D echocardiography allows direct planimetry measurement of the VC and direct anatomical measurement of the regurgitant orifice area. 3D TEE also gives the unambiguous location of the regurgitant jet in relation to the anterior and posterior scallops. In addition, obtaining good pulmonary vein Doppler signals to look for flow reversal can often be

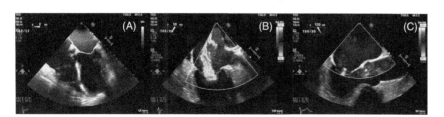

Figure 27.2   (a) Mid-esophageal view at 0°; (b) intercommissural view; (c) long-axis view.

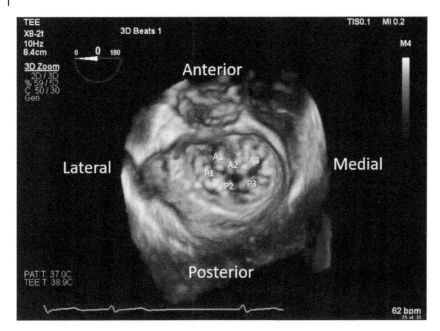

Figure 27.3 Surgeon's view.

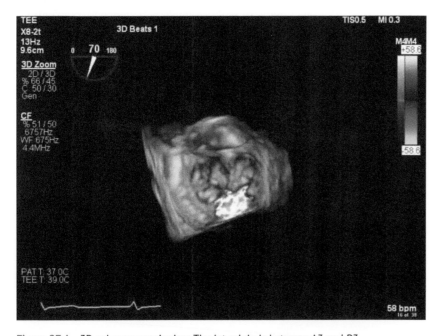

Figure 27.4 3D color surgeon's view. The jet origin is between A3 and P3.

challenging on TTE images, and excellent signals can be obtained consistently on TEE.

12. From the EVEREST trial, which anatomy is considered suitable?

Initially, the anatomical exclusion criteria for suitability of MitraClip were extrapolated from the EVEREST

(Endovascular Valve Edge-to-Edge Repair Study) trial as follows:

- Flail gap >10 mm
- Flail width >15 mm
- Coaptation depth >11 mm
- Coaptation length <2 mm
- Left ventricular end-systolic dimension >55 mm
- Mitral valve area <4.0 cm^2

Although these exclusion criteria are applied widely, they are not absolute contraindications and should be individualized case by case. Extended criteria have been studied with comparable results. Also, the new variations of the MitraClip device increased the ability to successfully deploy the clip with expanding criteria outside the EVEREST trial criteria.

13. Pair the figures with the appropriate measurements: (a) coaptation length, (b) coaptation depth, (c) flail gap, and (d) flail width.

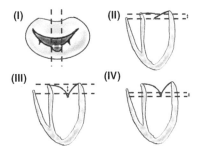

Answer: I: (d) Flail width. II: (c) Flail gap. III: (b) Coaptation depth. IV: (a) Coaptation length.

14. Which is the appropriate location for transseptal puncture?

The transseptal puncture location is paramount for a successful procedure and is mainly guided by TEE. Enough distance from the mitral annulus to the septal puncture site is necessary to manipulate the device into the mitral valve. It is unusual not to have enough interatrial septal length in the typical dilated left atrium for achieving this distance, but a suitable puncture site at least 4 cm from the mitral annulus should be documented.

The following views are useful to achieve the correct site (Figure 27.5):

- Bicaval view, for superior–inferior orientation. A length of 4 cm from the mitral annulus indicates enough interatrial septal distance for the procedure to be suitable.
- Four-chamber view to determine the height over the mitral valve.
- Short-axis view for anterior–posterior orientation.

The best site for puncture is usually located superiorly and posteriorly; it can be visualized as tenting of the interatrial septum.

Bibliography

1 Alfieri, O., Maisano, F., De Bonis, M. et al. (2001). The double-orifice technique in mitral valve repair: a simple solution for complex problems. *J. Thorac. Cardiovasc. Surg.* 122 (4): 674–681.
2 Aman, E. and Smith, T.W. (2019). Echocardiographic guidance for transcatheter mitral valve repair using edge-to-edge clip. *J. Echocardiogr.* 17 (2): 53–63.
3 Attizzani, G.F., Ohno, Y., Capodanno, D. et al. (2015). Extended use of percutaneous edge-to-edge mitral valve repair beyond EVEREST (Endovascular Valve Edge-to-Edge Repair) criteria: 30-day and 12-month clinical and echocardiographic outcomes from the GRASP (Getting Reduction of Mitral Insufficiency by Percutaneous Clip Implantation) registry. *JACC Cardiovasc. Interv.* 8 (1 Pt A): 74–82.
4 Faletra, F.F., Berrebi, A., Pedrazzini, G. et al. (2017). 3D transesophageal echocardiography: a new imaging tool for assessment of mitral regurgitation and for guiding

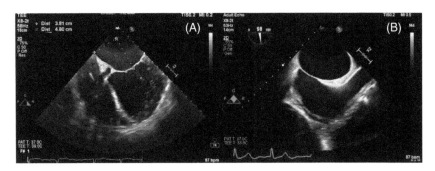

Figure 27.5 (a) Four-chamber view; (b) bicaval view.

percutaneous edge-to-edge mitral valve repair. *Prog. Cardiovasc. Dis.* 60 (3): 305–321.

5 Feldman, T., Foster, E., Glower, D.D. et al. (2011). Percutaneous repair or surgery for mitral regurgitation. *N. Engl. J. Med.* 364 (15): 1395–1406.

6 Flachskampf, F.A., Wouters, P.F., Edvardsen, T. et al. (2014). Recommendations for transoesophageal echocardiography: EACVI update 2014. *Eur. Heart J. Cardiovasc. Imaging* 15 (4): 353–365.

7 Grayburn, P.A., Sannino, A., and Packer, M. (2019). Proportionate and disproportionate functional mitral regurgitation: a new conceptual framework that reconciles the results of the MITRA-FR and COAPT trials. *JACC Cardiovasc. Imaging* 12 (2): 353–362.

8 Nyman, C.B., Mackensen, G.B., Jelacic, S. et al. (2018). Transcatheter mitral valve repair using the edge-to-edge clip. *J. Am. Soc. Echocardiogr.* 31 (4): 434–453.

9 Obadia, J.F., Messika-Zeitoun, D., Leurent, G. et al. (2018). Percutaneous repair or medical treatment for secondary mitral regurgitation. *N. Engl. J. Med.* 379 (24): 2297–2306.

10 Otto, C.M., Nishimura, R.A., Bonow, R.O. et al. (2021). 2020 ACC/AHA guideline for the Management of Patients with Valvular Heart Disease: a report of the American College of Cardiology/American Heart Association Joint Committee on Clinical Practice Guidelines. *Circulation* 143 (5): e72–e227.

11 Shah, M. and Jorde, U.P. (2019). Percutaneous mitral valve interventions (repair): current indications and future perspectives. *Front. Cardiovasc. Med.* 6: 88.

12 Sherif, M.A., Paranskaya, L., Yuecel, S. et al. (2017). MitraClip step by step; how to simplify the procedure. *Netherlands Heart J.* 25 (2): 125–130.

13 Stone, G.W., Lindenfeld, J., Abraham, W.T. et al. (2018). Transcatheter mitral-valve repair in patients with heart failure. *N. Engl. J. Med.* 379 (24): 2307–2318.

14 Zoghbi, W.A., Adams, D., Bonow, R.O. et al. (2017). Recommendations for noninvasive evaluation of native valvular regurgitation: a report from the American Society of Echocardiography developed in collaboration with the Society for Cardiovascular Magnetic Resonance. *J. Am. Soc. Echocardiogr.* 30 (4): 303–371.

28

Intra-procedural Transesophageal Echocardiography for Mitral Valve Structural Interventions

Pankaj Jain and Michael Fabbro, II

[1] *Department of Anesthesiology, University of Miami Miller School of Medicine, Miami, FL, USA*

1. Who is "qualified" to perform intra-procedural transesophageal echocardiography (TEE) for structural interventions on the mitral valve (MV)?

In 2019, an Expert Consensus Systems of Care document was published jointly by the major cardiac professional societies, including the American College of Cardiology (ACC), outlining recommendations and requirements for programs performing transcatheter mitral valve (MV) interventions. In this document, they advocate for having an accredited echocardiography laboratory, a Level 3 National Board of Echocardiography certified echocardiographer, and other cardiologists or cardiac anesthesiologists with training and experience in common echocardiographic modalities used for patients with MV disease. Level 3 competency is detailed by the American College of Cardiology Core Training Statement (COCATS) and is specific to cardiovascular medicine trainees. Most programs will have cardiology and cardiac anesthesia echocardiographers without level 3 competence providing many imaging services for these procedures, especially cardiac anesthesiologists, since this certification is not available to them. Experience among this group may vary widely as competencies are not as well defined. Most echocardiographers have either Adult Echocardiography or Advanced Perioperative Transesophageal Echocardiography (TEE) certification issued by the National Board of Echocardiography, but not all will. These certifications have no specific requirements regarding percutaneous mitral therapies.

2. Which structural mitral interventions is TEE most used for?

The most common TEE-driven percutaneous mitral procedure performed to date is the edge-to-edge repair. Transcatheter mitral valve replacement (TMVR) is also a growing field. The most robust TMVR experience is with valve-in-valve procedures. Native valve TMVR is more demanding and requires more nuanced echocardiography skills and therefore remains a growing field. Balloon valvuloplasty procedures are also frequently guided by TEE. The occasional percutaneous paravalvular leak (PVL) closure is also done with TEE guidance. Industry experts believe there is a sizeable unmet market demand for percutaneous mitral therapies, and their use is expected to grow significantly in the coming years.

3. What are the major views in 2D TEE used for MV structural interventions?

Guidelines for performing comprehensive TEE are published by the American Society of Echocardiography (ASE). This guideline document describes 28 tomographic views. During percutaneous interventions, non-standard views are frequently utilized, but these standard views provide a working foundation that most echocardiographers use. Almost all imaging for these procedures is performed from the mid-esophageal position. The most used views, degrees, and corollary procedural steps each view is most useful for are provided here:

- *Bicaval view* (90–110°) – *transseptal puncture* (TSP). The bicaval view allows for visualization of the superior vena cava, interatrial septum (IAS), and often the inferior vena cava. In this view, TSP can be directed in a superior or inferior direction. The ideal location is dependent upon the procedure type. This view also directs the identification and subsequent avoidance of a patent foramen ovale (PFO). Device guides used with the various mitral interventions are often best visualized in this view, which allows for determining the length of the guide extending into the left atrium (LA). Finally, this view can be used to evaluate residual interatrial defects and flow patterns following septal puncture.
- *Aortic valve short axis* (25–45°) – *TSP*. The aortic valve short axis allows for visualization of the IAS and demonstrates the location of a septal puncture device relative to the aortic valve. This allows the echocardiographer to direct the operator in an anterior and posterior direction prior to septal puncture.
- *Mitral commissural view* (50–70°) – *medial to lateral device positioning*. Visualizing the MV from the commissural view displays the valve from the medial A3/P3 commissure to the lateral A1/P1 commissure as you move from left to right on the screen. The echocardiographer uses this image to direct the operator, either medial or lateral, along the coaptation. This is important for several reasons during edge-to-edge mitral repair. First, it allows the operator to ensure that the device is positioned near the leaflet pathology or regurgitant jet and allows for placement of a clip device in a specific location along the coaptation. The view can also demonstrate a change in device position as it is advanced toward the valve. Following adequate tissue grasp, the commissural view with color flow Doppler is used during device closure to evaluate changes in jet characteristics. Finally, the commissural view in edge-to-edge repair helps understand where residual mitral regurgitation (MR) is, relative to an applied device. This information allows for consideration of moving the device before final deployment and facilitates relative positioning of additional devices when appropriate. In other types of structural mitral interventions, the commissural view can ensure crossing the valve in the more favorable A2/P2 position.
- *Aortic valve long axis* (120–140°) – *working view*. In edge-to-edge repair, the aortic valve long-axis view enables visualization of both anterior and posterior leaflets to ensure simultaneous grasp. In TMVR, the long-axis view is also paramount for assessing the position of the new valve and evaluating for left ventricular outflow tract obstruction (LVOTO).
- *Two-chamber view* (80–100°) – This view may help visualize the left atrial appendage (LAA). Many patients with MV disease have concomitant atrial fibrillation, and the LAA should be interrogated thoroughly to rule out the presence of a thrombus. This view also allows for visualization of the left upper pulmonary vein, which can be the target for wire placement and guide or device advancement in the early steps. This is done to avoid injuring the LA wall. Finally, the Coumadin ridge is seen well in the two-chamber view and is used to confirm clearance of the ridge when devices are moved from the left upper pulmonary vein position into the operating position.
- *Four-chamber view* (0–10°) – *Septal puncture distance to the mitral annulus*. From a procedural standpoint, the main purpose of the four-chamber view is to quantify the distance of a potential septal puncture (tenting) site to the mitral annulus. The tricuspid valve can also be evaluated, and the presence or enlargement of an existing pericardial effusion can be assessed from this view. Occasionally, leaflet grasp is performed and assessed using this view when long-axis views are suboptimal.

Several other views are used during structural mitral interventions. Each view can be used to thoroughly interrogate leaflet grasp, residual MR, paravalvular leaks, or valve-in-valve leaks. A systematic approach is used for each procedure to avoid complications.

4. Are there any advanced 2D imaging techniques that are useful in guiding structural heart interventions?

Bi-plane, also known as x-plane imaging, allows for simultaneous visualization of a structure in its 90° orthogonal plane. The movement of a line across the live image will change the newly displayed orthogonal image to match the plane the cursor bisects. Bi-plane imaging is particularly useful during TSP, where a short axis aortic valve and bicaval view can be simultaneously displayed, allowing for proper placement of the septal puncture along the IAS. Likewise, during edge-to-edge repairs, a commissural view and long-axis view can be simultaneously displayed during clip application. One important factor for the echocardiographer to consider is that any live image displayed over 90° will display an orthogonal plane greater than 180° during x-plane imaging, such that the new image will be inverted relative to its normal acquisition orientation. This can be managed by using corrective right–left invert features.

5. What are the major views in 3D TEE used for MV structural interventions?

3D TEE at this time is not standardized like 2D TEE, and the views are largely unnamed. Despite a lack of standardization, teams are incorporating more 3D imaging into their practice. For structural mitral cases, one of the most utilized 3D views is the en face view, which allows the team to rotate and see the mitral valve image from the so-called "surgeon's" view (i.e. with the aortic valve at the 12 o'clock position). In edge-to-edge repair, the arm orientation of the device is easily determined from this view. Devices below the valve can also be seen by reducing the gain or rotating the image to the left ventricular (LV) perspective. Medial and lateral orientation of devices relative to the mitral apparatus are also seen well in this view. Tissue bridges created by edge-to-edge repairs can also be evaluated. Finally, color Doppler with the 3D en-face view helps evaluate residual MR jets. 3D can also be used to visualize the IAS during septal puncture and can help ensure the proper puncture location for specific procedures. This will be discussed further under septal puncture.

6. Which 3D imaging modalities are most used in structural mitral interventions?

Multiple 3D imaging modalities are available. Large-volume or zoomed 3D datasets focusing on the MV, with or without color Doppler, can be acquired from the midesophagus and gated to the electrocardiogram over multiple beats. Large data sets and gating facilitate high-quality imaging but require acquisition and post-processing, which limits this imaging modality's use in real time. This is most useful for interrogating the valve during the pre-procedural planning stage for determining eligibility for structural heart interventions. The mitral valve area (MVA) and vena contracta area (3D VCA) measurements are often performed using these techniques. MVA is often measured by planimetry from the LV perspective during maximal valve opening. The 3D VCA is measured using multiplanar reconstruction by tracing the narrowest cross-section of the MR jet within the MV in early to mid-systole (Figure 28.1). The VCA obtained from individual jets are additive and enable direct measurement of the effective regurgitant orifice area (EROA) both pre- and post-procedurally. Authors have attempted to compare 3D-derived vena contracta parameters to predict suitability for edge-to-edge repairs. Live 3D TEE imaging modalities are ungated, smaller data set images that are used frequently. Zoomed or live 3D views of the MV in the en face orientation can be used to guide procedures in real time. This modality facilitates intra-procedural positioning and orientation of the MitraClip (Abbott) and evaluation for tissue bridges or "double orifice" following leaflet grasp. Live 3D images have also been used to guide septal puncture.

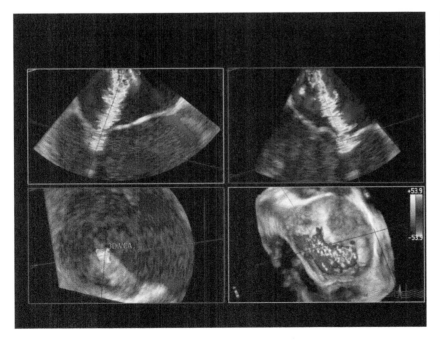

Figure 28.1 Measuring the 3D vena contracta (VCA) area using multiplanar reconstruction and planimetry of a 3D dataset.

Septal Puncture

7. How is TEE used to guide TSP?

The main 2D echocardiographic working views that enable targeted TSP are (i) the mid-esophageal bicaval view (ii) the mid-esophageal short-axis view. The bicaval view helps visualize the superior to inferior extent of the IAS, while the short-axis view provides an anterior to posterior perspective of the IAS. Used in conjunction, these two views guide the operator to an optimal TSP site. As noted, advanced echocardiographers often utilize bi-plane imaging to visualize both views at once (Figure 28.2). The mid-esophageal four-chamber view is utilized in assessing the height of the puncture site from the mitral annulus. Initial bicaval images are used to assess for a PFO, which is avoided during puncture.

Real-time 3D TEE has also been used to guide TSP. A zoomed 3D image of the IAS in the mid-esophageal bicaval view is obtained. The image is rotated on the z-axis to orient the superior vena cava (SVC) on the top of the screen and rotated again to visualize the IAS from the RA perspective. The TSP apparatus may then be directed to the appropriate location in reference to the fossa ovalis.

8. What are the procedural-specific considerations for the echocardiographer during TSP?

A mid to superior and posterior location along the IAS has traditionally been considered most suitable for edge-to-edge repair of the MV. This somewhat superior location enables optimal positioning of the clip delivery system in relation to the MV, while the posterior location along the IAS helps the operator stay clear of the aorta and ensure adequate distance or "height" from the mitral annulus, enhancing maneuverability of the delivery system. The four-chamber view helps confirm the appropriate height, usually 3.5–4.5 cm, with the reference point being either the mitral annulus (in primary MR) or coaptation point (in secondary MR).

Unlike in edge-to-edge repair, there are no definite recommendations for the optimal TSP site during TMVR. While a posterosuperior approach may be utilized, some authors prefer a posterior but inferior TSP site as it provides a direct path to the MV.

Edge-to-Edge Repair

9. What measurements are commonly made by echocardiography prior to an edge-to-edge repair?

Pre-procedural echocardiographic evaluation starts with an integrative assessment of MR severity using several qualitative and quantitative parameters as recommended by the ACC. An EROA of $0.4\,cm^2$ is the agreed-upon cut-off defining both primary and secondary severe MR and can be measured using the PISA method or 3D VCA. A MVA less than $4\,cm^2$ or a mean gradient across the MV exceeding $5\,mmHg$ increases the risk of post-procedural mitral

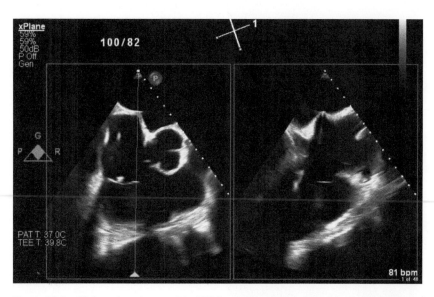

Figure 28.2 Biplane imaging used for TSP in edge-to-edge repair showing superior and posterior puncture sites.

stenosis (MS). For area measurements, the 2020 Guidelines for Management of Valvular Heart Disease support assessment by 2D and 3D planimetry or pressure half time. The continuity equation and proximal isovolumetric velocity derived area can be useful when encountering discordant measures. To minimize the risk of single leaflet device attachment (SLDA), a number of other measurements are also useful. A posterior leaflet length of least 6 and 9 mm is recommended for the MitraClip NTR and XTR devices, respectively. A flail gap of less than 10 mm and flail width of less than 15 mm is considered favorable for edge-to-edge repair in the setting of degenerative MR. The flail gap is measured from the tip of the flail leaflet to the point of coaptation. Flail width is simply measured by measuring the width of the flail segment from an en face view, typically in 3D.

10. What are the steps and imaging considerations for edge-to-edge repair?

These "steps" are from the perspective of the echocardiographer:

1. The first step is TSP, which has been covered in detail. A superior and posterior location along the IAS is considered optimal for the edge-to-edge repair device.
2. A wire is advanced through the septal puncture needle into the left upper pulmonary vein. This is usually done using the two-chamber view. The purpose of placing the wire in this position is to allow the device to be inserted in a direction facilitating maximal clearance of the LA wall.
3. The septal puncture needle is then exchanged for the edge-to-edge device steerable guide catheter (SGC) and dilator assembly. As the guide is advanced across the IAS, the amount of guide projecting into the LA is typically measured from the bicaval or a non-standard view. Bi-plane imaging can be helpful if the guide is not easily visualized from this view.
4. The device delivery system is inserted through the SGC toward the left upper pulmonary vein, during which the operators follow the fluoroscopy images and advance until "straddle" is achieved. This involves aligning radiopaque markers on both the SGC and device using fluoroscopy. Further advancement with medial and downward deflection ("M"ing) of the delivery system toward the MV is then performed under echocardiographic visualization while ensuring avoidance of LA wall and coumadin ridge. These maneuvers are guided via two-chamber and other non-standard views. Again,

bi-plane imaging can be helpful if the echocardiographer is uncertain where the tip of the device is located. Live 3D images can also be helpful. During this phase, the echocardiographer may need to return to the bicaval view to assess the amount of guide within the LA. Typically, 0.5 cm is the minimum amount required across the IAS.
5. Once above the MV, the device position in the medial-lateral and anterior–posterior extent of the MV is adjusted under the MV commissural and aortic valve long-axis view independently or simultaneously using bi-plane imaging. The device arms are typically opened above the MV, and an orientation perpendicular to the coaptation line can be achieved using these views as well. Live 3D en face imaging is also very useful in guiding device orientation. Color flow Doppler can be added in either 2D or 3D imaging to ensure that the device is above the targeted area (Figure 28.3a).
6. After proper positioning and orientation, the device is advanced across the valve into the LV. From this point, most of the imaging is done from a long-axis view focusing on the mitral leaflets. Live 3D imaging in the en face view, with lowered gain, can reconfirm the correct device orientation (Figure 28.3b). The operators then attempt to pull the device back toward the mitral leaflets, and the echocardiographer is tasked with identifying that both leaflet tips are within the device arms. This can be a tedious process requiring multiple small anterior and posterior movements of the device. Once both leaflets are on the device, the grippers are released to grasp the leaflets, and the device arms are partly closed. Adequate leaflet grasp is evaluated via multiple mid-esophageal 2D views, including long-axis, four-chamber, and mitral commissural views. Live 3D en-face views help confirm this by identifying a tissue bridge. Once confirmed, the mitral commissural view with color Doppler is focused on for final tightening, and the change in MR is evaluated. Each of the standard mid-esophageal images is finally evaluated to ensure leaflet insertion and grasp, grade residual MR, and measure the new mitral gradient. If the results are unsatisfactory with respect to residual MR, the commissural view with Doppler can help identify the location of the residual jet (whether medial or lateral to the device) for planning purposes. If the results are unsatisfactory or an additional device is being considered, the first device may have to be repositioned medially to allow for lateral placement of the next device. Additional devices are placed using the above steps; however, the arms are opened only after passage into LV. Fluoroscopy can be useful in helping guide a second device. The difficulty for the echocardiographer in multiple-clip cases is

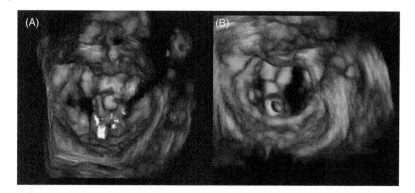

Figure 28.3 (a) Live 3D en-face mitral valve image with a color image to ensure the device is at the area of mitral regurgitation. (b) Live 3D en-face image with lowered gain to determine the arm orientation of device already across the mitral valve.

ensuring a bi-leaflet grasp with the additional devices. It is paramount to distinguish between previously deployed devices and the new device. Biplane imaging and the 3D en-face view can help make this distinction.

7. The final stages involve releasing the device completely and removing the delivery system. Once released, the same mid-esophageal views are used to re-evaluate the gradient, residual MR, and leaflet insertion. The delivery system is withdrawn under TEE guidance to ensure avoidance of the LA wall. The SGC is then retracted into the RA, and the bicaval view is assessed to determine the severity and direction of a residual shunt across the TSP site.

Frank Silvestry et al. provided one of the original documents describing their experience with the edge-to-edge device. This document holds up today and still provides a great resource for novice echocardiographers and operators.

11. What are the unique features of the different generations of MitraClip devices that echocardiographers should be familiar with?

The MitraClip NT was an improvement over the first-generation device in terms of steerability and leaflet grasp. The third generation offered further enhancement in SGC steerability and improved leaflet grasping ability and, for the first time, was available in two sizes: the NTR and the larger XTR. Although the XTR device is designed for improved leaflet grasp, echocardiographers should be aware that some investigators have reported increased SLDA with it. Fourth-generation (G4) devices added independent gripper controls for each arm and a wide-arm format to both the NT and XT, making the MitraClip available in four sizes (NTR, XTR, NTW, and XTW).

12. What are some common "tricks" that can be used to help with leaflet grasp during the clip procedure?

A number of tricks have been described to facilitate leaflet grasp in difficult cases, including rapid ventricular pacing, use of adenosine, and ventilatory maneuvers. Newer generations of clip devices (i.e. larger arms, independent arm movement) are designed to make it less likely for these maneuvers to be needed, but at times leaflet grasp will still remain challenging and these maneuvers should be utilized.

13. What are the key complications during MitraClip that echocardiographers need to consider?

SLDA remains one of the most important complications to avoid during edge-to-edge repair. Other complications echocardiographers should routinely assess for include MS, pericardial effusions, and right-to-left shunting at the septal puncture site.

TMVR

14. What is the role of the echocardiographer in TMVR?

Echocardiographers use TEE to aid in valve sizing, guide septal puncture and valve deployment, evaluate for paravalvular leaks and other complications, and evaluate for the risk or presence (after deployment) of LV outflow tract obstruction (LVOTO).

15. How do echocardiographers assist in sizing a valve during valve-in-valve and native valve TMVR?

Determining the appropriate transcatheter valve size during valve-in-valve TMVR is based on deriving the true internal diameter (ID) of the pre-existing bioprosthetic valve. This is typically done from patient records or manufacturer-derived information. Multi-detector computed tomographic (MDCT) and, to a lesser extent, echocardiography (TTE or TEE) may be of adjunctive value in obtaining the true ID. Gated full-volume data sets with post-processing provide the highest quality en face images for measuring the diameter, area, and perimeter of the bioprosthetic valve.

Sizing for the valve in native valve TMVR also uses the annular area and perimeter, as well as the intercommissural, intertrigonal, and septal-lateral distance. 3D TEE-derived measures using gated full-volume data sets and post-processing correlate well with CT in this situation and serve as a useful adjunct for valve sizing.

16. How do echocardiographers aid in valve deployment?

TSP is typically done in an inferior and posterior position using the techniques described in this chapter. When the transapical approach is elected, operators should obtain access under live echocardiographic visualization of the apex. For native valve TMVR, circumferential or near circumferential mitral annular calcium (MAC) should be confirmed. Aortic valve long-axis and live 3D en-face views in conjunction with fluoroscopy are used to advance the transcatheter valve into position. Fluoroscopy markers on the new valve are key during this step. Live 3D imaging is helpful during valve deployment, and color flow Doppler should be added to visualize paravalvular leaks post-deployment (Figure 28.4). Assessment with 2D TEE and color Doppler should be performed in multiple views. The pericardium should be assessed in transseptal cases for effusions.

17. Which echocardiographic parameters can predict LVOTO in native valve TMVR?

Echocardiography can provide information on the aortomitral angle, septal thickness, and anterior mitral leaflet length, which serve as predictors for LVOTO. Concerning features include aortomitral angle $<105°$, anterior mitral length $>24\,mm$, and predicted neo-LVOT area $<200\,mm^2$. Anterior leaflet length is usually measured from a long-axis AV view, and some authors have described dividing long anterior leaflets prior to valve deployment to prevent LVOTO. 3D reconstruction using full-volume data sets and proprietary post-processing software can provide the aortomitral angle. Traditionally, 2D measures of the aortomitral angle were done manually using annular lines and a protractor. Some software allows for offline aortomitral angle calculation using 2D images as well. MDCT is used to estimate the neo-LVOT area. LVOT gradients and color Doppler should be evaluated from mid-esophageal and deep transgastric views following deployment. LVOT gradients should not increase more than $10\,mmHg$ from baseline.

Balloon Valvuloplasty

18. Are there any special considerations the echocardiographer should be aware of during balloon valvuloplasty?

TTE is a class I indication for diagnosing, grading, and characterizing MS in patients with suspected rheumatic

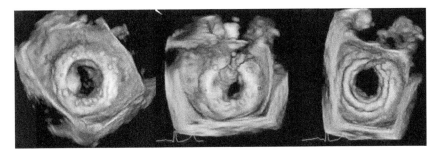

Figure 28.4 Valve-in-valve transcatheter mitral valve repair via the transseptal puncture approach. A 3D en face view confirms the positioning of the SAPIEN 3 transcatheter heart valve delivery system within the bioprosthetic valve in the mitral position. Deployed SAPIEN 3 valve demonstrates complete leaflet opening and absence of paravalvular leak.

mitral disease. Pre-procedural TEE is strongly recommended for further evaluation of valve characteristics and to rule out LA or LAA thrombus in patients being considered for percutaneous balloon mitral valvuloplasty (PBMV). In addition to grading MS severity (including gradients and MVA), the echocardiographer should pay special attention to (i) valve calcification, (ii) leaflet mobility, (iii) leaflet thickening, and (iv) subvalvular apparatus degeneration, as these characteristics form the basis of the Wilkins scoring system that predicts procedural success. Patients with a score of less than 8 are considered most suitable for PBMV. Commissural anatomy should also be carefully evaluated as patients with bilateral commissural fusion are known to obtain maximal procedural benefit. It is important to rule out the presence of moderate or severe MR, excess or bicommissural calcification, and concurrent aortic or tricuspid valve disease.

Intra-procedural TEE provides guidance for TSP in an inferior to mid-posterior position along the IAS. The intercommissural distance may serve as a reference for appropriate balloon size selection. 3D echocardiography is very useful for detailed pre-procedural anatomical characterization as well as pre and post MVA assessment using 3D planimetry. A post-procedural MVA of more than 1.5 mmHg, without moderate or severe MR, defines procedural success. Further attempts at dilatation should be avoided if there is a decrease in the transmitral pressure gradient, the occurrence of significant MR, or substantial splitting of the commissure.

19. What echocardiographic guided procedures are on the horizon?

Several devices other than the MitraClip are awaiting FDA approval. Some have approval in Europe and are being implanted there already. Several others are still in the early investigational stages. Broadly, these include percutaneous edge-to-edge repair systems, annuloplasty devices, TMVR systems, and chordal repair.

The PASCAL (Edwards Lifesciences) system is an edge-to-edge repair device. The system uses TEE guidance to deliver a spacer and grasp the mitral leaflets using paddles and independently adjustable clasps via a transfemoral, transseptal approach. The device is associated with favorable 30-day and one-year outcomes and has been approved for the treatment of MR in Europe. A prospective, multicenter, randomized controlled trial is currently underway to compare this device with the MitraClip in degenerative and functional MR.

Chief among the percutaneous annuloplasty devices for functional MR are the Cardioband (Edwards Lifesciences),

Carillon (Cardiac Dimension), and Mitralign (Edwards Lifesciences) systems. The Cardioband system is a direct annuloplasty device, delivered transseptally, that places a band on the posterior mitral annulus under echocardiographic guidance. The Carillon Mitral Contour is a coronary sinus-based indirect annuloplasty device delivered via the right internal jugular vein. Its use in the United States is currently investigational.

The non-TAVR TMVR systems being evaluated for use in native MV disease include transapical systems such as the Tendyne (Abbott), Tiara (Neovasc), and Intrepid (Medtronic). The transseptal systems, including the SAPIEN M3, Cephea, EVOQUE, Cardiovalve, Fortis, and CardiAQ (Edwards Lifesciences), are still in their early stages of investigation.

The Tendyne is the most extensively studied TMVR system and the first to obtain the European CE mark for commercial use. The valve has a unique apical tether that connects it to the apical epicardial surface via a pad and is designed for recapture if needed. Large, prospective, multi-centered randomized trials are currently ongoing.

The role of the echocardiographer in these novel devices mimics the considerations discussed in the TMVR section of this chapter.

The NeoChord DS1000 system enables neochord implantation to the affected scallop in degenerative MR through a transapical approach. Intra-procedural TEE (2D, x-plane, and 3D) guidance is vital for apex localization, grasping of the prolapsed scallop, adjustment of chord tension, and final evaluation of valve function. Approved for use in Europe, this device is currently undergoing clinical trials in the United States.

20. What are the health system implications of a growing field of structural heart interventions, as it relates to echocardiography?

The main health system implication from the echocardiographer's standpoint is being available and having the equipment to support these procedures. Many systems utilize cardiac anesthesiologists. This creates a resource strain since the cardiac anesthesia group supports numerous service lines within an organization, many of which are also expanding, such as heart failure programs. Some systems rely on a specific structural heart echocardiographer who performs the majority of echocardiographic studies for these patients, including planning and procedural studies. These are typically cardiologists, and this is a relatively new model. Cardiology fellowships across the country are increasingly offering structural heart echocardiography fellowships to their graduates. This is adding nationally to the resource pool of echocardiographers. One potential issue with this model is that it can leave a system with a smaller pool of echocardiographers for these cases. Some systems have addressed this, using hybrid models of cardiac anesthesiologists and cardiology-based structural heart echocardiographers.

Paravalvular Leak Closure

PVL closure can be applied to both mitral and aortic paravalvular leaks. Mitral PVL closure is typically done from

the transseptal approach, although transapical approaches have been used. TSP is typically mid-IAS, although its location can be modified based on the position of the leak. Steerable sheaths are typically used to approach the area of leak, and then a wire is advanced across the leak to guide the closure device. This step is best guided using live 3D imaging and can be tedious. Once wire access is obtained across the PVL, the closure device can be delivered and deployed. Careful assessment for residual leak should be carried out.

Bibliography

1 Aizer, A., Young, W., Saric, M. et al. (2015). Three-dimensional transesophageal echocardiography to facilitate transseptal puncture and left atrial appendage occlusion via upper extremity venous access. *Circ. Arrhythm. Electrophysiol.* 8 (4): 988–990.

2 Ali, M., Shreenivas, S.S., Pratt, D.N. et al. (2020). Percutaneous interventions for secondary mitral regurgitation. *Circ. Cardiovasc. Interv.* 13 (8): e008998.

3 Alter, E.J.H., Williams, M., and Saric, M. (2018). Imaging in MV interventions: MitraClip and beyond. *Expert Anal.* https://www.acc.org/latest-in-cardiology/articles/2018/08/06/13/25/imaging-in-mv-interventions.

4 Blanke, P., Naoum, C., Webb, J. et al. (2015). Multimodality imaging in the context of transcatheter mitral valve replacement: establishing consensus among modalities and disciplines. *JACC Cardiovasc. Imaging* 8 (10): 1191–1208.

5 Bonow, R.O., O'Gara, P.T., Adams, D.H. et al. (2020). 2019 AATS/ACC/SCAI/STS expert consensus systems of care document: operator and institutional recommendations and requirements for transcatheter mitral valve intervention: a joint report of the American Association for Thoracic Surgery, the American College of Cardiology, the Society for Cardiovascular Angiography and Interventions, and the Society of Thoracic Surgeons. *J. Am. Coll. Cardiol.* 76 (1): 96–117.

6 Calvert, P.A., Northridge, D.B., Malik, I.S. et al. (2016). Percutaneous device closure of paravalvular leak: combined experience from the United Kingdom and Ireland. *Circulation* 134 (13): 934–944.

7 Colli, A., Besola, L., Montagner, M. et al. (2018). Acute intraoperative echocardiographic changes after transapical off-pump mitral valve repair with NeoChord implantation. *Int. J. Cardiol.* 257: 230–234.

8 Fabbro, M. 2nd, Aljure, O.D., and Jain, P. (2019). Predicting the number of edge-to-edge repair devices needed to adequately treat mitral regurgitation using transesophageal echocardiography. *J. Cardiothorac. Vasc. Anesth.* 33 (10): 2647–2651.

9 Fernando, R.J., Shah, R., Yang, Y. et al. (2020). Transcatheter mitral valve repair and replacement: analysis of recent data and outcomes. *J. Cardiothorac. Vasc. Anesth.* 34 (10): 2793–2806.

10 Goldberg, S.L., Meredith, I., Marwick, T. et al. (2017). A randomized double-blind trial of an interventional device treatment of functional mitral regurgitation in patients with symptomatic congestive heart failure-trial design of the REDUCE FMR study. *Am. Heart J.* 188: 167–174.

11 Hensey, M., Brown, R.A., Lal, S. et al. (2021). Transcatheter mitral valve replacement: an update on current techniques, technologies, and future directions. *JACC Cardiovasc. Interv.* 14 (5): 489–500.

12 Khan, J.M., Babaliaros, V.C., Greenbaum, A.B. et al. (2019). Anterior leaflet laceration to prevent ventricular outflow tract obstruction during transcatheter mitral valve replacement. *J. Am. Coll. Cardiol.* 73 (20): 2521–2534.

13 Mackensen, G.B., Lee, J.C., Wang, D.D. et al. (2018). Role of echocardiography in transcatheter mitral valve replacement in native mitral valves and mitral rings. *J. Am. Soc. Echocardiogr.* 31 (4): 475–490.

14 Muller, D.W.M., Farivar, R.S., Jansz, P. et al. (2017). Transcatheter mitral valve replacement for patients with symptomatic mitral regurgitation: a global feasibility trial. *J. Am. Coll. Cardiol.* 69 (4): 381–391.

15 Nobuyoshi, M., Arita, T., Shirai, S. et al. (2009). Percutaneous balloon mitral valvuloplasty: a review. *Circulation* 119 (8): e211–e219.

16 Otto, C.M., Nishimura, R.A., Bonow, R.O. et al. (2021). 2020 ACC/AHA guideline for the management of patients with valvular heart disease: executive summary: a report of the American College of Cardiology/American Heart Association joint committee on clinical practice guidelines. *Circulation* 143 (5): e35–e71.

17 Paranskaya, L., Kische, S., Akin, I. et al. (2013). Combined use of rapid pacing and adenosine facilitates catheter based correction of severe bileaflet prolapse with the MitraClip system. *Can. J. Cardiol.* 29 (2): 255. e1–255-e3.

18 Praz, F., Braun, D., Unterhuber, M. et al. (2019). Edge-to-edge mitral valve repair with extended clip arms: early experience from a multicenter observational study. *JACC Cardiovasc. Interv.* 12 (14): 1356–1365.

19 Puchalski, M.D., Lui, G.K., Miller-Hance, W.C. et al. (2019). Guidelines for performing a comprehensive transesophageal echocardiographic: examination in children and all patients with congenital heart disease: recommendations from the American Society of Echocardiography. *J. Am. Soc. Echocardiogr.* 32 (2): 173–215.

20 Silvestry, F.E., Rodriguez, L.L., Herrmann, H.C. et al. (2007). Echocardiographic guidance and assessment of percutaneous repair for mitral regurgitation with the Evalve MitraClip: lessons learned from EVEREST I. *J. Am. Soc. Echocardiogr.* 20 (10): 1131–1140.

21 Singh, G.D., Smith, T.W., and Rogers, J.H. (2016). Targeted transseptal access for MitraClip percutaneous mitral valve repair. *Interv. Cardiol. Clin.* 5 (1): 55–69.

22 Webb, J.G., Hensey, M., Szerlip, M. et al. (2020). 1-year outcomes for transcatheter repair in patients with mitral regurgitation from the CLASP study. *JACC Cardiovasc. Interv.* 13 (20): 2344–2357.

23 Weir-McCall, J.R., Blanke, P., Naoum, C. et al. (2018). Mitral valve imaging with CT: relationship with transcatheter mitral valve interventions. *Radiology* 288 (3): 638–655.

24 Wunderlich, N.C. and Siegel, R.J. (2013). Peri-interventional echo assessment for the MitraClip procedure. *Eur. Heart J. Cardiovasc. Imaging* 14 (10): 935–949.

25 Zoghbi, W.A., Adams, D., Bonow, R.O. et al. (2017). Recommendations for noninvasive evaluation of native valvular regurgitation: a report from the American Society of Echocardiography developed in collaboration with the Society for Cardiovascular Magnetic Resonance. *J. Am. Soc. Echocardiogr.* 30 (4): 303–371.

29

Surgical Trials in Mitral Valvular Disease

Ali Ghodsizad[1], Matthias Loebe[1] and Tomas Salerno[2]

[1] *Miami Transplant Institute, University of Miami Miller School of Medicine, Miami, FL, USA*
[2] *Cardiothoracic Surgery, University of Miami Miller School of Medicine, Miami, FL, USA*

1. Describe the surgical therapy for acute MR.

Emergency mitral valve (MV) surgery, preferably mitral repair, can be lifesaving in symptomatic patients with acute severe primary MR. In patients with moderate MR, the heart may compensate as LV dilation enables lower filling pressure and increased cardiac output. Most patients with acute severe MR require surgical correction to maintain normal hemodynamics. In particular, patients with complete papillary muscle rupture can have very severe MR, which is poorly tolerated.

2. Discuss recent publications on mitral valve reconstruction being superior to replacement in chronic structural MR.

It is important to distinguish between chronic *primary* (degenerative) MR and chronic *secondary* (functional) MR. In chronic primary MR, components of the valve (leaflets, chordae tendineae, papillary muscles, annulus) can cause valve incompetence. The most common cause of chronic primary MR in high-income countries is MV prolapse. Younger populations present with severe myxomatous degeneration (Barlow's valve); alternatively, older populations present with fibroelastic deficiency disease, in which lack of connective tissue leads to chordal rupture. The differentiation of the etiology has therapeutic implications. Less common causes of chronic primary MR include endocarditis, connective tissue disorders, rheumatic heart disease, cleft MV, and radiation heart disease. Primary MR is a mechanical problem of the leaflet coaptation and requires mechanical MV intervention. The onset of symptoms comes with severe MR and predicts a worse prognosis even with normal LV function. So the onset of symptoms is an indication for MV surgery to correct the MR before starting LV systolic dysfunction (LVEF ≤60% or left ventricle end-systolic diameter [LVESD] ≥40 mm). Mitral valve repair is the procedure of choice for isolated severe primary MR limited to less than one-half of the posterior leaflet.

Surgical repair of primary MR has been successful. When only annuloplasty and repair of the posterior leaflet are required, MV repair has led to outcomes distinctly superior to those with biological or mechanical MV replacement: an operative mortality rate of <1%, long-term survival rate equivalent to that of the age-matched general population, and up to 95% freedom from reoperation and >80% freedom from recurrent moderate or severe (≥3) MR at 15–20 years following surgery. Posterior leaflet repair rather than MV replacement is the standard of care in this patient group.

Successful MV repair is the primary goal, but MV replacement is preferable to a poor repair. Patients with extensive degenerative disease, including rheumatic MV disease, have shown to be less suitable for mitral repair. The repair is limited by thickened and calcified leaflets and sub-valvular disease with chordal fusion and shortening. In rheumatic disease, freedom from reoperation at 20 years is in the 50–60% range. In a large series, repair was accomplished in 22% of cases operated on for rheumatic disease. Repair of rheumatic MV disease should be limited to less advanced disease and patients in whom a mechanical prosthesis cannot be used.

3. Discuss recent publications about MV replacement having similar and non-inferior results in patients with secondary MR.

There is no clear proof that surgical correction of chronic secondary MR improves survival. A sub-study of the randomized STICH (Comparison of Surgical and Medical Treatment for Congestive Heart Failure and Coronary Artery Disease) trial shows that it is wise to address the MV during coronary artery bypass surgery (CABG) when secondary MR is severe, provided hibernating myocardium is present. Recent publications comparing MV repair versus MV replacement in patients with severe ischemic secondary MR showed no difference between MV repair and MV replacement in survival rate and LV remodeling (two-year follow-up). The recurrence of moderate or severe MR was higher in the repair group compared to the replacement group. The repair group had a higher incidence of heart failure and repeat hospitalization. There is a lack of apparent benefit of valve repair over valve replacement in secondary MR versus primary MR. The results in the repair group were less durable in patients with secondary MR.

4. Describe two published randomized trials assessing the outcome of percutaneous MV repair using the MitraClip for therapy of secondary MR.

The two recently published trials were MITRA-FR (Percutaneous Repair with the MitraClip Device for Severe Functional/Secondary Mitral Regurgitation) and COAPT (Cardiovascular Outcomes Assessment of the MitraClip Percutaneous Therapy for Heart Failure Patients with Functional Mitral Regurgitation). The two randomized controlled trials assessed the efficacy and safety of MitraClip in patients with systolic heart failure and severe secondary MR. MITRA-FR presented more neutral results, whereas the COAPT trial presented definite positive results. Interventional techniques will be explicitly discussed in other sections.

5. What are the surgical indications for MV repair?

According to recent guidelines valvular heart disease surgery is indicated in cases of severe symptomatic primary MV regurgitation with LVEF >30%. In asymptomatic patients with LVESD ≤45 mm (or LVEF ≥60%), atrial fibrillation, or systolic pulmonary pressure ≥50 mmHg can benefit from surgery. Severe secondary MR in patients undergoing CABG with LVEF >30% can be another indication for surgery (class I; level C). In coronary heart disease (CHD) patients with severely reduced LVEF and evidence of myocardial viability, surgical repair should be considered (class IIa; level C). Symptomatic patients with low EF despite maximal advanced medical therapies have a low surgical risk (class IIb; level C). The primary goal, of course, is MV repair. In contrast to replacement, surgical MV repair has shown acceptable early-, mid-, and long-term results with a lower peri-operative mortality rate. As a clinical ground for long durability, an earlier repair should be intended. At 20 years, MR recurrence has been reported to be around 10%. Surgical repair for secondary MR has shown to be less durable, with high recurrence rates at two years. The Heart Team may consider this transcatheter option after carefully evaluating other strategies (i.e. left ventricular assistant devices or heart transplantation).

In patients with primary MR, mitral clip application is currently only approved for high-risk patients. Age remains a strong predictor of mortality in patients with MR undergoing MV repair. Increasing clinical experience with MV application will enable a stronger clinical approach. Future trials will look at the benefit of MitraClip application for moderate and low-risk patients compared to surgical MV repair.

6. Describe the "double-orifice" surgical repair technique described by Alfieri et al.

MV disease still is a clinically relevant valve disease. In the early 1980s, Carpentier et al. introduced the so-called "French correction," the first reproducible surgical technique to treat MV regurgitation, describing the reconstruction of the native valve anatomy mainly through resection of prolapsing tissue. Isolated prolapse of the posterior leaflet could be repaired with good results. Surgical valve repairs involving the anterior, bileaflet, and commissural lesions did not show the same excellent results. In 1991, Ottavio et al. introduced a surgical repair technique for patients with mitral regurgitation, "edge-to-edge" (later known also as the "Alfieri's stitch"), intending to keep the MV "functional." The free margins of the anterior and posterior leaflets (usually A2 and P2) are sutured and become visible as a "double-orifice" valve. The common indication for the edge-to-edge repair usually involves bileaflet prolapse in Barlow's disease. Given the risk of systolic anterior motion (SAM) of the anterior mitral leaflet, iatrogenic fusion of both leaflets by applying Alfieri's stitch reduces the fluctuation of the anterior leaflet toward the left ventricular outflow tract (LVOT). The concomitant use of a complete or partial prosthetic ring can decrease the tension on the edge-to-edge suture, allowing for stabilization of the annulus and enhancing the overall durability of the repair. In patients undergoing LVAD implantation with excessive MR, even a transapical Alfieri stitch can be attempted.

7. What are the surgical details of performing mitral ring annuloplasty?

A ring annuloplasty is a must to reinforce mitral repairs. The annuloplasty sutures can be placed to improve the exposure, starting with the posterior trigone and moving clockwise toward the other side by placing horizontal sutures without pledgets; it is important to involve the fibrous trigones. The coronary sinus along the right, the circumflex artery at the base, and the aortic valve on the left can be affected by deep stitches. In the case of a prolapsed posterior leaflet, depending on the amount of redundant leaflet tissue and height of the leaflets, quadrangular or triangular resection can be performed. An excessive amount of the tissue can be managed with a sliding annuloplasty after performing quadrangular resection. Anterior leaflet prolapse may require more challenging techniques with chordal transfer from posterior to anterior leaflet.

8. Should you resect the entire leaflet when replacing the valve?

The goal is not to resect too much tissue from the anterior leaflet, affecting the integrity of the annulus. The posterior leaflet should be left entirely in place when pliable. It is important not to resect too much to preserve the ventricular function. On the contrary, a wide-open LVOT, especially in a small left ventricular cavity in a hyperdynamic heart, can be a problem. Extensive decalcification may be necessary: atrial decalcification can be done safely, but the more you approach the ventricular calcium, the higher the risk of AV groove disruption and circumflex artery injury.

9. What is the ideal vascular access for VA extracorporeal membrane oxygenation (ECMO) implantation in patients undergoing mitral clip implantation?

The ideal scenario would start with an appreciation of the femoral artery, vein, and placement of introducer sheaths before the procedure. The placement of a 17F arterial cannula and a 19–23 venous cannula will enable fast and effective VA ECMO support.

10. What are the possible surgical complications during and/or post surgical MV insertion?

The majority of the currently used prosthetic MVs are tissue valves. A recently published animal model compared several different bioprosthetic valves with similar outcomes. Surgical MV reconstruction is the number-one choice compared to replacement. During MV replacement, complications can occur, the worst including the circumflex artery occlusion or damage and atrioventricular dissociation.

11. What size of surgical MV prosthesis placement enables later valve-in-valve implantation?

Ideally, the goal is to implant a 31 mm MV or larger. A mechanical mitral prosthesis is used in a very few cases and excludes future interventions, including valve-in-valve implantation.

12. Is persistent MR a negative predictive factor for patients requiring left ventricular assist device (LVAD) insertion?

No clear data shows persistent MR at the time of LVAD implantation to be a clear negative predictive factor. Hayashi and colleagues showed in their single-center study that concomitant atrial fibrillation and moderate to severe MR at the time of VAD insertion are associated with worse outcomes. Raake and colleagues described their experience on consequent LVAD insertion following mitral clip insertion, showing no disadvantage following their stepwise approach. Morgan and colleagues published opposing data on MR at the time of LVAD insertion showing patients with MR had no disadvantage when looking at follow-up data.

13. Why should the Heart Team discuss structural cases in detail before the procedure?

It is important for the surgical Heart Team to Understand the procedural steps during mitral clip deployment. Tailoring the right surgical and structural therapy to the right patient population can enable or limit future interventional or surgical therapeutic steps. As the cardiothoracic surgeon on call, you may be involved with clinical emergencies during the mitral clip placement, including having the tip of the wire being misplaced far into the left pulmonary vein or a ruptured left atrium. A concise discussion by the Heart Team is the key to success.

14. The Heart Team is consulted on a case with persistent atrial septal defect (ASD) and a left-to-right shunt following mitral clip placement. What is the therapeutic intervention?

Small persistent shunts following mitral clip placements usually do not require any steps. Unless the patient has extensive primary pulmonary hypertension, no other therapeutic steps are required. It still can become a clinically demanding situation when hypoxic blood starts shunting to the left atrium and needs to be managed more aggressively depending on the shunt fraction.

Bibliography

1 Baumgartner, H., Falk, V., Bax, J.J. et al. (2017). ESC scientific document group. 20 ESC/EACTS guidelines for the management of valvular heart disease. *Eur. Heart J.* 38: 2739–2791.

2 Braunberger, E., Deloche, A., Berrebi, A. et al. (2001). Very long-term results (more than 20 years) of valve repair with Carpentier's techniques in nonrheumatic mitral valve insufficiency. *Circulation* 104: I8–I119.

3 Carpentier, A. (1983). Cardiac valve surgery--the "French correction". *J. Thorac. Cardiovasc. Surg.* 86: 323–337.

4 Castillo, J.G., Anyanwu, A.C., Fuster, V. et al. (2012). A near 100% repair rate for mitral valve prolapse is achievable in a reference center: implications for future guidelines. *J. Thorac. Cardiovasc. Surg.* 144: 308–312.

5 Daneshmand, M.A., Milano, C.A., Rankin, J.S. et al. (2009). Mitral valve repair for degenerative disease: a 20-year experience. *Ann. Thorac. Surg.* 88: 1828–1837.

6 David, T.E., Armstrong, S., McCrindle, B.W., and Manlhiot, C. (2013). Late outcomes of mitral valve repair for mitral regurgitation due to degenerative disease. *Circulation* 127: 1485–1492.

7 David, T.E., David, C.M., Tsang, W. et al. (2019). Long term results of mitral valve repair for regurgitation due to leaflet prolapse. *J. Am. Coll. Cardiol.* 74: 1044–1053.

8 David, T.E., Ivanov, J., Armstrong, S. et al. (2005). A comparison of outcomes of mitral valve repair for degenerative disease with posterior, anterior, and bileaflet prolapse. *J. Thorac. Cardiovasc. Surg.* 130: 1242–1249.

9 Enriquez-Sarano, M., Tajik, A.J., Schaff, H.V. et al. (1994). Echocardiographic prediction of survival after surgical correction of organic mitral regurgitation. *Circulation* 90: 830–837.

10 Ghodsizad, A., Koerner, M.M., Brehm, C.E., and El-Banayosy, A. (2014). The role of extracorporeal membrane oxygenation circulatory support in the 'crash and burn' patient: from implantation to weaning. *Curr. Opin. Cardiol.* 29 (3): 275–280.

11 Goodwin, M., Nemeh, H.W., Borgi, J. et al. (2017). Resolution of mitral regurgitation with left ventricular assist device support. 104 (3): 811–818. Epub 2017 May 17.

12 Grigioni, F., Tribouilloy, C., Avierinos, J.F. et al. (2008). Outcomes in mitral regurgitation due to flail leaflets a multicenter European study. *JACC Cardiovasc. Imaging* 1: 133–141.

13 Hayashi, H., Naka, Y., Sanchez, J. et al. (2020). Consequences of functional mitral regurgitation and atrial fibrillation in patients with left ventricular assist devices. *J. Heart Lung Transplant.* 9 (12): 1398–1407.

14 Horstkotte, D., Schulte, H.D., Niehues, R. et al. (1993). Diagnostic and therapeutic considerations in acute, severe mitral regurgitation: experience in 42 consecutive patients entering the intensive care unit with pulmonary edema. *J. Heart Valve Dis.* 2: 512–522. cc.

15 Ji, Q., Zhao, Y., Shen, J. et al. (2020). Predictors of ischemic mitral regurgitation improvement after surgical revascularization plus mitral valve repair for moderate ischemic mitral regurgitation. *J. Card. Surg.* 35: 528–535.

16 Kang, D.-H., Kim, J.H., Rim, J.H. et al. (2009). Comparison of early surgery versus conventional treatment in asymptomatic severe mitral regurgitation. *Circulation* 119: 797–804.

17 Kopjar, T., Gasparovic, H., Mestres, C.A. et al. (2016). Meta-analysis of concomitant mitral valve repair and coronary artery bypass surgery versus isolated coronary artery bypass surgery in patients with moderate ischaemic mitral regurgitation. *Eur. J. Cardiothorac. Surg.* 50: 212–222.

18 Kreusser, M.M., Hamed, S., Weber, A. et al. (2020). MitraClip implantation followed by insertion of a left ventricular assist device in patients with advanced heart failure. *ESC Heart Fail.* 7 (6): 3891–3900. Ann. Thorac. Surg.

19 Geidel, S., Lass, M., Schneider, C. et al. Downsizing of the mitral valve and coronary revascularization in severe ischemic mitral regurgitation results in reverse left ventricular and left atrial remodeling. *Eur. J. Cardiothorac. Surg.* 27: 1011–1016.

20 Lazam, S., Vanoverschelde, J.-L., Tribouilloy, C. et al. (2017). Twenty-year outcome after mitral repair versus replacement for severe degenerative mitral regurgitation: analysis of a large, prospective, multicenter, international registry. *Circulation* 135: 410–422.

21 Mack, M.J., Abraham, W.T., Lindenfeld, J. et al. (2018). Cardiovascular outcomes assessment of the MitraClip in patients with heart failure and secondary mitral regurgitation: design and rationale of the COAPT trial. *Am. Heart J.* 205: 1–11.

22 Magne, J., Sénéchal, M., Dumesnil, J.G., and Pibarot, P. (2009). Ischemic mitral regurgitation: a complex multifaceted disease. *Cardiology* 112: 244–259.

23 Maisano, F., Torracca, L., Oppizzi, M. et al. (1998). The edge-to-edge technique: a simplified method to correct mitral insufficiency. *Eur. J. Cardiothorac. Surg.* 13: 240–246.

24 McClure, R.S., Athanasopoulos, L.V., McGurk, S. et al. (2013). One thousand minimally invasive mitral valve operations: early outcomes, late outcomes, and echocardiographic follow-up. *J. Thorac. Cardiovasc. Surg.* 145: 1199–1206.

25 Nanjappa, M.C., Ananthakrishna, R., Hemanna Setty, S.K. et al. (2013). Acute severe mitral regurgitation following balloon mitral valvotomy: echocardiographic features, operative findings, and outcome in 50 surgical cases. *Catheter. Cardiovasc. Interv.* 81: 603–608.

26 Otto, C.M., Nishimura, R.A., Bonow, R.O. et al. (2020). ACC/AHA Association Joint Committee on Clinical Practice Guidelines for the Management of Patients With Valvular Heart Disease. 2020 ACC/AHA Circulation 2020

27 Panza, J.A., Ellis, A.M., Al-Khalidi, H.R. et al. (2019). Myocardial viability and long-term outcomes in ischemic cardiomyopathy. *N. Engl. J. Med.* 381: 739–748.

28 Prasad, A., Ghodsizad, A., Brehm, C. et al. (2018). Refractory pulmonary edema and upper body hypoxemia during veno-arterial extracorporeal membrane oxygenation-a case for atrial septostomy. *Artif. Organs* 42 (6): 664–669.

29 Praz, F. and Windecker, S. (2019). Two-year outcomes of the MITRA-FR trial: towards an integrated approach in the evaluation of patients with secondary mitral regurgitation. *Eur. J. Heart Fail.* 21 (12): 1628–1631.

30 Rosenhek, R., Rader, F., Klaar, U. et al. (2006). Outcome of watchful waiting in asymptomatic severe mitral regurgitation. *Circulation* 113: 2238–2244.

31 Suri, R.M., Clavel, M.-A., Schaff, H.V. et al. (2016). Effect of recurrent mitral regurgitation following degenerative mitral valve repair: long-term analysis of competing outcomes. *J. Am. Coll. Cardiol.* 67: 488–498.

32 Suri, R.M., Vanoverschelde, J.-L., Grigioni, F. et al. (2013). Association between early surgical intervention vs watchful waiting and outcomes for mitral regurgitation due to flail mitral valve leaflets. *J. Am. Med. Assoc.* 310: 609–616.

33 Vassileva, C.M., Mishkel, G., McNeely, C. et al. (2013). Long- term survival of patients undergoing mitral valve repair and replacement: a longitudinal analysis of medicare fee-for- service beneficiaries. *Circulation* 127: 1870–1876.

34 Velazquez, E.J., Lee, K.L., Jones, R.H. et al. (2016). Coronary-artery bypass surgery in patients with ischemic cardiomyopathy. *N. Engl. J. Med.* 374: 1511–1520.

35 Virk, S.A., Tian, D.H., Sriravindrarajah, A. et al. (2017). Mitral valve surgery and coronary artery bypass grafting for moderate-to-severe ischemic mitral regurgitation: meta-analysis of clinical and echocardiographic outcomes. *J. Thorac. Cardiovasc. Surg.* 154: 127–136.

36 Wang, D.D., Caranasos, T.G., O'Neill, B.P. et al. (2021). Comparison of a new bioprosthetic mitral valve to other commercially available devices under controlled conditions in a porcine model. *J. Cardiac. Surg.* 36: 4654–4662.

37 Watanabe, N. (2019). Acute mitral regurgitation. *Heart* 05: 671–677.

38 Weiner, M.M., Hofer, I., Lin, H.-M. et al. (2014). Relationship among surgical volume, repair quality, and peri-operative outcomes for repair of mitral insufficiency in a mitral valve reference center. *J. Thorac. Cardiovasc. Surg.* 148: 2021–2026.

39 Wittwer, T., Wahlers, T., and Adams, D. (2008). *Operative Atlas Cardiac Surgery*. Lehmanns Media.

40 Yoran, C., Yecllin, E.L., Becker, R.M. et al. (1979). Mechanism of reduction of mitral regurgitation with vasodilator therapy. *Am. J. Cardiol.* 43: 773–777.

30

Surgical Techniques for Mitral Valve Repair

Corinne Aberle, Ahmed Alnajar and Joseph Lamelas

[1] *Division of Cardiothoracic Surgery, The DeWitt Daughtry Department of Surgery, University of Miami Miller School of Medicine, Miami, FL, USA*

1. What are the stages of primary mitral regurgitation (MR)?

Recent guidelines suggest categorizing the severity of chronic primary mitral regurgitation and other valvular diseases into four stages:

A. *At risk:* Patients with risk factors for the development of valvular disease. No mitral regurgitation (MR), or a small jet less than 20% of the atrium. Vena contracta <0.3.

B. *Progressive:* Patients with progressive valvular disease (mild to moderate severity and asymptomatic). Vena contracta <0.7, grade 1+ to 2+, effective regurgitant orifice (ERO) <0.4 cm^2, regurgitant fraction <50%.

C. *Asymptomatic severe:* Asymptomatic patients who have the criteria for severe valvular disease.
C.1. Asymptomatic patients with severe disease in whom the left ventricle (LV) or right ventricle (RV) remains compensated. MR can be holosystolic, angiographic grade 3+ or 4+, ERO >0.4 cm^2, vena contracta >0.7, regurgitant fraction >50%, MR jet >40% of the left atrium. C.2. Asymptomatic patients with severe valvular disease with decompensation of the LV or RV.

D. *Symptomatic severe:* Patients who have developed symptoms as a result of valvular disease, plus the same echo findings as asymptomatic severe.

2. When should patients be considered for surgical repair of their MR?

Any patient with severe and symptomatic MR warrants evaluation for surgical repair. Asymptomatic patients with severe MR and reduced ejection fraction (EF) or atrial fibrillation also warrant surgical evaluation. If patients have a normal EF and severe MR but are asymptomatic, a stress evaluation can be completed to see if they develop symptoms, as symptoms can often be masked or overlooked by changes in the patient's lifestyle. However, if the patient is truly asymptomatic, any patient with severe MR should be referred for surgical evaluation at a valve center of excellence if the chance of a durable repair is high.

3. Should mitral valves (MVs) be repaired or replaced? What are the advantages?

Whenever possible, attempts should be made to repair primary MR. The advantages of repair over replacement include, but are not limited to, reducing early and late mortality, better preservation of LV function, and greater freedom from thromboembolism, endocarditis, and anticoagulant-related hemorrhage, as well as excellent late durability reported for as long as 25 years. A repair can be completed with equally short bypass times; a flail leaflet is an example of primary MR, which is the ideal repair candidate.

4. What is SAM, and what are the risk factors for developing it?

SAM is the systolic anterior motion of the MV, which can lead to MR and obstruction of the LV outflow tract. SAM results from excess leaflet tissue obstructing the left ventricular outflow tract (LVOT). It was first reported in the 1960s as a feature of hypertrophic cardiomyopathy. In MV replacement (MVR), various transesophageal echocardiography (TEE) measurements pre-, intra-, and post-operative may indicate the risk of post-repair SAM and reveal its risk factors, such as:

(1) Presence of excessive leaflet tissue (Barlow's disease) with a tall posterior leaflet (>15 mm) (not a short posterior leaflet)
(2) Ratio of the heights of the anterior and posterior leaflets ≤1.3
(3) Aorto-mitral plane angle <120°
(4) Distance between the interventricular septum and mitral leaflet coaptation point <25 mm
(5) Thick basal interventricular septum (>15 mm)

5. What is the best initial step when SAM is identified while coming off cardiopulmonary bypass?

The first step for a patient coming off bypass with SAM is to reduce the heart rate, increase pre-load, and stop any inotropic support. During weaning from bypass, the patient's heart is often empty, and the patient may be on inotropic support, which exacerbates the potential for SAM. Often, these maneuvers alone will resolve the problem. Patients with SAM can be classified into different risk categories that range from minor chordal protrusion with minimal LVOT obstruction and trivial MR to more severe LVOT obstruction with severe MR leading to hemodynamic instability, low cardiac output syndrome, and intractable hypotension. Some procedure risk factors also predispose to SAM, such as anterior displacement of the papillary muscles, insertion of a small prosthetic ring, and inadequate reduction of the posterior leaflet height (which remains >15 mm). Depending on the severity of SAM and the hemodynamic status of the patient, attempts at re-repair with a larger ring or further leaflet height reduction may be necessary if initial maneuvers to fill the heart, slow the heart rate, and limit inotropes are not effective.

6. What should a surgeon do if SAM is still present after initial conservative measures to slow the heart rate and reduce inotropic support?

The surgeon should go back on bypass and re-repair the valve, possibly with a sliding plasty and a larger ring. SAM is a common problem following MV surgery and can be related to various factors, as discussed previously. According to Gillinov et al., "the only way to completely avoid SAM is to refrain from performing MV surgery." Usually, the initial steps for SAM include lowering the heart rate, increasing pre-load, and stopping inotropic use. However, this patient already has a slow heart rate and is not on inotropic support.

Additionally, the patient has hemodynamic compromise with outflow tract obstruction. This needs to be fixed. In general, every attempt should be made to achieve a durable repair. Therefore, replacing the valve is not the best option, and additional attempts at repair should be made. Measures to improve or avoid SAM center on moving the coaptation point posteriorly. The posterior leaflet height should be reduced by performing a posterior leaflet resection, sliding plasty, or folding plasty. Alternatively, the creation of short posterior leaflet chordae will effectively reduce the leaflet height and ensure that leaflet tissue does not move toward the LV outflow tract during systole. According to Alfieri et al., an aggressive SAM prevention strategy in the form of edge-to-edge repair (a.k.a. Alfieri stitch) can be considered if a second pump run has to be avoided with patients in poor condition. Finally, using an annuloplasty ring that is too small can create excessive leaflet tissue and move the coaptation point too far anteriorly, creating SAM. Therefore, re-repair with a larger ring may be indicated.

7. Describe standard surgical approaches to the MV

Standard approaches include minimally invasive right thoracotomy, upper hemi sternotomy, full sternotomy, and even left thoracotomy. While sternotomy has long been considered the standard, minimally invasive approaches have shown outstanding long-term results, including a 94% freedom from reoperation at 10 years. However, excellent results have been achieved for other approaches as well, and thus no approach has been proven to be generally superior to the others. The choice of approach mainly depends on the patient's preference and the surgeon's skill and comfort level following the learning curve. The ability to perform minimally invasive approaches was demonstrated at different complexity levels. However, safety comes first. While we prefer right mini-thoracotomy for all comers, other surgeons may be more comfortable with traditional sternotomy in the following cases:

(1) With significant LV or RV dysfunction, shorter ischemic times to allow for ventricular recovery may be achieved with the traditional familiar approach.

(2) Moderate or more aortic regurgitation may preclude adequate antegrade cardioplegia delivery and increase concerns about adequate myocardial protection.

(3) The presence of an inferior vena cava filter may preclude femoral perfusion. Although it may be crossed directly via femoral cannulas, or alternative peripheral perfusion sites can be utilized, the filter may prove problematic for novice surgeons.

(4) Complex MV pathology thatrequires a complex repair, as these can be very challenging techniques to complete minimally invasively.

8. Which patients should be considered for MitraClip or other transcatheter edge-to-edge repair?

Patients with reduced EF and severe secondary MR while on goal-directed medical therapy should be considered for intervention on their MV. MV surgery may be considered if a concomitant procedure (atrial fibrillation requiring a maze procedure) or revascularization (with coronary artery bypass graft [CABG]) is indicated. Additionally, if the patient is lower risk or if the EF is preserved (>50%), then MV surgery should be pursued. In cases of secondary MR, MV replacement is recommended, as repair in these situations has a high recurrence rate. Transcatheter MV intervention was introduced more than 10 years ago, but it is less advanced than transcatheter aortic valve implantation, mostly because of the complexity of the MV. The MitraClip technique aims at replicating the surgical edge-to-edge technique, creating a "double-orifice" MV. Various studies, including the EVEREST II (Percutaneous Repair or Surgery for Mitral Regurgitation), COAPT (Cardiovascular Outcomes Assessment of the MitraClip Percutaneous Therapy for Heart Failure Patients With Functional Mitral Regurgitation), and MITRA-FR (Percutaneous Repair with the MitraClip Device for Severe Functional/Secondary Mitral Regurgitation) trials, have been completed to evaluate patients with secondary MR. They showed that:

(1) In experienced centers, MitraClip is a safe procedure with a low rate of complications.

(2) It is effective in reducing MR with very high procedural success.

(3) It improves symptoms and quality of life.

(4) Mortality outcomes remain uncertain (COAPT may have shown survival benefits, while the other trials did not).

9. When should a surgeon consider a MV replacement? What techniques should be used?

Patients with severe ischemic MR are candidates for MV replacement rather than repair, especially if undergoing concomitant heart surgery. In a randomized controlled trial of MV repair versus replacement in a patient with severe ischemic MR, there was no difference in survival between repair and replacement at two years. However, there was a significantly higher recurrence rate of moderate to severe MR in the repair group, which resulted in a higher incidence of heart failure and repeat hospitalizations. For this reason, MV replacement is recommended. Additionally, chordal sparing techniques should be employed to preserve ventricular geometry and improve outcomes following replacement.

10. What is a papillary muscle sling, and when may it be of benefit?

A papillary muscle sling uses a PTFE graft at the base of the papillary muscles in the LV to reapproximate the papillary muscles. This technique is typically used in conjunction with an annuloplasty ring on the MV (the so-called "ring and sling" procedure) for MV repair in cases of ischemic MR. As discussed earlier, recurrence rates of MR following repair of ischemic MR are high. This is hypothesized to be secondary to ventricular dilation and papillary muscle displacement. In this high-risk cohort, the ventricular papillary muscle sling has shown to benefit in terms of both ventricular function and reduction of MR recurrence rates. The reduction in lateral inter-papillary muscle separation and LV volume provided by this technique is expected to improve ventricular function, limit progression of ventricular dilation, and avoid progression of MR even when performed without MV annuloplasty. A recent clinical trial was launched to investigate this matter (NCT04475315: Papillary Muscle Sling).

11. How much MR is acceptable following a mitral repair?

Any MR greater than mild is unacceptable for mitral repair. Any residual MR left after the operation is likely to progress and require re-intervention. After confirming a failed repair with a careful TEE study, attempts at re-repair should be made. A repair has proven to be superior in terms of morbidity and mortality compared to mitral replacement for primary MR. For this reason, replacement is not the best next option.

12. When is the appropriate time to assess the success of MV repair?

A surgeon must always inspect the quality of the mitral repair prior to completing the operation. As discussed earlier, any MR more than mild is unacceptable. Ideally, the patient is off cardiopulmonary bypass and in sinus rhythm at the time of the evaluation. The evaluation should be completed before giving protamine and before removing the cannulas for cardiopulmonary bypass if additional repair attempts are required. However, it is important to confirm that LV function has returned to its baseline level before assessing the quality of the repair. A central or anteriorly directed jet of MR may occur with reduced LV function or pacing, both of which can occur when weaning from cardiopulmonary bypass. This trivial MR almost always resolves with the recovery of LV function and may require the administration of inotropes for a better assessment. Therefore, ventricular recovery should be considered before the final TEE assessment.

13. What are the advantages of a Heart Team and center of excellence?

Optimal management of MV disease occurs in heart valve centers with a dedicated Heart Team. The specialized team approach was found to be valuable for patient selection and for triaging patients into different treatment modalities, proposing all therapeutic alternatives with good efficacy and safety. Furthermore, specialists in each modality have shown improved outcomes. Specifically, heart failure specialists managing goal-directed medical therapy can reduce LV volumes and reduce the severity of secondary MR. Surgical mortality is reduced at centers that perform at least 50 mitral repairs per year. This specialized team approach resulted in lower than expected in-hospital mortality for MitraClip patients and high four-year survival rates for patients undergoing surgical or percutaneous repair of isolated primary MR. Nevertheless, while higher-volume centers have consistently reported better outcomes due to higher rates of mitral repair to replacement, low-volume centers may achieve comparable outcomes when they employ repair techniques in a safe and effective matter. The probability of mitral repair over replacement and the improved outcome is surgeon-specific rather than institution-specific.

Bibliography

1 Alfieri, O. and Lapenna, E. (2015). Systolic anterior motion after mitral valve repair: where do we stand in 2015? *Eur. J. Cardio-Thorac. Surg.* 48: 344–346.

2 Braunberger, E., Deloche, A., Berrebi, A. et al. (2001). Very long-term results (more than 20 years) of valve repair with Carpentier’s techniques in nonrheumatic mitral valve insufficiency. *Circulation* 104: I-8-I-11.

3 Chikwe, J., Toyoda, N., Anyanwu, A.C. et al. (2017). Relation of mitral valve surgery volume to repair rate, durability, and survival. *J. Am. Coll. Cardiol.* 69: 2397–2406.

4 Dumont, E., Gillinov, A.M., Blackstone, E.H. et al. (2007). Reoperation after mitral valve repair for degenerative disease. *Ann. Thorac. Surg.* 84: 444–450. discussion 450.

5 Elmahdy, H.M., Nascimento, F.O., Santana, O., and Lamelas, J. (2013). Outcomes of minimally invasive triple valve surgery performed via a right anterior thoracotomy approach. *J. Heart Valve Dis.* 22: 735–739.

6 Giraldo-Grueso, M., Sandoval-Reyes, N., Camacho, J. et al. (2018). Mitral valve repair, how to make volume not matter; techniques, tendencies, and outcomes, a single center experience. *J. Cardiothorac. Surg.* 13: 108.

7 Glauber, M., Miceli, A., Canarutto, D. et al. (2015). Early and long-term outcomes of minimally invasive mitral valve surgery through right minithoracotomy: a 10-year experience in 1604 patients. *J. Cardiothorac. Surg.* 10: 181–181.

8 Heuts, S., Olsthoorn, J.R., Hermans, S.M.M. et al. (2019). Multidisciplinary decision-making in mitral valve disease: the mitral valve heart team. *Neth. Heart J.* 27: 176–184.

9 Külling, M., Corti, R., Noll, G. et al. (2020). Heart team approach in treatment of mitral regurgitation: patient selection and outcome. *Open Heart* 7: e001280.

10 Lamelas, J. (2015). Minimally invasive concomitant aortic and mitral valve surgery: the "Miami method". *Ann. Cardiothorac. Surg.* 4: 33–37.

11 Lamelas, J., Aberle, C., Macias, A.E., and Alnajar, A. (2020). Cannulation strategies for minimally invasive cardiac surgery. *Innovations* 15: 261–269.

12 Lamelas, J. and Alnajar, A. Commentary: the role of less-invasive mitral valve surgery when the mitral

annulus is calcified: when less is more. *Semin. Thorac. Cardiovasc. Surg.* 34: 510–511.

13 Lamelas, J., Sarria, A., Santana, O. et al. (2011). Outcomes of minimally invasive valve surgery versus median sternotomy in patients age 75 years or greater. *Ann. Thorac. Surg.* 91: 79–84.

14 Levine, R.A., Vlahakes, G.J., Lefebvre, X. et al. (1995). Papillary muscle displacement causes systolic anterior motion of the mitral valve. *Circulation* 91: 1189–1195.

15 Luckie, M. and Khattar, R.S. (2008). Systolic anterior motion of the mitral valve—beyond hypertrophic cardiomyopathy. *Heart* 94: 1383–1385.

16 Mihos, C.G., Santana, O., Pineda, A.M. et al. (2014). Right anterior minithoracotomy versus median sternotomy surgery for native mitral valve infective endocarditis. *J. Heart Valve Dis.* 23: 343–349.

17 Modi, P., Hassan, A., and Chitwood, W.R. Jr. (2008). Minimally invasive mitral valve surgery: a systematic review and meta-analysis. *Eur. J. Cardio-Thorac. Surg.* 34: 943–952.

18 Mohty, D., Orszulak, T.A., Schaff, H.V. et al. (2001). Very long-term survival and durability of mitral valve repair for mitral valve prolapse. *Circulation* 104: I-1-I-7.

19 Otto, C.M., Nishimura, R.A., Bonow, R.O. et al. (2021). 2020 ACC/AHA guideline for the management of patients with valvular heart disease: A report of the American College of Cardiology/American Heart Association joint committee on clinical practice guidelines. *Circulation* 143: e72–e227.

20 Santana, O., Solenkova, N.V., Pineda, A.M. et al. (2014). Minimally invasive papillary muscle sling placement during mitral valve repair in patients with functional mitral regurgitation. *J. Thorac. Cardiovasc. Surg.* 147: 496–499.

21 Shuhaiber, J., Isaacs, A.J., and Sedrakyan, A. (2015). The effect of center volume on in-hospital mortality after aortic and mitral valve surgical procedures: a population-based study. *Ann. Thorac. Surg.* 100: 1340–1346.

22 Suri, R.M., Burkhart, H.M., Daly, R.C. et al. (2011). Robotic mitral valve repair for all prolapse subsets using techniques identical to open valvuloplasty: establishing the benchmark against which percutaneous interventions should be judged. *J. Thorac. Cardiovasc. Surg.* 142: 970–979.

23 Suri, R.M., Schaff, H.V., Dearani, J.A. et al. (2006). Survival advantage and improved durability of mitral repair for leaflet prolapse subsets in the current era. *Ann. Thorac. Surg.* 82: 819–826.

24 Zegdi, R., Sleilaty, G., Latrémouille, C. et al. (2008). Reoperation for failure of mitral valve repair in degenerative disease: a single-center experience. *Ann. Thorac. Surg.* 86: 1480–1484.

31

Structural Interventions for Mitral Stenosis

Napatt Kanjanahattakij[1], Aditya Bakhshi[1], Igor F. Palacios[2] and Christian Witzke[1]

[1] *Department of Cardiology, Albert Einstein Medical Center, Philadelphia, PA, USA*
[2] *Cardiology, Massachusetts General Hospital, Harvard Medical School, Boston, MA, USA*

1. What are the current classification criteria for mitral stenosis (MS)?

The 2020 American College of Cardiology/American Heart Association (ACC/AHA) Guidelines for the Management of Valvular Heart Disease classifies MS into four stages: A, B, C, and D (Table 31.1). The stages are defined by symptoms, valve anatomy, valve hemodynamics, and the consequences of valve obstruction.

At a mitral valve area (MVA) of $>1.5\,cm^2$, MS is generally asymptomatic. Once MS has progressed to an MVA of $\leq1.5\,cm^2$, cardiac output may decrease at rest and be unable to increase during exercise, resulting in symptomatic MS. Therefore, mitral valve (MV) intervention should be considered in this valve area to improve symptoms. However, obtaining an accurate MVA by echocardiography can be challenging, limiting assessment with the current classification system. Alternatively, the transmitral gradient (TMG) can be obtained from simple Doppler echocardiography. A TMG of 6–10 mmHg (at a normal heart rate and stroke volume) generally corresponds to a MVA $<1.5\,cm^2$. However, the TMG can be highly influenced by stroke volume and heart rate. In a study by Kato et al., the authors proposed a formula to project TMG, correcting for heart rate and stroke volume. This corrected TMG has a better correlation with MVA and clinical outcomes.

2. What are the current indications and contraindications for percutaneous MV intervention in rheumatic MS?

Percutaneous mitral balloon valvuloplasty (PMV) is indicated in patients with symptomatic (New York Heart Association [NYHA] Class II to IV), severe rheumatic MS (stage D) who have favorable valve morphology, defined as a Wilkins score of ≤8.

PMV can be considered in patients with asymptomatic, severe rheumatic MS (stage C) with favorable valve morphology and the following conditions:

- Pulmonary artery systolic pressure >50 mmHg (Class IIa)
- New-onset atrial fibrillation (Class IIb)
- Hemodynamically significant MS, defined as pulmonary artery wedge pressure >25 mmHg or mean MV gradient >15 mmHg during exercise (Class IIa)

PMV can also be considered in patients with severe, symptomatic MS (stage D) who have suboptimal valve anatomy but are at high risk for surgery.

PMV is contraindicated in patients with at least moderate mitral regurgitation (MR) or left atrial thrombus.

3. What are the predictors of successful/failed PMV?

A successful PMV has been arbitrarily defined as a resultant MVA of $>1.5\,cm^2$ without producing significant MR. Anatomical features of the MV, such as the lack of commissural calcification seen on fluoroscopy, have been used in the past to predict successful PMV. However, due to the complexity of the MV apparatus and the mechanics of balloon valvuloplasty causing commissural splitting, more complex scoring systems have been developed to predict both acute and long-term success.

The most common scoring system currently used is the Wilkins score. This scoring system evaluates leaflet mobility, valvular thickening, valvular calcification, and subvalvular thickening. Each component is scored from 0 to 4, with higher scores suggesting unfavorable valve anatomy.

Table 31.1 Current classification of mitral stenosis.

Stage	Definition	Valve anatomy	Valve hemodynamics	Hemodynamic consequences	Symptoms
A	At risk of MS	Mild valve doming during diastole	Normal transmitral flow velocity	None	None
B	Progressive MS	Rheumatic valve changes with commissural fusion and diastolic doming of the MV leaflets MVA by planimetry >1.5 cm^2	Increased transmitral flow velocities MVA > 1.5 cm^2 Diastolic pressure half-time <150 ms	Mild to moderate LA enlargement Normal pulmonary pressure at rest	None
C	Asymptomatic severe MS	Rheumatic valve changes with commissural fusion and diastolic doming of the MV leaflets MVA by planimetry ≤1.5 cm^2	MVA ≤ 1.5 cm^2 Diastolic pressure half-time ≥150 ms	Severe LA enlargement Elevated PASP >50 mmHg	None
D	Symptomatic severe MS	Rheumatic valve changes with commissural fusion and diastolic doming of the MV leaflets MVA by planimetry ≤1.5 cm^2	MVA ≤ 1.5 cm^2 Diastolic pressure half-time ≥150 ms	Severe LA enlargement Elevated PASP >50 mmHg	Decreased exercise tolerance Exertional dyspnea

LA, left atrial; MS, mitral stenosis; MV, mitral valve; MVA, mitral valve area; PASP, pulmonary artery systolic pressure. *Source:* Otto et al. (2021) / Wolters Kluwer Health.

The most recent ACC/AHA guidelines considered patients with a Wilkin's score of ≤8 to have "favorable" valve morphology for PMV. Studies have demonstrated that a Wilkins score of ≤8 predicts good immediate and long-term outcomes after PMV, while a score of >8 portends worse outcomes. A Wilkins score of ≤8 is associated with an 82% five-year event free survival in patients who underwent successful PMV.

While the Wilkins score is widely used, it has limitations. Although the grading system is relatively simple, it is semi-quantitative and subject to observer variability. Commissural morphology is not included in the scoring system, and, more importantly, the score does not predict post-procedural MR.

Padial et al. developed an echocardiographic scoring system that can be used to predict the possibility of severe MR after PMV. The score has components including valvular thickening (each leaflet scored separately), commissural calcification, and subvalvular disease. Each component is scored from 1 to 4, with a maximum score of 16. Increased thickening, calcification, and uneven distribution of pathology correspond to higher scores. A score of ≥10 predicts severe post-PMV MR with a sensitivity of 90% and specificity of 97%. Although the scoring

system is appealing for use in clinical practice, the Padial score was derived from a retrospective study with a small sample size.

Nunes et al. have proposed a quantitative scoring system that also incorporates commissural morphology and leaflet displacement. Scores are assigned to parameters including MVA ≤ 1 cm^2 (2 points), maximum leaflet displacement ≤12 mm (3 points), commissural area ratio ≥ 1.25 (3 points), and subvalvular involvement (3 points). Based on the cumulative score, patients are stratified into low (0–3 points), intermediate (5 points), and high (6–11 points) risk groups. The result of PMV in these groups was found to be sub-optimal in 17%, 56%, and 74% of patients, respectively. This score more accurately predicts both acute and long-term outcomes after PMV when compared to the Padial score and Wilkins score.

The risk scoring systems are summarized in Table 31.2.

4. What are the techniques for PMV?

Currently, the Inoue balloon is the most widely used technique worldwide for the percutaneous treatment of rheumatic MS. This technique was preceded by the use

Table 31.2 Summary of available scores to predict success and complications after percutaneous mitral balloon valvuloplasty.

Scoring system	Leaflet mobility	Valvular thickening	Valvular calcification	Sub-valvular thickening
Wilkins score: Score of ≤8 predicts good immediate and long-term outcome after PMV	– Normal (0 points) – Highly mobile with restriction of leaflet tip (1 point) – Leaflet mid and base portions have normal mobility (2 points) – Leaflets move forward in diastole mainly at the base (3 points) – No or minimal forward movement of the leaflets in diastole (4 points)	– Normal (0 points) – Near normal 4–5 mm thickness (1 point) – Mid leaflet thickening, marked thickening of the margin (2 points) – Thickening of the entire leaflet 5–8 mm (3 points) – Marked thickening of the entire leaflet >8-10 mm (4 points)	– Normal (0 points) – Single area of increased echo brightness (1 point) – Scattered areas of brightness confined to leaflet margins (2 points) – Brightness extending into the leaflet midportion (3 points) – Extensive brightness throughout most of the leaflet (4 points)	– Normal (0 points) – Minimal thickening of chordal structures just below the valve (1 point) – Thickening of chordae up to one-third of the chordal length (2 points) – Thickening extends to the distal third of the chordae (3 points) – Extensive thickening and shortening of all chordae down to the papillary muscles (4 points)
Padial et al.: Score ≥ 10 predicts severe MR after PMV		Score each leaflet separately: – Leaflet near normal 4–5 mm (1 point) – Leaflet fibrotic/calcified with even distribution, no thin area (2 points) – Leaflet fibrotic/calcified with uneven distribution; thinner segments are mildly thickened 5–8 mm (3 points) – Leaflet fibrotic/calcified with uneven distribution; thinner segments are near normal	Commissural calcification: – Fibrosis/ calcium in one commissure (1 point) – Both commissures mildly calcified/fibrotic (2 points) – Calcium in both commissures; one markedly affected (3 points) – Calcium in both commissures; both markedly affected (4 points)	– Minimal thickening of chordal structures just below the valve (1 point) – Thickening of chordae extending up to one-third of the chordal length (2 points) – Thickening up to distal third of the chordae (3 points) – Extensive thickening and shortening of all chordae extending down to the papillary muscle (4 points)
Revised Echo Score by Nunes et al.: Risk of sub-optimal PMV 0–3 points: 17% 5 points: 56% 6–11 points: 74%	Mitral valve area ≤ 1 cm² (2 points) Maximum leaflet displacement ≤12 mm (3 points) Commissural area ratio ≥ 1.25 (3 points) Sub-valvular involvement (3 points)			

MR, mitral regurgitation; PMV, percutaneous mitral valvuloplasty.

of a regular valvuloplasty balloon, where a single balloon was placed across the MV via transseptal puncture. Due to the size limitations of a single valvuloplasty balloon, the technique evolved to use two valvuloplasty balloons.

With the development of the Inoue balloon, the PMV technique has been markedly simplified by returning to the use of a single transseptal puncture and a single balloon with the ability to efficiently dilate the MV commissures.

The technique has minimized peri-procedural complications and reduced the duration of the procedure.

From a historical perspective, the metallic commissurotomy technique was developed by Cribier et al. The advantage of this technique is the use of a detachable metallic cylinder attached to a disposable catheter, allowing reuse of the device and thus reducing cost. The technique was used only in a few countries worldwide and was never approved in the US.

Mitral Balloon Valvuloplasty

Currently, there are two main balloon valvuloplasty techniques used to manage rheumatic MS. As stated previously, the Inoue technique is the most widely used, leaving the double-balloon technique to a few high-volume operators worldwide.

The Inoue technique requires the use of a specially designed Inoue balloon, available in 26, 28, and 30 mm sizes. This single-balloon technology facilitates access to the left atrium (LA) with increased ease and safety while crossing the MV. Stepwise inflation of the balloon, guided by echocardiography with color Doppler, ensures optimal results and reduces post-PMV MR.

The double-balloon technique requires the creation of a left ventricle (LV) loop to prevent balloon watermelon seeding and LV perforation. Although observational studies suggest larger valve-areas post valvuloplasty, the long-term outcomes of the Inoue technique are comparable. It is important to note that the life-threatening LV perforation seen in the double-balloon technique is extremely rare when using the Inoue balloon.

5. What are the steps to perform PMV with the Inoue technique?

Equipment List

1. 6F arterial access.
2. Transseptal puncture equipment. We normally use an SL1 transseptal sheath; however, any transseptal equipment can be used to access the LA. The Baylis transseptal sheath allows transseptal puncture using electrocauterization, making the transseptal puncture safer on certain occasions (e.g. in the presence of interatrial septal aneurysms).
3. Intracardiac echocardiography (ICE) equipment. Transseptal puncture under ICE guidance increases the safety of the interatrial puncture. Alternatively, fluoroscopy-guided transseptal puncture can be utilized. Finally, transesophageal echocardiography (TEE)-guided transseptal puncture can be performed; however, it requires endotracheal intubation and general anesthesia for patient comfort.
4. 6F pigtail catheter for hemodynamic assessment and left ventricular cineangiography.
5. Swan Ganz catheter for diagnostic hemodynamic assessment.
6. Diluted contrast (saline-contrast ratio of 4 : 1).
7. Two hemodynamic transducers.
8. Power injector with non-diluted contrast.
9. Inoue balloon (Toray) kit (Figure 31.1):
   a. The Inoue balloon is attached to the end of a 12F polyvinyl chloride catheter 70 cm in length. The balloon is made of two layers of latex with polyester micromesh in between. Proximally, there are two stopcocks for balloon inflation and catheter venting.
   b. A 14F, 70 cm tapered dilator can be used to dilate the femoral vein and interatrial septum (IAS).
   c. A stainless-steel 0.025 in. diameter, 175 cm guide wire with spring coil tip for delivery of the balloon to the LA.
   d. A stainless-steel 19-gauge, 80 cm tube inserted through the middle port of the catheter to stretch and slenderize the balloon before insertion.
   e. A stainless-steel 0.038 in. diameter, 80 cm stylet to help steer the balloon to facilitate access to the LV.

The balloon has three portions, each with slightly different compliance. The balloon is inflated with diluted contrast media (saline-contrast ratio of 4 : 1). As volume is gradually added, the distal portion inflates (Figure 31.2a), followed by the proximal portion, forming an hourglass shape (Figure 31.2b). This unique shape allows the fixation of the balloon in the proper position across the valve. When further volume is added, the middle portion expands at the level of the commissure, resulting in the splitting of the fused commissure (Figure 31.2c).

Balloon Selection

Three balloon sizes are available (PTMC-30, PTMC-28, PTMC-26). The number indicates the maximum diameter of the balloon in millimeters. A simple formula (height [cm]/10 + 10) has been proposed for balloon selection based on height. However, the relationship between height and mitral orifice diameter is not always linear. Balloon size can also be selected by directly measuring the mitral annular diameter via 2D echocardiography. The diameter of the mitral annulus is best measured in apical four-chamber and two-chamber views during mid- to end-systole. The reference balloon size is chosen based on the smallest measured diameter to avoid the risk of complications. A study comparing both methods showed that echocardiography-based reference balloon size resulted in larger MVA and less MR.

Procedure Detail

Pre-PMV coronary angiography should be performed in patients aged 40 years and older. At our institution, we

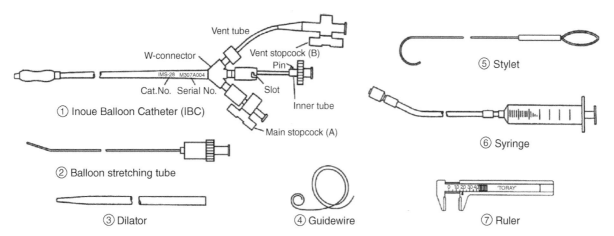

Figure 31.1 Equipment needed for percutaneous balloon valvuloplasty: (1) Inoue balloon; (2) balloon-stretching tube used to elongate and slenderized the balloon; (3) dilator used to dilate the femoral and septal puncture site; (4) guidewire; (5) stylet inserted into the inner tube to steer the balloon across the valve; (6) calibrated syringe for balloon inflation; (7) ruler used to confirm the size of the balloon. *Source:* Toray Industries, Inc., Tokyo, Japan, with permission.

normally perform diagnostic coronary angiography immediately prior to the planned valvuloplasty. Before placing the patient on the procedure table, TEE should be performed to rule out LA thrombus. We normally do not exclude patients from a PMV based on the degree of MR seen on TEE unless it is severe.

The procedure can be done under moderate sedation when using ICE or fluoroscopy guidance for transseptal puncture. On occasion, we place the patient under general anesthesia and perform the procedure under TEE guidance.

We prefer using the femoral artery to have sufficient arterial access in case of peri-procedural complications, specifically acute MR post-PMV. An intra-aortic balloon pump (IABP) could rapidly be placed if severe, acute MR occurred after the PMV. We generally prefer the left femoral arterial access, leaving the right inguinal area for the valvuloplasty procedure. Alternatively, the radial artery can be used, which minimizes bleeding complications. Once arterial access is obtained, we proceed with transseptal puncture. At our institution, we administer heparin to target an ACT

>300 seconds once arterial and venous access are obtained. If ICE is used, we place a catheter from the left femoral vein.

Using the SL1 or the transseptal system of choice, transseptal puncture is performed, and access to the LA is obtained. If a patent foramen ovale (PFO) is present, entry to the LA through the PFO *should be avoided* at any cost: it will bias the valvuloplasty equipment anteriorly, making posterior manipulation of the balloon extremely difficult. From the left femoral venous access, right-heart catheterization is performed to assess hemodynamic parameters, including pulmonary artery pressures and cardiac output. Using a 6F pigtail catheter, simultaneous LV-LA pressure is recorded, with the calculation of the MVA using the Gorlin equation. Left ventricular angiography is then performed to assess the presence of MR. If ≥2+ MR is seen on LV gram, the procedure is aborted, and surgical MVR should be considered.

Once the hemodynamic parameters are obtained and significant MR is ruled out by LV angiography, we proceed with the valvuloplasty. The coiled-tip Inoue guide wire is inserted through the transseptal catheter into the LA. Care

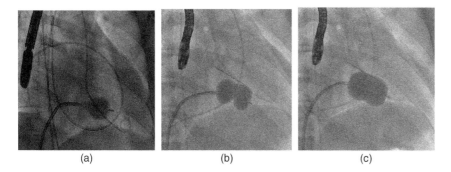

Figure 31.2 Inoue balloon when (a) the distal balloon is inflated and pulled back to the commissure; (b) the balloon is partially inflated into an hourglass shape within the commissure (the indentation of the balloon indicates commissural fusion); (c) the balloon is fully inflated, causing commissural splitting.

should be taken when advancing this wire into the LA, as we have seen micro-perforations from the wire. This wire will take 2½ loops in the LA before giving the straight configuration across the IAS. The transseptal catheter is then removed, and a 14F dilator, included in the Inoue equipment box, is advanced over the wire to dilate the femoral vein and the IAS. Occasionally the patient can develop a transient vagal response with subsequent bradycardia and/or advanced AV block.

Once the dilator is retrieved, the Inoue balloon catheter system (straightened by the stainless-steel tube) is advanced over the 0.025″ guide wire into the LA. Once the tip of the balloon reaches the mid-LA, the stainless-steel tube is fixed, and the balloon catheter is further advanced a few centimeters into the LA. The balloon is then fully deployed by separating the most distal portion from the polyvinyl chloride catheter. The stainless steel tube is completely withdrawn, and the distal balloon is partially inflated. Inflating the distal portion of the balloon prevents unintentional loss of the transseptal puncture and facilitates the manipulation of the balloon when crossing the MV.

The 0.038″ stylet is placed in the inner lumen of the balloon to give the curvature needed to cross the MV. The balloon is then rotated counterclockwise and slowly pulled back to cause prolapse into the LV. In cases when the LA is markedly dilated and the balloon does not reach the MV annulus, a clockwise rotation to loop the catheter in the LA will bring the balloon anterograde (en face) to the MV annulus. The right anterior oblique projection helps identify the correct plane of the MV. Once the MV is crossed with the balloon, the stylet can be partially retrieved. The distal balloon is then fully inflated. To ensure that the balloon is free in the LV, we move the balloon catheter back and forth in the LV before pulling back to fully engage the MV. Once the distal balloon is anchored at the MV, we proceed with the complete inflation of the balloon. On fluoroscopy, the mid-waist of the balloon will inflate prior to the inflation of the most proximal portion of the balloon. The balloon is then fully deflated.

After each dilation, the left ventricular and left atrial pressure should be obtained simultaneously. Echocardiography should also be performed following each balloon inflation to evaluate the MVA and MR. A special assessment of commissural splitting should follow each balloon inflation to maximize results and prevent complications. At our institution, we start with low-volume inflation and increase by 1 cc after each inflation until a defined endpoint is achieved.

After PMV, a diagnostic oxygen shunt run should be performed to determine the presence of a significant left-to-right shunt across the atrial septum.

6. What are the steps to perform PMV with the antegrade double-balloon technique?

Balloon Selection

Choosing the appropriate balloon size to achieve an effective balloon dilatation area (EBDA) corrected by body surface area of 3.1 to $4 \, cm^2/m^2$ is key to ensuring the maximum increase in MVA and preventing significant MR. We use a previously published balloon combination chart (Table 31.3) to determine the combination to achieve a specific EBDA.

Procedure Detail

As previously described, arterial and venous access, transseptal puncture, and hemodynamic assessment are obtained. Once access to the LA is obtained, the MV is crossed with an 8F balloon wedge catheter (Arrow). The catheter is then looped in the LV and placed in the descending aorta. Using the inner lumen of the balloon catheter, two 0.035″ J-wires are placed into the ascending aorta. The selected balloon-dilating catheters are then advanced over each guide wire. The balloon is placed across the MV, parallel to the longitudinal axis of the LV. The balloons are inflated until the indentation is no longer seen.

7. What is the follow-up protocol after PMV?

Echocardiography and hemodynamic measurements are usually done after the procedure to evaluate the change in gradients and valve area and detect MR or other potential complications. The valve area is most accurately evaluated with planimetry, as pressure half-time is inaccurate after PMV. 3D echocardiography is also helpful in evaluating the anatomy and detection of MR. In our institution, we obtain 2D transthoracic echocardiography the day after the procedure and then again at 30 days.

8. What are the potential complications of PMV?

The overall mortality in patients undergoing PMV is less than 1%. Most complications associated with this procedure occur during transseptal puncture, balloon manipulation, and commissurotomy.

Table 31.3 Effective dilating diameter of the two balloons for the double-balloon valvuloplasty technique. Balloon sizes are labeled in bold. The intersection of balloons 1 and 2 represents effective dilating diameter when these two balloons are inflated simultaneously.

Balloon 1	5	6	7	8	9	10	11	12	13	14	15	16	17	18	19	20	21	22	23	24	25	Balloon 2
5	8.2	9.0	9.9	10.7	11.6	12.5	13.5	14.4	15.3	16.2	17.2	18.1	19.1	20.0	21.0	21.9	22.9	23.9	24.8	25.8	26.8	**5**
6		9.8	10.7	11.5	12.4	13.3	14.1	15.1	16.0	16.9	17.8	18.7	19.7	20.6	21.6	22.5	23.5	24.4	25.4	26.3	27.3	**6**
7			11.5	12.3	13.1	14.0	14.9	15.8	16.7	17.6	18.5	19.4	20.3	21.2	22.2	23.1	24.1	25.0	25.9	26.9	27.8	**7**
8				13.1	13.9	14.8	15.8	16.5	17.4	18.3	19.2	20.1	21	21.9	22.8	23.7	24.7	25.6	26.5	27.5	28.4	**8**
9					14.7	15.6	16.4	17.2	18.1	19.0	19.9	20.8	21.7	22.6	23.5	24.4	25.3	26.2	27.2	28.1	29	**9**
10						16.4	17.2	18.0	18.9	19.7	20.6	21.5	22.4	23.3	24.2	25.1	26.0	26.9	27.8	28.8	29.7	**10**
11							18.0	18.8	19.7	20.5	21.4	22.2	23.1	24.0	24.9	25.8	26.7	27.6	28.5	29.4	30.3	**11**
12								19.7	20.5	21.3	22.1	23.0	23.9	24.7	25.6	26.5	27.4	28.3	29.2	30.1	31.0	**12**
13									21.3	22.1	22.9	23.8	24.6	25.5	26.4	27.2	28.1	29.0	29.9	30.8	31.7	**13**
14										22.9	23.7	24.6	25.4	26.3	27.1	28.0	28.9	29.7	30.6	31.5	32.4	**14**
15											24.5	25.4	26.2	27.0	27.9	28.8	29.6	30.5	31.4	32.2	33.1	**15**
16												26.2	27.0	27.8	28.7	29.5	30.4	31.2	32.1	33.0	33.9	**16**
17													27.8	28.6	29.5	30.3	31.2	32.0	32.9	33.7	34.1	**17**
18														29.5	30.3	31.1	32.0	32.8	33.6	34.5	35.4	**18**
19															31.1	31.9	32.7	33.6	34.4	35.3	36.1	**19**
20																32.7	33.6	34.4	35.2	36.1	36.0	**20**
21																	34.4	35.2	36.0	36.9	37.7	**21**
22																		36	36.8	37.7	38.5	**22**
23																			37.6	38.5	39.3	**23**
24																				39.3	40.1	**24**
25																					40.9	**25**

Source: Adapted from Radtke, W., Keane, J.F., Fellows, K.E. et al. (1986). Percutaneous balloon valvotomy of congenital pulmonary stenosis using oversized balloons. *J. Am. Coll. Cardiol.* 8: 909–915.

Hemopericardium

Hemopericardium/cardiac tamponade occurs in up to 4% of patients, most commonly during transseptal puncture. Manipulation of the transseptal needle may cause injury to adjacent structures, including the ascending aorta. Rarely, perforation of the LA appendage, pulmonary vein, or LV can occur by a guide wire and balloon manipulation.

Mitral Regurgitation

An undesirable increase in MR (≥ 2) can occur in up to 10% of patients and is usually well tolerated. Severe MR occurs in 3–4% of patients. Only 1% of these patients will need an emergent (<24 hours) surgical MV replacement. The other 3% of the patients who develop severe MR post-PMV require surgery within 30 days due to the persistence of symptoms.

There are several proposed mechanisms of MR after PMV: excessive tearing of the leaflets at the commissure or non-commissure area, incomplete closure of the calcified leaflets, or localized rupture of the subvalvular apparatus.

Worsening MR primarily occurs in patients with unfavorable anatomy. Uneven distribution of calcification/thickening of the leaflet, commissure, and subvalvular disease have been associated with the development of severe post-PMV MR.

Iatrogenic Interatrial Septal Defect

Left-to-right shunt occurs in up to 16% of patients. The size of the shunt is usually small (Qp:Qs < 2 : 1), without hemodynamic significance. The defect spontaneously closes in the majority of these patients.

On very rare occasions, the iatrogenic interatrial septal defect must be closed: specifically, in patients who develop a right-to-left shunt or large left-to-right shunt, or patients with pulmonary hypertension and/or poor right ventricular function.

9. What is the role of transcatheter therapy for rheumatic MS in women who are pregnant or contemplating pregnancy?

As with most stenotic valve diseases, severe rheumatic MS is poorly tolerated during pregnancy. Pregnant women with severe rheumatic MS are at increased risk of adverse maternal outcomes. The most recent ACC/AHA guidelines recommend PMV in the following situations.

Before Pregnancy

In patients with severe, asymptomatic rheumatic MS with favorable valve morphology who are considering pregnancy, PMV is reasonable before pregnancy (Class IIa).

During Pregnancy

In pregnant women with severe MS and favorable valve morphology, PMV is reasonable during pregnancy if the patient has symptomatic NYHA Class III or IV heart failure despite maximum medical therapy (Class IIa).

A recent meta-analysis including 745 pregnancies showed that PMV can be safely performed during pregnancy. Most of the procedures were performed in the second trimester. The fluoroscopy time was usually <8 minutes. Maternal death was reported in approximately 0.01% of patients. Procedure failure occurred in 5.7% of patients, with nearly half of the procedure failures occurring in patients with severe subvalvular disease. The most common complication was new-onset or worsening MR (12.7%). Stillbirth was reported in 0.9% of patients.

10. What is the role of PMV in patients with aortic regurgitation?

Patients with rheumatic MS often also have aortic valve involvement. In patients with rheumatic MS who were referred for PMV, approximately 46% had at least mild AR.

In patients with both severe MS and severe AR, correction of both pathologies with replacement of both valves, or PMV with subsequent aortic valve replacement, should be performed. If the AR is mild at the time of MV intervention, the chance of progressing to severe AR is low. In patients with moderate AR undergoing PMV, the presence of moderate AR has not been associated with worse outcomes. Thus, patients with mild to moderate AR remain good candidates for PMV. However, patients with moderate AR have an increased chance of requiring subsequent AVR (13%) within 4–5 years.

11. What is the role of PMV in patients with concomitant severe tricuspid regurgitation?

Concomitant tricuspid regurgitation (TR) can occur in patients with rheumatic MS due to rheumatic involvement of the tricuspid valve or functional TR from significant pulmonary hypertension. In patients with severe rheumatic MS undergoing PMV, the degree of TR can be a marker of disease severity. The presence of severe TR is associated with unfavorable morphology, calcified MV, severe symptoms, and smaller MVA. Severe TR is also associated with suboptimal immediate results and worse outcomes overall. However, in up to 30% of patients undergoing PMV with severe TR, the regurgitation lesion improved in severity after successful valvuloplasty. The improvement of the TR is most likely related to a decrease in the pulmonary pressure and improvement in RV performance. In rare cases where the TR jet is medially directed, post-PMV hypoxemia due to right-to-left shunt can be seen. In these cases, the iatrogenic atrial septal defect should be closed after the procedure.

12. Should PMV be attempted in patients with MV calcification?

As previously described, significant mitral calcification is associated with a lower success rate and increased risk of severe MR post-PMV. Patients with commissural and leaflet calcification tend to be older and have lower pre-PMV MVA. Performing PMV in this population remains a point of debate, as achieving procedural success is believed to be less likely.

A retrospective study by Dreyfus et al. compared post-PMV outcomes between patients with no calcification, leaflet calcification without commissural calcification, and patients with significant commissural calcification. Good immediate results were achieved in a significant number of patients with leaflet calcification (78%) or commissural calcification (73%), although still less successful compared to patients without calcification (88%). Thus, MV calcification should not be a contraindication of PMV.

13. Can PMV be done in patients with previous PMV?

Multiple studies have shown that redo-PMV in patients with MV restenosis led to good immediate and long-term outcomes. This was particularly seen in patients with favorable valve anatomy and in the absence of comorbid diseases. The immediate procedural success of repeat PMV is approximately 75–77%, with overall survival of approximately 70% three years after the procedure. Quality of life and symptoms improved significantly.

14. What are the roles of transcatheter intervention in patients with nonrheumatic calcific MS?

Compared to rheumatic MS, patients with nonrheumatic calcific MS are often older with more comorbidities. The pathogenesis of MS in these patients is different from rheumatic MS. Calcification of the annulus extending into the leaflet bases results in narrowing of the annulus and rigidity of the leaflets. The leaflet tips are generally not involved, and commissural calcification is rare. Thus, these patients are not ideal candidates for PMV. Shockwave balloon valvuloplasty has been utilized to facilitate PMV in patients with degenerative MS. In one case report, rapid pacing was used to optimize balloon position, and a carotid filter device was used to prevent a cerebro-embolic event. The use of a Shockwave balloon is still experimental, and more data is needed regarding safety and efficacy for the treatment of calcific MS.

According to the most recent ACC/AHA guidelines, percutaneous MV intervention may be considered in patients with severe symptomatic calcific MS after discussing the procedure risk (Class IIa). However, transcatheter intervention in nonrheumatic MS is experimental due to the lack of long-term outcome data. The available devices are limited to compassionate use or clinical trials.

15. What are the current and future transcatheter therapies for nonrheumatic MS?

Transcatheter Mitral Valve Replacement (TMVR) Using Balloon-Expandable Transcatheter Aortic Valves in Mitral Position

The TMVR in Mitral Annular Calcification (MAC) Global Registry data included 116 patients at high surgical risk with severe MAC who subsequently underwent TMVR. Balloon-expandable valves originally designed for transcatheter aortic valve replacement (TAVR) were used for TMVR. The majority of the valves were Edwards SAPIEN XT (45%) and SAPIEN 3 (49%). The procedures were predominantly done through the transapical and transseptal approaches. Procedure-related LVOT obstruction with hemodynamic compromise occurred in 11% of the patients. Although technical success was achieved in 76% of the patients, the procedure is associated with poor 30-day (25%) and one-year all-cause mortality (53%).

However, of the patients who survived past 30 days, 63% were alive at one year, and 72% of the patients who were alive at one year had good functional class. TMVR using TAVR valves is being studied in the MITRAL (Mitral Implantation of Transcatheter Valves) trial.

Future Directions of TMVR in Non-rheumatic MS

The Tendyne (Abbott Vascular) TMVR system has demonstrated a high implant success rate in patients with severe MR. The device has also shown promising results in small studies of patients with severe MAC. The SUMMIT (Clinical Trial to Evaluate the Safety and Effectiveness of Using the Tendyne Mitral Valve System for the Treatment of Symptomatic Mitral Regurgitation) trial (NCT03433274) is ongoing to further investigate the effectiveness of the Tendyne valve. Patients with severe MAC (including patients with severe MS from MAC) will be included in the MAC cohort of the trial. A pilot study using the Intrepid TMVR system (Medtronic) demonstrated acceptable results in patients with severe MR. In this study, 34% of the patients had at least mild MAC. The APOLLO (Transcatheter Mitral Valve Replacement With the Medtronic Intrepid TMVR System in Patients With Severe Symptomatic Mitral Regurgitation) trial (NCT03243642) is currently ongoing to further investigate the feasibility of Intrepid. The study includes up to 300 patients with significant MAC (severe MR with MAC or moderate MR with moderate MS). It will be interesting to see the results of both SUMMIT and APOLLO and how they can be applied to patients with MS from severe MAC.

Bibliography

1 Abascal, V.M., Wilkins, G.T., O'shea, J.P. et al. (1990). Prediction of successful outcome in 130 patients undergoing percutaneous balloon mitral valvotomy. *Circulation* 82: 448–456.

2 Bapat, V., Rajagopal, V., Meduri, C. et al. (2018). Early experience with new transcatheter mitral valve replacement. *J. Am. Coll. Cardiol.* 71: 12–21.

3 Baumgartner, H., Hung, J., Bermejo, J. et al. (2009). Echocardiographic assessment of valve stenosis: EAE/ASE recommendations for clinical practice. *J. Am. Soc. Echocardiogr.* 22: 1–23. Quiz 101-2.

4 Chen, C.R. and Cheng, T.O. (1995). Percutaneous balloon mitral valvuloplasty by the Inoue technique: a multicenter study of 4832 patients in China. *Am. Heart J.* 129: 1197–1203.

5 Chen, Z.Q., Hong, L., Wang, H. et al. (2015). Application of percutaneous balloon mitral valvuloplasty in patients of rheumatic heart disease mitral stenosis combined with tricuspid regurgitation. *Chin. Med. J. (Engl)* 128: 1479–1482.

6 Chmielak, Z., Klopotowski, M., Kruk, M. et al. (2010). Repeat percutaneous mitral balloon valvuloplasty for patients with mitral valve restenosis. *Catheter. Cardiovasc. Interv.* 76: 986–992.

7 Choudhary, S.K., Talwar, S., Juneja, R., and Kumar, A.S. (2001). Fate of mild aortic valve disease after mitral valve intervention. *J. Thorac. Cardiovasc. Surg.* 122: 583–586.

8 Cribier, A., Eltchaninoff, H., Carlot, R. et al. (2000). Percutaneous mechanical mitral commissurotomy with the metallic valvulotome: detailed technical aspects and overview of the results of the multicenter registry on 882 patients. *J. Interv. Cardiol.* 13: 255–262.

9 Dreyfus, J., Cimadevilla, C., Nguyen, V. et al. (2014). Feasibility of percutaneous mitral commissurotomy in patients with commissural mitral valve calcification. *Eur. Heart J.* 35: 1617–1623.

10 Eng Marvin, H., Villablanca, P., Wang Dee, D. et al. (2019). Lithotripsy-facilitated mitral balloon valvuloplasty for senile degenerative mitral valve stenosis. *JACC Cardiovasc. Interv.* 12: E133–E134.

11 Guerrero, M., Urena, M., Himbert, D. et al. (2018). 1-year outcomes of transcatheter mitral valve replacement in patients with severe mitral annular calcification. *J. Am. Coll. Cardiol.* 71: 1841–1853.

12 Kato, N., Pislaru Sorin, V., Padang, R. et al. (2021). A novel assessment using projected transmitral gradient improves diagnostic yield of Doppler hemodynamics in rheumatic and calcific mitral stenosis. *JACC Cardiovasc. Imaging* 14: 559–570.

13 Lau, K.W. and Hung, J.S. (1994). A simple balloon-sizing method in Inoue-balloon percutaneous transvenous mitral commissurotomy. *Catheter. Cardiovasc. Diagn.* 33: 120–129. Discussion 130-1.

14 Leon, M.N., Harrell, L.C., Simosa, H.F. et al. (1999). Comparison of immediate and long-term results of mitral balloon valvotomy with the double-balloon versus Inoue techniques. *Am. J. Cardiol.* 83: 1356–1363.

15 Nobuyoshi, M., Arita, T., Shirai, S.-I. et al. (2009). Percutaneous balloon mitral valvuloplasty. *Circulation* 119: E211–E219.

16 Nunes, M.C., Tan, T.C., Elmariah, S. et al. (2014). The echo score revisited: impact of incorporating commissural morphology and leaflet displacement to the prediction of outcome for patients undergoing percutaneous mitral valvuloplasty. *Circulation* 129: 886–895.

17 Otto, C.M., Nishimura, R.A., Bonow, R.O. et al. (2021). 2020 ACC/AHA guideline for the management of patients with valvular heart disease: a report of the American College Of Cardiology/American Heart Association joint committee on clinical practice guidelines. *Circulation* 143: E72–E227.

18 Padial, L.R., Freitas, N., Sagie, A. et al. (1996). Echocardiography can predict which patients will develop severe mitral regurgitation after percutaneous mitral valvulotomy. *J. Am. Coll. Cardiol.* 27: 1225–1231.

19 Palacios, I.F. and Arzamendi, D. (2012). Percutaneous mitral balloon valvuloplasty for patients with rheumatic mitral stenosis. *Interven. Cardiol. Clin.* 1: 45–61.

20 Palacios, I.F., Sanchez, P.L., Harrell, L.C. et al. (2002). Which patients benefit from percutaneous mitral balloon valvuloplasty? *Circulation* 105: 1465–1471.

21 Pathan, A.Z., Mahdi, N.A., Leon, M.N. et al. (1999). Is redo percutaneous mitral balloon valvuloplasty (PMV) indicated in patients with Post-PMV mitral restenosis? *J. Am. Coll. Cardiol.* 34: 49–54.

22 Post, J.R., Feldman, T., Isner, J., and Herrmann, H.C. (1995). Inoue balloon mitral valvotomy in patients with severe valvular and subvalvular deformity. *J. Am. Coll. Cardiol.* 25: 1129–1136.

23 Radtke, W., Keane, J.F., Fellows, K.E. et al. (1986). Percutaneous balloon valvotomy of congenital pulmonary stenosis using oversized balloons. *J. Am. Coll. Cardiol.* 8: 909–915.

24 Sagie, A., Schwammenthal, E., Newell, J.B. et al. (1994). Significant tricuspid regurgitation is a marker for adverse outcome in patients undergoing percutaneous balloon mitral valvuloplasty. *J. Am. Coll. Cardiol.* 24: 696–702.

25 Sanchez-Ledesma, M., Cruz-Gonzalez, I., Sanchez, P.L. et al. (2008). Impact of concomitant aortic regurgitation on percutaneous mitral valvuloplasty: immediate results, short-term, and long-term outcome. *Am. Heart J.* 156: 361–366.

26 Sorajja, P., Gössl, M., Babaliaros, V. et al. (2019). Novel transcatheter mitral valve prosthesis for patients with severe mitral annular calcification. *J. Am. Coll. Cardiol.* 74: 1431–1440.

27 Sreerama, D., Surana, M., Moolchandani, K. et al. (2020). Percutaneous balloon mitral valvotomy during pregnancy: a systematic review and meta-analysis. *Acta Obstet. Gynecol. Scand.* 100: 666–675.

28 Tastan, A., Ozturk, A., Senarslan, O. et al. (2016). Comparison of two different techniques for balloon sizing in percutaneous mitral balloon valvuloplasty: which is preferable? *Cardiovasc. J. Africa* 27: 147–151.

29 Zhang, L., Hou, J., Duan, Y. et al. (2019). Study on the long-term curative effect of repeat percutaneous balloon mitral valvuloplasty in patients with mitral restenosis. *Medicine (Baltimore)* 98: E16790.

32

Transcatheter Edge-to-Edge Repair Trials

The EVEREST and COAPT Trials

Felipe N. Albuquerque[1] and Ashvin Zachariah[2]

[1] *Division of Interventional Cardiology and Structural Heart Diseases, Holy Cross Hospital, Fort Lauderdale, FL, USA*
[2] *Division of Internal Medicine, Holy Cross Hospital, Fort Lauderdale, FL, USA*

Edge-to-Edge Mitral Valve Repair (EVEREST Trials)

1. What is the difference between primary and secondary mitral regurgitation?

The overarching categories of mitral regurgitation (MR) are primary (degenerative) MR and secondary (functional) MR. Primary MR is caused by disease in the valve itself. The most common causes of primary MR are leaflet prolapse or flail leaflet. Secondary MR is more commonly caused by abnormal left ventricular structure or function.

2. What is the basis of edge-to-edge mitral valve (MV) repair?

Edge-to-edge surgical MV repair was pioneered by Alfieri et al. in 1991 as an alternative to the previously described technique for repair proposed by Carpentier et al. The concept behind this form of repair lies in functional rather than anatomical repair and involves suturing the diseased leaflet to the opposing leaflet at exactly the position where the regurgitant jet is located. When a central jet is present, this form of repair can result in a double orifice structure of the MV. This form of repair also serves as the basis for percutaneous transcatheter edge-to-edge repair.

3. What was the purpose of the EVEREST Phase I clinical trial?

The Endovascular Valve Edge-to-Edge Repair Study (EVEREST) aimed to evaluate the safety and feasibility of edge-to-edge MV repair using the percutaneous MitraClip (Abbott) system. The study population consisted of patients with symptomatic moderate-to-severe or severe functional or degenerative MR or asymptomatic patients with moderate-to-severe or severe MR with diminished left ventricular function (defined as ejection fraction [EF] <60% or end-systolic left ventricular dimension >45 mm) (Table 32.1).

A total of 107 patients were chosen based on specific severity and anatomic criteria (Figure 32.1). The regurgitant jet in these patients was localized between the A2 and P2 segments. For patients with functional MR, the minimum leaflet coaptation length was 2 mm, with a coaptation depth of less than 11 mm. For patients with flail leaflet, the flail gap was less than 10 mm and the flail width was less than 15 mm (Figure 32.1). Functional MR was present in 21% of the patients; the remainder had either degenerative or a combination of degenerative and functional MR.

4. What were the results of EVEREST Phase 1?

Acute procedural success (APS) was defined as the reduction of MR to ≤2+ following clip implantation. APS was achieved in 79 of 107 (74%) patients.

Table 32.1 Inclusion and exclusion criteria for EVEREST Phase I.

Key inclusion criteria
Candidate for mitral valve repair or replacement surgery
Moderate to severe (3+) or severe (4+) chronic mitral valve regurgitation and symptomatic with LVEF >25% and LV internal diameter during systole
LVEF >25–60%
LVID-s ≥40–55 mm
New onset of atrial fibrillation
Pulmonary hypertension defined as pulmonary artery systolic pressure > 50 mm Hg at rest or >60 mm Hg with exercise

Key exclusion criteria
Recent myocardial infarction
Any interventional/surgical procedure within 30 days of the index procedure
Mitral valve orifice area < 4cm^2
Renal insufficiency, endocarditis, rheumatic heart disease
Previous mediastinal surgery in the first 27 patients

LVEF, left ventricular ejection fraction; LVID, left ventricular internal diameter.
Source: Feldman et al. 2009 / With permission of Elsevier.

Safety: The primary safety endpoint was freedom from 30-day major adverse events (MAEs), which consisted of death, myocardial infarction, nonelective cardiac surgery, renal failure, transfusion of >2 units of blood, reoperation for failed surgery, stroke, gastrointestinal complications requiring surgery, ventilation for >48 hours, deep wound infection, septicemia, and new-onset or permanent atrial fibrillation. Ten patients (9.1%) experienced a MAE. A single death occurred: a patient who did not receive a clip and had a relatively high Society of Thoracic Surgeons (STS) operative mortality score.

Efficacy: The primary composite efficacy endpoint was freedom from MR >2+, freedom from cardiac surgery for valve dysfunction, and freedom from death at 12 months. The efficacy endpoint was reached in 50 of 76 patients (66%). Of note, of the 79 treated patients with APS, 3 did not have an echocardiogram performed at 12 months.

The majority of patients required only one clip implantation (65 patients) vs. two clips (31 patients). The remaining 11 patients did not receive a clip. Of these 11 patients, 8 did not receive a clip due to inability to reduce MR, and 3 did not receive a clip due to transseptal complications.

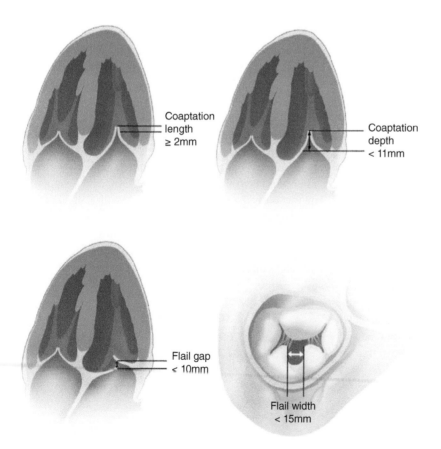

Figure 32.1 Anatomic criteria for placement of MitraClip device in EVEREST Phase 1. *Source:* Feldman et al. (2009) / with permission of Elsevier.

Significant MR reduction was achieved in 90% of the patients by successful clip placement or MV surgery following the clip attempt.

5. What was the basis of the EVEREST II trial?

Once feasibility and safety were established in Phase I, EVEREST II was developed to compare outcomes between percutaneous MV repair and surgical MV repair.

6. Describe the patient population in EVEREST II

Patients were enrolled in the trial if they had grade 3+ or 4+ chronic MR. Symptomatic patients required an EF greater than 25% and an end-systolic left ventricular diameter of 55 mm or less. Asymptomatic patients qualified if they met at least one of the following criteria: EF of 25–60%, end-systolic left ventricle (LV) diameter of 40–55 mm, new atrial fibrillation, or pulmonary hypertension.

Furthermore, the patients satisfied anatomical criteria such that the regurgitant jet originated from poor coaptation of the middle scallops of the anterior and posterior leaflets.

7. What were the endpoints for comparison used in EVEREST II?

The primary endpoint for efficacy was a composite outcome consisting of lack of death, MV surgery, and grade 3+ or 4+ MR at 12 months.

The primary safety endpoint was the same composite safety endpoint used in EVEREST Phase I consisted of the 30-day MAE rate and a composite of several components including death, myocardial infarction, stroke, renal failure, sepsis, new-onset or permanent atrial fibrillation, deep wound infection, mechanical ventilation for greater than two days, gastrointestinal complication requiring surgery, repeat operation for failed MV surgery, cardiovascular surgery, or transfusion of greater than two units of blood.

8. What were the results of EVEREST II?

Patients were randomized in a 2:1 ratio to receive either percutaneous MV repair or surgical repair.

The primary efficacy endpoint was reached by 55% of patients in the percutaneous repair group at 12 months and 73% of patients in the surgical repair group (p-value = 0.007).

The primary safety endpoint of MAEs by 30 days was reached in 15% of patients in the percutaneous repair group and 48% of patients in the surgical repair group.

41 patients (23%) in the percutaneous repair group had grade 3+ or 4+ MR before hospital discharge and were referred for surgery. However, all of the patients in the surgical group maintained MR severity of 2+ or less prior to discharge.

There was a greater reduction in the severity of MR in the surgery group than in the percutaneous repair group (p-value <0.001). Also important to note was that the reduction of MR to 1+ or less in the surgery group was more common after valve replacement than after valve repair.

In terms of quality of life, New York Heart Association (NYHA) functional class III or IV heart failure (HF) was present in 2% of patients in the percutaneous repair subgroup and 13% of those in the surgery subgroup at 12 months. Furthermore, quality of life improved from baseline in both groups but was transient at 30 days in the surgery group.

9. What are the takeaway messages of EVEREST II?

Although perhaps less effective at reducing MR, percutaneous edge-to-edge MV repair maintains a better safety profile than surgical repair and was associated with improved NYHA functional class and quality of life.

Secondary MR and Transcatheter Repair (COAPT Trial)

10. What was the purpose of the COAPT trial?

In heart failure with reduced ejection fraction (HFrEF), left ventricular dilation can result in displacement of the papillary muscles and chordae tendinae and lead to inadequate leaflet coaptation and ultimately secondary (functional) MR. Secondary MR carries a significant burden of decreased quality of life, increased hospitalizations for HF, and shorter survival.

Although the efficacy of surgical repair of primary MR is well established, surgical repair or replacement had not yet been shown to improve outcomes or mortality in patients with secondary MR.

The Cardiovascular Outcomes Assessment of the MitraClip Percutaneous Therapy for Heart Failure Patients with Functional Mitral Regurgitation (COAPT) trial was designed to assess whether percutaneous MV repair using the MitraClip device reduces hospitalizations and/or mortality among patients with moderate-to-severe or severe mitral regurgitation due to HFrEF (functional MR).

11. Describe the patient population of the COAPT trial.

The study population consisted of patients with ischemic or nonischemic cardiomyopathy and left ventricular EF of 20–50% with moderate-to-severe (3+) or severe (4+) secondary MR, who were symptomatic despite maximally tolerated medical therapy and/or cardiac resynchronization therapy if indicated.

Each participating site included a Heart Team consisting of a heart-failure specialist, an interventional cardiologist, and a cardiothoracic surgeon who assessed eligibility for device placement in each patient and confirmed that each patient was not a surgical candidate. A central committee assessed that each patient met enrollment criteria and would not undergo MV surgery, and categorized the patient's risk for surgical complications. Patients were assessed using the STS score for risk of death within 30 days after MV replacement, with high risk as 8% or higher or the presence of features portending high operative stroke risk or death.

Patients were randomly assigned to undergo transcatheter MV repair with guideline-directed medical therapy or to receive guideline-directed medical therapy alone.

12. What were the endpoints of the COAPT trial?

Efficacy: The primary efficacy endpoint was hospitalizations for HF within 24 months of follow-up. This included recurrent events in patients with multiple hospitalizations.

Safety: The primary safety endpoint was freedom from complications in relation to the MitraClip device at 12 months. Such complications included single leaflet attachment, embolization of the device, endocarditis leading to surgery, mitral stenosis leading to MV surgery, implantation of a left ventricular assist device, heart transplantation, or any device-related event leading to cardiovascular surgery.

Secondary endpoints: Secondary endpoints included MR grade 2+ or lower at 12 months, death from any cause at 12 months, death or hospitalization for HF within 24 months, change in Kansas City Cardiomyopathy Questionnaire (KCCQ) from baseline to 12 months, change in distance of six-minute walk test from baseline to 12 months, all hospitalizations for any reason within 24 months, NYHA class of I or II at 12 months, change in LV end-diastolic volume from baseline to 12 months, death from any cause within 24 months, and freedom from death from any cause/stroke/myocardial infarction/nonelective cardiovascular surgery for device-related complication at 30 days.

13. What were the results of the COAPT trial?

A total of 514 patients were enrolled, 302 in the device group and 312 in the control group. The etiology of cardiomyopathy was ischemic in 60.7% of patients and nonischemic in 39.3% of patients. Mean left ventricular EF was $31.3+/-9.3\%$, and MR grade was 3+ in 52.2% and 4+ in 47.8%.

Device implantation was attempted in 293 of the 302 (97%) patients, with one or more clips implanted in 98% of the 293 patients.

At the time of discharge, in the 260 patients in which echocardiography was performed, MR was 1+ or lower in 214 patients (82.3%), 2+ in 33 (12.7%), 3+ in 9 patients (3.5%), and 4+ in 4 patients (1.5%). The device group faced a 30-day rate of death of 2.3% and stroke of 0.7%:

- *Primary efficacy endpoint:* The device group had 160 total hospitalizations (in 92 patients) for HF within 24 months. The control group experienced 283 total hospitalizations (in 151 patients) for HF within 24 months (p-value <0.001).
- *Primary safety endpoint:* The rate of freedom from device complications at 12 months was 96.6% (p-value <0.001).
- *Secondary endpoints:* All-cause mortality was significantly lower in the device group compared to the control (29.1% vs. 46.1%, p <0.001). Quality of life, as assessed by change in KCCQ score and NYHA functional class, was also noted to be significantly better in the device group. Functional capacity measured through the six-minute walk test was better in the device group as well.

Mitral regurgitation grade of 2+ or lower was maintained in 94.8% of patients in the device group, as compared to 46.9% of patients in the control group (p < 0.001).

Subgroup analysis revealed a consistent treatment effect (lower rates of hospitalization for HF, death, and composite of death or hospitalization for HF) in the device group across all the examined subgroups. There was no noted interaction between the trial group and events according to age, sex, MR severity, LV function or volume, etiology of cardiomyopathy, or risk of surgery-related complications/ risk of death at baseline.

14. What are the takeaway messages from the COAPT trial?

The COAPT trial found that transcatheter MV repair in patients with HF with reduced EF and moderate-to-severe or severe secondary MR who were symptomatic despite guideline-directed medical therapy resulted in lower mortality, lower rate of hospitalization for HF, and improved functional status and quality of life within 24 months of follow-up compared to medical therapy alone. Furthermore, the goal of freedom from device-related complications was met.

15. What are the guidelines for transcatheter MV repair in secondary MR?

First-line therapy for secondary MR relies on guideline-directed medical therapy for HFrEF, both pharmacologic therapy and cardiac resynchronization therapy (if indicated). Assessment and treatment of coexisting coronary artery disease are also essential, including revascularization if necessary. In patients with moderate to severe or severe chronic secondary MR with left ventricular ejection fraction (LVEF) <50% who are symptomatic (NYHA II, III, or IV) while on optimal guideline-directed medical therapy for HF, transcatheter MV repair should be considered for patients with appropriate anatomy as determined on transesophageal echocardiography and with LVEF between 20% and 50%, LV end-systolic diameter ≤70 mm, and pulmonary artery systolic pressure ≤70 mmHg (Class 2A).

Bibliography

1 Alfieri, O., Maisano, F., De Bonis, M. et al. (2001). The double-orifice technique in mitral valve repair: a simple solution for complex problems. *J. Thorac. Cardiovasc. Surg.* 122: 674–681.

2 Asgar, A.W., Mack, M.J., and Stone, G.W. (2015). Secondary mitral regurgitation in heart failure: pathophysiology, prognosis, and therapeutic considerations. *J. Am. Coll. Cardiol.* 65: 1231–1248.

3 De Bonis, M. and Alfieri, O. (2010). The edge-to-edge technique for mitral valve repair. *Hsr Proceedings In Intensive Care & Cardiovascular Anesthesia* 2: 7–17.

4 Feldman, T., Foster, E., Glower, D.D. et al. (2011). Percutaneous repair or surgery for mitral regurgitation. *N. Engl. J. Med.* 364: 1395–1406.

5 Feldman, T., Kar, S., Rinaldi, M. et al. (2009). Percutaneous mitral repair with the MitraClip system: safety and midterm durability in the initial EVEREST (Endovascular Valve Edge-To-Edge REpair Study) cohort. *J. Am. Coll. Cardiol.* 54: 686–694.

6 Goar, F.G.S., Fann, J.I., Komtebedde, J. et al. (2003). Endovascular edge-to-edge mitral valve repair. *Circulation* 108: 1990–1993.

7 O'gara, P.T. and Mack, M.J. (2020). Secondary mitral regurgitation. *N. Engl. J. Med.* 383: 1458–1467.

8 Otto, C.M., Nishimura, R.A., Bonow, R.O. et al. (2021). 2020 ACC/AHA guideline for the management of patients with valvular heart disease: A report of the American College Of Cardiology/American Heart Association joint committee on clinical practice guidelines. *Circulation* 143: E72–E227.

9 Stone, G.W., Lindenfeld, J., Abraham, W.T. et al. (2018). Transcatheter mitral-valve repair in patients with heart failure. *N. Engl. J. Med.* 379: 2307–2318.

33

Mitral Valve TEER

The MitraClip Procedure

Sibi Krishnamurthy, Kelley N. Benck and Carlos E. Alfonso

Department of Medicine, Division of Cardiovascular Medicine, University of Miami Miller School of Medicine, Miami, FL, USA

Introduction

Mitral valve transcatheter edge-to-edge repair (TEER) was developed based on the analogous surgical Alfieri stitch procedure for surgical correction of mitral insufficiency. The MitraClip (Abbott Vascular) device was the first device to attain the CE mark and was approved by the US FDA in 2013 for transcatheter treatment of mitral valve regurgitation (Figure 33.1). During the TEER procedure, a clip is attached to both the anterior and posterior leaflets of the mitral valve, approximating the leaflets and thereby reducing the degree of mitral insufficiency. The MitraClip is delivered from venous access using a transseptal approach across the atrial septum into the left atrium. Initially validated for the treatment of degenerative mitral valve disease, subsequent studies have now proven safety and efficacy for the use in functional mitral valve insufficiency. Therefore, a broader subset of patients is now eligible for treatment with TEER.

1. What are the anatomical and pathophysiologic considerations of the mitral valve in evaluating patients for TEER?

The mitral valve is a bileaflet valve with an anteromedial leaflet and a posterolateral leaflet and has a complex subvalvular apparatus, including the chordae tendinae and papillar muscles. Mitral insufficiency can occur because of pathology involving the valve leaflets or the subvalvular apparatus. Degenerative mitral disease may result in redundancy and thickening of leaflets. Mitral insufficiency may occur because of either congenital disease such as prolapse, Barlow's or fibroelastic deficiency, or acquired valvular heart disease, such as in endocarditis, rheumatic, and ischemic heart disease. Carpentier proposed a classification system of mitral regurgitation (MR) into three types based on the function and pathophysiologic etiology of mitral insufficiency:

- *Type I:* Normal leaflet motion; annular dilation or leaflet perforation.
- *Type II:* Increased leaflet motion secondary to leaflet prolapse, chordal elongation, and/or rupture related to myxomatous disease, Ehlers-Danlos, Marfan's, or acute rupture from myocardial infarction (MI), traumatic injury, acute rheumatic insufficiency, or endocarditis.

- *Type IIIa:* Restricted leaflet motion during systole and diastole; subvalvular involvement with leaflet thickening, commissural or chordal fusion and shortening. Seen with rheumatic heart disease, Ergot lesions, Hurler disease, systemic erythematous lupus (SLE), radiation injury, infiltrative disease, antiphospholipid syndrome, or hypereosinophilia.
- *Type IIIb:* Restricted leaflet motion in systole; leaflet tethering by dyskinetic myocardial segments as seen in ischemic MR and secondary, FMR from dilated cardiomyopathy. It has been estimated that the largest number of people with MR fall into this category.

Mastering Structural Heart Disease, First Edition. Edited by Eduardo J. de Marchena and Camilo A. Gomez.
© 2023 John Wiley & Sons Ltd. Published 2023 by John Wiley & Sons Ltd.
Companion website: www.wiley.com/go/deMarchena/Mastering-Structural-Heart-Disease

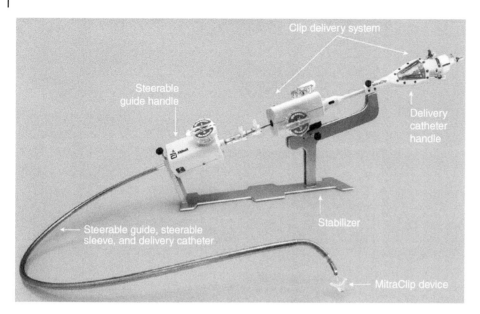

Figure 33.1 The components of the MitraClip system include the steerable guide catheter, the clip delivery system and handle, and the MitraClip device. The system is mounted on a stabilizer during the case. The clip delivery system is fed through the port on the back end of the steerable guide catheter. The clip delivery system can be articulated medial (M) or lateral (L) by the use of the M/L knob. The current generation delivery catheter handle allows for independent control of the gripper arms using the gripper lever and controls the clip locking using the lock lever. The opening/closing of the clip arms on the MitraClip is controlled via the white knob. The activation knob on the end is used during the release, and the release pin is removed during the final steps of clip release. *Source:* Sherif et al. (2017), Springer Nature, CC BY 4.0.

2. What is the difference between primary mitral valve insufficiency related to degenerative mitral valve disease and secondary functional mitral insufficiency?

In primary degenerative mitral regurgitation (DMR) valve pathology, there is a structurally abnormal or damaged valve, e.g. such as in myxomatous mitral valve disease, mitral valve prolapse, and fibroelastic deficiency or acquired as in rheumatic heart disease. Other causative factors of acquired primary MR include chordal rupture, flail leaflets, or endocarditis. Primary valvular insufficiency has traditionally been treated with surgical valve repair. Secondary or functional mitral regurgitation (FMR) occurs in the absence of leaflet pathology. Inadequate leaflet coaptation in FMR is primarily related to annular dilation, left ventricular dysfunction, and/or chordal tethering, leading to restricted leaflet motion. Surgical mitral repair is feasible in the setting of MR with ischemic disease or annular dilation, particularly if surgical coronary revascularization is planned, although the long-term outcomes are more variable.

3. What is the Heart Team approach to evaluation for mitral valve therapies?

Similar to the current evolution of the treatment of other structural heart pathologies, the management of mitral valve disease is best accomplished using a multidisciplinary team. The team includes interventional cardiologist(s), cardiothoracic surgeon(s), cardiac imaging specialists and echocardiographer(s), cardiac anesthesiologist(s), heart failure specialist(s), and ancillary staff including valve coordinator(s). The pre-procedural evaluation of potential patients determines their candidacy for TEER or if they would be better served with alternative treatments for mitral insufficiency. For patients with DMR, a surgical evaluation is essential, and patients with low to intermediate surgical risk may be better served with surgical valve repair. Unlike with transcatheter aortic valve replacement (TAVR), it is not necessary or required to have the surgeons directly involved with the transcatheter procedure. For patients with functional mitral valve insufficiency, the heart failure (HF) specialist is instrumental in ensuring that the patient is on guideline medical therapy while still evaluating candidacy for further therapies that may improve outcomes.

4. What patients are appropriate to consider for surgical mitral valve repair vs. the TEER procedure using the MitraClip device?

Patient selection is an important part of successful TEER. TEER has been evaluated for patients with symptomatic severe mitral valvular insufficiency. Surgical mitral valve repair remains a viable treatment and the standard for patients with symptomatic DMR with low to intermediate surgical risk. However, for those patients deemed at high or prohibitive risk for surgery, TEER using the MitraClip has been shown to be an effective treatment. Unlike with degenerative mitral valvular disease, in patients with FMR, the surgical data is more limited and less optimal. TEER with the MitraClip successfully reduces MR severity in patients with FMR.

5. What are the current indications for the TEER procedure using the MitraClip device?

TEER using the MitraClip is currently indicated for the reduction of symptomatic MR ($\geq$ 3+) for both DMR and FMR. TEER is indicated for patients with DMR at high or prohibitive risk for mitral valve surgery, with favorable anatomy, and without severe comorbidities that would diminish the benefit of TEER. MitraClip intervention also has a Class IIa recommendation in the ACC/AHA Guidelines for FMR when persistent heart failure symptoms are present despite optimal medical therapy and there is concomitant left ventricular systolic dysfunction with reduced left ventricle ejection fraction (LVEF) between 20% and 50% and a left ventricular end-systolic diameter (LVESD) $\leq$ 70 mm, with a pulmonary artery (PA) systolic pressure $\leq$ 70 mmHg.

6. Are there any absolute contraindications to TEER?

There are a few absolute contraindications to TEER, including:

- Severe mitral stenosis (MS)
- Patients with left atrial and/or left atrial appendage thrombus

- Active endocarditis or rheumatic disease of the mitral valve
- Intracardiac, inferior vena cava (IVC), or femoral venous thrombus
- Patients with an allergy or hypersensitivity to anticoagulation or antiplatelet regimens or clip components (nickel, titanium, cobalt, chromium, polyester), or a contrast sensitivity
- Comorbidities that limit life expectancy to <1 year

7. Aside from the absolute contraindications, what are the relative contraindications to be aware of for TEER?

While not contraindicated, patients with anticipated challenges with TEER include those with a difficult anatomical substrate that may preclude safely treating the patient with TEER or lead to long-term adverse outcomes. Therefore, some relative contraindications or considerations prior to TEER include:

- Mild to moderate MS
- Difficult transseptal access
- Small left atrium (LA)

8. Is the presence of a transcatheter atrial septal defect (ASD) occlusion device a contraindication for TEER?

While the presence of a prior ASD closure device may make the transseptal puncture technique more challenging, it is not an absolute contraindication for TEER or other "left-sided" structural heart interventions. Transseptal puncture for left-heart structural interventions remains feasible with a detailed understanding of the anatomical considerations and multimodality imaging for the transseptal puncture.

9. What are the important aspects and key questions in the pre-procedural imaging during the pre-operative evaluation for TEER?

Pre-procedural transesophageal imaging is critical for the evaluation of the mitral valve apparatus in patients being considered for TEER. Initially, it was important to differentiate the etiology of mitral valve pathology, i.e. whether the insufficiency was related to degenerative valve disease or secondary FMR, given that TEER was initially only approved for primary degenerative valve pathology. The approval of TEER for treatment of FMR has made this somewhat of a moot point. Nonetheless, a better understanding of the pathophysiology of valve disease remains critically important.

Factors that are critical to assess during pre-operative transesophageal echocardiography (TEE) include:

- Presence of LA or left atrial appendage (LAA) thrombus
- Mitral annular dimensions and mitral valve area (MVA)
- Adequacy of the atrial septum for transseptal puncture
- Location of mitral valve pathology
- Posterior leaflet size and/or restriction

10. In degenerative valve disease including mitral valve prolapse and/or flail mitral valve leaflets, what are the important aspects to assess during the pre-procedural TEE?

The coaptation depth is important to assess. It is also important to assess the flail gap in patients with severe prolapse and/or flail leaflets. In addition, the location of the prolapse is important to help guide clip deployment. A2-P2 prolapses are ideal for treatment, whereas more medial or lateral prolapses may be more difficult to treat.

11. What are the anatomical considerations for percutaneous TEER?

Based on the anatomic eligibility criteria for TEER from the EVEREST (Endovascular Valve Edge-to-Edge Repair Study) II trial, certain anatomical factors are predictive of favorable outcomes, including:

- A2-P2 pathology
- Coaptation length > 2 mm
- Coaptation depth < 11 mm
- Flail gap < 10 mm
- Flail width < 15 mm
- Mobile leaflet length > 1 cm

While many patients who fall outside the criteria have been successfully treated with TEER, certain anatomical findings are associated with less favorable outcomes,

including commissural lesions, short posterior leaflet, severe asymmetric tethering, calcification, severe annular calcification, mitral clefts, severe LV dilation and annular remodeling, a large extension of the regurgitant jet, and multi-scallop prolapse.

12. What are the minimal MVA requirements for TEER?

The presence of MS at baseline is a relative contraindication for TEER, as TEER can further reduce the effective MVA. Further small annular dimensions can increase the risk of development of iatrogenic MS during a mitral TEER. Generally, the recommended minimal MVA requirements for safe TEER without causing significant MS is > 4.0 mm^2.

13. What are the important aspects in the assessment of the atrial septum for adequate transseptal access?

Obtaining an adequate transseptal puncture is critically important for a successful TEER. For TEER, the ideal septal puncture should occur posterior and superior, at an adequate distance from the mitral valve annulus to allow optimal device delivery. Generally, at least 4.0–4.5 cm^2 are recommended distance between the mitral annular plane and the transseptal access point to ensure that the device can be delivered (Figure 33.2).

14. What are the current literature and trial results using TEER for the treatment of degenerative mitral valve insufficiency?

The EVEREST I trial was the first feasibility trial validating the use of the MitraClip to treat degenerative mitral valve insufficiency. In the EVEREST II trial, the MitraClip device was successfully placed in 96% of 78 patients, reducing MR in these high-risk surgical patients, which was associated with improvement in clinical symptoms as well as significant left ventricular reverse remodeling over 12 months as compared to a matched comparator group. The five-year results from the EVEREST II study show that beyond six months, the rates of surgery and moderate to severe MR were comparable between groups, and the five-year mortality was 26.8% in the percutaneously treated group as compared to 20.8% in

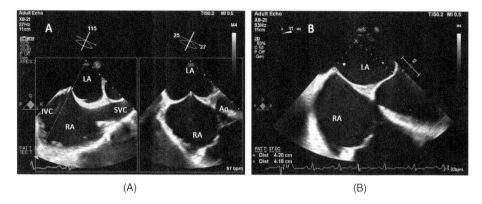

(A)   (B)

Figure 33.2 (a) Transesophageal echocardiography images during transseptal puncture demonstrating the bicaval and short-axis views and the right atrium (RA), left atrium (LA), aorta (Ao), superior vena cava (SVC), and inferior vena cava (IVC). The transseptal puncture should aim to be posterior and superior. (b) In a four-chamber view, the distance (height) between the tenting and the mitral annulus and coaptation plane is measured and should be 4–4.5 cm to allow for adequate device maneuvering in the LA.

the conventional mitral valve surgery group. The long-term safety and efficacy of the MitraClip in a cohort of high-surgical-risk patients were maintained for five years.

15. What are the current data for the treatment of functional mitral valve insufficiency?

There are currently two randomized controlled trials evaluating the safety and efficacy of TEER using the MitraClip for the treatment of secondary, functional mitral insufficiency: MITRA-FR (Percutaneous Repair with the MitraClip Device for Severe Functional/Secondary Mitral Regurgitation) and COAPT (Cardiovascular Outcomes Assessment of the MitraClip Percutaneous Therapy for Heart Failure Patients with Functional Mitral Regurgitation). The MITRA-FR trial was a European study that assigned patients with severe secondary MR, LVEF between 15% and 40%, and symptomatic heart failure to medical therapy alone versus medical therapy + TEER. TEER failed to demonstrate any decrease or benefit in the primary endpoint of death from any cause or unplanned hospitalization for heart failure at 12 months.

The COAPT trial was a multicenter, randomized, controlled, parallel-group, open-label trial of TEER with the MitraClip device in symptomatic patients with heart failure and moderate-to-severe or severe MR. A total of 614 patients were enrolled in the trial and had ischemic or nonischemic cardiomyopathy with a LVEF between 20% and 50%, moderate-to-severe (grade 3+) or severe (grade 4+) secondary MR, and New York Heart Association (NYHA) functional class II, III, or IVa congestive heart failure.

Whereas in the MITRA-FR study, the rate of death or unplanned hospitalization for heart failure at one year did not differ, the COAPT trial was able to demonstrate a benefit for TEER at two years. In the COAPT study, compared to maximal guideline-directed medical therapy alone, the addition of TEER for patients with symptomatic heart failure and severe secondary MR resulted in a lower rate of hospitalization for heart failure and lower all-cause mortality within 24 months.

16. Why do the results from the MITRA-FR and COAPT studies differ so significantly?

The clinical differences and conclusions between the two studies have been attributed to a few differences in study design. Even though the COAPT study had much stricter enrollment criteria for patients, its sample size was double the MITRA-FR study. The COAPT study's narrower inclusion criteria resulted in the enrollment of patients with greater MR severity but significantly less left ventricular damage, whereas the patients in MITRA-FR had larger LV end-diastolic volumes and a larger proportion of patients with moderate mitral insufficiency. Major procedural differences included an overall greater number of clips implanted per patient in the COAPT study, possibly leading to the higher prevalence of sustained MR reduction. Finally, the timing of medical therapy optimization is a noteworthy difference between the trials. The MITRA-FR study allowed adjustments in medical therapy to be made during follow-up to mimic real-world practice, while the COAPT study made the use of guideline-directed medical therapy (GDMT) an inclusion criterion, allowing for optimization to occur at baseline.

17. What are the real-world experience and outcomes using the MitraClip for TEER?

The COAPT trial showed device efficacy and long-term improvement in outcomes; however, its strict eligibility criteria raise questions of real-world applicability. A post-market surveillance study to evaluate the real-world clinical effectiveness and safety of TEER in the US based on data from the STS TVT registry demonstrated similar outcomes, with acute procedure success occurring in 91.8% and with low in-hospital mortality at 2.7%. The mortality at 30 days and one year were estimated at 5.2% and 25.8% for those patients with available linked data. Two further retrospective registry analyses have compared participants who would and wouldn't meet the COAPT trial's inclusion criteria. Both studies looked at patients with secondary MR and reported similar procedural success between the two groups but better long-term mortality outcomes for the COAPT-eligible group. Adamo et al. further investigated what components of the COAPT exclusion criteria were more likely to lead to adverse outcomes with MitraClip use. COAPT-ineligible patients with LV impairment had a higher risk of all-cause death at five years compared to COAPT-eligible patients, and those with right ventricular impairment and/or pulmonary hypertension had a greater incidence of mortality at two years. In a retrospective review of a real-world cohort of 1022 patients treated with TEER in the EuroSMR registry (European Registry of Transcatheter Repair for Secondary Mitral Regurgitation), the application of adapted COAPT enrollment criteria successfully identified a phenotype with lower mortality rates in these "COAPT-eligible" patients.

Although these studies support the efficacy of the MitraClip for COAPT-eligible patients, in some circumstances, COAPT-ineligible patients may benefit from the treatment as well. For example, a recent unpublished study reported better one-year survival for COAPT-ineligible patients compared to those treated with medical therapy alone, with survival at one year of 91.9%, which was similar to the COAPT-eligible patients who received the MitraClip. More recently, it has been suggested that the degree of secondary MR can be classified as proportionate or disproportionate, with those patients with a disproportionately large degree of MR when compared with the degree of LV dilatation benefiting most from TEER. Overall, the data from real-world registries consistently demonstrate a similar sustained reduction in MR severity, improved functional capacity, and lower mortality rates. Future data may continue to refine which patients may benefit more or less from TEER, and ultimately treatment decisions should continue to be made through a multidisciplinary Heart Team.

The MitraClip Device

18. What are the components of the MitraClip catheter system?

The Mitral Clip catheter system consists of the steerable guide catheter (SGC), the clip delivery system (CDS), and the MitraClip device (Figure 33.1). Once the device is introduced, it is positioned and secured within the stabilizer. The SGC can be rotated anterior or posterior (A vs. P) and has a knob (+/−), which allows for catheter deflection and steering during introduction into the body and across the septum. The CDS is introduced through a secure, air-tight seal at the back of the SGC. The CDS has a knob allowing for medial (M) vs. lateral (L) positioning. The implantable MitraClip features cobalt-chromium construction and a polyester cover that is designed to promote tissue growth and is delivered via the CDS. The delivery catheter handle has an independent gripper handle, a clip handle, and an activator knob for the final clip release mechanism.

19. What are the differences between the currently available clips?

The chief difference between the first-generation NT and next-generation XT mitral clips is the length of the clip arms. The G4 NT and NTW have clip arms measuring 9 mm and an overall tip-to-tip diameter of 17 mm. The current generation G4 XT and XTW have longer clip arms, each measuring 12 mm (instead of 9 mm), and an overall tip-to-tip diameter of 22 mm. In addition, the newer clips have a controlled gripper actuation (CGA) that gives the option to move the grippers simultaneously or independently, allowing for independent leaflet grasping.

20. Are there any evidence-based recommendations for using the NTR vs. XTR clips?

Real-world data from the EXPAND study demonstrated that in primary MR, the XTR clip, compared to the NTR, was associated with improved MR reduction for severe baseline MR, smaller annular dimensions, larger prolapse gaps, and complex disease in primary MR. Conversely, for secondary MR, there was no evidence of advantage for either clip.

Echocardiographic Imaging

21. What is the role of echocardiography and TEE during TEER?

TEER remains a largely echocardiographic-guided procedure. As such, procedural imaging and guidance during TEER are critical and essential both during the pre-procedural evaluation and throughout the procedure. During the procedure, intra-procedural imaging with TEE should be done by a dedicated physician with expertise in TEE and structural imaging of the mitral valve. The TEE operator can be a dedicated cardiologist with structural TEE experience or a cardiac anesthesiologist with a similar appropriate level of expertise with TEER and structural imaging. The exact make-up of the team may vary between institutions. The interventional cardiologist should also be familiar with the key images and views necessary during different stages of the TEER procedure and how to apply these effectively and interpret the images.

22. What are the essential TEE views to obtain during TEER?

There are various essential TEE views to be familiar with during TEER. The typical views are obtained from the mid-esophageal position by rotating and changing the omniplane angle. The views include:

- *Bicaval view* (90–120°): Allows for superior-inferior orientation of the atrial septum to guide transseptal puncture and demonstrates the superior vena cava (SVC) and IVC, right atrium (RA), and LA with a superior and inferior orientation of the atrial septum. While biplane imaging can provide simultaneous bicaval and short-axis views, it should be recognized that these views are not completely orthogonal and should be used with caution (Figure 33.2)
- *Short axis:* Provides a medial-lateral view of the atrial septum, which allows for adequate anteroposterior positioning during transseptal puncture.
- *Four chamber view* – (0–20°) – During the transseptal puncture, the four-chamber view allows for measuring the distance between septal tenting and the coaptation plane to ensure the adequate height of puncture prior to transseptal puncture.
- *Commissural view* (60–90°): Provides medial-lateral positioning of the clip during TEER. It cuts through the P1,

A2, and P3 scallops as you go from the anterolateral to posteromedial aspects.
- *Long-axis LV outflow tract* (LVOT) view (120°): Provides a view of both anterior and posterior mitral valve leaflets. Used for anterior/posterior positioning and for grasping, as the gripper arms should only be visible in the long-axis view.
- *En face mitral valve view* (0–30°): Allows for viewing all three scallops of both the anterior and posterior mitral leaflets in a surgeon's view. Additional 3D TEE imaging allows for better characterization, and while the typical view is from the LA perspective, it can be done from either an LA or LV perspective; The en face view allows for orienting the clip perpendicular to the mitral orifice and positioning the clip in the affected area during TEER; it also is used to confirm that an adequate tissue bridge is present after grasping.

Procedure

23. What are the steps involved in TEER?

The approach involved with TEER includes a sequential series of maneuvers, including:

1. Vascular access
2. Transseptal crossing, guide, and delivery system insertion
3. Steering and advancing the clip into the LA
4. Clip alignment to the line of coaptation
5. Leaflet grasping
6. Clip deployment and removal

24. What are the preferred access site and vascular closure approaches during TEER?

Right common femoral vein access is preferred and remains the primary access point for TEER. Best practice for vascular access involves the use of ultrasound-guided vascular access. The SGC is a large-bore 24F system. Vascular closure can be obtained with a suture-mediated pre-closure technique using the Perclose ProGlide (Abbott Vascular) device, a "figure 8" suture technique, or manual compression.

25. What equipment is necessary for transseptal puncture for TEER?

The transseptal puncture can be performed with a regular, standard transseptal needle such as a Brockenbrough needle and Mullins sheath, although more specialty sheaths and needles have been developed to facilitate the transseptal puncture. Equipment includes:

- *Transseptal sheath*
  - Mullins sheath and dilator
  - Agilis NxT steerable introducers (St. Jude Medical)
  - Terumo Nagare steerable sheath
  - Acutus Medical AcQCross™ transseptal access system

- *Transseptal needles*
  - Standard Brockenbrough needle (BRK, St. Jude Medical)
  - BRK series of transseptal needles (BRK, BRK-1, and BRK-2)
  - HEARTSPAN (Biosense Webster)
  - Baylis radiofrequency transseptal needle – (Baylis Medical)

The Agilis NxT steerable introducers are specialized catheters with adjustable curves that may be particularly suitable for complex anatomy. Application of a surgical Bovie (Bovie Medical) to the BRK needle can be used to assist in crossing and cauterizing the way through the septum. The Bovie technique or a Baylis radiofrequency needle may be particularly useful in difficult cases such as a hyperelastic or thickened septum. The Baylis transseptal needle uses radiofrequency energy to facilitate crossing. In addition, the VersaCross (Baylis Medical) system, which combines a transseptal needle with radiofrequency on a shaped and curved wire for positioning in the LA, reduces the number of wire exchanges and may reduce procedural time.

26. What is the procedure for transseptal puncture for TEER?

A well-positioned transseptal puncture is a critical first step to an overall successful TEER procedure. A transseptal puncture can be performed via the conventional procedure. After initial venous access, a multipurpose (MP) catheter can be advanced over a 0.032″ wire to the SVC under fluoroscopic guidance. Afterward, the catheter and sheath are removed, and a transseptal sheath and dilator are advanced into the SVC. The transseptal needle is advanced to the distal tip of the dilator, and the system is oriented to the 4 to 5 o'clock position.

Under both fluoroscopic and TEE guidance, the sheath/needle system is slowly pulled down from the SVC junction into the RA. Two subtle drops can be felt as the needle pulls back into the RA and then the fossa ovalis, respectively. TEE imaging during puncture is critically important at this point to obtain an adequate postero-superior transseptal position.

27. What are the optimal TEE views during transseptal puncture?

The typical optimal views used during transseptal puncture include:

- Short-axis aortic valve view (medial-lateral view)
- Bicaval view (superior-inferior view)
- Four-chamber view

During the pullback, the TEE is focused on a bicaval view, which provides a superior-inferior orientation of the septum as the needle and sheath pull back from the SVC to the RA. The short-axis aortic valve view then provides an anterior/posterior orientation of the atrial septum (Figure 33.2). The aortic valve sits anteriorly; thus, with gentle tenting of the septum in a short-axis view, the transseptal needle is moved away from the aortic valve in a posterior direction by rotating the needle clockwise. This will give the puncture more height and increase the distance from the transseptal puncture to the mitral annular plane. The four-chamber view is finally used to measure the annular distance from the puncture site and eventual CDS crossing to the coaptation plane.

28. What is the optimal positioning for transseptal puncture for TEER?

The optimal position is a posterior superior position on the interatrial septum. The height of the puncture above the annular plane of the mitral valve may depend on the type of pathology. For FMR, a height of 3.5–4 cm from the transseptal puncture is adequate, given that the line of coaptation is often below the annulus. For degenerative MR, a height of 4–4.5 cm is recommended and higher for flail leaflets. During transseptal puncture, a clockwise rotation of the needle moves the tip posterior, away from the mitral valve plane, and increases transseptal height. This allows for the necessary distance to position the clip optimally. Once adequate positioning is confirmed, the transseptal puncture is performed and the transseptal needle is advanced into the LA. Heparin should be administered at this point to maintain an adequate activated clotting time (ACT).

29. How is the delivery system advanced into the LA?

After the transseptal sheath is advanced into the LA, an Amplatz wire is advanced into the L superior pulmonary vein. A multipurpose catheter can be used to direct a stiff 0.035-in. guidewire into the left upper pulmonary vein (Figure 33.3a,b). Alternatively, a Toray or ProTrack wire can be looped in the LA. The VersaCross wire facilitates this step as the wire is pre-shaped with loops that stabilize the LA position and prevention migration back across the septum; therefore, once positioned in the LA, no further manipulation is necessary. It is over this guidewire that the transseptal sheath is exchanged out for the SGC. The guide should be positioned posteriorly toward the L superior pulmonary vein, as this allows for the longest distance in the LA. The guide is pulled back to keep above 1 cm of guide across the septum (Figure 33.3c,d). The guidewire and dilator are then retracted and removed in tandem to avoid introducing air into the system.

30. How is the delivery system advanced into the LA and directed toward the mitral valve leaflets?

Afterward, with the sheath positioned across the septum, the delivery system and clip are advanced into the guide

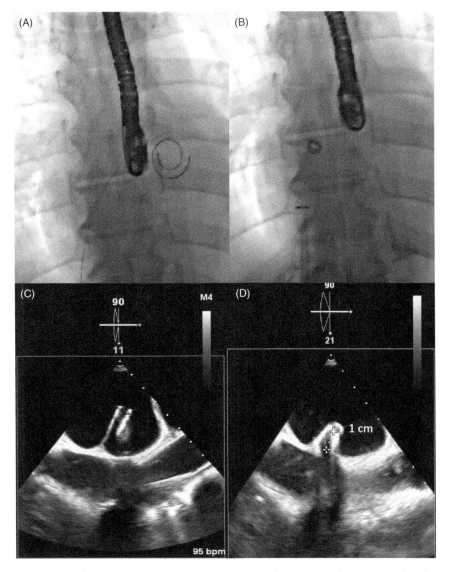

Figure 33.3 After transseptal puncture is performed, the transseptal needle and sheath are advanced into the left atrium, and (a) a stabilization wire such as the TORAYGUIDE or VersaCross wire is advanced in the left atrium. (b) The delivery sheath is then advanced over the wire. (c) The delivery sheath can be seen by transesophageal echocardiography and (d) is pulled back across the septum, allowing for approximately 1 cm to remain across the atrial septum.

sheath. The clip is externalized in the LA and then slowly advanced toward the left upper pulmonary vein (Figure 33.4). The delivery device is straddled across the guide sheath by observing that the markers on the CDS are positioned on either side of the SGC. Then medial rotation is applied using the M knob, actuating the device to bend away from the upper pulmonary vein, past the "coumadin ridge" and LA appendage, and toward the mitral annulus. Gentle repositioning of the system (advancing or retracting) may be needed during this step to adjust the device and clip position within the LA. The en face view of the mitral valve can be used to determine the medial lateral position of the clip along the mitral annulus and the orientation of the clip in relation to the mitral valve prior to advancing the clip across the valve.

31. What are the steps for grasping the leaflets with the MitraClip?

A 3D en face view on TEE is used to visualize the open clip and position it perpendicular to the coaptation line (Figure 33.5). The handle can be rotated clockwise with simultaneous short, rapid, back-and-forth movements to orient the clip perpendicular to the mitral opening at the intended grasping position. Positioning should be optimized while still in the LA, as repositioning in the LV can cause chordal entrapment. Once adequately positioned and oriented, the clip is advanced into the LV and reexamined with imaging to ensure that no rotational movement has occurred. The LVOT view on TEE is used, as it provides superior visualization and spatial resolution of the clip arms, grippers, and insertion of valve leaflets. The clip arms are opened, positioned at a 120° angle, and pulled back until the leaflets are firmly captured (Figure 33.6). The newer device allows for independent leaflet grasping in difficult anatomy. Once both leaflets are adequately grasped, the clip is gradually closed, and the grasp is assessed.

32. Prior to deployment, how is the MitraClip assessed to ensure adequate position, grasp, and results?

After leaflet grasping, the residual regurgitation is assessed by color Doppler with the clip arms fully closed. If significant regurgitation is still present, the leaflets can be released and the clip repositioned following the same procedure. Optimal positioning and grasp are also assessed to confirm an adequate tissue bridge and a lack of significant motion of the leaflets (Figure 33.6). Excessive motion may indicate inadequate grasp and signal an increased risk of clip detachment. Once secure, the clip is released, and the CDS handle is removed.

33. How do you assess mitral valve stenosis during clip deployment?

Prior to deployment, it is also important to assess the degree of MS with the clip attached (Figure 33.7). Measurement of MS can best be done by measuring the mitral diastolic gradients using pulse wave Doppler across the mitral valve. An optimal result will yield mean mitral gradients ≤4 mmHg. If significant MS with gradients ≥8 mmHg occurs, then consideration should be given to repositioning and regrasping or removing the clip altogether.

34. What should you do if the device becomes entrapped in the chordal apparatus during TEER?

During TEER, advancement of the system across the mitral valve can sometimes lead to chordal entrapment. Chordal entrapment can cause worsening MR or other injuries requiring surgical fixation. If suspected, avoid rotating the system. TEE and fluoroscopy should be used to assess the position of the device. Once confirmed, invert the clip, raise and lower the grippers, and carefully retract the device into the LA. If this fails, surgery may be required.

35. After deployment, how is the adequacy of the edge-to-edge repair assessed?

Intra-procedure TEE is used to assess the degree of residual MR. The stability of the deployed clip is assessed in multiple views, with the 3D en-face view in particular useful to assess an adequate tissue bridge. MV gradients should be assessed to avoid significant MS (>5 mmHg), which would prevent further clip deployments. Continuous LA pressure monitoring can be a useful adjunct to TEE for real-time assessment. The degree of LA v-wave reduction has been

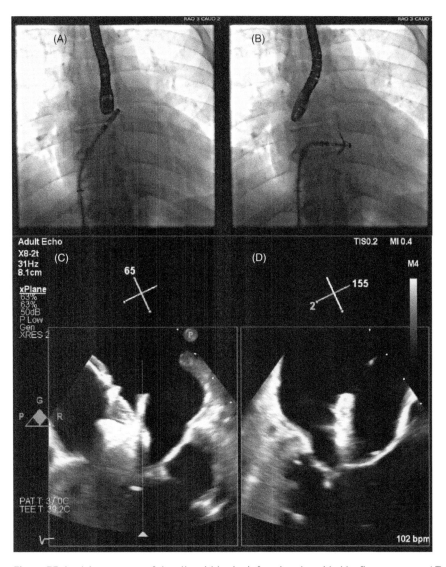

Figure 33.4 Advancement of the clip within the left atrium is guided by fluoroscopy and Transesophageal echocardiography (TEE). (a) The clip is advanced through the delivery system, and the handle is "straddled" across the delivery sheath. (b) The clip is then articulated medially by using the M knob toward the valve plane. (c) On TEE imaging, the open clip arms can be seen. (d) In the commissural view, the medial/lateral positioning of the clip is confirmed prior to crossing the mitral valve.

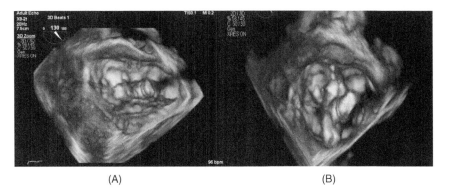

Figure 33.5 (a) The 3D surgeon's en face view of the valve also allows for positioning of the clip at the appropriate medial/lateral position along the mitral coaptation plane, usually at the A2/P2 position. (b) Rotating the handle clockwise or counterclockwise adjusts the orientation of the clip arms perpendicular to the valve leaflets prior to advancement into the left ventricle.

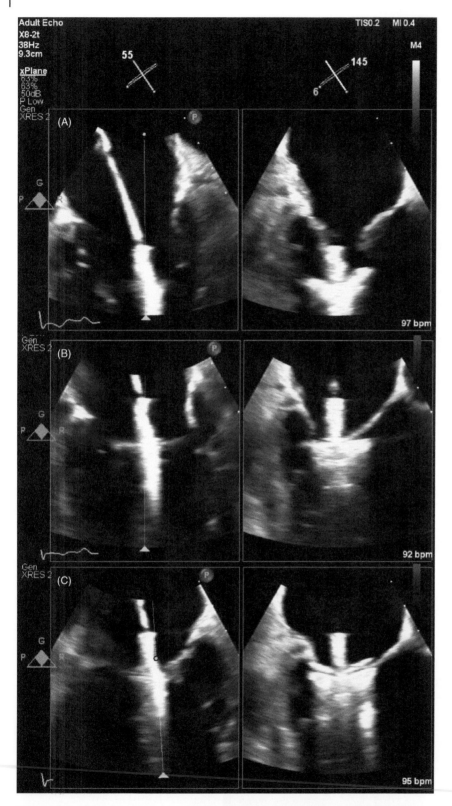

Figure 33.6 Clip advancement and leaflet grasping. (a) In the left ventricular outflow tract view, the clip arms and both posterior and anterior mitral leaflets are visible. (b) The clip is gradually pulled back with the arms in the open position and rotated posterior or anterior to engage both mitral valve leaflets. (c) Once the leaflets are engaged, the gripper arms are dropped down to grasp both leaflets between the clip arm and the gripper.

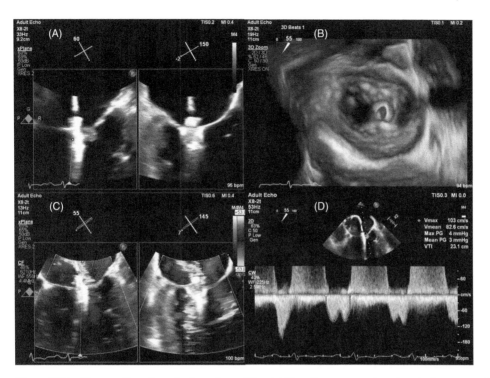

Figure 33.7 Final confirmation of adequate position. (a) The clip arms are closed and adequate position and leaflet grasp are confirmed in the commissural and LVOT views. (b) The en face view allows confirming an adequate tissue bridge. (c) Color Doppler across the valve can assess the degree of residual dysfunction. (d) Pulse wave Doppler across the mitral valve is performed to assess the degree of mitral stenosis, and confirm that the mean mitral gradients remain <7 mmHg.

shown to predict improvement of 6-minute walk distance at 30 days post-procedure.

36. If there is residual MR after the initial MitraClip, can additional clips be placed? How does the operator decide when and how to deliver additional clips during TEER?

Additional clips can be placed, especially if there is still significant regurgitation and the anatomy is favorable for more clips. The clips should be placed as close to each other as possible, and the successive clips are usually easier to deploy lateral to the prior one. To minimize interference with the first clip, the second clip should be advanced from LA into LV, either closed or at an angle no greater than 60°. Fluoroscopy can also be used to assess the positioning of the clips next to each other. Development of MS (MV gradients > 5 mmHg) post-clip deployment has been associated with increased all-cause mortality and should limit the placement of more clips.

Special Patient Subgroups and Considerations

37. Can TEER still be used in patients with complex mitral valve pathology?

Significant anatomical mitral pathologies remain highly challenging for TEER cases and require thorough pre-procedural imaging and planning. Most of these cases have only been performed in patients who are prohibitive for surgical intervention. Recent advances in clip design, including longer arms, have led to some improved outcomes in some of these subsets of patients. The presence of MS at baseline should be carefully assessed, particularly when the annular dimensions are small. In these cases, careful assessment is required as the risk of worsening MS is significant during TEER. During the procedure, it is advisable to check mitral valve gradients after each clip prior to deployment and, if significant MS is noted, to remove and not deploy the clip.

38. Can TEER still be used in patients with mitral valve and/or mitral annular calcification?

Calcification of the mitral valve leaflets may be of concern for the MitraClip as significant mitral leaflet calcification has been found to be a poor predictor of MitraClip outcomes. However, recent studies show that if the calcifications are limited to just the annulus, despite moderate to severe MAC, TEER is feasible and can be used safely with similar procedural success and one-year outcomes. Therefore, if the mitral calcification is limited to MAC without concomitant leaflet calcification, it should not preclude a patient from being considered for TEER.

39. What are the applications and limitations of TEER in patients with restricted posterior mitral valves, mitral valve clefts, and/or flail mitral valve leaflets?

In patients with small, tethered, and restricted posterior leaflets, ensuring adequate posterior leaflet grasping during TEER is a challenge. While the independent grasping technology may facilitate leaflet grasping, it remains paramount to ensure that an adequate amount of tissue is grasped. For optimal MitraClip use in the restricted posterior leaflet population, the length should at least be 7 mm in order to obtain a good grasp by the device.

Regarding patients with Barlow pathology of the mitral valve, while TEER is feasible, the procedure is technically more challenging with perhaps less favorable long-term outcomes. Given the significant tissue redundancies and atypical anatomy of Barlow disease, procedure times were noted to be longer with more device implants, lower durability of procedural results,

and a trend toward more hospitalization with heart failure at three years.

While the EVEREST II trial excluded patients with large flails (flail segment width ≥ 15 mm or flail gap ≥ 10 mm), the newer and longer clips have facilitated the use of TEER for flail leaflets, and good outcomes have been achieved. An anchor technique can be used in which an initial clip stabilizes the valve and flail segment for implantation of a second clip for extremely flail segments. Acute mitral valve insufficiency following myocardial infarction (MI) has been successfully treated with TEER. Therefore, the presence of a flail segment, or recent MI with acute MR, should not exclude patients from being considered for TEER, but these cases should be carefully evaluated on a case-by-case basis. There has been no significant use of TEER for leaflet perforations. Isolated case reports have described the use of TEER in combination with a transcatheter Amplatzer cribriform device in isolated cases at prohibitive surgical risk. The long-term outcomes of TEER for mitral insufficiency in the case of perforation remain undetermined and largely experimental.

Conclusion

Mitral clip edge-to-edge repair with the MitraClip system has proven effective for treating both primary and secondary functional mitral insufficiency with excellent acute procedural results and short- to intermediate-term clinical outcomes. The TEER procedure is performed by following best practices and a sequential stepwise approach. Transesophageal echocardiographic intra-procedural imaging remains key throughout the procedure to ensure safe and appropriate transseptal puncture, guide optimal clip positioning, and assess the immediate procedural results and reduction of mitral insufficiency. Future modifications may continue to improve applications, results, and applicability to complex anatomy and patient subsets.

Bibliography

1 Adamo, M., Grasso, C., Capodanno, D. et al. (2019). Five-year clinical outcomes after percutaneous edge-to-edge mitral valve repair: insights from the multicenter GRASP-IT registry. *Am. Heart J.* 217: 32–41.

2 Carpentier, A. (1983). Cardiac valve surgery – the "French correction". *J. Thorac. Cardiovasc. Surg.* 86 (3): 323–337.

3 Cheng, R., Tat, E., Siegel, R.J. et al. (2016). Mitral annular calcification is not associated with decreased procedural

success, durability of repair, or left ventricular remodelling in percutaneous edge-to-edge repair of mitral regurgitation. *EuroIntervention* 12 (9): 1176–1184.

4 De Bonis, M., Al-Attar, N., Antunes, M. et al. (2015). Surgical and interventional management of mitral valve regurgitation: a position statement from the European Society of Cardiology Working Groups on Cardiovascular Surgery and Valvular Heart Disease. *Eur. Heart J.* 37 (2): 133–139.

5 de Marchena, E., Badiye, A., Robalino, G. et al. (2011). Respective prevalence of the different carpentier classes of mitral regurgitation: a stepping stone for future therapeutic research and development. *J Cardiac Surg.* 26 (4): 385–392.

6 Estévez-Loureiro, R., Shuvy, M., Taramasso, M. et al. (2021). Use of MitraClip for mitral valve repair in patients with acute mitral regurgitation following acute myocardial infarction: effect of cardiogenic shock on outcomes (IREMMI Registry). *Catheter. Cardiovasc. Interv.* 97 (6): 1259–1267.

7 Feldman, T.,.K.S.,.R.M. et al. (2009). Percutaneous mitral repair with the MitraClip system: safety and midterm durability in the initial EVEREST (Endovascular Valve Edge-to-Edge REpair Study) cohort. *J. Am. Coll. Cardiol.* 54 (8): 686–694.

8 Feldman, T., Kar, S., Elmariah, S. et al. (2015). Randomized comparison of percutaneous repair and surgery for mitral regurgitation: 5-year results of EVEREST II. *J. Am. Coll. Cardiol.* 66 (25): 2844–2854.

9 Fernández-Peregrina, E., Pascual, I.P., Freixa, X.F. et al. (2021). Percutaneous edge-to-edge mitral repair in the presence of mitral annulus calcification. *EuroIntervention* .

10 Flint, N., Price, M.J., Little, S.H. et al. (2021). State of the art: transcatheter edge-to-edge repair for complex mitral regurgitation. *J. Am. Soc. Echocardiogr.* 34 (10): 1025–1037.

11 Gheorghe, L.L., Mobasseri, S., Agricola, E. et al. (2021). Imaging for native mitral valve surgical and transcatheter interventions. *JACC Cardiovasc. Imaging* 14 (1): 112–127.

12 Glower, D.D., Kar, S., Trento, A. et al. (2014). Percutaneous mitral valve repair for mitral regurgitation in high-risk patients: results of the EVEREST II study. *J. Am. Coll. Cardiol.* 64 (2): 172–181.

13 Grayburn, P.A., Sannino, A., and Packer, M. (2019). Proportionate and disproportionate functional mitral regurgitation: a new conceptual framework that reconciles the results of the MITRA-FR and COAPT trials. *JACC: Cardiovasc. Imaging* 12 (2): 353–362.

14 Iliadis, C., Metze, C., Korber, M.I. et al. (2020). Impact of COAPT trial exclusion criteria in real-world patients undergoing transcatheter mitral valve repair. *Int. J. Cardiol.* 316: 189–194.

15 Inohara, T., Gilhofer, T., Luong, C. et al. (2022). VersaCross radiofrequency system reduces time to left atrial access versus conventional mechanical needle. *J. Interv. Card. Electrophysiol.* 63 (1): 9–12.

16 Kar, S., Feldman, T., Qasim, A. et al. (2019). Five-year outcomes of transcatheter reduction of significant mitral regurgitation in high-surgical-risk patients. *Heart* 105 (21): 1622–1628.

17 Koell, B., Orban, M., Weimann, J. et al. (2021). Outcomes Stratified by Adapted Inclusion Criteria After Mitral Edge-to-Edge Repair. *J. Am. Coll. Cardiol.* 78 (24): 2408–2421.

18 Maisano, F. (2020). Clip selection strategy and outcomes with MitraClip™ (NTR/XTR): Evidence-based recommendations from the global EXPAND study. PCR 2020.

19 Maisano, F., Torracca, L., Oppizzi, M. et al. (1998). The edge-to-edge technique: a simplified method to correct mitral insufficiency. *Eur. J. Cardiothorac. Surg.* 13 (3): 240–246.

20 Nishimura, R.A. and Bonow, R.O. (2018). Percutaneous repair of secondary mitral regurgitation — A tale of two trials. *N. Engl. J. Med.* 379 (24): 2374–2376.

21 Obadia, J.F., Messika-Zeitoun, D., Leurent, G. et al. (2018). Percutaneous repair or medical treatment for secondary mitral regurgitation. *N. Engl. J. Med.* 379 (24): 2297–2306.

22 Otto, C.M., Nishimura, R.A., Bonow, R.O. et al. (2021). 2020 ACC/AHA guideline for the management of patients with valvular heart disease: executive summary: a report of the American College of Cardiology/American Heart Association Joint Committee on clinical practice guidelines. *Circulation* 143 (5): e35–e71.

23 Paulsen, J.M. and Smith, T.W. (2016). Echocardiographic imaging of the mitral valve for transcatheter edge-to-edge repair. *Interv. Cardiol. Clin.* 5 (1): 17–31.

24 Pibarot, P., Delgado, V., and Bax, J.J. (2019). MITRA-FR vs. COAPT: lessons from two trials with diametrically opposed results. *Eur. Heart J. Cardiovasc. Imag.* 20 (6): 620–624.

25 Singh, G.D., Smith, T.W., and Rogers, J.H. (2015). Multi-MitraClip therapy for severe degenerative mitral regurgitation: "Anchor" technique for extremely flail segments. *Catheter. Cardiovasc. Interv.* 86 (2): 339–346.

26 Sorajja, P., Vemulapalli, S., Feldman, T. et al. (2017). Outcomes with transcatheter mitral valve repair in the United States: an STS/ACC TVT registry report. *J. Am. College Cardiol.* 70 (19): 2315–2327.

27 Stone, G.W., Lindenfekd, J., Abraham, W.T. et al. (2018). Transcatheter mitral-valve repair in patients with heart failure. *N. Engl. J. Med.* 379 (24): 2307–2318.

28 Thaden, J.J., Malouf, J.F., Nkomo, V.T. et al. (2018). Mitral valve anatomic predictors of hemodynamic success with transcatheter mitral valve repair. *J. Am. Heart Assoc.* 7 (2): e007315.

29 Whitlow, P.L., Feldman, T., Pedersen, W.R. et al. (2012). Acute and 12-month results with catheter-based mitral valve leaflet repair: the EVEREST II (Endovascular Valve Edge-to-Edge Repair) High Risk Study. *J. Am. Coll. Cardiol.* 59 (2): 130–139.

30 Zancanaro, E., Buzzatt, N., Denti, P. et al. (2019). Applicability of the COAPT trial in the real world. PCR London Valves., November 17, London, England.

34

TEER Challenging Anatomy and MitraClip Tips and Tricks

Houman Khalili[1,2], Hamza Lodhi[1,2], Adithya Mathews[1,2] and Brijeshwar Maini[1,2]

[1] Department of Cardiovascular Diseases, Florida Atlantic University, Boca Raton, FL, USA
[2] Cardiology, Delray Medical Center, Delray Beach, FL, USA

Introduction

1. What are the Alfieri stitch and transcatheter edge-to-edge repair techniques?

Alfieri described a simple surgical edge-to-edge stitch technique for anterior mitral valve (MV) prolapse by apposing the middle scallops of the anterior and posterior leaflets, thereby creating a double-orifice valve. Although the surgical technique was mostly utilized as a bailout strategy for surgical repair of the MV, it provided the idea for a catheter-based technique to achieve a similar anatomical result. During the past two decades, transcatheter edge-to-edge repair (TEER) techniques have steadily grown as the percutaneous method of choice and have revolutionized the treatment of mitral regurgitation (MR). MitraClip (Abbott) remains the only FDA-approved device in the United States for this application and has widespread use both in the United States and Europe. The EVEREST-II (Endovascular Valve Edge-to-Edge Repair Study) and COAPT (Cardiovascular Outcomes Assessment of the MitraClip Percutaneous Therapy for Heart Failure Patients with Functional Mitral Regurgitation) trials provide the evidence for the use of MitraClip in patients with degenerative and functional MR.

2. What is the MitraClip system?

The MitraClip system includes a steerable guide catheter (SGC) (24 Fr tapers to 22 Fr) and a clip delivery system (CDS), which houses the detachable clip. The clip is a two-armed Nitinol mechanical device covered with a Dacron polyester fabric; it is opened and closed by a complex set of mechanisms contained in the CDS. The inner portion of the clip contains a U-shaped barbed gripper for each arm that can be raised and lowered and help capture and secure each leaflet. The Dacron polyester fabric aids with the endothelialization and healing of the valve and maintains the two leaflets' coaptation.

The initial anatomical criteria for the use of MitraClip – based on the EVEREST-II clinical trial inclusion and exclusion criteria – was restricted to mid-A2/P2 pathologies with sufficient coaptation and excluded complex MV anatomies (Table 34.1). However, there have been several iterations of the MitraClip system over the past several years. These improvements provide more responsive steering and grasping, an independent gripper mechanism, and clip arms with varying sizes to accommodate more complex anatomies: myxomatous valves, flail leaflets with large gaps, and calcified MV.

Despite the availability of newer-generation devices to treat complex MV lesions, operator experience plays an important role in procedural and clinical success. All factors need to be considered when determining eligibility for the MitraClip procedure (Table 34.2).

MitraClip for the Myxomatous Mitral Valve

3. What are the anatomical findings of myxomatous mitral valve disease?

Diffuse myxomatous degeneration (DMD; i.e. Barlow's) is characterized by disruption of the leaflet matrix structure.

Table 34.1 Inclusion and exclusion criteria for the EVEREST-II trial.

Inclusion criteria

Grade ≥3 MR

Symptomatic or asymptomatic with one or more of the following:

Recent-onset atrial fibrillation

LVEF between 25 and 60%

LVESD >40 mm

Pulmonary hypertension (resting PASP >50 mmHg or >60 mmHg with exercise)

Candidate for MV surgery

Primary regurgitant jet originating from the A2-P2 scallops; secondary jet clinically insignificant

Exclusion criteria

No MI in the prior 12 wk

MV orifice area <4 cm^2

LVEF <25% or LVESD >55 mm

Flail segment width ≥15 mm or flail gap ≥10 mm

Leaflet tethering with coaptation depth >11 mm or coaptation length <2 mm

Severe MAC

Calcifications at the grasping area

Significant cleft

Bileaflet flail or severe bileaflet prolapse

Prior MV surgery

LVEESD, left ventricular end-systolic diameter; LVEF, left ventricular ejection fraction; MAC, mitral annular calcification; MI, myocardial infarction; MR, mitral regurgitation; PASP, pulmonary artery systolic pressure.

Expansion of the spongiosa layer leads to thickening of the leaflets and prolapse of multiple leaflet segments and scallops. Multiple MV lesions typically account for the resulting mitral regurgitation (MR) in patients with DMD. Although a flail leaflet due to chordal rupture may account for the largest MR jet, MV prolapse due to chordal elongation, large coaptation gap due to severe annular dilatation, and presence of calcification may lead to the presence of multiple jets. Moreover, leaflet grasp of the flail segment can be difficult due to thickened leaflets and a large coaptation gap. DMD anatomy was an exclusion criterion in the original EVEREST-II trial; however, treatment of DMD patients using the new iterations of the MitraClip system is feasible. Following are several considerations that may aid in treating DMD with TEER.

Table 34.2 Anatomical considerations for patient selection.

Beginner case	Intermediate experience	High-volume center
Central A2/P2	Commissural	Grasping zone with calcium
No calcification	Calcium at annulus but none at grasping zone	MVA <3 cm^2
MVA >4 cm^2	MVA >3 cm^2	Posterior leaflet <7 mm and presence of cleft
Posterior leaflet >10 mm	Posterior leaflet 7–10 mm or presence of cleft	Carpentier IIIA, rheumatic
Tenting height, 10 mm	Tenting height >10 mm	Multiple segments prolapse, Barlow
Normal leaflets and mobility	Carpentier IIIB	
Flail gap <10 mm, flail width <15 mm	Flail width >15 mm	

MVA, mitral valve area.
Both anatomical factors and individual operator and center experience should be considered to maximize procedural success.

4. Where are some key strategies to increase success in TEER treatment of DMD?

First, careful attention should be paid to obtaining transseptal puncture, as sufficient height (4.5–5.0 cm) is needed for grasping the high coaptation points in DMD. An inferior and posterior puncture may be needed to accommodate a medial A3/P3 lesion.

Second, the lesion accounting for the largest MR jet needs to be targeted first. This is usually a flail or leaflet segment with the highest mobility/prolapse. Leaflet height, high flail gap (>10 mm), and bileaflet prolapse can also be challenging to treat in this patient population. The longer and wider G4 NTW, XT, and XTW clips (Figure 34.1) can accommodate more tissue, reducing leaflet tension across a greater surface area. This may reduce the risk of acute or long-term leaflet injury and tear. The EXPAND registry data showed that the XTR is the preferred clip for treatment of prolapse (not published).

Third, using end-expiratory hold or rapid pacing may aid grasping in anatomies with wide coaptation gaps.

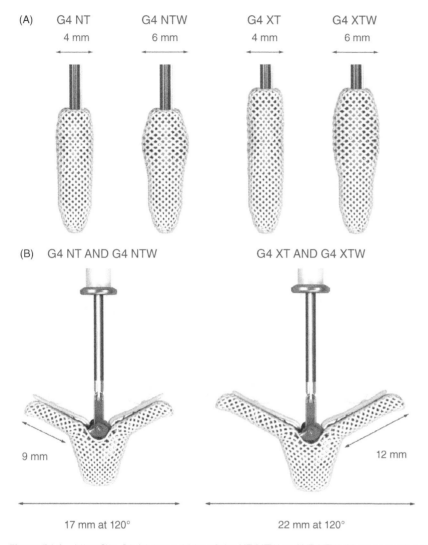

(A) G4 NT — 4 mm   G4 NTW — 6 mm   G4 XT — 4 mm   G4 XTW — 6 mm

(B) G4 NT AND G4 NTW — 9 mm — 17 mm at 120°   G4 XT AND G4 XTW — 12 mm — 22 mm at 120°

Figure 34.1 MitraClip G4. (a) Arm widths of the NT/NTW and XT/XTW. (b) Arm length and grasping width of the NT/NTW and XT/XTW systems. *Source:* Courtesy of Abbott Structural Heart.

Although this technique was first described with the older-generation MitraClip devices, extreme anatomies can still prove difficult with XT clip platforms. A word of caution that independent grasping of the anterior or posterior leaflets with the G4 system to overcome these anatomical challenges should be a last resort, as this technique invariably places excessive stress on the leaflets and may lead to injury and tear. Alternatively, the anchoring technique stabilizes a flail segment by placing a clip immediately adjacent to the lesion with the wide coaptation gap/flail, which then allows treatment of the primary lesion.

Fourth, if multiple jets are noted across the coaptation line without a "main" lesion, targeting mid-A2-P2 with the primary clip should be considered. The implantation of additional clips can then target the residual jets ("zip and clip"). Given the high tensile force exerted by the leaflets in DMD,

placement of additional stabilizing clips was common with the older-generation devices. However, with the introduction of XTR and XTW, a single clip may be sufficient.

5. When should an additional clip be placed?

Placement of additional clips should be driven by (i) residual MR burden by echocardiography, (ii) left atrial (LA) hemodynamic, (iii) pulmonary venous (PV) return Doppler, and (iv) trans-mitral gradient. Of note, given leaflet thickening and tissue redundancy, the edge-to-edge approximation may lead to new open indentation and pseudo-cleft lesions. Release and re-grasping may aid in "unrolling" these new lesions, although additional clips are frequently needed (Figure 34.2).

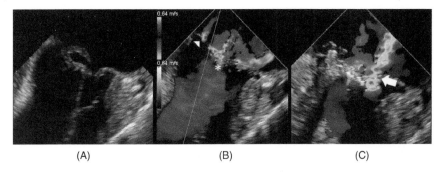

Figure 34.2 (a) Severely myxomatous valve with flail medial P2. (b) Single A2/P2 clip (asterisk) resulted in a significant reduction in mitral regurgitation and mild residual jets (arrowhead). However, placement of a "stabilizing" clip at medial A1/P1 led to an open indentation and a new mitral regurgitation jet laterally.

MitraClip for Wide Flail Leaflets

6. What is considered a wide flail MV prolapse?

The EVEREST-II trial excluded patients with large flail, defined as flail width ≥15 mm or flail gap ≥10 mm. However, transcatheter treatment of flail MV pathologies is especially important, given the association of flail leaflet with excessive mortality. Moreover, flail MV pathology is a strong predictor of improvement in LA hemodynamics post-MitraClip.

7. What are the technical considerations when treating wide flail mitral leaflets?

Like the treatment of DMD lesions, careful attention must be paid to transseptal puncture. Sufficient height (4.5–5.0 cm) is needed for grasping, and height must be measured to the MV plane. Grasping wide flail gaps is challenging, particularly using the older-generation MitraClip devices. Anchoring, as described previously, was the technique of choice for the treatment of these lesions when grasping the target lesion was unsuccessful. Other techniques such as end-expiratory hold and rapid pacing can also aid with grasping. Additional clips for treatment of residual regurgitation and stabilization of the clip were also often required, given the significant mobility of the clip at the site of the flail.

However, the MitraClip G4 system allows treatment of the target lesion using the longer and wider clip arms without resorting to anchoring or zipping techniques. XT and XTW are the devices of choice to treat wide flail gaps. Independent grasping of the leaflets is an additional tool afforded by the G4 system that may be used as a *last resort*

for grasping. Another important consideration when treating flail leaflets is to advance the clip into the left ventricle with the arm closed to avoid interaction of the flail leaflet with the grippers.

Noncentral and Commissural Lesions

8. How common is noncentral MR, and can it be treated using TEER?

The EVEREST-II trial included only lesions in the A2-P2 "chordal-free zone." Patients with lesions in noncentral areas were excluded due to concern about device entanglement and chordal rupture near the commissures, given the higher number and complexity of subvalvular chordae. Nonetheless, noncentral lesions constitute a significant portion of MR patients and account for over 20% of MitraClip cases in the Society of Thoracic Surgeons/ American College of Cardiology Transcatheter Valve Therapy Registry (STS-ACC /TVT). Multiple single- and multi-center studies have demonstrated the safety and efficacy of MitraClip in the treatment of noncentral lesions. Nonetheless, there are several considerations when treating these pathologies.

9. Where should the transseptal puncture be positioned for medial mitral regurgitant lesions?

For medial lesions, a high transseptal puncture is crucial to provide adequate height for grasping. End-expiratory hold provides additional medial position during grasping (conversely, end-inspiratory hold shifts the system laterally). Given the anatomical complexity of the subvalvular apparatus near the commissures together with shorter P1 and

P2 scallop lengths, the use of shorter arm clips (i.e. NT, NTW) is preferred.

10. How is the optimal MitraClip arm angle determined?

The angle of the clip arm should be perpendicular to the MV coaptation plane for optimal grasping. Although the clip arm angle is usually established relative to the aorta in a three-dimensional (3D) en face view and grasping view (LV outflow tract view ~130–150° angle) for central A2-P2 lesions, a higher or lower angle is needed to visualize clip arms and tissue grasp for lateral and medial lesions, respectively (Figure 34.3). Alternatively, a transesophageal echocardiogram system with live 3D multiplanar reconstruction capability can aid in finding the optimal view.

11. What are the strategies to avoid and deal with entanglement?

With truly commissural lesions, consider advancing the clip into the left ventricle with the arm closed and then opening the arms just beneath the leaflets to avoid entanglement. Consider avoiding the use of longer arm XT/XTW to reduce the risk of entanglement and chordal rupture. Avoid excessive maneuvers while in the ventricle. If entanglement is encountered, fully the invert the clip and gently withdraw into the left atrium. If retraction is still unsuccessful, consider undoing the maneuvers performed in the ventricle step by step in reverse fashion before the withdrawal. Avoid forceful pullback, which may lead to chordal rupture or leaflet laceration.

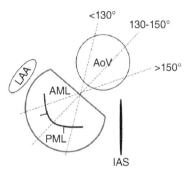

Figure 34.3 Perpendicularity of the clip arm relative to the line of coaptation can be achieved in the three-chamber grasp view at ~130–150°, with clip arms lined up with the aorta. For medial lesions, perpendicularity is achieved at a more counterclockwise orientation, and the clip can be visualized at imaging planes <130°. For lateral lesions, clip arms should be oriented more clockwise and can be visualized at imaging planes >150°.

12. How can vascular plugs and cardiac occluders be used to treat commissural lesions?

Commissural lesions should be treated before placing additional clips toward the center ("outside-in"). Treating residual commissural lesions after placement of adjacent clips is more difficult, with a likely higher risk of entrapment and complication. However, *residual* commissural lesions that cannot be safely treated with an additional clip have been treated using the Amplatzer Vascular Plug II (AVP-II; St. Jude Medical) or a CARDIOFORM Septal Occluder (Gore Medical) with a lower risk of hemolysis. In addition to residual commissural MR, AVP-II has been used to successfully treat paraclip, interclip, and leaflet perforations.

Calcified Mitral Valve

13. Did the EVEREST and COAPT trials include patients with calcification of the MV?

These trials excluded patients with severe mitral annular calcification (MAC) or leaflet calcification near or at the grasp zone. These patients were excluded due to concern for mitral stenosis (MS) after TEER, poor tissue elasticity and tear, and inadequate leaflet visualization, particularly with posterior MAC.

14. Is TEER feasible in patients with calcified MV apparatus?

Despite the previously described limitations, the use of TEER for treatment of inoperable patients with calcified MAC or MV leaflets is feasible provided (i) at least 7 mm of noncalcified tissue is available for grasp, (ii) the estimated MV area is >4 cm^2, and (iii) optimal TEE imaging is available to evaluate leaflet tissue and guide TEER.

Additionally, the use of NTR is preferred over XTR clips, given the shorter arms and likely less tension on calcified leaflets with reduced elasticity. Transthoracic echocardiography or intracardiac echocardiogram can complement TEE images if significant acoustic shadowing, particularly involving the posterior shelf, hinders grasp confirmation. With severe subvalvular calcification, consider advancing the clip into the left ventricle with the arms closed and then opening the arms immediately beneath the leaflets (Figure 34.4).

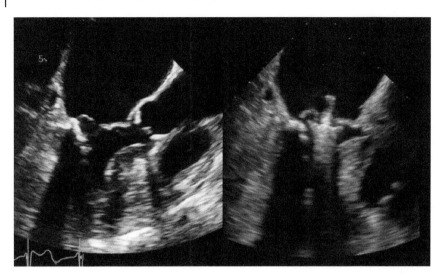

Figure 34.4 A 92-year-old patient was referred for the MitraClip. (a) Baseline transesophageal echocardiography revealed P2 prolapse with a shelf of calcium encroaching into the mitral outflow below the posterior leaflet. Despite elevated baseline gradient at baseline (7 mmHg), the mitral regurgitation was successfully treated with the clip arms advanced carefully below the leaflets and opened immediately above the calcium shelf. Final mean gradient: 6 mmHg.

The transvalvular gradient needs to be meticulously measured before release to avoid mitral stenosis (mean gradient [MG] <7 mmHg). If the resting heart rate is low, consider 3D MV area measurement or reevaluating mitral gradients with pacing or dobutamine infusion.

Secondary Mitral Regurgitation

15. What are the anatomical considerations of secondary MR?

Unlike primary MR, which is a disease of the MV leaflets, secondary MR is a disease of the left ventricle or left atrium. Secondary MR in ischemic and non-ischemic cardiomyopathy can be due to ventricular dilation and lateral displacement of the papillary muscles, mitral annular dilation with leaflet malcoaptation, and dyssynchrony due to bundle branch block. There are no MV leaflet abnormalities in non-ischemic cardiomyopathy with resulting central MR; however, in ischemic cardiomyopathy, regional wall motion abnormalities may lead to asymmetrical chordal traction (for example, posterior leaflet tethering with anterior leaflet override) and a posteriorly directed jet. Severe atrial dilation may also lead to significant annular dilation and mitral leaflet malcoaptation with central MR (atrial functional MR). Finally, secondary MR is more likely to have a wide jet than primary MR.

16. What are the key strategies to success in treating secondary MR?

Treatment of secondary MR routinely required the "zip-and-clip" technique using multiple first iterations of MitraClip. However, with the introduction of the wider G4 MitraClip, a single wide clip may be adequate to achieve a sufficient reduction in MR. In ischemic cardiomyopathy with restricted posterior leaflet and leaflet length <9 mm, G4 NTW or NT clips are favored.

17. When should an additional clip be placed?

As noted earlier, placement of additional clips should be driven by (i) residual MR burden by echocardiography, (ii) left atrial (LA) hemodynamic, (iii) pulmonary venous (PV) return Doppler, and (iv) trans-mitral gradient. Although achieving less residual final MR is clinically favorable, this should be balanced against the development of significant mitral stenosis. In the analysis of the two-year COAPT data, death or heart failure hospitalization was similar for moderate (2+) versus trace or mild (1+) residual MR at 30 days. Approximately 84% of patients with acceptable MR reduction (≤2+) had a durable result at 30 days, and the only anatomical predictor of worsening MR was significant anterior leaflet tethering.

Bibliography

1 Alfieri, O., Maisano, F., De Bonis, M. et al. (2001). The double-orifice technique in mitral valve repair: a simple solution for complex problems. *J. Thorac. Cardiovasc. Surg.* 122: 674–681.

2 Avierinos, J.F., Tribouilloy, C., Grigioni, F. et al. (2013). Impact of ageing on presentation and outcome of mitral regurgitation due to flail leaflet: a multicentre international study. *Eur. Heart J.* 34: 2600–2609.

3 El Sabbagh, A., Reddy, Y.N.V., and Nishimura, R.A. (2018). Mitral valve regurgitation in the contemporary era: insights into diagnosis, management, and future directions. *JACC Cardiovasc. Imaging* 11: 628–643.

4 Estevez-Loureiro, R., Franzen, O., Winter, R. et al. (2013). Echocardiographic and clinical outcomes of central versus noncentral percutaneous edge-to-edge repair of degenerative mitral regurgitation. *J. Am. Coll. Cardiol.* 62: 2370–2377.

5 Feldman, T., Foster, E., Glower, D.D. et al. (2011). Percutaneous repair or surgery for mitral regurgitation. *N. Engl. J. Med.* 364: 1395–1406.

6 Flint, N., Price, M.J., Little, S.H. et al. (2021). State of the art: transcatheter edge-to-edge repair for complex mitral regurgitation. *J. Am. Soc. Echocardiogr.* 34: 1025–1037.

7 Gavazzoni, M., Taramasso, M., Zuber, M. et al. (2020). Conceiving MitraClip as a tool: percutaneous edge-to-edge repair in complex mitral valve anatomies. *Eur. Heart J. Cardiovasc. Imaging* 21: 1059–1067.

8 Kar, S., Mack, M.J., Lindenfeld, J. et al. (2021). Relationship between residual mitral regurgitation and clinical and quality-of-life outcomes after transcatheter and medical treatments in heart failure: COAPT trial. *Circulation* 144: 426–437.

9 Lodhi, H.A., Mathews, A., Bansal, P. et al. (2021). Feasibility of transcatheter mitral valve repair for non-A2P2 mitral regurgitation. *J. Invasive Cardiol.* 33: E968–E969.

10 Nakajima, Y. and Kar, S. (2018). First experience of the usage of a GORE CARDIOFORM septal occluder device for treatment of a significant residual commissural mitral regurgitation jet following a MitraClip procedure. *Catheter. Cardiovasc. Interv.* 92: 607–610.

11 Niikura, H., Bae, R., Gossl, M. et al. (2019). Transcatheter therapy for residual mitral regurgitation after MitraClip therapy. *EuroIntervention* 15: e491–e499.

12 Patzelt, J., Zhang, Y., Seizer, P. et al. (2016). Effects of mechanical ventilation on heart geometry and mitral valve leaflet coaptation during percutaneous edge-to-edge mitral valve repair. *JACC Cardiovasc. Interv.* 9: 151–159.

13 Raphael, C.E., Malouf, J.F., Maor, E. et al. (2019). A hybrid technique for treatment of commissural primary mitral regurgitation. *Catheter. Cardiovasc. Interv.* 93: 692–698.

14 Singh, G.D., Smith, T.W., and Rogers, J.H. (2015). Multi-MitraClip therapy for severe degenerative mitral regurgitation: "anchor" technique for extremely flail segments. *Catheter. Cardiovasc. Interv.* 86: 339–346.

15 Sorajja, P., Mack, M., Vemulapalli, S. et al. (2016). Initial experience with commercial transcatheter mitral valve repair in the United States. *J. Am. Coll. Cardiol.* 67: 1129–1140.

16 Stone, G.W., Lindenfeld, J., Abraham, W.T. et al. (2018). Transcatheter mitral-valve repair in patients with heart failure. *N. Engl. J. Med.* 379: 2307–2318.

17 Thaden, J.J., Malouf, J.F., Nkomo, V.T. et al. (2018). Mitral valve anatomic predictors of hemodynamic success with transcatheter mitral valve repair. *J. Am. Heart Assoc.* 7.

35

MitraClip Complications

Prevention and Management

Raviteja R. Guddeti[1] and Santiago Garcia[2]

[1]Valve Science Center at the Minneapolis Heart Institute Foundation, Abbott Northwestern Hospital, Minneapolis, MN, USA
[2]Structural Heart Program and Harold C. Schott Foundation Endowed Chair for Structural and Valvular Heart Disease The Carl and Edyth Lindner Center for Research and Education at The Christ Hospital. Cincinnati, OH

Introduction

Ever since it received CE mark approval in 2008 and FDA approval in 2013, MitraClip (Abbott Vascular) has been used with increasing frequency to treat severe mitral regurgitation (MR), both degenerative mitral regurgitation (DMR) and functional mitral regurgitation (FMR). Both the European and the American College of Cardiology guidelines on valvular heart diseases endorse transcatheter edge-to-edge repair (TEER; class IIa) for patients with severe MR and favorable anatomy. For DMR patients, a high or prohibitive surgical risk is required, whereas for FMR patients, medical therapies should be optimized prior to TEER. So far, more than 100 000 procedures have been performed worldwide.

The MitraClip system consists of a 24 Fr steerable guide catheter and a clip delivery system (CDS) that hosts the grippers and the clip. The five steps of the MitraClip procedure include (i) large-bore venous access, (ii) transseptal puncture, (iii) device navigation in the left atrium (LA), (iv) leaflet grasping, and (v) device deployment. Serious procedure-related complications after MitraClip are rare and are estimated at <5%, of which major bleeding needing blood transfusions constitutes the majority. Device-related complications account for about 1.4% based on data from the TVT registry. Enhanced operator experience is associated with a significantly improved procedural success rate and lower complication rates (Table 35.1).

1. What is the incidence of vascular complications from the MitraClip procedure?

The MitraClip procedure requires 24 Fr access through the femoral vein. Access is preferably obtained under ultrasound guidance. Although vascular complications following large-bore venous access are infrequent compared to arterial access, injury to the femoral artery may occur due to the close proximity of the artery to the vein. Prior surgical procedures to the groin and inflammatory processes can increase the likelihood of vascular complications from the formation of fibrotic tissue around the vessels. A thorough review of the history of inferior vena cava (IVC) filter placement is important prior to

Table 35.1 MitraClip complications and prevention.

	What could go wrong?	Best practice
Venous access	Vessel injury, bleeding	Pre close with ProGlide, figure-eight
Transseptal puncture	Perforation, aortic injury, pericardial effusion	"Targeted" TS puncture, TEE-guided, learning curve
Left atrial navigation	Air embolism, atrial fibrillation, perforation	Optimal device preparation and handling, TEE and fluoroscopic guidance, communication with the imaging specialist
Leaflet grasping	SLDA, chordal entanglement	TEE guidance, communication with the imaging specialist
Device deployment	Iatrogenic MS, residual MR, iatrogenic ASD	Careful hemodynamic and TEE assessment

ASD, atrial septal defect; MR, mitral regurgitation; MS, mitral stenosis, SLDA, single leaflet device attachment; TEE, transesophageal echocardiography; TS, transseptal.

Mastering Structural Heart Disease, First Edition. Edited by Eduardo J. de Marchena and Camilo A. Gomez.
© 2023 John Wiley & Sons Ltd. Published 2023 by John Wiley & Sons Ltd.
Companion website: www.wiley.com/go/deMarchena/Mastering-Structural-Heart-Disease

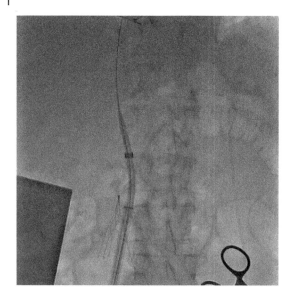

Figure 35.1 Inferior vena cava filter and MitraClip steerable guide catheter.

proceeding with the procedure, although the presence of a filter in the IVC does not preclude the MitraClip procedure (Figure 35.1). Major bleeding requiring blood transfusion was seen in about 13.4% of patients in the EVEREST (Endovascular Valve Edge-to-Edge Repair Study) high-risk cohort. Analysis from the TVT registry noted an incidence of 3.9% for major bleeding. Similar findings were noted from the ACCESS EU registry.

2. How can you prevent vascular complications during the MitraClip procedure?

Using ultrasound guidance for access, preclose the access site using a ProGlide (Abbott Vascular) closure device and/or figure-eight sutures to help prevent bleeding complications from the venous access site. Take care not to use excessive force while advancing the 24 Fr guide catheter, which could result in kinking.

Transseptal Puncture Complications

3. What are the complications of a transseptal puncture during the MitraClip procedure?

A targeted transseptal puncture (TS) is key for a successful MitraClip procedure. TS puncture is ideally performed in a posterior and superior location in the interatrial septum to allow sufficient height above the mitral annulus for device navigation (Figure 35.2). A good TS puncture is critical to the overall success of the procedure. Inadvertent advancement of the TS needle may result in left atrial perforation and cardiac tamponade. The incidence of cardiac tamponade during the MitraClip procedure is about 1–2%.

Rarely, a thickened or fibrotic interatrial septum may be encountered in some patients, which can lead to challenges in attaining TS puncture. This can be overcome by using radiofrequency needles (Baylis Medical), large-curved needles (BRK-1), or needle-wire systems (SafeSept Transseptal Guidewire, Pressure Products). Occasionally, if the interatrial septum is floppy and aneurysmal, significant tenting can occur while performing the TS puncture, thereby reducing the distance between the needle tip and the posterior wall of the LA. Utmost care should be taken while advancing the needle in such scenarios to avoid puncturing the left atrial posterior wall. Gentle twisting movements of the sheath and needle assembly use of specialized TS puncture systems such as a radiofrequency needle or needle-wire systems may help minimize the risk of adverse complications.

Inadvertent puncture and sheath placement in the aorta during TS puncture is an extremely rare complication that can lead to fatal outcomes. This is secondary to a very anterior puncture and can be identified on short-axis transesophageal echocardiography (TEE) views. Because of the location of the interatrial septum in close proximity to the non-coronary cusp (Figure 35.3), inadvertent puncture of the aorta may allow for percutaneous device closure without interfering with coronary access. If this complication occurs, it is important to maintain the guide wire and sheath position in the aorta until all treatment options are considered (device closure vs. open surgical repair) rather than pulling the equipment into the atria.

Complications from Device Navigation in the Left Atrium: Air Embolism and Thrombus Formation

4. What are the complications of device navigation in the LA?

Air embolism and thrombus formation are rare complications of the MitraClip procedure. Air embolism can occur during device manipulation due to inadequate device preparation and can cause myocardial ischemia, typically manifested as inferior ST-segment elevation and hemodynamic

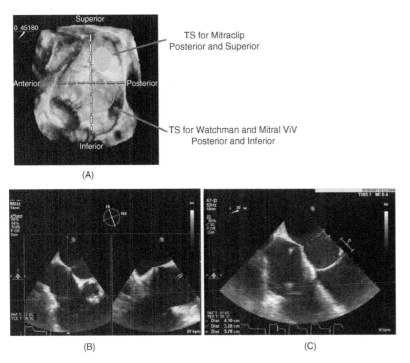

Figure 35.2 (a) Targeted transseptal puncture for the MitraClip procedure performed in a posterior and superior location in the interatrial septum. (b, c) Targeted TS is key for a successful MitraClip procedure. It is ideally performed in a posterior and superior location in the interatrial septum to allow sufficient height above the mitral annulus for device navigation.

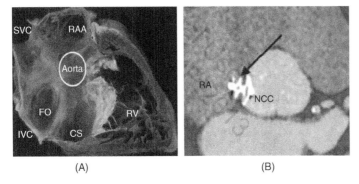

Figure 35.3 (a) Anatomy of the atrial septum. *Source:* Reprinted from Mohamad Alkhouli, Charanjit S. Rihal, David R. Holmes, Transseptal Techniques for Emerging Structural Heart Interventions, *JACC: Cardiovascular Interventions*, Volume 9, Issue 24, 2016, Pages 2465–2480, ISSN 1936-8798, Figure 2. https://doi.org/10.1016/j.jcin.2016.10.035. (b) Inadvertent puncture of the aorta due to a very anterior transseptal puncture, repaired with an Amplatzer closure device. Contrast computed tomography. Angled transverse section demonstrating the Amplatzer closure device (identified by arrow) deployed between the right atrium (RA) and the non-coronary cusp (NCC) of the aorta and its anterior relationship to the left atrium (LA). *Source:* Reproduced with permission from HMP Global: Webber MR, Stiles MK, Pasupati S. Percutaneous repair of aortic puncture with Amplatzer closure device during attempted transseptal puncture. *J Invasive Cardiol.* 2013;25(4):E110-E113, Figure 6.

instability. This is treated immediately with 100% oxygen and supportive therapies (vasopressors and fluids). Proper de-airing techniques should be used to minimize the risk of air embolism.

In patients with severe MR, atrial fibrillation and co-existent mitral stenosis (MS) are common; thereby, thrombus formation may occur. Cases have been reported on thrombus formation at the TS puncture site and spontaneous echo contrast formation in the LA immediately post MitraClip implantation. In addition, endothelial injury at the TS puncture site, presence of a foreign body in the LA, very low cardiac output, inadequate anticoagulation, and prolonged duration of the procedure may further contribute to thrombus formation. It is crucial to maintain activated clotting time (ACT) between 250 and 300 seconds for the duration of the procedure.

Care should be taken while navigating the clip in the LA. Deliberate small adjustments should be made, complemented by TEE imaging, to position the clip in the desired location prior to grasping the leaflets.

Complications from Leaflet Grasping

5. What complications may occur during leaflet grasping?

Leaflet grasping by MitraClip may damage the MV leaflets. The risk of damage increases significantly with a greater number of grasping attempts and unfavorable anatomies. Severe leaflet prolapse, degenerative leaflets, and thickened and calcified leaflet tips are more prone to damage during grasping attempts.

Chordal entrapment of the MitraClip device can result in worsening MR requiring surgical intervention (Figure 35.4, Video 35.1 [See Online]). Therefore, it is recommended to perform clip orientation in the LA before advancing the clip to the left ventricle (LV). However, the torque stored in the CDS may result in a change in orientation during advancement into the LV. The longer clip arms of the XTR and XTW devices make maneuverability difficult, especially in the presence of another clip, and increase the risk of chordal entrapment. This is minimized by obtaining sufficient height on the TS puncture and avoiding clip manipulations while in the LV. Ideally, the MitraClip is positioned approximately 10 mm above the leaflets and perpendicular to the line of coaptation until ready to grasp and advanced slowly into the LV under TEE guidance and placed below

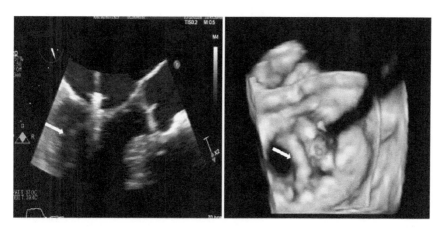

Figure 35.4 Transesophageal echocardiogram showing chordal entanglement of MitraClip.

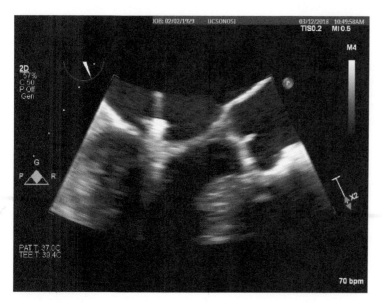

Video 35.1 MitraClip chordal entanglement.

the leaflets to prevent chordal entanglement. For the new G4 MitraClip, the gripper orientation (anterior or posterior) should be checked in the LA prior to advancing into the LV under TEE. Careful assessment of fluoroscopy and TEE is important while removing an entrapped clip. Inverting the clip, raising and lowering the grippers, and slowly retracting the clip into the LA can help prevent chordal rupture and worsening MR. Undoing the maneuvers that led to chordal entrapment in a reverse sequence tends to work well. For example, if the guide was torqued anteriorly and the M-knob was turned clockwise, leading to chordal entanglement, turning the M-knob counterclockwise and the guide posterior would release the clip. At this point, it should be pulled back to the LA for reorientation.

6. What is a single leaflet device attachment?

Single leaflet device attachment (SLDA), defined as loss of insertion of one leaflet from the MitraClip with continued insertion of the opposite leaflet (Figure 35.5a, b), was seen in 2.2% of patients in the EVEREST high-risk registries and 4.8% of patients in the ACCESS EU registry. On the other hand, data from the TVT registry showed only a 1.5% rate of SLDA. In most cases, SLDA is noted acutely during the procedure or shortly after. However, it can also occur several months after the index procedure. Clinically, SLDA can lead to a recurrence of severe MR.

7. How is SLDA treated?

Options for managing SLDA include placement of an additional clip (Figure 35.5c,d), referral to surgical MV repair, and medical management. Data from the ACCESS EU registry showed that of the 27 patients who had SLDA out of 567, 10 underwent a second MitraClip procedure, 6 underwent surgical MV repair or replacement, and 11 were treated medically. If SLDA is noticed during the index procedure, placing a second clip is always a reasonable option if the gradients allow it.

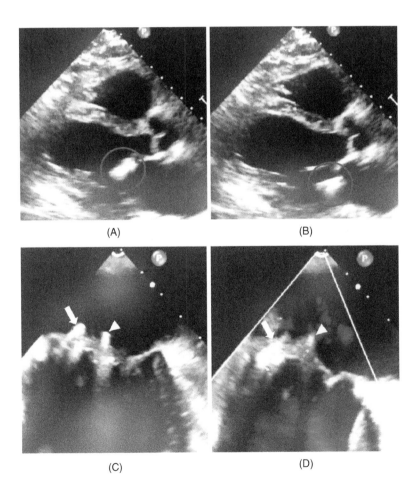

(A) (B) (C) (D)

Figure 35.5 (a, b) Single leaflet attachment of the MitraClip (red circle) to the anterior mitral leaflet, (c, d) which was treated by a second MitraClip (white arrow) medial to the prior clip (white arrowhead).

8. How is SLDA prevented?

Meticulous TEE assessment during leaflet grasping and device deployment helps prevent SLDA. Appropriate leaflet grasping should be confirmed in multiple TEE views, including the long-axis view prior to device deployment. Particularly in degenerative MR with redundant leaflets, where the MitraClip XTW device may be preferred, care should be taken to ensure that enough leaflet tissue is grasped before releasing the clip. Leaflet insertion should occur in at least two-thirds of the clip arms, which means 6 mm minimum leaflet insertion for an XT device and 9 mm for an XT device (Figure 35.5). Partial leaflet insertion and grasping may lead to SLDA.

9. What is the incidence of MitraClip embolization?

Embolization of MitraClip is an extremely rare complication that is infrequently reported in the literature (Figure 35.6, Video 35.2 [See Online]). While there were no cases of device embolization in the ACCESS EU registry, its incidence was 0.4% in the TVT registry. Clip embolization is usually recognized immediately during the index procedure. However, late clip embolization weeks to months after the index procedure has been reported in some cases. An embolized clip can migrate into the arterial system and potentially cause ischemia in the territory involved.

10. How can you manage clip embolization?

Emergent surgical MV repair or replacement should be considered if clip embolization is noted at the time of the index procedure. In asymptomatic patients, continued monitoring can be considered depending on the location of the clip in the arterial system. In symptomatic cases, retrieval of the clip can be performed using a snare. A surgical cutdown of the arteriotomy site will be required to completely retrieve the clip from the arterial system. Extreme caution must be maintained while snaring an embolized clip from the LV as the clip may embolize and cause a stroke.

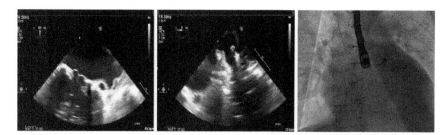

Figure 35.6 Transesophageal echocardiogram and fluoroscopy demonstrating embolization of MitraClip into the left upper pulmonary vein (white arrow).

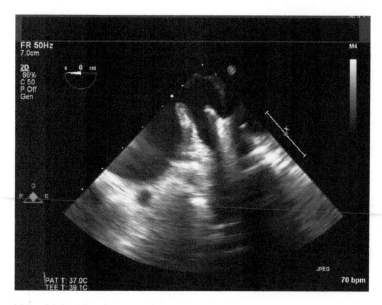

Video 35.2 MitraClip embolization.

Complications from Device Deployment

11. What is the incidence of residual MR after the MitraClip procedure?

MitraClip procedural success is defined as ≥1 grade reduction in MR, compared to baseline, to a degree ≤ moderate MR. The incidence of more than moderate (>2+) MR was 7% in the commercial TVT registry. Significant residual MR after MitraClip implantation is associated with worse clinical outcomes (higher all-cause mortality, heart failure readmissions, and need for MV surgery). Reichart et al. demonstrated that patients with ≥2+ residual MR at discharge had significantly lower survival rates than those with ≤1+ residual MR. Moreover, MR grade ≥2+ at the end of the procedure is associated with a higher risk of ≥3+ recurrent MR at follow-up.

Adequate patient selection is key to preventing suboptimal results. The A2-P2 area of the MV apparatus is a relatively chordal-free zone. In patients with a central MR jet or pathology involving A2-P2 segments, the proceduralist must ensure that the clip is placed in this zone. Commissural MR poses unique anatomic challenges due to a dense network of chordae in this area. Due to the increased risk of chordal entrapment, an NT device is recommended for commissural MR. The presence of a leaflet cleft at the grasping site can significantly increase the risk of having ≥2+ residual MR.

12. How is residual MR treated?

Treatment of post-procedure residual MR is challenging. In most cases, it can be treated by placing additional clips if the transmitral gradients and anatomy allow. However, placing additional clips can sometimes be technically challenging due to the complex MV anatomy and limited space to maneuver the second clip and position it in the desired location. The second clip should be placed and deployed close to the first to ensure maximal coaptation reserve.

Transcatheter occluder devices have been used as a bail-out strategy in cases where the placement of additional clips is not feasible either between clips or between a clip and the commissure. Taramasso et al. first reported a case where residual "inter-clip" MR was successfully treated using the Amplatzer Vascular Plug II. Kubo et al. reported a series of nine patients who successfully received the Amplatzer Duct Occluder II for treatment of significant ≥3+ residual MR. Of the nine patients, seven received the occluder device during the index MitraClip procedure while the other two were during follow-up. At one-month post-procedure follow-up, all patients were alive and had NYHA functional class I or II. Device embolization and hemolysis are some potential complications of this approach.

13. What is the incidence of iatrogenic MS after MitraClip implantation?

Incidence of iatrogenic MS, defined as a mean diastolic gradient across the MV as >5 mmHg (Figure 35.7), post clip implantation occurs in about 25–35%. Data from the German TRAMI registry showed an incidence of 0.5% for clinically relevant iatrogenic MS in patients undergoing the MitraClip procedure. A pre-procedure MV area of ≥4 cm² is recommended prior to MitraClip implantation. Predictors of elevated MV gradients post-MitraClip include pre-procedural MV area < 4.0 cm², more than one clip implantation, and elevated baseline mean MV gradients.

Mean Gradient 6 mmHg, TEE, HR: 56 bpm   Mean Gradient 15 mmHg, TTE, HR: 96 bpm

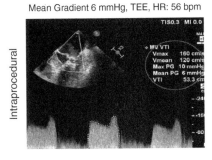 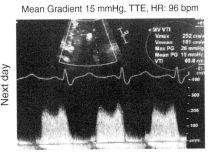

Figure 35.7 Iatrogenic mitral stenosis. Post-procedural mitral gradients after MitraClip are often elevated compared to intra-procedural gradients.

14. What are the complications of elevated mean MV gradients post-MitraClip implantation?

A mean diastolic gradient of >5 mmHg across the MV after MitraClip implantation is associated with worse outcomes, including all-cause mortality. Neuss et al. demonstrated that among patients who underwent the MitraClip procedure, those with post-procedure MV gradients >5 mmHg had a significantly higher rate of a combined endpoint of all-cause mortality, LV assist device placement, MV replacement, and redo procedure. A recent analysis from the COAPT (Cardiovascular Outcomes Assessment of the MitraClip Percutaneous Therapy for Heart Failure Patients with Functional Mitral Regurgitation) trial stratified patients into quartiles of MV gradients and showed no difference in heart failure hospitalizations or death across the spectrum of residual gradients. However, caution is warranted when extrapolating these results to clinical practice, given the small number of patients with gradients >10 mmHg.

15. How can you prevent iatrogenic MS?

Appropriate pre-procedural imaging, patient selection, and minimizing the number of clip implantations by measuring mean MV gradients and MR grades after each clip implantation can help prevent iatrogenic MS. A balance between the degree of MR reduction and MV gradients should be maintained throughout the procedure. If the mean gradient across the MV is >5 mmHg and the MV area is <4 cm^2, additional MitraClips should not be placed. It is reasonable to leave the procedure with some residual MR rather than compromise the MV gradients, especially in patients at higher risk of iatrogenic MS, as outcomes are worse with elevated gradients compared to having a residual ≤2+ MR, and MV gradients are likely to increase post-procedure under physiology conditions.

16. What is the incidence of iatrogenic atrial septal defects post-MitraClip procedure?

The MitraClip device uses a 24 Fr steerable guide catheter with a cross-sectional diameter of 22 Fr at the level of the inter-atrial septum. TS puncture is specifically performed more posteriorly in the fossa ovalis to have more room for steerability of the MitraClip delivery system and improve trajectory to the valve. The majority of these iatrogenic atrial septal defects (iASDs) close spontaneously or leave no clinical sequelae and therefore do not require further intervention. Studies have shown that the incidence of persistent iASD post-MitraClip procedure is about 24–50% which is similar to that after other transcatheter heart procedures involving a septal puncture.

17. What are the clinical implications of persistent iASD?

The potential clinical implications of persistent iASD are a topic of debate, with some studies showing worse clinical outcomes at follow-up compared to those without iASD, while others demonstrate similar outcomes. Acute right-heart failure from a significant left-to-right shunt is rare. Persistent iASD can lead to right-heart enlargement, greater severity of tricuspid regurgitation, and pulmonary hypertension, all secondary to left-to-right shunting. Oxygen desaturation can be noticed immediately after the procedure if there is a significant right-to-left shunt, especially in patients with severe pre-procedure pulmonary hypertension and/or right-heart volume overload. Toyama et al. demonstrated higher re-hospitalization rates for heart failure at follow-up in patients with persistent iASD compared to those without. In addition, patients with iASD had greater severity of tricuspid regurgitation at follow-up but no difference in MR grades. On the other hand, Smith et al. noted more residual MR at follow-up in patients with iASD. At 12 months, more patients with iASD had MR grade > 2+. Persistent iASD was associated with higher mortality rates and less improvement in six-minute walking distance, and presented more often with NYHA functional class >II at six months in one study.

18. What are the indications for device closure of persistent iASD?

There are currently no specific guidelines for the management of iASD. Oxygen desaturation immediately after the MitraClip procedure is an indication for closure of iASD at the time of the index procedure if a causal relationship is established using TEE. Indications for closure of a persistent iASD include right-to-left shunt with evidence of oxygen desaturation or concerns of paradoxical embolism. Device closure of iASD may preclude additional clipping or other left-sided percutaneous valve therapies. Therefore, patient selection is vital before considering the closure of iASD. Baseline hemodynamic assessment prior to

MitraClip may help identify patients with high pulmonary vascular resistance in whom closure may not be indicated. Use of pressure-volume loops before and after balloon occlusion of the defect may help assess right ventricle (RV) and LV workload changes and help determine candidacy for closure. In addition, if balloon occlusion of the defect results in severely elevated left atrial or pulmonary capillary wedge pressure, then closure may not be indicated.

Bibliography

1 Feldman, T., Kar, S., Elmariah, S. et al. (2015). Randomized comparison of percutaneous repair and surgery for mitral regurgitation: 5-year results of Everest II. *J. Am. Coll. Cardiol.* 66: 2844–2854.

2 Obadia, J.F., Messika-Zeitoun, D., Leurent, G. et al. (2018). Percutaneous repair or medical treatment for secondary mitral regurgitation. *N. Engl. J. Med.* 379: 2297–2306.

3 Stone, G.W., Lindenfeld, J., Abraham, W.T. et al. (2018). Transcatheter mitral-valve repair in patients with heart failure. *N. Engl. J. Med.* 379: 2307–2318.

4 Baumgartner, H., Falk, V., Bax, J.J. et al. (2018). 2017 ESC/EACTS guidelines for the management of valvular heart disease. *Rev. Esp. Cardiol. (Engl. Ed.)* 71: 110.

5 Otto, C.M., Nishimura, R.A., Bonow, R.O. et al. (2021). 2020 ACC/AHA guideline for the management of patients with valvular heart disease: a report of the American College Of Cardiology/American Heart Association joint committee on clinical practice guidelines. *Circulation* 143: E72–E227.

6 Sorajja, P., Mack, M., Vemulapalli, S. et al. (2016). Initial experience with commercial transcatheter mitral valve repair in the United States. *J. Am. Coll. Cardiol.* 67: 1129–1140.

7 Chhatriwalla, A.K., Vemulapalli, S., Szerlip, M. et al. (2019). Operator experience and outcomes of transcatheter mitral valve repair in the United States. *J. Am. Coll. Cardiol.* 74: 2955–2965.

8 Sorajja, P., Vemulapalli, S., Feldman, T. et al. (2017). Outcomes with transcatheter mitral valve repair in the United States: an STS/ACC TVT registry report. *J. Am. Coll. Cardiol.* 70: 2315–2327.

9 Maisano, F., Franzen, O., Baldus, S. et al. (2013). Percutaneous mitral valve interventions in the real world: early and 1-year results from the ACCESS-EU, a prospective, multicenter, nonrandomized post-approval study of the MitraClip therapy in Europe. *J. Am. Coll. Cardiol.* 62: 1052–1061.

10 Bilge, M., Saatci Yasar, A., Ali, S., and Alemdar, R. (2014). Left atrial spontaneous echo contrast and thrombus formation at septal puncture during percutaneous mitral valve repair with the MitraClip system of severe mitral regurgitation: a report of two cases. *Anadolu Kardiyol. Derg.* 14: 549–550.

11 Glower, D.D., Kar, S., Trento, A. et al. (2014). Percutaneous mitral valve repair for mitral regurgitation in high-risk patients: results of the Everest II study. *J. Am. Coll. Cardiol.* 64: 172–181.

12 Alozie, A., Westphal, B., Kische, S. et al. (2014). Surgical revision after percutaneous mitral valve repair by edge-to-edge device: when the strategy fails in the highest risk surgical population. *Eur. J. Cardiothorac. Surg.* 46: 55–60.

13 Bilge, M., Alsancak, Y., Ali, S. et al. (2016). An extremely rare but possible complication of MitraClip: embolization of clip during follow-up. *Anatol. J. Cardiol.* 16: 636–638.

14 Chitsaz, S., Jumean, M., Dayah, T. et al. (2016). Late MitraClip embolization: a new cause of ST-segment-elevation myocardial infarction. *Circ. Cardiovasc. Interv.* 9.

15 Rahhab, Z., Kortlandt, F.A., Velu, J.F. et al. (2017). Current MitraClip experience, safety and feasibility in the Netherlands. *Neth. Heart J.* 25: 394–400.

16 Buzzatti, N., De Bonis, M., Denti, P. et al. (2016). What is a "good" result after transcatheter mitral repair? Impact of 2+ residual mitral regurgitation. *J. Thorac. Cardiovasc. Surg.* 151: 88–96.

17 Reichart, D., Kalbacher, D., Rubsamen, N. et al. (2020). The impact of residual mitral regurgitation after MitraClip therapy in functional mitral regurgitation. *Eur. J. Heart Fail.* 22: 1840–1848.

18 Kubo, S., Cox, J.M., Mizutani, Y. et al. (2016). Transcatheter procedure for residual mitral regurgitation after MitraClip implantation using Amplatzer duct Occluder II. *JACC Cardiovasc. Interv.* 9: 1280–1288.

19 Taramasso, M., Zuber, M., Gruner, C. et al. (2016). First-in-man report of residual "intra-clip" regurgitation between two MitraClips treated by Amplatzer vascular plug II. *Eurointervention* 11: 1537–1540.

20 Neuss, M., Schau, T., Isotani, A. et al. (2017). Elevated mitral valve pressure gradient after MitraClip implantation deteriorates long-term outcome in patients with severe mitral regurgitation and severe heart failure. *JACC Cardiovasc. Interv.* 10: 931–939.

21 Toggweiler, S., Zuber, M., Surder, D. et al. (2014). Two-year outcomes after percutaneous mitral valve repair with the MitraClip system: durability of the procedure and predictors of outcome. *Open Heart* 1: E000056.

22 Van Riel, A.C., Boerlage-Van Dijk, K., De Bruin-Bon, R.H. et al. (2014). Percutaneous mitral valve repair preserves right ventricular function. *J. Am. Soc. Echocardiogr.* 27: 1098–1106.

23 Eggebrecht, H., Schelle, S., Puls, M. et al. (2015). Risk and outcomes of complications during and after MitraClip implantation: experience in 828 patients from the German transcatheter mitral valve interventions (TRAMI) registry. *Catheter. Cardiovasc. Interv.* 86: 728–735.

24 Halaby, R., Herrmann, H.C., Gertz, Z.M. et al. (2021). Effect of mitral valve gradient after MitraClip on outcomes in secondary mitral regurgitation: results from the COAPT trial. *JACC Cardiovasc. Interv.* 14: 879–889.

25 Schueler, R., Ozturk, C., Wedekind, J.A. et al. (2015). Persistence of Iatrogenic atrial septal defect after interventional mitral valve repair with the MitraClip system: a note of caution. *JACC Cardiovasc. Interv.* 8: 450–459.

26 Toyama, K., Rader, F., Kar, S. et al. (2018). Iatrogenic atrial septal defect after percutaneous mitral valve repair with the MitraClip system. *Am. J. Cardiol.* 121: 475–479.

27 Smith, T., Mcginty, P., Bommer, W. et al. (2012). Prevalence and echocardiographic features of Iatrogenic atrial septal defect after catheter-based mitral valve repair with the MitraClip system. *Catheter. Cardiovasc. Interv.* 80: 678–685.

28 Von Roeder, M., Rommel, K.P., Blazek, S. et al. (2016). Pressure-volume-loop-guided closure of an iatrogenic atrial septal defect for right heart failure following MitraClip-implantation. *Eur. Heart J.* 37: 3153.

36

CT Imaging for TMVR

Pedro Engel Gonzalez, Pedro Villablanca, Brian P. O'Neill, Tiberio Frisoli, James C. Lee, William W. O'Neill and Dee Dee Wang

Division of Cardiology, Center for Structural Heart Disease, Henry Ford Hospital, Detroit, MI, USA

1. What are the important components of the mitral valve apparatus that are important to know for TMVR planning?

The mitral valve apparatus is a complex anatomical structure. Detailed pre-procedural and intra-procedural imaging is necessary to ensure successful transcatheter mitral valve replacement (TMVR). The mitral domain is composed of the annulus, anterolateral and posteromedial commissures, anterior and posterior leaflets, chordae tendineae, and anterolateral and posteromedial papillary muscles. The annulus has a parabolic geometry with peaks toward the anterior and posterior edges and is sometimes referred to as saddle-shaped. The mitral annulus is a dynamic structure that experiences physical deformations during the cardiac cycle. The deformation of the annulus is a significant challenge for device anchoring and stability in TMVR. The fibrous nature of the anterior mitral annulus (also known as the aortic mitral curtain) makes it less prone to pathological remodeling, whereas the predominantly muscular posterior portion of the annulus is more prone to remodeling.

Knowledge of adjacent annular structures is critical to planning successful TMVR interventions. The mitral leaflets attach to the mitral annulus at the anterolateral and posteromedial commissures. The posterior leaflet borders the free cardiac wall and covers approximately one-third of the annular opening (Figure 36.1). The posterior leaflet has marked indentations, also called scallops, which are named from lateral to medial: P1, P2, and P3. The anterior leaflet similarly is divided, typically into three portions named from lateral to medial: A1, A2, and A3. Anatomical standardization of nomenclature of leaflet scallops optimizes intraprocedural device navigation and team communication.

The papillary muscles are located anterolaterally and posteromedially, as indicated by their names, and originate from the middle to apical region of the left ventricle (LV). The anterolateral papillary muscle has a dual blood supply from the circumflex and left anterior descending coronary artery. In turn, the posteromedial papillary muscle is most frequently supplied only by the right coronary artery, which makes it more prone to ischemic pathological changes. Extending from the tip of each papillary muscle are chords known as chordae tendineae, which attach to the leaflet. Each papillary muscle distributes chords to the ipsilateral side of both leaflets. Primary chords are thinner and attach to the free edge of the leaflet, maintaining leaflet apposition and valve closure. Dysfunction of these primary cords results in acute mitral regurgitation. Secondary chords attach to the ventricular surface of the leaflet and function to maintain the left ventricular size and shape of the LV rather than help with leaflet apposition. Understanding the anchoring of mitral annular and leaflet pathology allows for optimal patient anatomical selection based on specific device design and anchor mechanisms.

2. What is the role of echocardiography in TMVR?

2D transthoracic echocardiography (TTE) is the first-line imaging tool utilized to diagnose and assess the severity of underlying mitral pathophysiology. Real-time imaging capabilities coupled with high spatial resolution by TTE allows for assessment of the geometry and dimensions of the mitral annulus, presence of annular calcification, valve leaflet morphology, leaflet motion, anatomy of subvalvular apparatus, and left ventricular size and

Mastering Structural Heart Disease, First Edition. Edited by Eduardo J. de Marchena and Camilo A. Gomez.
© 2023 John Wiley & Sons Ltd. Published 2023 by John Wiley & Sons Ltd.
Companion website: www.wiley.com/go/deMarchena/Mastering-Structural-Heart-Disease

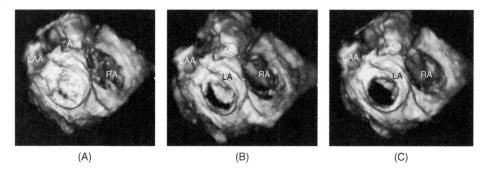

(A)   (B)   (C)

Figure 36.1 Changes in deformation of the mitral annulus and atrial structures during cardiac contractility. (a) Closure of anterior and posterior mitral annulus scallops is appreciated in end-systole from a 3D transesophageal echocardiographic acquired surgeon's view of the left atrium. (b) During early diastole, the leaflet scallop opening of the respective anterior and posterior mitral leaflets is appreciated in a crescentic fashion along the mitral leaflet coaptation plane. (c) During end-diastole, the maximal opening of the mitral leaflets demonstrates a parabolic shape to the mitral leaflet opening area with tenting of the anterior mitral leaflet secondary to restriction of its full movement into the left ventricular outflow tract secondary to tethering by anterior leaflet chordal apparatus.

function. Transesophageal echocardiography (TEE) provides a more detailed evaluation of valvular anatomy and function in comparison to TTE given the imaging is obtained from the esophagus, immediately posterior to the cardiac silhouette (Figure 36.2). 3D TEE and TTE images allow for multi-planar reconstruction not afforded by traditional 2D technologies.

Current limitations of echocardiography in pre-procedural planning for TMVR therapies revolve around the inability to accurately simulate transcatheter heart valve implantation and generate predictive left ventricular outflow tract (LVOT) obstruction risk assessment. Additionally, the small sector field of echocardiographic image acquisition limits its role in peri-procedural planning evaluations of extracardiac structures that may be susceptible to injury

(i.e. complex transseptal punctures, anomalous left circumflex artery course, location of coronary sinus relative to proposed device implants).

3. What are the advantages of utilizing multi-detector computed tomography (MDCT) in TMVR planning?

TEE remains the mainstay of intraprocedural TMVR image guidance. However, the utility of pre-procedural TEE is limited by the anatomic complexity of each patient's anatomy and the skillset of the physician performing the TEE. Multi-detector computed tomography (MDCT)

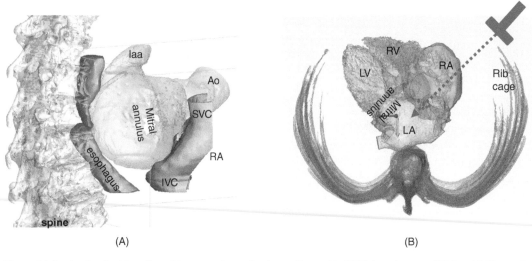

(A)   (B)

Figure 36.2 Anatomical location of transesophageal echocardiographic (TEE) imaging capabilities. (a) The typical esophageal tract courses posterior to the left atrium and provides an optimal window into the left heart chambers. Placement of the TEE probe into the esophagus provides optimal proximity for human cardiac imaging. (b) Red upside-down letter T depicts the location of a surface ultrasound probe to the cardiac silhouette demonstrating increased distance to travel for optimal endocardial and left-sided cardiac structure chamber visualization.

image acquisition allows physicians to overcome the limitation of variability in pre-procedural TEE physician-operator skillsets and anatomical difficulties to accurately assess whether a patient is a candidate for TMVR. Reduction in the inter-observer variability by CT enhances procedural success and multi-disciplinary heart team confidence in the feasibility of a study. This level of reproducibility, accuracy, and validation of CT in TMVR pre-procedural planning is critical for the safe scalability of TMVR procedures.

CT provides additional incremental value as an imaging tool with its high isotropic spatial resolution, large field of view, multi-planar reconstruction capabilities, and rapid turnaround time. Whereas ultrasound image technologies are limited to the small-sector field array of interest, multi-planar CT allows for evaluation of cerebral protection, transapical access planning, and potential large cardiac vessel anatomies simultaneously with the valvular anatomy of interest. This large sector field provides enhanced guidance for device sizing and procedural planning since it can simulate virtual delivery systems, prosthesis positioning, neo-LVOT assessment, as well as risk assessment of adjacent cardiac structures that may interfere with procedural success.

4. What are the basic CT scanner image acquisition concepts and technical protocols required for obtaining a usable mitral CT?

Clinical sites with experience in performing coronary cardiac CT are best equipped to start imaging for pre-TMVR structural evaluation. At a minimum, a 64-slice CT scanner with a cardiac package is required for basic structural CT image acquisition. Modern-day 128-slice or higher CT scanners are recommended for improved image quality with the added benefit of less radiation exposure to the patient (Figure 36.3).

Prior to the patient's arrival for their structural CT, they are instructed to take their cardiac medications as prescribed to optimize their heart rate control. Despite modern-day CT scanner capabilities, heart rate variations > 30–40 heartbeats in a three-second window can greatly impair the quality and interpretability of a mitral CT scan. Hence, at minimum, a 64-slice cardiac CT scanner is recommended, with high-volume sites pivoting to dual-source CT scanner technologies with the fastest gantry times.

At the time of CT scan acquisition, there are a few key patient preparation parameters. First, patients must be able to follow breath-hold instructions. All structural CT scans are performed with a shallow inspiratory breath-hold to prevent lung artifact motion from impacting the assessment of cardiac chamber sizes. Second, stable EKG gating tracking should be noted by the CT technologists prior to scan acquisition to prevent the loss of image datasets. Mitral CT scans should be performed with retrospectively gated ECG image acquisition to allow full volume acquisition of cardiac chamber size analysis, cine imaging of the cardiac chambers and valvular apparatus, and accurate planning for neo-LVOT prediction modeling and device sizing.

The optimal timing of mitral CT scans is when patients are as close as possible to their euvolemic state. In patients with end-stage renal disease requiring intermittent hemodialysis, mitral CT should be performed after the patient has completed dialysis. Mitral CT neo-LVOT prediction modeling aims to anticipate the worst-case scenario for patients and their risk profile for LVOT obstruction. Hence, for hypervolemic patients, this condition would best be met when they have exited their acute systolic heart failure exacerbation. This is also true for patients with atrial fibrillation

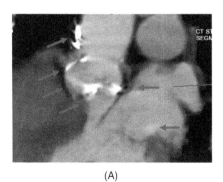
(A)

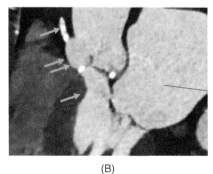
(B)

Figure 36.3 Impact of gantry speed on structural computed tomography (CT) image quality. (a) Image acquired on a scanner greater than 10 years old with a gantry speed >0.3 seconds. (b) Image acquired on the same patient on a Siemens dual-source CT scanner with a gantry speed <0.3 seconds and shorter data acquisition time, demonstrating enhanced temporal resolution and more accurate depiction of cardiac structures of interest.

or atrial flutter. Optially, image acquisition and assessment should be performed when they are no longer in rapid ventricular response to allow for true loading condition ejection fraction and volumetric state assessment. In general, sublingual nitrates are not required for cardiac CT imaging of the mitral annulus, unlike coronary CT, for which they are utilized to enhance visualization of the coronary vasculature.

5. How is the TMVR landing zone sized and evaluated?

Current TMVR devices are being studied in clinical trials to treat multiple different mitral valve pathologies. The sizing and evaluation of the mitral valve or TMVR device landing zone are unique to the underlying patient anatomy and device design. Each TMVR device currently used in a commercial or clinical trial setting is unique. Every TMVR device has different deformation properties, metal properties, and stent cell configurations. Even though a discussion of each specific device is beyond the scope of this chapter, it is important to understand the basic concepts in TMVR CT planning.

Most clinical trial TMVR device designs for mitral regurgitation require an anchoring mechanism within the LV. This includes subvalvular chordae encircling mechanisms, transapical device tethering, or leaflet capture mechanisms. Sizing for each of these devices involves test fitting the TMVR design to prevent para-prosthesis leak post-implantation and evaluating whether there is sufficient room within the LV to seat the ventricular portion of the TMVR. In traditional balloon-expandable valves used for TMVR in mitral annulus calcification (MAC), the mitral landing zone is defined as the point of maximal constraint between the anterior and posterior mitral annulus with sufficient calcification for anchoring the TMVR device. With transseptal delivery of TMVR becoming the most common route for this procedure, the TMVR device mitral landing zone has expanded to a more ventricular region of the LV with deeper ventricular protrusion than traditional open-heart surgical mitral valve prosthesis. Understanding the nuances and engineering behind each TMVR device design is critical to planning accurate device sizing. Inaccurate sizing can have devastating consequences since undersizing can lead to device embolization, and oversizing can result in annular rupture.

6. What is the neo-LVOT?

CT planning for TMVR has led to the new concept of the neo-LVOT (or new LVOT). Soon after the first-in-human

fully percutaneous TMVR, a feared and possibly lethal procedural complication was recognized: acute LVOT obstruction, which is an important cause of morbidity and mortality following TMVR. In TMVR, the neo-LVOT is defined as any part of the basal-mid-anteroseptal wall of the LV that directly interacts with the TMVR frame (Figure 36.4). It is important to understand that the LVOT is a dynamic structure. Depending on the patient's anatomy, the location and severity of their basal to mid-anteroseptal left ventricular wall hypertrophy directly affect cardiac CT phase selection for modeling LVOT obstruction risk, TMVR device positioning, and device sizing (Figure 36.5). Optimal evaluation for TMVR LVOT prediction modeling should be done in the mid-end systolic phases of the cardiac CT acquisition phases.

It is important for clinical teams to recognize that LVOT obstruction is not limited to the TMVR device frame. A secondary mechanism for LVOT obstruction occurs when the placement of the TMVR device causes deflection of the anterior mitral leaflet into the LVOT, thereby decreasing the neo-LVOT area for systolic blood flow. In patients where the native anterior mitral leaflet exceeds the distal strut of the TMVR device by ≥5 mm, this inherent risk of invagination of the anterior mitral leaflet tips into either the TMVR device or the neo-LVOT should be recognized during pre-procedural CT planning. Loading conditions can also result in changes to the LVOT. Severe right ventricular volume overload and patients on hemodialysis will have different LVOT sizes depending on the amount of chamber volume at the time of cardiac CT scan

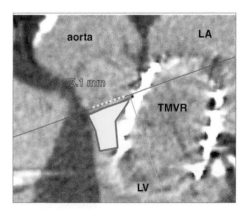

Figure 36.4 Definition of neo-LVOT in TMVR. In the TMVR space, the neo-LVOT is analogous to any part of the left ventricle that interacts with the TMVR frame (area in yellow enclosed with red outline). It does not correlate to traditional echocardiographic or TAVR CT measurements obtained at a level of 5 mm infra-annular to the aortic annulus (yellow dotted line). LVOT, left ventricular outflow tract; TAVR, transcatheter aortic valve replacement; TMVR, transcatheter mitral valve repair. *Source:* Wang et al. (2021), with permission from John Wiley & Sons.

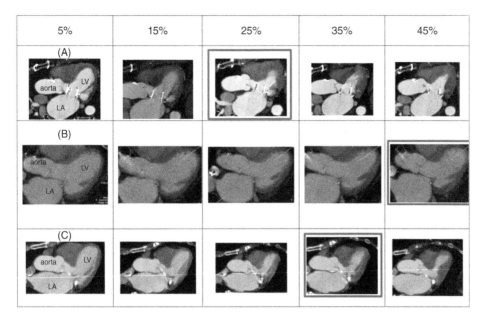

Figure 36.5 Cardiac computed tomography (CT) phase selection. (a–c) Three distinct patient LVOT anatomies. Given the variation of location and presence or absence of basal to mid-anteroseptal left ventricular wall hypertrophy (as demonstrated by the red rectangular boxes), the optimal systolic cardiac phase selection by CT varies for each patient. *Source:* Wang et al. (2021), with permission from John Wiley & Sons.

acquisition. Therefore, CT evaluation of the neo-LVOT requires integrating cardiac physiology, echocardiography, and hemodynamics into accurate peri-procedural TMVR planning.

7. How can neo-LVOT be predicted?

CT modeling is used to estimate the size and anticipated neo-LVOT, and it can simulate a virtual prosthesis, a 3D model that matches the shape and dimensions of a specific TMVR prosthesis. This modeling allows for the prediction of potential obstruction of the LVOT. Neo-LVOT prediction modeling involves planning for optimal and worst-case scenario TMVR implantation. Neo-LVOT prediction modeling and device sizing are performed during static phases of the cardiac cycle since, as of now, commercial CT software packages do not allow for computational fluid modeling. Optimal LVOT prediction modeling requires not only evaluating the landing zone but also understanding of the catheter delivery mechanisms. Virtual simulation of device implantation can be performed using computer-aided design software (Mimics, Materialise Leuven) of the patient's left atrium (LA) and LV cavity, modeling different ventricular depths of TMVR implantation: 60% ventricular/40% atrial, or 80% ventricular/20% atrial for TMVR in native mitral annulus or TMVR in the mitral ring (and at 0% with distal strut marker of surgical mitral bioprosthesis and 20% ventricular distal to surgical strut marker for valve-in-valve TMVR procedures)

(Figure 36.6). Understanding the method of anchoring allows for simulation of the virtual device landing zone and identification of the area at greatest risk of LVOT obstruction post-implantation.

Current cutoffs for neo-LVOT prediction modeling are based on an analysis by Wang et al. Data was collected over five years, assessing pre- and post-TMVR cardiac CT procedural images and intraprocedural catheterization LV pigtail catheter hemodynamic gradients before and after TMVR implantation. Receiver operator characteristic (ROC) curve generation demonstrated a predicted neo-LVOT $\leq 189.4\,mm^2$ had 100% sensitivity and 96.8% specificity for identifying the risk of LVOT obstruction. This LVOT prediction modeling algorithms currently apply to single-unit close-cell TMVR device technologies and may not apply to all open-cell technologies that utilize external docking systems with an inner valve.

8. What factors make neo-LVOT prediction modeling complex?

Even though the correlation between pre- and post-cardiac CT TMVR neo-LVOT prediction modeling is excellent ($R^2 = 0.8169$, $P < 0.0001$), there are inherent limitations in catheters and TMVR design technologies that are difficult to account for in prediction model algorithms. First, in the absence of a steerable catheter for TMVR device delivery, the delivery sheath can only articulate in two orthogonal

CT LVOT prediction modeling (systolic phase):			
valve	Position	Baseline LVOT surface area (mm²)	Predicted neo-LVOT surface area (mm²)
S3 26	0%	464.1	246.5
	20% ventricular	547.9	170.5

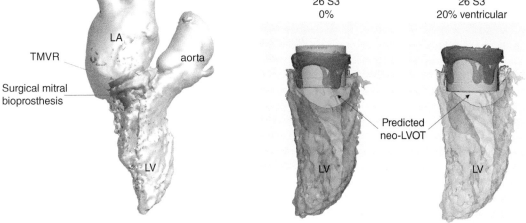

Figure 36.6 TMVR valve-in-valve neo-LVOT modeling. The THV is positioned first at 0% or flush with the most distal portion of the surgical mitral bioprosthesis for neo-LVOT prediction modeling (surgical bioprosthesis depicted in purple). The THV is then positioned 20% ventricular to the distal edge of the surgical mitral bioprosthesis to anticipate the worst-case scenario if the proposed THV experienced intra-procedural difficulty obtaining full coaxiality with the surgical mitral bioprosthesis during implantation. LVOT, left ventricular outflow tract; THV, transcatheter heart valve; TMVR, transcatheter mitral valve replacement.

planes. In some patients, this limitation in catheter design inhibits the TMVR device from reaching optimal coaxiality during implantation (Figure 36.7). Second, in transseptal TMVR, canting of the atrial portion of the transcatheter heart valve (THV) toward the septum and away from the appendage is not uncommon. In the LV, the anterior

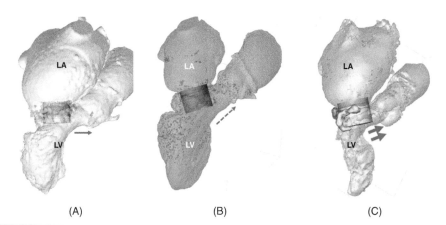

(A) (B) (C)

Figure 36.7 Variations in human anatomy affect the TMVR delivery system and device positioning. (a) Positioning the basal anteroseptal wall ventricular (red arrow) to the deployment zone of the TMVR device does not impact the delivery system trajectory and allows for optimal coaxiality of the final TMVR device in a 12:00 pm to 6:00 pm orientation. (b) In a patient with prior aortic root surgery and surgical mitral bioprosthesis implant with underlying RV dysfunction, septal flattening of the basal anteroseptal portion of the left ventricular wall (as depicted by the red dotted arrow) coupled with non-horizontal surgical implantation of the surgical mitral bioprosthesis results in a canted valve-in-valve TMVR delivery system implanting a THV biased toward the aorta and away from the LV apex. (c) In a patient with severe basal anteroseptal hypertrophy (double red arrows), the valve cannot be deployed at an 80/20 LV : LA configuration due to the small LV cavity size, resulting in limited landing zone options. LA, left atrium; LV, left ventricle; RV, right ventricle; THV, transcatheter heart valve; TMVR, transcatheter mitral valve replacement.

portion of the TMVR device seats deeper than the posterior portion. This correlates with the trajectory of the catheter during transseptal crossing and maneuvering into the LV. Finally, peri-procedural CT modeling and 3D printing demonstrate variation in the size and location of the fossa ovalis for each patient. Variation in the fossa ovalis width, height, and amount of surface area covered contributes to the complexity and nonlinearity of device delivery between pre- and post-CT neo-LVOT prediction modeling.

9. Which type of TMVR is at greatest risk of LVOT obstruction: valve-in-valve, valve-in-ring, or valve-in-MAC?

CT imaging has demonstrated that MAC is typically sub-annular or ventricular to the patient's native mitral annulus. This sub-annular growth of MAC makes the TMVR landing zone of devices for MAC more ventricular in placement than devices for noncalcified mitral landing zones (Figure 36.8). This is why valve-in-MAC TMVR is associated with a significantly higher risk of LVOT obstruction. In valve-in-MAC TMVR, the THV positions itself within the mitral landing zone according to the path of least resistance: that is, the area of mitral landing zone without calcification. The question of how much this affects the predicted neo-LVOT modeling and the long-term impact of this deformation change of the TMVR device in the mitral landing zone space are yet not well understood.

Other factors that affect neo-LVOT size can be both device-specific and patient-specific. For example, the risk of neo-LVOT obstruction is greater with flaring, protrusion, and skirt size of the device. Patient-specific characteristics that increase the risk of LVOT obstruction include but are not limited to basal-mid anteroseptal left ventricular wall thickness $\geq 10\,mm$, redundant anterior mitral leaflet length (>30 mm), and severely enlarged right ventricle. Device-specific risk profiles for TMVR LVOT obstruction include large ventricular footprint designs, absence of anterior mitral leaflet capturing mechanisms, and varying device-specific deformation and conformation properties within the mitral annular landing zone.

10. How can CT imaging estimate the coplanar fluoroscopic angle?

During TMVR deployment, it is essential to have a fluoroscopic angle that is perpendicular to the mitral annulus (coplanar angle) for accurate coaxial deployment. Any obliquity in the fluoroscopic angle can lead to an inaccurate

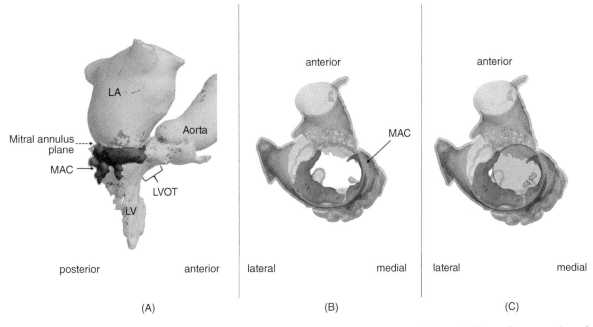

Figure 36.8 Location of mitral annulus calcification in one patient. (a) Three-chamber left ventricular outflow tract view of the left heart demonstrates MAC to be ventricular to the native mitral annulus plane (dashed black arrow). (b) Surgeon's view of the LA also demonstrates mitral annulus calcification to be located mainly (or predominantly) posterior of the mitral native annulus. (c) Surgeon's view of the LA demonstrates virtual THV positioning biased toward mitral annulus positioning in a location away from the calcification or point of least MAC. LA: left atrium; MAC: mitral annulus calcification; LVOT: left ventricular outflow tract; LV: left ventricle; THV, transcatheter heart valve.

deployment, which can increase the risk of LVOT obstruction, device embolization, severe paravalvular leakage (PVL), and prolonged fluoroscopy times for the patient and implanting team. The coplanar fluoroscopic angle can be estimated by CT (Figure 36.9). CT post-processing software can generate a coplanar curve specific to the patient. This curve has a sinusoidal path that the C-arm follows as it rotates around the patient, providing a tangential view of the valve and allowing coaxial deployment with optimal visualization of the mitral annulus plane and aortic outflow tract.

11. What are other relevant adjacent structures to consider in CT planning for TMVR?

The left circumflex artery and the coronary sinus are in close proximity to the mitral annulus and are at theoretical risk of compression with TMVR device oversizing. Using CT, the course of the left circumflex artery and coronary sinus relative to the mitral annulus and virtual prosthesis can be simulated. Some TMVR devices can interfere with the left atrial appendage and subvalvular apparatus. TMVR devices with supra-annular components can occlude the left atrial appendage ostium. The distance between the mitral annular plane and the left atrial appendage ostium can be measured on volumetric CT images. There are no specific cutoffs, but clinical experience demonstrates that the smaller the distance between the left atrial appendage ostium and the mitral annulus landing zone, the greater the risk of ostial

left atrial appendage partial occlusion. On the other hand, devices that extend into the left ventricular chamber, such as the Tendyne (Abbott) and Intrepid (Medtronic) TMVR systems, may interfere with chordae tendineae and papillary muscles. The distance from the mitral annulus plane to the papillary muscles, the distance between the papillary muscles, and the separation between the papillary muscles and the ventricular wall should be obtained to help predict sub-valvular apparatus interference. The mechanism of device delivery and final device positioning should all be considered in pre-procedural CT planning. Balloon-expandable devices require an assessment of the distal apical LV volumes in mid-end systole to anticipate whether the LV cavity will accommodate a fully inflated balloon for TMVR device coaxiality (Figure 36.7).

12. What are the important measurements and characteristics to define prior to the transseptal approach for TMVR?

There is a growing interest in the transseptal approach for TMVR since it is the least invasive mechanism for TMVR device delivery and has been demonstrated to be feasible and safe. CT can help characterize the interatrial septum and determine the optimal site for puncture. The preferred puncture site is mid-posterior with respect to the mitral annulus landing zone to achieve the most coaxial alignment of the THV with the mitral annulus. As with MitraClip (Abbott Vascular) delivery systems, adequate

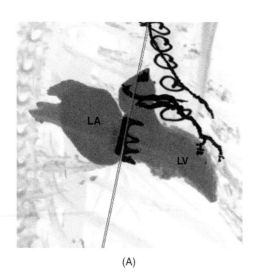

(A)

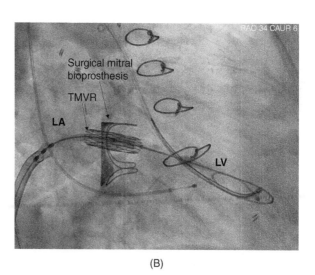

(B)

Figure 36.9 Fluoroscopic CT-generated C-arm angles provide optimal guidance for intra-procedural device coaxiality positioning. (a) Pre-procedural CT-generated fluoroscopic C-arm angle: RAO 34 CRA 9. (b) Intra-procedural fluoroscopic C-arm angle: RAO 34 CAU 6. (a) Pre-procedural CT-generated fluoroscopic angle: RAO 34 CRA 9. (b) Intra-procedural fluoroscopic C-arm angle: RAO 34 CAU 6. CAU, caudal; CRA, cranial; CT, computed tomography; RAO, right anterior oblique.

heights >3.5 cm are required for current TMVR transseptal delivery systems to navigate the interatrial crossing to achieve optimal landing zone coaxiality. The distance from the puncture to the mitral valve can be estimated with CT procedural planning. The thickness of the atrial septum may also be assessed with an evaluation documenting the presence or absence of an existing interatrial septal defect, patent foramen ovale, lipomatous hypertrophy, and septal aneurysm to account for necessary intra-procedural equipment supply lists before the date of the planned procedure.

13. What are the important measurements and characteristics to define prior to the transapical approach for TMVR?

CT images can be used to identify the intercostal space closest to the LV apex best suited for a transapical approach. It is essential to deliver the device perpendicular to the mitral annulus to avoid canting, obstruction, and PVL. Additionally, the fluoroscopic angle for optimal transapical coaxial alignment can be simulated with CT. Post-processing software can project the mitral annulus central axis, left ventricular central axis, angle between these axes, and true left ventricular apex. Key measurements for percutaneous transapical planning include finding a 10 mm window for transapical micropuncture that is free from adjacent coronary vasculature. Lung fields and papillary muscles cannot be in the zone of transapical access. LV cavity dimensions from the mitral annulus plane to the distal endocardial LV apex need to be measured to

ensure adequate room for the full length of the pre-specified TMVR delivery system.

14. What is the role of CT in post-procedural imaging?

Post-mitral CT is clinically indicated in the setting of changes in New York Heart Association (NYHA) classification post-hospitalization discharge. Post-mitral CT is complementary and additive to surveillance transthoracic echocardiogram, the latter of which is typically performed before discharge and then one month after discharge. Cine CT image generation of post-TMVR devices help characterize dynamic TMVR-induced LVOT narrowing, potential hypo-attenuation leaflet thickening of implanted devices, and potential size and location of PVL identified by post-surveillance echocardiographic studies. CT can also identify left ventricular pseudoaneurysms, which are rare complications following TMVR. These pseudoaneurysms are depicted on CT images as a focal contrast material-filled outpouching from the LV with a narrow neck. CT is also key for helping characterize the anatomic suitability for advanced catheter-based closure of atrial septal defects and PVL. CT can characterize PVL, which appears as contrast material-opacified tunnels around the TMVR connecting the left atrial and LV. CT can also help define the position and the size of the PVL and determine the suitability for percutaneous closure. Of note, the PVL location is usually described based on its clock position relative to the mitral annulus in the surgeon's view of the left atrium, with the aorta at the 12 o'clock position (Figure 36.10).

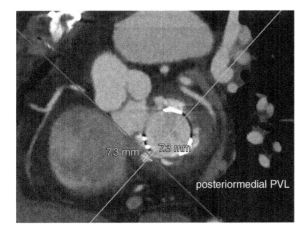 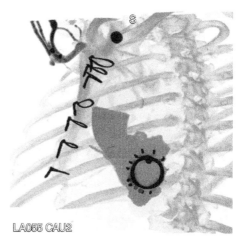

Figure 36.10 PVL assessment for a surgical mitral bioprosthesis. (a) Posteromedial PVL sized at 7.3 × 7.3 mm in dimensions. CT pre-procedural planning depicts the PVL with two pink dots in the 7 pm position of the surgical mitral bioprosthesis for fluoroscopic-guided defect crossing. CT, computed tomography; PVL, paravalvular leakage.

Conclusion

TMVR is a safe and feasible option for selected patients with severe native mitral valve disease or a failed bioprosthetic valve or ring. Given the complexity of the mitral valve apparatus, TMVR devices have been developed with different characteristics and delivery systems/strategies. Due to the complexity of pre-procedural planning, CT imaging has emerged as the pivotal imaging modality. Pre-procedural CT provides critical information on the sizing of the transcatheter heart valve, landing zone, neo-LVOT obstruction risk, fluoroscopic angles, location/relationship of adjacent structures, and access-specific concerns. TMVR clinical outcomes have significantly improved with increasing adaptation and understanding of the value of integrating multi-modality imaging tools by physicians for patient-centric anatomy evaluation.

Bibliography

1 Greenbaum, A.B., Condado, J.F., Eng, M. et al. (2018). Long or redundant leaflet complicating transcatheter mitral valve replacement: case vignettes that advocate for removal or reduction of the anterior mitral leaflet. *Catheter. Cardiovasc. Interv.* 92: 627–632.

2 Guerrero, M., Greenbaum, A., and O'Neill, W. (2014). First in human percutaneous implantation of a balloon expandable transcatheter heart valve in a severely stenosed native mitral valve. *Catheter. Cardiovasc. Interv.* 83: E287–E291.

3 Guerrero, M., Urena, M., Himbert, D. et al. (2018). 1-year outcomes of transcatheter mitral valve replacement in patients with severe mitral annular calcification. *J. Am. Coll. Cardiol.* 71: 1841–1853.

4 Hahn, R.T., Mahmood, F., Kodali, S. et al. (2019). Core competencies in echocardiography for imaging structural heart disease interventions: an expert consensus statement. *JACC: Cardiovasc. Imaging* 12: 2560–2570.

5 Ho, S.Y. (2002). Anatomy of the mitral valve. *Heart* 88 (Suppl 4): iv5–iv10.

6 Khan, J.M., Lederman, R.J., Devireddy, C.M. et al. (2018). LAMPOON to facilitate tendyne transcatheter mitral valve replacement. *JACC: Cardiovasc. Interv.* 11: 2014–2017.

7 Korsholm, K., Berti, S., Iriart, X. et al. (2020). Expert recommendations on cardiac computed tomography for planning transcatheter left atrial appendage occlusion. *JACC: Cardiovasc. Interv.* 13: 277–292.

8 Leipsic, J., Norgaard, B.L., Khalique, O. et al. (2019). Core competencies in cardiac CT for imaging structural heart disease interventions: an expert consensus statement. *JACC: Cardiovasc. Imaging* 12: 2555–2559.

9 McCarthy, K.P., Ring, L., and Rana, B.S. (2010). Anatomy of the mitral valve: understanding the mitral valve complex in mitral regurgitation. *Eur. J. Echocardiogr.* 11: i3–i9.

10 Muller, D.W.M., Sorajja, P., Duncan, A. et al. (2021). 2-year outcomes of transcatheter mitral valve replacement in patients with severe symptomatic mitral regurgitation. *J. Am. Coll. Cardiol.* 78: 1847–1859.

11 Silbiger, J.J. and Bazaz, R. (2009). Contemporary insights into the functional anatomy of the mitral valve. *Am. Heart J.* 158: 887–895.

12 Wang, D.D., Eng, M., Greenbaum, A. et al. (2016). Predicting LVOT obstruction after TMVR. *JACC: Cardiovasc. Imaging* 9: 1349–1352.

13 Wang, D.D., Eng, M.H., Greenbaum, A.B. et al. (2018). Validating a prediction modeling tool for left ventricular outflow tract (LVOT) obstruction after transcatheter mitral valve replacement (TMVR). *Catheter. Cardiovasc. Interv.* 92: 379–387.

14 Wang, D.D., Geske, J., Choi, A.D. et al. (2018). Navigating a career in structural heart disease interventional imaging. *JACC: Cardiovasc. Imaging* 11: 1928–1930.

15 Wang, D.D., Geske, J.B., Choi, A.D. et al. (2019). Interventional imaging for structural heart disease: challenges and new frontiers of an emerging multi-disciplinary field. *Struct. Heart* 3: 187–200.

16 Wang, D.D., Guerrero, M., Eng, M.H. et al. (2019). Alcohol septal ablation to prevent left ventricular outflow tract obstruction during transcatheter mitral valve replacement: first-in-man study. *JACC Cardiovasc. Interv.* 12: 1268–1279.

17 Wang, D.D., Guerrero, M., O'Neill, B. et al. (2021). CT planning for TMVR and predicting LVOT obstruction. In: *Transcatheter Mitral Valve Therapies* (ed. R. Waksman and T. Rogers), 63–73. Wiley.

18 Wang, D.D., O'Neill, B.P., Caranasos, T.G. et al. (2021). Comparative differences of mitral valve-in-valve implantation: a new mitral bioprosthesis versus current mosaic and epic valves. *Catheter. Cardiovasc. Interv.* 14: 854–866.

19 Webb, J.G., Murdoch, D.J., Boone, R.H. et al. (2019). Percutaneous transcatheter mitral valve replacement: first-in-human experience with a new transseptal system. *J. Am. Coll. Cardiol.* 73: 1239–1246.

20 Wojakowski, W., Smolka, G., Piazza, N. et al. (2021). Transseptal implantation of HighLife self-expandable mitral valve in a patient with severe secondary mitral regurgitation and heart failure. *Kardiol. Pol.* 79: 708–709.

37

Transcatheter Mitral Valve Replacement

Transcatheter Mitral Valve-in-Valve (ViV), Valve-in-Ring (ViR), and Valve-in-MAC (ViMAC)

Yashasvi Chugh[1] and Santiago Garcia[2]

[1] Valve Science Center at the Minneapolis Heart Institute Foundation, Abbott Northwestern Hospital, Minneapolis, MN, USA
[2] Structural Heart Program and Harold C. Schott Foundation Endowed Chair for Structural and Valvular Heart Disease The Carl and Edyth Lindner Center for Research and Education at The Christ Hospital. Cincinnati, OH

1. What is the best way to approach a patient with a failing bioprosthetic mitral valve?

Bioprosthetic valves in the mitral position are at the greatest risk of degenerating (stenosis, regurgitation, or both) over time compared to valves in other positions. According to the Valve-in-Valve International Data (VIVID) registry, the median time to bioprosthetic mitral valve failure was nine years (interquartile range [IQR] 5–12 years). Therapy for these patients is limited to redoing the surgical valve replacement or a percutaneous transcatheter valve-in-valve procedure, the latter being a less invasive alternative, especially in the setting of multiple comorbidities and high surgical risk patients. It is important to recognize that the risk of a second mitral valve operation is significantly higher than the first. Once the mechanism of valve failure (stenosis, regurgitation, or mixed disease) has been established by transesophageal echocardiography (TEE), it is prudent to know (i) the valve type and (ii) the valve size, which will aid with transcatheter heart valve (THV) selection and procedure planning. Other important considerations prior to ViV procedures include

assessing the septal anatomy (previous patent foramen ovale [PFO] or atrial septal defect [ASD] devices) and the presence of a left atrial appendage clot on TEE (Figure 37.1).

The valve type (usually only stented bioprostheses are used in the mitral position, unlike the aortic) and size can be obtained from the operative report or valve manufacturer or on fluoroscopic identification. Once that is obtained, finding the true internal diameter (ID) is the next step (Figure 37.2). The true ID is the mechanical internal diameter and is calculated as follows. If the bioprosthetic valve is made of porcine leaflets, true ID = stent ID – 2 mm, where the stent ID is the external diameter of the sewing ring and is provided by the manufacturers. If the bioprosthetic valve is made of pericardial leaflets, true ID = stent ID – 1 mm. The ViV Aortic app also has true IDs for most commercially available valves.

Once the true ID is known, a THV can be selected. Balloon-expandable valves are preferred for such cases (SAPIEN 3 [Edwards Lifesciences]). A 2–3 mm oversize over the true ID is preferred due to higher closing pressure (in systole, unlike the aortic valve, which closes in diastole so that 1 mm oversize is preferred) and to minimize the risk of embolization.

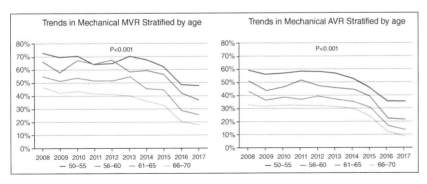

Figure 37.1 Trends in the use of mechanical valves for mitral and aortic valve disease in the United States (2008–2017). *Source:* Alkhouli et al. (2021) / with permission of American Heart Association, Inc.

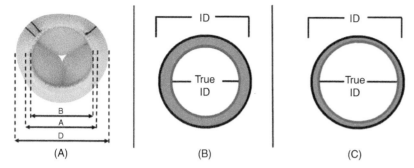

Figure 37.2   Relationship of the external diameter of the sewing ring to the true internal diameter (ID). (a) A: stent outer frame diameter, B: stent frame inner diameter, D: external diameter of the sewing ring. (b) Porcine leaflets: true ID = stent ID – 2 mm. (c) Pericardial leaflets: true ID = stent ID – 1 mm. *Source:* Pirelli et al. (2021) / with permission of AME Publishing Company.

2.   What are the important anatomic variables on cardiac computerized tomography to consider when evaluating a patient for TMVR suitability?

Obtaining a computerized tomography (CT) scan of the mitral valve is also crucial (if renal function permits) to assess the sub-valvular apparatus and left ventricular outflow tract. The following variables are important when evaluating these CT scans:

- *Annular size* (diameter, perimeter, shape) to evaluate the size of THV needed and percent oversizing desired to decrease the risk of paravalvular leakage (PVL).
- Knowing the anterior *leaflet length* is important when determining the risk of left ventricular outflow tract obstruction (LVOTO). Anterior leaflet length > 2.5 cm increases the risk of LVOTO.
- Using CT scan modeling of virtual valves, the *neo-(LVOT)* can be predicted. The neo-LVOT is a dynamic three-dimensional structure; measurements are usually taken in mid-systole. Patients with predicted neo-LVOT areas <180–200 mm^2 are usually considered high risk for LVOTO.
- *Transseptal vs. transapical*: In the absence of anatomic contraindications (previous device in the interatrial septum or unfavorable angles), transseptal (TS) access is preferred. CT allows identification of optimal crossing anatomic plane for TS puncture and implantation fluoroscopic angles that can facilitate optimal coaxial deployment. CT also allows evaluation of the left ventricle (LV) apex for suitability for transapical access (thin, scarred, and aneurysmal apex are poor characteristics for transapical access).

3.   What is the best way to approach and evaluate a patient with a failing mitral ring in preparation for a ViR procedure?

Once the mechanism of ring failure has been determined via echocardiography, it is prudent to know (i) the ring type, (ii) the size, and (iii) the characteristics of the anterior mitral leaflet. Ring types can be classified as (i) complete or incomplete and (ii) rigid, semirigid, or flexible.

Favorable characteristics of a surgical ring are as follows.

- *Ability to become circular*: This ability is possessed by complete rings and semi-rigid or flexible rings. ViR performed in rigid rings (e.g. St. Jude Saddle Ring) is associated with poor outcomes as the THV is usually under-expanded or deformed, increasing the risk of early THV degeneration and PVL.
- *Ability to provide a good anchor*: Semirigid (and complete) rings (e.g. Sorin Memo 3D) provide the best anchoring for THVs compared to incomplete rings or flexible rings, which may not provide good anchoring, increasing the risk of device embolization. However, certain flexible rings can provide a good anchor when stretched.
- *Ring sizes* usually vary from 28 to 40 mm, and available SAPIEN valves vary from 20 to 29 mm; thus rings with label sizes more than 34 may not be suitable for ViR. A majority of rings are kidney-shaped and become circular after ViR; the information provided by manufacturers (area and diameter) is based on the ring's original shape and must be taken into consideration when planning ViR procedures.
- *Radio-opacity* (discussed further in a later question) is important for adequate THV positioning, in the absence of which the intra-procedural TEE visualization is crucial.

4. What are the ideal rings in the market for ViR procedures?

Ideal rings include Memo 3D (Sorin Freedom), Duran AnCore (Medtronic), Sovering (Corcym), Physio 1 and 2 (Carpentier-Edwards), CG Future (Medtronic), AnnuloFlex (CarboMedics), and Simulus (Medtronic).

5. What fluoroscopic landmarks are important for positioning THVs for ViV and ViR procedures?

The ideal place for THV deployment (10–15% in the left atrium) is at the narrowest portion of the failing bioprosthesis, which usually corresponds to the sewing ring. Some bioprosthesis valves have markers at the sewing ring (e.g. Epic mitral valve [St. Jude]), and others have them at the stent frame or stent posts (e.g. Mosaic mitral valve [Medtronic]), making identification of the sewing ring more difficult. Mitral valve rings have different degrees of radio-opacity. The less-radio-opaque rings are poorly visualized on fluoroscopy, so device placement depends on TEE guidance. THV placement is ideally performed in a steep right anterior oblique view.

6. What are the available treatment options for severe mitral annular calcification?

Patients with mitral annular calcification (MAC) and severe mitral regurgitation are usually at the highest surgical risk. The balloon-expandable transcatheter valves (Edwards Lifesciences) have been used off-label for ViMAC. The largest reported registry (TMVR in MAC Global Registry) of extreme surgical risk patients (n = 116) with an Society for Thoracic Surgery (STS) score of 15.3± 11.6% found a one-year, all-cause mortality rate of 53.7%. Even though feasible, ViMAC with balloon-expandable THVs carries a very high mortality rate. Due to an unmet need in treating these patients, there are novel valve systems currently under study, including the Intrepid (Medtronic) and Tendyne (Abbott) valves.

The APOLLO (Transcatheter Mitral Valve Replacement with the Medtronic Intrepid TMVR System in Patients with Severe Symptomatic Mitral Regurgitation) trial is currently evaluating the Intrepid valve in a non-randomized arm for surgery-ineligible patients (n = 300) with severe mitral regurgitation (MR) and MAC or moderate MR with mitral stenosis (MS) and MAC. The primary endpoints of the trial are all-cause mortality and heart failure hospitalization at one year.

The SUMMIT (Safety and Effectiveness of Using the Tendyne Mitral Valve System for the Treatment of Symptomatic Mitral Regurgitation) Tendyne trial also has a non-randomized MAC cohort consisting of patients with severe MAC and ≥Grade III MR, or Severe MS, or Moderate MR and MS, rendering them unsuitable for mitral valve surgery. The primary endpoint is survival free from heart failure hospitalization at 12 months, and the trial is currently enrolling.

In the initial feasibility study of the first 100 patients with primary or secondary MR, the Tendyne valve showed promising results. Device implantation was associated with a 96% technical success rate and 0% perioperative mortality, with a majority of patients having a significant resolution in MR grade and left ventricular volumes and improved quality of life at 30-day and one-year follow-up. The first-in-human case series of compassionate use of Tendyne in five patients at prohibitive surgical risk with severe primary or secondary mitral regurgitation did well at two-year follow-up, with a significant reduction in their heart failure symptoms and complete resolution of their MR.

7. What are favorable characteristics for transcatheter valve anchoring in severe mitral annular calcification?

Adequate valve anchoring is paramount to avoid complications associated with valve migration following ViMAC. The pattern and distribution of annular calcium are important to consider. Four variables have been identified as predictive of good anchoring: calcium thickness, degree of arc distribution along the annular circumference, and trigone and leaflet involvement. The presence of circumferential calcification is not mandatory; however, in the presence of non-circumferential calcification, involvement of the posterior leaflet and parts of the medial and lateral annulus is necessary for appropriate anchoring. Calcification of the anterior annulus may not be necessary. Specifically, on CT, the following features are associated with the lowest risk of valve embolization: (i) calcium thickness ≥ 5 mm, (ii) >270° arc of distribution along the annular circumference, (iii) trigone calcification, and (iv) leaflet calcification. Using these variables, a scoring system (MAC score) is available; a score of ≥7 is associated with favorable valve anchoring (Figure 37.3).

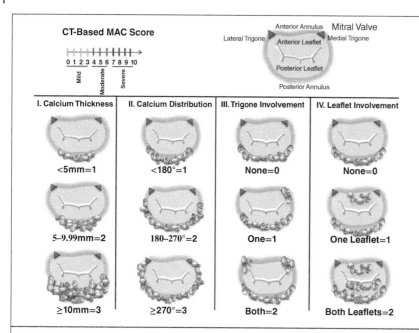

Figure 37.3 Mitral annular calcification scoring system (MAC score). *Source:* Guerrero et al. (2020) / With permission of Elsevier.

8. What is the ideal location for a transseptal puncture for TMVR?

The ideal transseptal puncture site is posterior-inferior, 3–4 cm from the mitral valve annulus, similar to left atrial appendage (LAA) closure procedures.

9. What are the indications to close the transseptal septostomy site after TMVR?

The presence of residual significant bidirectional shunt or right to left shunt is an accepted indication for closure.

10. What are the steps taken to perform the procedure?

Once the transseptal sheath is in the left atrium, a 0.032-in. exchange wire, e.g. Inoue wire (Toray Medical) or 0.035-in. Safari wire (Boston Scientific), is placed in the left atrium. The transseptal sheath is exchanged with a steerable Agilis (St. Jude Medical) catheter over the wire and positioned over the mitral orifice with the assistance of TEE and fluoroscopy (right anterior oblique cranial or caudal projection). The mitral orifice is then crossed with a 0.035-in. J wire and

5-F catheter (pigtail or multipurpose). Once in the LV, the pigtail is exchanged for a stiff guidewire (Amplatz Super Stiff [Cook Medical), Safari, or Confida [Medtronic]). Following this, atrial septostomy is performed, typically using a 12 mm (for S3 23 or 26) or 14 mm (S3 29) balloon. At this point, the Agilis catheter is withdrawn and the THV's designated sheath is inserted. The valve is mounted on the balloon in opposite orientation to that in TAVR (SAPIEN 3) with the sealing skirt away from the nose cone (Figure 37.4). Once the valve is mounted on the balloon, the delivery system is rotated 180 degrees° prior to crossing the septum, which allows flexing of the delivery system and coaxial alignment. The valve is deployed slowly to allow for minor adjustments under rapid pacing with the goal of achieving a final 10–20% atrial and 80–90% ventricular position.

11. What are potential complications associated with TMVR and the solutions to managing them?

The following are a list of potential complications and their solutions:

- *Valve embolization from improper positioning:* At times, a second valve can be used to secure the first. However,

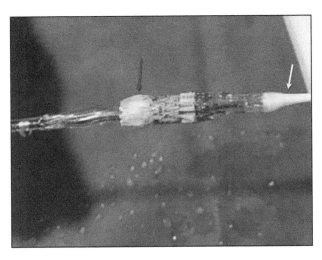

Figure 37.4 For mitral procedures with SAPIEN 3, the valve is loaded in the opposite direction relative to transcatheter aortic valve replacement procedures with the sealing skirt (red arrow) away from the nose cone (yellow arrow). *Source:* Pirelli et al. (2021) / with permission of AME Publishing Company.

emergent surgery may be needed to remove the embolized valve. The risk of mortality is high.

- *PVL:* If the valve was deployed high (atrial), significant PVL may have to be treated with a second valve. When the leak is circumferential around a valve, despite proper positioning and deployment, post-dilation may be necessary. If there is a significant and persistent PVL (despite adequate positioning and expansion of the valve), percutaneous PVL closure may be indicated.
- *MR:* For central MR persisting after removal of the stiff wire, a second valve may be needed.
- *High transmitral gradients:* If the mechanism is incomplete valve expansion, post-dilation is required. It is important to consider patient-prosthesis mismatch when small surgical valves are treated. Bioprosthetic valve fracture (BVF) prior to valve implantation is emerging as a potential solution, but more data is needed regarding the safety of this approach. The largest non-compliant balloon used for BVF (True balloon) is 28 mm.
- *Leaflet stuck or abnormal motion:* Remove the stiff wire first; if the issue persists, a second valve may be needed.
- *Severe hypotension:* Suspect vascular complication, tamponade (source could be transseptal puncture or LV perforation), LVOT obstruction (can consider rescue alcohol septal ablation if a prominent septal bulge is present or implantation of a self-expanding aortic prosthesis in more ventricular position), or severe MR (due to displacement and impingement of anterior leaflet).

12. What are the contraindications for ViV or ViR procedures?

The presence of significant PVL, infective endocarditis, or partial bioprosthetic (valve or ring) dehiscence affecting > 50% of the circumference. These patients are best served with surgical treatment.

13. What are the procedural success rates and complications associated with TMVR?

There are no randomized trials available for mitral ViV or ViR interventions. However, various registries report success and complication rates, as shown in Table 37.1. Technical success was notably highest among ViV cases and lowest in ViMAC cases, with 30-day mortality also being highest for ViMAC. The risk of LVOTO was higher in ViR vs. ViV but highest with ViMAC cases. The need for a second valve was higher in ViR cases vs. ViV.

Valve embolization rates were higher after ViR vs. ViV (7 vs. 2.4% from the VIVID registry, p < 0.001, 2.4 vs. 0.1% from the STS/TVT registry, 1.4 vs. 0.9% from the TMVR registry, and 0% in the MITRAL [Mitral Implantation of Transcatheter Valves] trial). Because the MV is subjected to higher closing pressure in systole, this may lead to reduced anchoring and thus a higher risk of embolization.

Given the variability in ring types, shapes and dimensions (as discussed in a previous question), the utilization of THVs designed for aortic valve interventions in the mitral space increases the risk of paravalvular leaks and mitral regurgitation. The presence of moderate or greater residual MR was higher after ViR compared to ViV (16.6 vs. 3.1%, p < 0.001 VIVID registry, 10.6 vs. 2.5% STS/TVT, 10% vs 0% MITRAL trial, and 12.6% vs 3.3% TMVR registry). Higher residual MR was associated with a later need for repeat TMVR and higher all-cause mortality. It can also be postulated that poor valve hemodynamics may lead to decreased THV durability.

14. What factors are responsible for left ventricular outflow tract obstruction (LVOTO) after ViV and ViR?

LVOTO is a dynamic structure and is considered an Achilles heel of TMVR (Figure 37.5). Predicting LVOTO is challenging. Certain characteristics adapted from

Table 37.1 Summary of published transcatheter mitral valve replacement registries.

Study/total patients	Study duration	STS score	Technical success	Conversion to surgery	Need for second valve	LVOTO	CVA	30-day mortality
TMVR registry n = 521 (322 ViV, 141 ViR, 58 ViMAC)	2009–2018	9.0 ± 7.0	94.4% ViV, 80.9% ViR, 62.1% ViMAC*	0.9% ViV, 2.8% ViR, 8.6% ViMAC*	2.5% ViV, 12.1% ViR, 5.2% ViMAC*	2.2% ViV, 5.0% ViR, 39.7% ViMAC*	2.3% ViV, 0% ViR, 3.9% ViMAC	6.2% ViV, 9.9% ViR, 34.5% ViMAC*
VIVID registry n = 1079 (857 ViV, 222 ViR)	2006–2020	8.6 (5.4–14.1)	93.5% ViV, 82% ViR*	N/A	2.8% ViV, 10.1% ViR*	1.8%, 5.9%*	1.4% ViV, 0.5% ViR	6.5% ViV, 8.6% ViR
Guerrero et al. (STS/ACC/TVT registry) N = 903 (680 ViV, 123 ViR, 100 ViMAC)	2013–2017	10 (6.5–16)	90.9% ViV, 82.9% ViR, 74% ViMAC*	1.3% ViV, 2.4% ViR, 2% ViMAC	1.5% ViV, 7.3% ViR, 14% ViMAC	0.7% ViV, 4.9% ViR, 10% ViMAC*	1.6% ViV, 1.6% ViR, 4% ViMAC	8.1% ViV, 11.5% ViR, 21.8% ViMAC*
MITRAL trial (ViV arm)	2016–2017	9.4 (5.8–12.0)	93.3%	0%	0%	0%	6.7%	3.3%
MITRAL Trial (ViR arm)		7.6 (5.1–11.8)	66.7%	0%	0%	0%	3.3%	6.7%

TMVR, transcatheter mitral valve replacement; LVOTO, left ventricular outflow tract obstruction; VIVID, Valve in Valve International Data; STS, Society of Thoracic Surgeons; ACC, American College of Cardiology; TVT, Transcatheter Valve Therapy registry; ViV, valve in valve; ViR, valve in ring; ViMAC, valve in mitral annular calcification.
* = p-value is significant.

pre-procedural CT and echocardiographic planning may be utilized to predict LVOTO: (i) aorto-mitral angle – less obtuse angles are associated with a greater risk (<110°); (ii) septal thickness – septal bulging or asymmetric septal hypertrophy may increase the risk (>2 cm); (iii) length of anterior mitral leaflet – once the valve is deployed, the anterior leaflet will be displaced toward the LVOT, increasing the risk of LVOTO: anterior mitral leaflet length > 2.5 cm is associated with a considerable risk of LVOTO; (iv) depth of THV implantation – the deeper the THV, the higher the LVOTO risk; (v) degree of THV flaring – greater THV flare in the LV is associated with an increased risk of LVOTO; (vi) small LVOT; (vii) small LV cavity; (vii) heavily calcified sub-valvular apparatus.

ViR has an increased risk of LVOTO (as the anterior mitral leaflet is intact). With ViV, the risk is more with peri-cardial valves (taller, and covering the THV more) than the porcine valves (short leaflets) but overall is considered low as the anterior leaflet is removed during mitral valve replacement surgery. The degree of tolerable residual LVOT (or neo-LVOT) after ViV or ViR is unclear. In patients where the risk of LVOTO is high and prohibitive for redo surgery, pre-TMVR alcohol septal ablation or Laceration of the Anterior Mitral leaflet to Prevent Outflow ObtructioN (LAMPOON) can be considered.

There is no formal neo-LVOT cut-off value; however, an area of 1.7 cm² for the estimated neo-LVOT after ViV-TMVR has predicted LVOT obstruction accurately, with sensitivity and specificity values of 96.2 and 92.3%, respectively.

15. What is the anticoagulation/antiplatelet strategy after TMVR?

Current guidelines recommend three to six months of anti-coagulation with a vitamin K antagonist after bioprosthetic mitral valve implantation (in patients without an indication for long-term anticoagulation). However, data on anti-coagulation after TMVR is limited, and the utilization of antiplatelet or antithrombotic regimens post-TMVR has not been standardized. The large TMVR registry reported 10 cases (out of 322) with valve thrombosis after ViV or ViR, with timing varying from one day to two years post-procedure. The one-year cumulative valve thrombosis rates were higher in patients treated with antiplatelet vs. anticoagulant therapy (60.6 vs. 1.6%, p 0.019). Another recent study reported a two-year cumulative THV thrombosis rate of 14.4% (n = 91 patients) undergoing ViV, ViR, or ViMAC.

For ViV and ViR cases, the interplay between the THV and degenerated bioprosthesis may play a role in

		Favorable	Unfavorable
(A)	Depth of Implant	a	b
(B)	Degree of flaring	c	d
(C)	AMA angle	e	f
(D)	Septal bulge	g	h

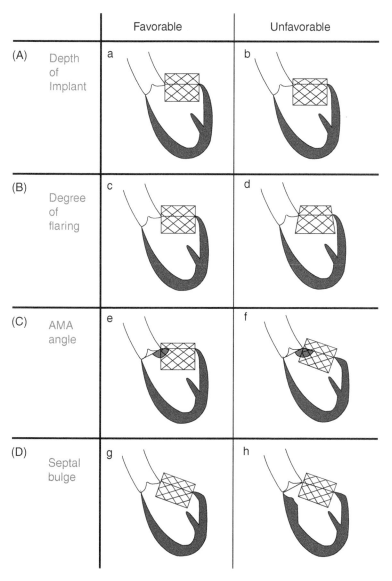

Figure 37.5 Factors influencing left ventricular outflow tract obstruction. (a) Depth of implantation, (b) degree of flaring, (c) aorto-mitra angle, (d) septal bulge. *Source:* Adapted from Pirelli, L. et al. (2021). Mitral valve-in-valve and valve-in-ring: tips, tricks, and outcomes. *Ann. Cardiothorac. Surg.* 10 (1): 96.

thrombotic risk. There is a higher reported rate of THV thrombosis in ViV of stented porcine valves relative to pericardial valves. For ViR cases, the presence of low flow in the perivalvular spaces could also predispose to turbulent flow and stasis.

The most ideal clinical or echocardiographic follow-up after ViV or ViR is unknown. Using serial CT scans for surveillance may not be cost-efficient and exposes patients to radiation and contrast. If the clinical suspicion is high – i.e. new heart failure,troke, or echocardiogram revealing thick valve leaflets, new gradient, or restricted leaflet mobility – further workup is warranted. Certain cases may need prolonged anticoagulation (beyond three to six months) based on the balance of their embolic and bleeding risks.

16. What cases are better performed transseptal vs transapical?

The VIV International Data (VIVID) registry showed transapical utilization in 81% of ViV cases and 68% of ViR cases (25.4% transseptal for both ViV and ViR). We have also learned that transapical access is associated with worse clinical outcomes and impairment in myocardial function. However, transseptal access is limited by poor co-axiality and a residual atrial septal defect that may require closure. There are certain scenarios where either approach may be favored, as described in Table 37.2.

Table 37.2 Clinical scenarios favoring transseptal versus transapical approach for transcatheter mitral valve replacement.

Favors transseptal	Favors transapical
Shorter hospital stay	Challenging atrial septal anatomy or peripheral venous system anomaly
Left ventricular systolic dysfunction or apical scar	Need for precise valve positioning
Severely calcified and bulky sub-valvular apparatus	Small surgical valves or poor fluoroscopic markers
Combined mitral and pulmonary/tricuspid implantation	Combined mitral and aortic implantation

Conclusion

There has been a shift away from mechanical surgical valves in favor of bioprosthetic valves, motivated by a desire to avoid the long-term risks of anticoagulation therapy. However, bioprosthetic valves degenerate, and when they do, the pro and cons of redo surgery and transcatheter TMVR need to be considered. Understanding the characteristics of the first implanted device and mitral valve anatomy with TEE and CT planning is crucial for adequate patient selection, procedural planning, and good clinical outcomes.

Bibliography

1 Beller, J.P., Rogers, J.H., Thourani, V.H. et al. (2018). Early clinical results with the Tendyne transcatheter mitral valve replacement system. *Ann. Cardiothorac. Surg.* 7 (6): 776.

2 Blanke, P., Naoum, C., Dvir, D. et al. (2017). Predicting LVOT obstruction in transcatheter mitral valve implantation: concept of the neo-LVOT. *JACC Cardiovasc. Imaging* 10 (4): 482–485.

3 Case, B.C., Lisko, J.C., Barbaliaros, V. et al. (2021). LAMPOON techniques to prevent or manage left ventricular outflow tract obstruction in transcatheter mitral valve replacement. *Ann. Cardiothorac. Surg.* 10 (1): 172–179.

4 Duncan, A., Daqa, A., Yeh, J. et al. (2017). Transcatheter mitral valve replacement: long-term outcomes of first-in-man experience with an apically tethered device – a case series from a single Centre. *EuroIntervention* 13 (9): e1047–e1057.

5 Dvir, D. (2016). Transseptal instead of transapical valve implantation: making mitral great again?*. *J. Am. Coll. Cardiol. Intv.* 9 (11): 1175–1177.

6 Eleid, M.F., Cabalka, A., Williams, M.R. et al. (2016). Percutaneous transvenous transseptal transcatheter valve implantation in failed bioprosthetic mitral valves, ring annuloplasty, and severe mitral annular calcification. *JACC Cardiovasc. Interv.* 9 (11): 1161–1174.

7 Ge, Y., Gupta, S., Fentanes, E. et al. (2021). Role of cardiac CT in pre-procedure planning for transcatheter mitral valve replacement. *JACC Cardiovasc. Imaging* .

8 Ghatak, A., Bavishi, C., Cardoso, R.N. et al. (2015). Complications and mortality in patients undergoing transcatheter aortic valve replacement with Edwards SAPIEN & SAPIEN XT valves: a meta-analysis of world-wide studies and registries comparing the transapical and transfemoral accesses. *J. Interv. Cardiol.* 28 (3): 266–278.

9 Grube, E. and Sinning, J.M. (2021). Transcatheter mitral valve therapies. *Intrepid* 299–307.

10 Guerrero, M., Urena, M., Himbert, D. et al. (2018). 1-year outcomes of transcatheter mitral valve replacement in patients with severe mitral annular calcification. *J. Am. Coll. Cardiol.* 71 (17): 1841–1853.

11 Guerrero, M., Pursnani, A., Narang, A. et al. (2021). Prospective evaluation of transseptal TMVR for failed surgical bioprostheses. *J. Am. Coll. Cardiol. Intv.* 14 (8): 859–872.

12 Guerrero, M., Vemulapalli, S., Xiang, Q. et al. (2020). Thirty-day outcomes of transcatheter mitral valve replacement for degenerated mitral bioprostheses (valve-in-valve), failed surgical rings (valve-in-ring), and native valve with severe mitral annular calcification (valve-in-mitral annular calcification) in the United States. *Circ. Cardiovasc. Interv.* 13 (3): e008425.

13 Guerrero, M., Wang, D.D., Pursnani, A. et al. (2020). A cardiac computed tomography–based score to categorize mitral annular calcification severity and predict valve embolization. *Cardiovasc. Imaging* 13 (9): 1945–1957.

14 Guerrero, M., Wang, D.D., Pursnani, A. et al. (2021). Prospective evaluation of TMVR for failed surgical annuloplasty rings. *J. Am. Coll. Cardiol. Intv.* 14 (8): 846–858.

15 Mehaffey, H.J., Hawkins, R.B., Schubert, S. et al. (2018). Contemporary outcomes in reoperative mitral valve surgery. *Heart* 104 (8): 652–656.

16 Naoum, C., Leipsic, J., Cheung, A. et al. (2016). Mitral annular dimensions and geometry in patients with functional mitral regurgitation and mitral valve prolapse:

implications for transcatheter mitral valve implantation. *JACC Cardiovasc. Imaging* 9 (3): 269–280.

17 Otto, C.M., Nishimura, R.A., Bonow, R.O. et al. (2021). 2020 ACC/AHA guideline for the management of patients with valvular heart disease: a report of the American College of Cardiology/American Heart Association joint committee on clinical practice guidelines. *J. Am. Coll. Cardiol.* 77 (4): e25–e197.

18 Pirelli, L., Hong, E., Steffen, R. et al. (2021). Mitral valve-in-valve and valve-in-ring: tips, tricks, and outcomes. *Ann. Cardiothorac. Surg.* 10 (1): 96.

19 Simonato, M., Whisenant, B., Ribeiro, H.B. et al. (2021). Transcatheter mitral valve replacement after surgical repair or replacement: comprehensive midterm evaluation of valve-in-valve and valve-in-ring implantation from the VIVID registry. *Circulation* 143 (2): 104–116.

20 Sorajja, P., Moat, N., Badhwar, V. et al. (2019). Initial feasibility study of a new transcatheter mitral prosthesis: the first 100 patients. *J. Am. Coll. Cardiol.* 73 (11): 1250–1260.

21 Urena, M., Himbert, D., Brochet, E. et al. (2017). Transseptal transcatheter mitral valve replacement using balloon-expandable transcatheter heart valves. *J. Am. Coll. Cardiol. Intv.* 10 (19): 1905–1919.

22 Vinayak, B. (2014). Valve-in-valve apps: why and how they were developed and how to use them. *EuroIntervention* 10: U44–U51.

23 Yoon, S.-H., Whisenant, B.K., Bleiziffer, S. et al. (2019). Outcomes of transcatheter mitral valve replacement for degenerated bioprostheses, failed annuloplasty rings, and mitral annular calcification. *Eur. Heart J.* 40 (5): 441–451.

38

Transseptal Transcatheter Mitral Valve-in-Valve Replacement (TS MViV)

Technical Considerations and Step-by-Step Procedure

Camilo A. Gomez[1] and Eduardo J. de Marchena[2]

[1] Department of Cardiology,, Jackson Memorial Health System, Miami, FL, USA
[2] Division of Cardiovascular Medicine, University of Miami Miller School of Medicine, University of Miami Hospital, Miami, FL, USA

1. What are the important pre-procedural considerations in transseptal mitral valve-in-valve replacement ?

In transseptal (TS) mitral valve-in-valve (MViV) replacement, an extensive and cautious pre-procedure workup is essential, as described in previous chapters. The most important parts of the workup include identifying the mechanism of bioprosthetic mitral valve failure, characterizing the bioprosthetic mitral valve type and size, assessing the risk of left ventricular outflow tract (LVOT) obstruction with the use of cardiac tomography reconstruction, and accurately selecting a transcatheter heart valve (THV). A careful review of the case by the Heart Team is mandatory to elaborate a procedure plan for each anatomical and patient characteristic.

2. What are the important recommendations for patient preparation and the room setting for the TS MViV procedure?

All the materials for the procedure should be available in the room; a pre-procedural list is always helpful. The procedure should be performed in a hybrid room with enough space for the nursing staff and interventional, surgery, and anesthesia teams. Patient preparation does not differ from that used for the transcatheter aortic valve replacement (TAVR) procedure. The procedure is performed under general anesthesia, and transesophageal echocardiography (TEE) guidance is mandatory to increase the levels of safety and success.

3. What steps should be followed for a successful TS MViV procedure?

Our recommendations and steps to follow for a successful procedure are outlined in questions 4–15. They can be modified to fit each operator's preferences.

4. What is important for vascular access during TS MViV?

Vascular access should be obtained using fluoroscopic landmarks and ultrasound guidance to prevent vascular complications. It is recommended to use the right femoral vein as the primary access for ergonomic comfort and easier manipulation of the system by the implanter. Left femoral venous access should be obtained for temporary pacemaker implantation and left femoral arterial access for left-heart catheterization. The size of the sheaths is operator independent. We use a 7 Fr short sheath for the right femoral vein, a 7 Fr 23 cm sheath in the left femoral vein for easier advancement of the temporary pacemaker, and a 6 Fr short sheath in the left femoral artery; radial access can be used for arterial access if preferred.

5. Should the femoral vein access be pre-closed?

The right femoral venous access can be pre-closed with 1 or 2 ProGlide (Abbott Vascular) if desired, but doing so is not mandatory. Another alternative is to use a figure-eight tissue stitch at the end for hemostasis.

Mastering Structural Heart Disease, First Edition. Edited by Eduardo J. de Marchena and Camilo A. Gomez.
© 2023 John Wiley & Sons Ltd. Published 2023 by John Wiley & Sons Ltd.
Companion website: www.wiley.com/go/deMarchena/Mastering-Structural-Heart-Disease

6. How do you obtain baseline LVOT hemodynamics during TS MViV?

The short 6 Fr arterial sheath is exchanged for a 45 cm destination sheath to facilitate simultaneous pressure recording in the aorta (Ao). If radial arterial access is selected for arterial access, a radial destination sheath is used to reach the Ao and record simultaneous pressures. The aortic valve is crossed with the usual technique, and a 5 Fr pigtail catheter is advanced into the left ventricle (LV). Simultaneous LV-Ao pressures are recorded, obtaining a baseline LVOT gradient in the absence of aortic stenosis. In high-risk cases of LVOT obstruction, the pigtail can be left in the LV for the duration of the procedure to assess for LVOT obstruction during valve deployment.

7. How do you perform a safe transseptal puncture at an optimal location for TS MViV?

TEE guidance is mandatory to determine the optimal puncture site. The ideal transseptal puncture (TP) location is inferior and posterior, 3 to 4 cm from the mitral valve annulus plane; this allows maneuvering of the equipment in the left atrium (LA) and favors the crossing of the system into the LV. When the TP is performed, the transseptal sheath (TS) is advanced into the LA; at that moment, anticoagulation should be administered, and the recommended dose is 70–100 units per Kg of heparin for a target activated clotting time (ACT) of 300–350. Once the TS has entered the LA, a 0.032 in. Inoue wire (Toray Medical) is advanced into the LA. The coiled design provides optimal safety and prevents accidental pullback into the right atrium (RA). Another option on the market is the 0.025 in. ProTrack pigtail wire (Baylis Medical): it is integrated into the Baylis transseptal system, saving some time by requiring one less step.

8. When do you insert the Edwards E sheath?

The Edwards eSheath (Edwards Lifesciences) should be inserted once the patient receives the full dose of anticoagulant. It can be advanced either after the TP over the Toray wire or later in the procedure after crossing into the LV over any of the pre-shaped stiff wires.

9. How do you cross the surgical mitral valve into the LV?

A steerable sheath is advanced to the LA, and the simultaneous LA-LV pressure is recorded to obtain a baseline mitral gradient. The steerable sheath needs an inner lumen diameter of at least 8.5 Fr; the available sheaths on the market are the Agilis Steerable Introducer (Abbott), the SureFlex steerable guiding sheath (Baylis Medical), the Nagare Steerable Sheath (Terumo Interventional Systems), the DiRex Steerable Sheath (Boston Scientific), and the FlexCath Advance Steerable Sheath (Medtronic) (Figure 38.1a). Atrial septostomy dilation with an 8 mm balloon catheter is sometimes required to advance the steerable sheath.

TEE guidance and fluoroscopy are important in a projection perpendicular to the mitral annulus; most cases are right anterior oblique (RAO) with either cranial or caudal angulation. The steerable sheath is oriented toward the mitral valve, and an antegrade crossing is performed using a 0.035 in. J wire in a pigtail catheter (5–7 Fr) (Figure 38.1b, c). If the crossing is unsuccessful, other catheters can be used, such as a Multipurpose or Amplatz. The steerable catheter should be advanced and positioned close to the mitral valve to provide support and prevent prolapse of the system into the LA (prolapse can happen at the moment of the wire exchange with the pre-shaped stiffer wire). Using a large, curved Agilis sheath may give additional support for wire advancement. The pigtail is positioned at the apex, a pre-shaped stiff wire (Safari [Boston Scientific], Confida [Medtronic], or Amplatz [Cook Medical]) is advanced through the pigtail with cautious positioning of the wire loop "facing down" in the LV (the opposite of the wire position in TAVR) (Figure 38.2), and then the pigtail is removed. Some operators advance a second "safety" wire, but it is important to retrieve it before the THV implantation.

10. How do you perform atrial septostomy dilation?

The septum is dilated with a 12–14 mm peripheral balloon. The balloon is advanced through the steerable sheath that is still in the LA to facilitate crossing through the septum; then it is "unsheathed" by pulling the steerable sheath back to the RA. TEE and fluoroscopy are used to confirm the position in the septum. The balloon is inflated and flossed over; multiple inflations are recommended to guarantee a successful THV crossing and prevent mechanical tearing of the septum or system entrapment. Once an adequate septostomy is obtained, the balloon should be

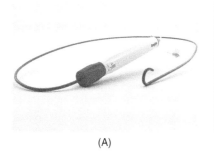

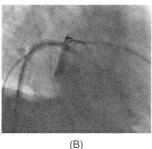

(A)   (B)

Figure 38.1 (a) SureFlex steerable guiding sheath (Baylis Medical). (b) Crossing the mitral valve with a pigtail catheter. The image shows the steerable sheath, the pigtail catheter crossing the mitral valve, and a pigtail catheter in the left ventricle from the aortic valve. (c) Transesophageal echocardiography images guiding the crossing into the left ventricle with the steerable sheath and pigtail catheter.

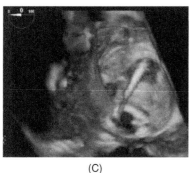

(C)

advanced to the mitral valve to check the pathway trackability and anticipate any potential obstacles (Figure 38.3).

11. How do you prepare the transcatheter valve for the TS MViV?

The THV is prepared following the standard process, except that it is mounted in the opposite orientation of that in TAVR. This is the most important step and should be confirmed multiple times, because failure to mount the valve correctly can be catastrophic. The THV is mounted on the balloon for antegrade implantation with the sealing skirt away from the nose cone. It is recommended to add an extra 2–3 cc to the inflation syringe to obtain adequate anchoring and avoid atrial migration of the THV (see Figure 37.4 in the previous chapter of this book).

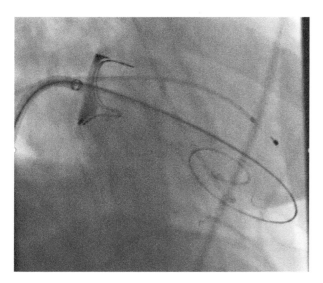

Figure 38.2 Steerable catheter positioned close to the mitral valve, and pre-shaped stiff wire positioned with the wire loop facing down in the left ventricle.

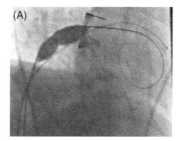

(A)

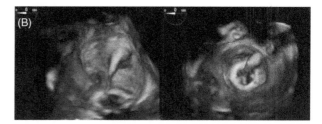

(B)

Figure 38.3 (a) Atrial septostomy with a 14 × 40 mm balloon. (b) Transesophageal echocardiography images of the balloon atrial septostomy.

12. Should the surgical mitral valve be pre-dilated?

It is recommended to avoid pre-dilation because there is a risk of fracture of the old calcified leaflets and embolization of degenerated material. The only instance where pre-dilation can be considered is for an uncrossable valve, but it must be performed with extreme caution using an undersized balloon that is briefly inflated. Consider the use of embolic protection devices in very calcified or degenerated valves.

13. How do you advance and position the delivery system?

Before advancing the system, do a second check of the valve orientation. After the system is introduced, the balloon is loaded, and the valve is aligned in the inferior vena cava. The delivery system is rotated 180° (E logo oriented down) to allow flexion of the delivery system toward the mitral valve.

14. How do you cross the septum and the mitral valve with the delivery system and THV?

Once the valve is in the RA, flex should be added before crossing the septum. The septum is crossed and guided by fluoroscopy and TEE. Three operators are required, and the technique is performed with perfect coordination between them. Operator 1 advances the system in a smooth push until the THV covers the ventricular edge of the surgical valve. Operator 2 adds more flex to the system appropriate to orient the THV into the mitral valve. Operator 3 maintains the wire with subtle push-pull movements to maintain adequate support and railing of the THV into the mitral valve: continuous attention is required to prevent any ventricular injury or loss of the wire position.

15. How do you position and implant the THV during TS MViV?

The THV is positioned and deployed in a projection perpendicular to the frame of the surgical mitral bioprosthesis. The delivery system pusher is pulled back to the most distal marker to maintain the directability of the THV. The exact THV marker landmark position differs depending on the surgical bioprosthesis, but the valve is positioned with a final target of 10–20% atrial and 80–90% ventricular. The THV is deployed under rapid pacing with mechanical ventilation on hold. A test "pacing cine run" is recommended to confirm an adequate pacer capture and THV position. At deployment, slow inflation is performed to allow for minor adjustments, followed by full deployment of the inflation syringe with an extra 2–3 cc's to secure anchoring and prevent THV migration during systole (Figure 38.4).

16. What is important in the post–valve deployment assessment?

Once the THV is deployed, the delivery system is withdrawn. TEE images evaluate the THV position, leaflet mobility, presence of leaks, transmitral gradients, LVOT gradients, and presence of mitral regurgitation or pericardial effusion. Immediate post-deployment hemodynamics are measured with LV-Ao for the LVOT gradient, and the final LA–LV pressure can be obtained using a Multipurpose catheter in the LA.

17. When should atrial septostomy closure be considered?

The atrial septostomy or iatrogenic atrial septal defect (ASD) size and flow direction are evaluated with TEE. Closure with an ASD closure device should be considered when there is either severe pulmonary hypertension with right-to-left shunting along with hypoxemia or significant left-to-right shunting with right ventricular failure and dysfunction.

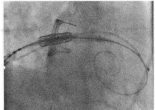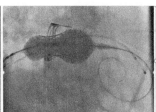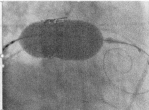

Figure 38.4 Sequence of positioning and deploying the transcatheter heart valve during the transseptal mitral valve-in-valve procedure.

18. How do you obtain adequate hemostasis at the vascular access site?

The large-bore femoral venous access can be closed by tightening the pre-deployed ProGlide sutures if the access site was pre-closed. If not, a figure-eight stitch can be used, which usually provides adequate hemostasis.

Potential Obstacles and Bailout Strategies

19. What can be done if the THV is not crossing the septum?

When crossing the septum, if some resistance is felt, the delivery system should not be pushed forcefully. Instead, the system should be retracted into the RA, and another attempt should be made with the catheter in a different orientation. TEE is helpful in evaluating the point of resistance and mechanical interaction of the THV.

20. What can be done if the THV is not crossing the mitral orifice?

Gentle manipulations of the catheter in combination with push-pull movements of the wire support are performed to find the ideal orientation to cross. If still unable to cross, another technique is to unlock the catheter and pull the pusher back, enabling engagement into the mitral orifice.

Bibliography

1 Chris Malaisrie, S., Ricciardi, M.J., and Davidson, C.J. (2018). Chapter 27: Transfemoral/Transseptal mitral valve-in-valve using Sapien 3. In: *Transcatheter Heart Valve Handbook: A Surgeons' and Interventional Council Review* (ed. A. Iribarne, A.C. Stefanescu Schmidt and T.C. Nguyen). American College of Cardiology.

2 Otto, C.M., Nishimura, R.O., Bonow, R.O. et al. (2021). 2020 ACC/AHA guideline for the management of patients with valvular heart disease: a report of the American College of Cardiology/American Heart Association Joint Committee on Clinical Practice Guidelines. *J. Am. Coll. Cardiol.* 77 (4): e25–e197.

3 Pirelli, L., Hong, E., Vahl, T.P. et al. (2021). Mitral valve-in-valve and valve-in-ring: tips, tricks, and outcomes. *Ann. Cardiothorac. Surg.* 10 (1): 96.

4 Urena, M., Himbert, D., Brochet, E. et al. (2017). Transseptal Transcatheter mitral valve replacement using balloon-expandable Transcatheter heart valves. *J. Am. Coll. Cardiol. Intv.* 10 (19): 1905–1919.

39

Transseptal Systems for TMVR and Transcatheter Devices for Mitral Annuloplasty

Sergio A. Perez[1,2] and Eberhard Grube[3, 4, 5]

[1] Cardiovascular Service, Baptist Health Medical Center, Montgomery, AL, USA
[2] Jackson Health System, Miami, FL, USA
[3] Center of Innovative Interventions in Cardiology (CIIC), University Hospital Bonn, Bonn, Germany
[4] Division of Cardiovascular Medicine, Stanford University School of Medicine, Stanford, CA, USA
[5] INCOR Heart Institute of the University of São Paulo, São Paulo, São Paulo, Brazil

1. Is there any role for percutaneous treatment of mitral valve disease?

Although approximately two-thirds of all heart valve operations are for aortic valve replacement, mitral valve (MV) disease is more common than aortic stenosis (AS), and mitral regurgitation (MR) in particular is the most common valve disease. Considering the significant drop in the prevalence of rheumatic valve disease in the United States (US) and Europe over the last several decades because of primary prevention of rheumatic fever and increased life expectancy, with the growing incidence of ischemic heart disease, the relative incidence of MR compared to other valve lesions is only expected to increase.

In general, valve intervention should be considered for patients with functional disability and asymptomatic patients with progressive left ventricular (LV) remodeling with deterioration of function or increasing dimensions. As per current guidelines, surgery remains the principal treatment modality for patients with primary or degenerative MR (DMR). These recommendations are based on observational data that demonstrated improved survival with surgery, particularly with repair. However, operative mortality rates of 3–9% are common in many centers, and some patients are denied surgery because of prohibitive risk. Furthermore, the indications for MV surgery are less clear for secondary or functional MR (FMR), where retrospective data have failed to show a survival benefit compared to medical therapy. Hence, catheter-based interventions have become a fundamental treatment option in patients with secondary or FMR in addition to optimal medical therapy and have some role in managing non-surgical patients with primary or DMR. Transcatheter edge-to-edge MV repair (TEER), discussed in a separate chapter, has a Class 2a recommendation for symptomatic patients with FMR despite optimal medical therapy with favorable anatomy and also a Class 2a recommendation for symptomatic patients with DMR and high or prohibitive surgical risk as per last American College of Cardiology/American Heart Association (ACC/AHA) guidelines for the management of valvular heart disease.

The mitral apparatus is complex. It incorporates the leaflets, chordae tendinae, papillary muscles, annulus, left atrium, and left ventricle (LV). Although the MitraClip was the first approved and remains the most widely used transcatheter therapy for MV disease, isolated leaflet repair remains limited compared to the extensive armamentarium available to the mitral surgeon when considering the complexity of the MV apparatus. Technologies addressing different elements of a dysfunctional valve are needed if transcatheter therapies for MV are to develop to their full potential. Moreover, specific catheter-based technologies would be more suitable for treating primary than secondary MR and vice versa or could be used in non-surgical patients with isolated MV stenosis or combined stenosis and regurgitation.

2. What are the different transcatheter MV techniques?

As mentioned, the MV apparatus is very complex, and transcatheter interventions of the MV can be broadly grouped depending on their approach or the valvular element they address. The two primary catheter-based interventions of the MV are transcatheter mitral valve replacement (TMVR) and transcatheter mitral valve repair (TMVr). TMVr techniques can be classified as transcatheter edge-to-edge leaflet repair (TEER), indirect or direct transcatheter annuloplasty, and chordal repair. Other technologies use miscellaneous approaches such as LV remodeling or hybrid surgery. This chapter will focus on TMVR using a transseptal approach, transcatheter annuloplasty, and miscellaneous devices. TEER with the MitraClip is covered in a separate chapter of this book. Table 39.1 summarizes different devices for percutaneous treatment of MV disease. At the time of writing this chapter, only the MitraClip device (Abbott Vascular) is approved by the Food and Drug Administration (FDA) for clinical use in the US. In Europe, several devices have received the CE mark. An extensive list of devices is still under investigation or in early safety and feasibility trials.

3. What is transcatheter mitral valve replacement (TMVR), and how does it differ from transcatheter aortic valve replacement (TAVR)?

After the dramatic success of transcatheter aortic valve replacement (TAVR), transcatheter mitral valve replacement (TMVR) quickly became an area with growing interest to study. Nevertheless, the development of TMVR has not been easy, and further refinements in technology and clinical results will be required before it becomes the standard of care like its aortic counterpart. In addition, extrapolating the surgical preference of MV repair over replacement, some interest shifted to transcatheter technologies for repair. Despite this, TMVR may mature as a promising option for non-surgical patients without anatomy suitable for repair. Furthermore, some conflicting

Table 39.1 Transcatheter mitral valve devices.

Transcatheter mitral valve replacement (TMVR)				
Device	**Manufacturer**	**Description**	**Access**	**Development status**
EVOQUE	Edwards Lifesciences	Nitinol self-expanding trileaflet valve	Transapical/transseptal	Investigational
SAPIEN M3	Edwards Lifesciences	Nitinol docking system and a modified SAPIEN 3 valve	Transseptal	Investigational
Intrepid	Medtronic	Nitinol self-expanding	Transapical/transseptal	Investigational
Caisson	Caisson Interventional	Nitinol self-expanding	Transseptal	Investigational
Cardiovalve	Cardiovalve	Dual Nitinol frame	Transseptal	Investigational
Tendyne	Abbott Vascular	Nitinol double-frame stent	Transapical	CE mark
Tiara	Neovasc	Nitinol self-expanding	Transapical	Investigational
FORTIS	Edwards Lifesciences	Nitinol self-expanding	Transapical	Investigational
MValve	Boston Scientific	Docking system combined with Lotus heart valve	Transapical	Investigational

Transcatheter mitral valve repair (TMVr)				
Device	**Manufacturer**	**Anatomic target**	**Description**	**Development status**
MitraClip	Abbott Vascular	Leaflets	Edge-to-edge repair	FDA/CE mark
PASCAL	Edwards Lifesciences	Leaflets	Edge-to-edge repair	CE mark
Carillon	Cardiac Dimensions	Mitral annulus	Indirect annuloplasty	CE mark
ARTO	MVRx	Mitral annulus	Indirect annuloplasty	Investigational
Cerclage	Tau-PNU	Mitral annulus	Indirect annuloplasty	Investigational
Cardioband	Edwards Lifesciences	Mitral annulus	Direct annuloplasty	CE mark
Millipede	Millipede	Mitral annulus	Direct annuloplasty	Investigational
AccuCinch	Ancora Heart	Mitral annulus/left ventricle	Direct annuloplasty	Investigational
NeoChord	NeoChord	Chordal apparatus	Artificial chordal	CE mark
Harpoon	Edwards Lifesciences	Chordal apparatus	Artificial chordal	Investigational
V-Chordal	Valtech Cardio	Chordal apparatus	Artificial chordal	Investigational

data suggest less difference between repair and replacement, particularly in higher-risk patients, and higher rates of MR recurrence with both surgical and transcatheter repair, leaving some roles to be played by TMVR.

Much of the early experience with transcatheter mitral replacement has come from using aortic transcatheter heart valves (THVs) in mitral prostheses (valve-in-valve), rings (valve-in-ring), or severely calcified valves (valve-in-MAC [mitral annular calcification]). Given the knowledge we have obtained from the development of TAVR, it may be helpful to recognize some challenges of TMVR compared to TAVR.

First, there may be differences in patient demographics. Age, life expectancy, and valve durability are relevant issues given that many patients in need of MV surgery are younger than patients needing aortic valve surgery for aortic stenosis (AS) and that mitral bioprostheses are exposed to greater hemodynamic stress and degenerate more frequently than aortic bioprostheses. Also, patients with FMR are more likely to have cardiac abnormalities associated with heart failure, such as atrial fibrillation, pulmonary hypertension, and tricuspid regurgitation.

Mitral THVs and delivery systems for TMVR are larger than those used for TAVR, requiring larger vascular access. TAVR is usually performed from arterial transfemoral access, and although infrequent, alternative accesses can be used when needed. For TMVR, the THV can be delivered using a venous transfemoral/transseptal, transapical, or transatrial approach. Transapical and transatrial approaches offer a more direct and easier way to reach the MV at the expense of myocardial damage because they are more invasive. Transfemoral/transseptal access is less invasive, but maneuverability and positioning of catheters can be impaired. This chapter will focus on TMVR devices that use a transfemoral/transseptal approach.

Significant anatomic differences between a more complex MV and the aortic valve are additional challenges. The mitral annulus is larger, D-shaped, and often not calcified, and it offers less support and anchoring than the tubular, rigid, often calcified aortic root. These factors play a role in potential differences in the rate of perivalvular leak (PVL) between TAVR and TMVR. Structures surrounding the mitral annulus should also be carefully taken into consideration. The risk of left ventricular outflow tract (LVOT) obstruction is one of the most critical challenges in TMVR. The size and position of the THV, the MV/LVOT angle, and the thickness of the basal interventricular septum are some predictors of LVOT obstruction.

Finally, underlying etiology and disease process can undoubtedly impact the results of TMVR. For example, valve replacement in a patient with DMR may not yield the same results as in another patient with FMR and progressive LV and annular dilation.

4. What TMVR devices are available?

Compared to TAVR devices, most TMVR technologies are still under investigation or in safety and feasibility studies. Therefore, comparison with surgical devices is lacking. Early clinical results have been predominantly reported for devices delivered using a transapical approach. Clinical data for devices that use a transfemoral/transseptal approach remains limited. To date, only the Tendyne (Abbott Vascular) has been approved for use in Europe.

The list of devices is growing; Figure 39.1 illustrates some of them. Devices that use a transfemoral/transseptal approach include the CardiAQ-EVOQUE (Edwards Lifesciences), SAPIEN M3 (Edwards Lifesciences), Caisson (LivaNova), Cardiovalve, and Cephea (Cephea Valve Technologies). Conversely, the Tiara (Neovasc), Fortis (Edwards Lifesciences), Tendyne, AltaValve (4C Medical Technologies), NaviGate, and MValve use a transapical approach. The Intrepid (Medtronic and HighLife also have a primary transapical approach but a transseptal approach under development.

The initial CardiAQ was a self-expanding trileaflet bovine pericardial valve mounted on a Nitinol stent frame with polyurethane foam-covered anchors to grasp the leaflets and chords. The new version of the device was renamed EVOQUE. It incorporates an intra-annular

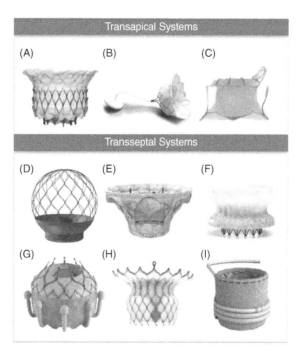

Figure 39.1 Transcatheter mitral valve replacement (TMVR) systems: (a) Intrepid, (b) Tendyne, (c) Tiara, (d) AltaValve, (e) Cardiovalve, (f) Cephea, (g) EVOQUE, (h) HighLife, and (i) SAPIEN M3. *Source:* Hensey et al. (2021), Elsevier.

sealing skirt to minimize PVL. In addition, it offers two valve sizes (44 and 48 mm) and has an overall lower profile, allowing a transfemoral approach via a 28 French delivery system (it also offers a transapical approach) and decreasing ventricular projection and risk of LVOT obstruction. The MISCEND (Edwards EVOQUE Eos Mitral Valve Replacement: Investigation of Safety and Performance After Mitral Valve Replacement with Transcatheter Device) study has an estimated primary completion date of December 2022. Results of early experience were presented at the ACC in 2020, including 14 patients treated under compassionate use in Canada or in the US Early Feasibility Study. Procedural success was high (93%) with an acceptable safety profile (one patient died at 30 days) and significant MR reduction.

The SAPIEN M3 system resulted from substantial experience with MV-in-valve, valve-in-ring, and valve-in-MAC using the balloon-expandable SAPIEN 3 transcatheter heart valve. This device combines a modified SAPIEN 3 TAVR valve and a coiling Nitinol docking system. The SAPIEN M3 valve is identical to the 29 mm diameter SAPIEN 3 aortic THV with an external knitted polyethylene terephthalate (PET) seal. The size of this system is suitable for a relatively broad range of anatomies. The Nitinol dock is composed of a leading turn with a larger diameter (37 mm) to capture the chords and subsequent functional turns with a smaller diameter. The knitted PET skirt facilitates sealing between the native MV and the dock and prevents migration. Because the dock encircles the mitral chords, it exerts a variable annuloplasty effect. The most updated results of the US Early Feasibility Study were presented at the Transcatheter Cardiovascular Therapeutics (TCT) meeting in 2019. Among 35 patients, the success rate was 88.6% and 30-day all-cause mortality was 2.9%, with a resolution of MR < 1+ of 87.9%.

The Intrepid MV is a trileaflet bovine pericardial valve with a self-expanding Nitinol frame. It is composed of a circular outer fixation frame (43, 46, or 50 mm diameter) that engages the dynamic MV anatomy and a circular inner stent frame (27 mm) that houses the leaflets. The outer frame has different degrees of radial stiffness along its axial length and small cleats, facilitating anchoring. It was first studied with transapical delivery; however, a new generation 35-F transfemoral access system that enables transseptal delivery is now under investigation. The early feasibility study of the Intrepid transseptal system was recently published. Fifteen patients underwent the study procedure. The device was successfully implanted in 14 patients. At 30 days, outcomes were favorable, including the absence of mortality, stroke, reintervention, or new pacemaker implantation. The major adverse events were driven by access site bleeding. At follow-up, all 14 patients with successful implantation had trace or no MR. Larger trials with longer follow-up are underway.

5. What is transcatheter MV repair?

Based on the surgical principle of "repair over replacement," the device industry and investigators have invested significant effort and resources in developing TMVr technologies. Moreover, positive results of TEER in trials such as COAPT (Cardiovascular Outcomes Assessment of the MitraClip Percutaneous Therapy for Heart Failure Patients with Functional Mitral Regurgitation) have boosted interest in and optimism about other repair techniques, not only from interventional cardiologists and surgeons but also from heart failure specialists who are joining the journey. With TEER as a standard of care, it may become the comparator for other mitral innovations in the future; and given the magnitude of the results, its safety and efficacy may be challenging to replicate. Although experience with TMVr devices is limited except for the MitraClip, these devices seem to show a good safety profile. However, improvements in ease of use and efficacy are still needed. Current devices can target different elements of the MV apparatus: leaflets, chordae, or annulus.

The selection of a technique for a specific patient should be based on a comprehensive evaluation of the patient, anatomy, and mechanism of MV disease. For instance, annuloplasty is best fitted for FMR with enlarged annuli, chordal repair is indicated for flail or prolapse of the posterior leaflet, and TEER could work for both DMR and FMR, provided the anatomy is suitable for adequate grasping of the leaflets.

6. What is transcatheter MV annuloplasty?

Surgical annuloplasty can be performed alone or combined with leaflet resection or augmentation, edge-to-edge repair, or artificial chords. Transcatheter MV annuloplasty is probably the most surgical-like option to treat MR in non-surgical patients. The fundamental principle of MV annuloplasty is to improve leaflet coaptation length by decreasing the size of the annulus with the use of an undersized ring.

Transcatheter MV annuloplasty devices can be classified as indirect or direct. Indirect annuloplasty devices are deployed in the venous structures of the heart, taking advantage of the proximity of the distal coronary sinus and the great cardiac vein to the posterior mitral annulus. The attractiveness of an easy venous procedure created much early interest; however, it was later realized that MR reduction with these devices might be limited as compared to surgery because of multiple factors, including the cranial location of the coronary sinus relative to the actual mitral annulus, the ability to perform only partial and not complete annular remodeling, and individual anatomic variability. Nonetheless, MR reduction can be significant and beneficial in some patients with favorable anatomy.

The Carillon XE2 (Cardiac Dimension) is the only indirect device that has obtained CE mark approval. Other indirect annuloplasty devices under investigation include Cerclage (Tau-PNU Medical), the ARTO system (MVRx), and Kardium MR. Unfortunately, the Viacor percutaneous transvenous mitral annuloplasty (PTMA), MONARC (Edwards Lifesciences), and similar devices have failed and are no longer in use.

To overcome some of the limitations of indirect annuloplasty, some devices have been designed for remodeling the annulus itself or the LV more directly. This list includes devices such as the Cardioband (Edwards Lifesciences), Millipede IRIS, and AccuCinch (Ancora Heart, among others).

7. What are some devices for transcatheter indirect MV annuloplasty?

The Carillon mitral contour system is a self-expanding Nitinol transcatheter device designed to reshape the anatomy of the mitral apparatus from the coronary sinus using proximal and distal anchors that are connected by a ribbon and, once in place, cinched and tethered, reducing the annular circumference (Figure 39.2). The coronary sinus is accessed via a transjugular or transfemoral venous approach using a 9 French delivery catheter. It is also

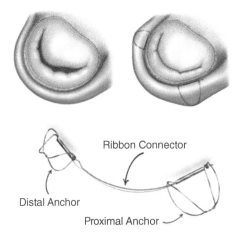

Figure 39.2 The Carillon mitral contour system. *Source:* Modified from the Cardiac Dimensions website (https://cardiacdimensions.com/physicians).

recapturable and retrievable prior to release. One appeal of this design is that it does not compromise future treatment options. However, this device has required several modifications due to suboptimal initial results. Of particular concern is the risk of compression of the left circumflex artery. AMADEUS (CARILLON Mitral Annuloplasty Device European Union Study), TITAN (Tighten the Annulus Now), and TITAN II were the initial studies to evaluate feasibility, safety, and efficacy. REDUCE FMR (CARILLON Mitral Contour System for Reducing Functional Mitral Regurgitation) is the first sham-controlled randomized trial of any catheter-based therapy for patients with valvular heart disease. A total of 120 patients were randomized to the treatment device (87 patients) or a sham procedure (33 patients). This study showed that Carillon could safely and effectively reduce FMR. The proportion of patients judged to have a significant improvement in the grade of MR at one year was higher in patients allocated to treatment than in those allocated to control (50.0 vs. 20.0%, respectively; p = 0.02); moreover, there was evidence of reverse remodeling with a significant decrease in LV end-diastolic volume (LVEDV) in patients allocated to treatment versus an increase in those allocated to control (−10.4 ml [95% confidence interval (CI):−18.5 to −2.4] vs. 6.5 ml [95%CI:−5.1 to 18.2], respectively; p = 0.03). There was only one myocardial infarction in the treatment arm associated with coronary artery compression of an AV groove branch of the circumflex coronary artery. Recently, the launch of the EMPOWER study (The Carillon Mitral Contour System in Treating Heart Failure With at Least Mild FMR) was announced, a US pivotal trial that is expected to randomize 300 patients at up to 75 sites. The Carillon system received CE mark approval in September 2011, but even though it has been implanted in more than 1000 patients around the world, it is still approved only for investigational use in the US.

Cerclage is a four-component catheter system that intends to create a complete circumferential annuloplasty irrespective of the rotational orientation of the mitral commissure in relation to the coronary sinus and of high atrial variants of the coronary sinus by reducing the septal-lateral dimension (Figure 39.3). A suture is placed from the coronary sinus through a basal septal perforator vein across a segment of interventricular septum into the right ventricle and then returning across a tricuspid valve commissure into the right atrium. The guidewire is snared and externalized. Tension is applied in a closed purse-string fashion to reduce the mitral annular dimension to the desired level. The system incorporates an arch-like device to protect entrapped coronary arteries against compression. At the end of the procedure, the tension is locked in a left sub-clavicular pocket and the skin incision is

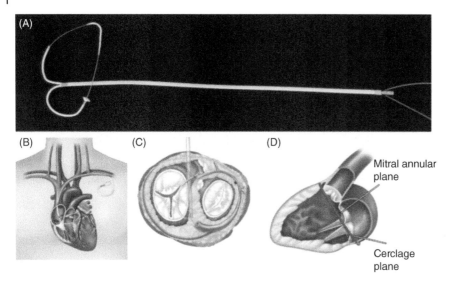

Figure 39.3 Mitral loop cerclage. (a) All four elements of the mitral loop cerclage implants assembled. (b) Device positioning. (c) The bridge device straddles the tricuspid valve between the coronary sinus and right ventricular septum. (d) Discordant planes of the mitral annulus and cerclage. *Source:* Park et al. (2017) / with permission of Elsevier.

closed. First-in-human results were reported in a small feasibility study in 2017. The device was successful in four out of five patients.

The ARTO system shortens the mitral annulus's anteroposterior (AP) diameter. It consists of two anchors deployed over the lateral wall of the left atrium via the coronary sinus (CS) and in the atrial septum, connected by a tether that traverses the left atrial chamber. The length of these sutures can be adjusted by applying tension to them. This device requires coronary sinus cannulation and a transseptal puncture. In 2021, the two-year outcomes of the MAVERIC (MitrAl ValvE RepaIr Clinical) trial were published. Among 45 patients, there was a sustained reduction in MR, left ventricular end-diastolic volume index, and anteroposterior diameter.

8. What are some devices for transcatheter direct MV annuloplasty?

The Cardioband is the closest transcatheter device to a surgical prosthetic ring. It is a direct annuloplasty adjustable and suture-less device implanted on the posterior mitral annulus under fluoroscopic and transesophageal echocardiographic (TEE) guidance. The implant is a Dacron tube anchored from commissure to commissure by a series of stainless-steel anchors (Figure 39.4). The device is available in six lengths to cover a wide range of annulus sizes. Once anchored, the device is cinched with a wire to obtain a controlled reduction in MV annulus dimensions. The

device is inserted using a 24 French delivery system from the left femoral vein and a transseptal approach similar to the MitraClip system.

Based on a multicenter prospective study, this device received the CE mark in September 2015. Two-year follow-up results of the European CE trial were presented in PCR London Valves in 2018. Survival was 79%, and 96% showed a sustained reduction in MR < 2+ and septal-lateral annular reduction. Unfortunately, technical success in this early experience was only 78.3% due to anchor disengagement. Recent device iterations aim to improve this complication.

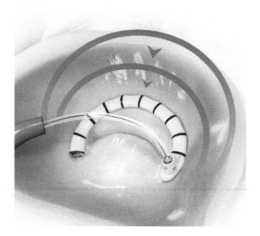

Figure 39.4 The Cardioband mitral valve reconstruction system. *Source:* Edwards Lifesciences LLC, Irvine, CA. Edwards, Edwards Lifesciences, the stylized E logo, CardiAQ, CardiAQ-Edwards, Cardioband and CardioCath are trademarks of Edwards Lifesciences Corporation.

The device has not yet received FDA approval, and the ACTIVE (Edwards Cardioband System ACTIVE Pivotal Clinical Trial) trial is ongoing in the US. The MiBAND (Edwards Cardioband European Post-Market Study) trial is a prospective, multicenter, single-arm European post-market study designed to assess safety and efficacy; it is currently enrolling patients.

The Millipede IRIS device is a complete annuloplasty ring delivered via a transfemoral or transseptal approach with a 23 French delivery system. It is a semi-rigid Nitinol ring with eight pre-attached helical anchors in the base and tensioning sliding collars at the top (Figure 39.5). Each anchor can be maneuvered and rotated independently and is directly attached to the annulus. When tensioning one of the sliding collars, the two adjacent anchors are pulled closer together. A unique feature of this technology is the possibility of using an integrated intracardiac echocardiography (ICE) catheter through the central lumen of the delivery catheter, facilitating device anchoring. The initial in-human clinical report demonstrated proof of concept in seven patients. Every patient demonstrated a reduction of MR and improvement in New York Heart Association (NYHA) class without significant procedural complications. Currently, there is an ongoing feasibility trial outside of the US. This device has not received CE mark or FDA approval at the time of writing this chapter.

AccuCinch is a ventricular restoration system designed to treat FMR by decreasing the circumference of a dilated LV and, therefore, the mitral annulus. It is a form of transcatheter ventricular remodeling. The device consists of anchors with self-expanding Nitinol arms that fix the anchor into the myocardium. Although the anchors were placed in the annulus in original attempts, they are now positioned in the basal LV sub-annular space 10–20 mm below the MV plane. A cable that connects the anchors is cinched to bring them together (Figure 39.6). The system catheter is delivered to the LV via a retrograde femoral

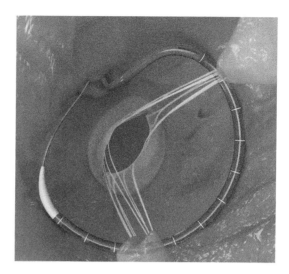

Figure 39.6 The AccuCinch system. *Source:* Modified from ANCORA HEART, INC.

arterial approach over a guidewire placed behind the chordae. The CorCinch FMR (Early Feasibility Study of the AccuCinch® Ventricular Repair System) and CorCinch HF (Clinical Evaluation of the AccuCinch Ventricular Restoration System in Patients Who Present With Symptomatic Heart Failure With Reduced Ejection Fraction) trials are currently ongoing, and promising early data was presented at 2019 Transcatheter Cardiovascular Therapeutics scientific meeting. At this time, this device has not received CE mark, nor is it FDA approved.

9.   What are some other devices for transcatheter MV repair?

Many other devices under investigation target different elements of the MV or use approaches not addressed in the chapter. For instance, the NeoChord DS1000 (NeoChord) and HARPOON TDS-5 (Edwards Lifesciences) are two of many chordal repair devices; the Cardinal ring (Valtech Cardio) and the enCor Dynaplasty ring (MiCardia) are examples of hybrid surgically implanted and transcatheter adjustable devices.

10.   What is the future of transcatheter treatment of MV disease?

The lag in the success of transcatheter MV therapies compared to TAVR is somewhat less than expected, given the variability and complexity in MV anatomy and disease etiology. It is complicated to develop one device that will fit all

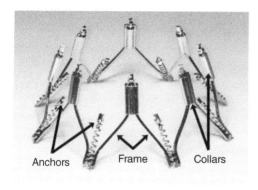

Anchors   Frame   Collars

Figure 39.5 The transcatheter Millipede IRIS device. *Source:* Rogers et al. (2019), Elsevier.

patients and anatomies. Instead, the complex structure has required an extensive array of techniques and technologies to match the large toolkit available to the mitral surgeon. Nevertheless, the success of TEER and TAVR has reignited interest in the field. With a long journey ahead, transcatheter MV devices have shown promising results. Increasing experience, technological improvements, clinical trial results, and the creation of programs and specialized centers, among many other things, will spur the development of successful transcatheter MV therapies.

Bibliography

1 Acker, M.A., Parides, M.K., Perrault, L.P. et al. (2014). Mitral-valve repair versus replacement for severe ischemic mitral regurgitation. *N. Engl. J. Med.* 370: 23–32.

2 Alperi, A., Granada, J.F., Bernier, M. et al. (2021). Current status and future prospects of transcatheter mitral valve replacement: JACC state-of-the-art review. *J. Am. Coll. Cardiol.* 77: 3058–3078.

3 Bapat, V., Rajagopal, V., Meduri, C. et al. (2018). Early experience with new transcatheter mitral valve replacement. *J. Am. Coll. Cardiol.* 71: 12–21.

4 Enriquez-Sarano, M., Schaff, H.V., Orszulak, T.A. et al. (1995). Valve repair improves the outcome of surgery for mitral regurgitation. A multivariate analysis. *Circulation* 91: 1022–1028.

5 Hensey, M., Brown, R.A., Lal, S. et al. (2021). Transcatheter mitral valve replacement: an update on current techniques, technologies, and future directions. *JACC Cardiovasc. Interv.* 14: 489–500.

6 Herrmann, H.C. and Maisano, F. (2014). Transcatheter therapy of mitral regurgitation. *Circulation* 130: 1712–1722.

7 Kim, J.H., Kocaturk, O., Ozturk, C. et al. (2009). Mitral cerclage annuloplasty, a novel transcatheter treatment for secondary mitral valve regurgitation: initial results in swine. *J. Am. Coll. Cardiol.* 54: 638–651.

8 Miller, M., Thourani, V.H., and Whisenant, B. (2018). The Cardioband transcatheter annular reduction system. *Ann. Cardiothorac Surg.* 7: 741–747.

9 Nishimura, R.A., Otto, C.M., Bonow, R.O. et al. (2017). 2017 AHA/ACC focused update of the 2014 AHA/ACC guideline for the Management of Patients with Valvular Heart Disease: a report of the American College of Cardiology/American Heart Association task force on clinical practice guidelines. *J. Am. Coll. Cardiol.* 70: 252–289.

10 Park, Y.H., Chon, M.K., Lederman, R.J. et al. (2017). Mitral loop cerclage annuloplasty for secondary mitral regurgitation: first human results. *JACC Cardiovasc. Interv.* 10: 597–610.

11 Piazza, N., Treede, H., Moat, N. et al. (2015). The Medtronic transcatheter mitral valve implantation system. *EuroIntervention* 11 (Suppl W): W80–W81.

12 Poncelet, A.J. (2003). Recurrence of mitral valve regurgitation after mitral valve repair in degenerative valve disease. *Circulation* 108: e125. author reply e125.

13 Rogers, J.H., Boyd, W.D., Smith, T.W., and Bolling, S.F. (2018). Early experience with Millipede IRIS transcatheter mitral annuloplasty. *Ann. Cardiothorac. Surg.* 7: 780–786.

14 Rogers, J.H., Boyd, W.D., Smith, T.W., and Bolling, S.F. (2019). Transcatheter mitral valve direct annuloplasty with the millipede IRIS ring. *Interv. Cardiol. Clin.* 8: 261–267.

15 Rogers, J.H., Thomas, M., Morice, M.C. et al. (2015). Treatment of heart failure with associated functional mitral regurgitation using the ARTO system: initial results of the first-in-human MAVERIC trial (mitral valve repair clinical trial). *JACC Cardiovasc. Interv.* 8: 1095–1104.

16 Schofer, J., Siminiak, T., Haude, M. et al. (2009). Percutaneous mitral annuloplasty for functional mitral regurgitation: results of the CARILLON Mitral Annuloplasty Device European Union study. *Circulation* 120: 326–333.

17 Sorajja, P., Leon, M.B., Adams, D.H. et al. (2017). Transcatheter therapy for mitral regurgitation clinical challenges and potential solutions. *Circulation* 136: 404–417.

18 Testa, L., Popolo Rubbio, A., Casenghi, M. et al. (2019). Transcatheter mitral valve replacement in the transcatheter aortic valve replacement era. *J. Am. Heart Assoc.* 8: e013352.

19 Witte, K.K., Lipiecki, J., Siminiak, T. et al. (2019). The REDUCE FMR trial: a randomized sham-controlled study of percutaneous mitral annuloplasty in functional mitral regurgitation. *JACC Heart Fail* 7: 945–955.

20 Zahr, F., Song, H.K., Chadderdon, S.M. et al. (2022). 30-day outcomes following transfemoral transseptal transcatheter mitral valve replacement: intrepid TMVR early feasibility study results. *JACC Cardiovasc. Interv.* 15: 80–89.

40

Transcatheter Mitral Valve Replacement

The Tendyne System

Michael P. Rogers and Lucian Lozonschi

Division of Cardiothoracic Surgery, Department of Surgery, University of South Florida Morsani College of Medicine, Tampa, FL, USA

1. What is the rationale for the Tendyne transcatheter mitral valve replacement system?

Mitral regurgitation (MR) is a leading cause of valvular heart disease, with a 9.3% prevalence of at least moderate MR in patients over 75 years of age. However, only a small proportion of patients with MR are treated with surgical mitral repair or replacement, leaving a large unmet need in patients at high or prohibitive surgical risk. Transcatheter mitral valve repair technology (i.e. transcatheter edge-to-edge repair [TEER]) has attempted to address this cohort, but often with not enough reduction of MR. Minimally invasive solutions have been sought that result in the elimination of MR, superior to any existing transcatheter repair techniques. An evolution of transcatheter mitral technology has been realized over the last decade, with remarkable results in animal models. Difficulties in adapting transcatheter replacement technologies to the mitral valve (MV) have included the lack of fixed landmarks and annular calcification for valve anchoring, the anatomy of the valve being intra-cardiac, challenging transseptal mitral access, vascular access complications, valve malposition, paravalvular leak (PVL), and the inability to use radial force due to the possibility of left ventricular outflow tract (LVOT) obstruction. Despite these hurdles, the Tendyne transcatheter mitral valve replacement (TMVR) system (Abbott Structural) evolved from the concept of the, Lutter Lozonschi valve, which employed a unique solution of securing the valve stent to the left ventricle (LV) wall to overcome the challenges described (Figure 40.1).

The Tendyne TMVR system is a fully repositionable and retrievable device that consists of two self-expanding Nitinol frames and a tri-leaflet porcine pericardial valve.

The two available valve configurations with multiple sizes allow for a customized fit to individual patient anatomies with respect to both the LVOT geometry and native mitral annular dimensions. The valve is available in multiple sizes (13 commercial sizes available currently), with two sealing height configurations, the Standard Profile "SP" and Low Profile "LP." The SP valve has an effective orifice area (EOA) of approximately 3.0 cm^2. The LP valve has an EOA of approximately 2.2 cm^2 (equivalent EOA to a 33 mm mitral bioprosthesis). The LP valve is designed to accommodate patients with smaller native annulus dimensions and to reduce LVOT obstruction. The valve size and sealing height configuration are selected to provide proper fit for paravalvular sealing, device stability, and LVOT area. The outer stent is designed in a D-shape configuration to mimic the native mitral annulus, with the straight and longer edge of the atrial cuff resting along the atrial wall on the aorto-mitral continuity (Figure 40.2). The system also contains an apical tether connected to the distal Nitinol stem of the Tendyne valve, which is secured to a pad that rests on the epicardial surface. The system is delivered via a 36 Fr transapical sheath with access by left anterior thoracotomy.

Early feasibility studies, including a multinational, non-randomized, prospective early feasibility study of 100 patients with at least moderate MR (grade $\geq$ 3+) at high or prohibitive surgical risk (mean Society for Thoracic Surgery Predictor of Mortality [STS PROM] 7.8%), have demonstrated excellent results. Sorajja and colleagues reported the largest published study on TMVR in native valves to date, with 96% successful device implantation and three intra-operative device retrievals (one related to LVOT obstruction, the second from a non-orthogonal access location and inability to deploy the valve within the annulus,

From Lutter-Lozonschi Valve to Tendyne

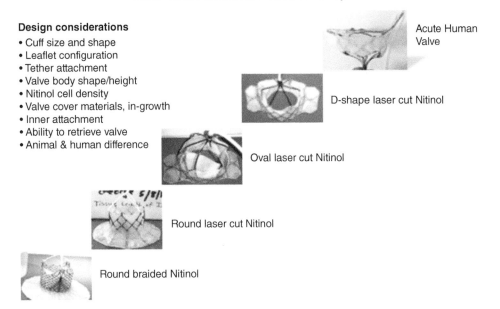

Design considerations
- Cuff size and shape
- Leaflet configuration
- Tether attachment
- Valve body shape/height
- Nitinol cell density
- Valve cover materials, in-growth
- Inner attachment
- Ability to retrieve valve
- Animal & human difference

Acute Human Valve

D-shape laser cut Nitinol

Oval laser cut Nitinol

Round laser cut Nitinol

Round braided Nitinol

Figure 40.1 Evolution of mitral valve technology with design considerations.

and the third for mal-positioning of the valve during the implant – in this procedure, a second valve was successfully implanted following successful retrieval of the first valve). One patient had PVL treated with percutaneous closure at three months. Major bleeding was seen in only 1% of patients. Four patients underwent valve re-intervention. The one-year survival in this cohort was 72.4%, with 88.5% of surviving patients reported with New York Heart Association (NYHA) Class I/II symptoms and improvements in six-minute walk distance and quality-of-life score for the entire study population. In a two-year follow-up

report, sustained MR elimination was reported in 93% of patients.

Tendyne is investigational in the United States and is currently being evaluated in the SUMMIT trial (Clinical Trial to Evaluate the Safety and Effectiveness of Using the Tendyne Mitral Valve System for the Treatment of Symptomatic Mitral Regurgitation), enrolling adult patients not suitable for surgery with moderate-to-severe or severe MR, or those with symptomatic MV disease due to severe mitral annular calcification. The study has three cohorts: a randomized arm for patients suitable for both

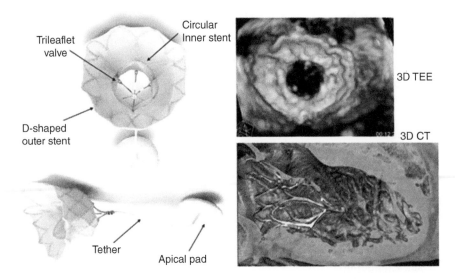

Trileaflet valve

Circular Inner stent

D-shaped outer stent

Tether

Apical pad

3D TEE

3D CT

Figure 40.2 Components of the Tendyne TMVR system with positioning by three-dimensional transesophageal echocardiogram (TEE) and computed tomography (CT).

transcatheter replacement or repair, a non-randomized arm for patients deemed not suitable for TEER, and a severe mitral annular calcification (MAC) arm.

2. What are the indications and contraindications for considering TMVR with the Tendyne system?

Current indications for use include treatment of the native MV in adult patients without prior valve intervention with moderate-to-severe or severe MV regurgitation (MR grade ≥ 3+), a life expectancy less than five years, left ventricular ejection fraction (LVEF) ≥30%, left ventricular end-diastolic dimension (LVEDD) ≤7.0 cm, and deemed not suitable for surgical repair or replacement by a multidisciplinary Heart Team who (i) have primary MR, are deemed not suitable for transcatheter repair, and have a left ventricular end-systolic dimension ≥3.0 cm; or (ii) have secondary MR and are symptomatic despite maximal guideline-directed therapy.

Contraindications include patients with a small neo-LVOT, those unable to tolerate procedural anticoagulation or a post-procedural antiplatelet/anticoagulation regimen, and those with sepsis (including active endocarditis), evidence of left ventricular or atrial thrombus, vegetation or mass on the MV, thin or fragile cardiac apex unsuitable for transapical access, anterior MV leaflet at risk for systolic anterior motion (SAM), hypersensitivity to nickel or titanium, and prior mitral intervention.

3. What are the anatomic variables to consider on pre-operative imaging when evaluating a patient for TMVR using Tendyne?

Pre-operative planning is paramount to successful device implantation. Contrast-enhanced gated full-cycle cardiac computed tomography (CT) should be obtained to assess valve geometry and the anatomy of surrounding structures. CT segmentation of the native mitral annulus with Tendyne valve simulation in the systolic and diastolic phases must be performed. The associated measurements should include the septal-lateral diameter, inter-commissural diameter, aorto-mitral angle, anterior MV leaflet length, and LVOT dimensions. The ideal location for apical access is determined by the orthogonal trajectory to the D-shaped mitral annular segmentation plane (trigone to trigone line and posterior MV perimeter). This method is described by Blanke and colleagues.

Using pre-operative imaging, the following conditions are recommended at both end-systole and end-diastole:

- A minimum neo-LVOT area of 250 mm^2.
- At least 5 mm of tether length within the ventricle.
- The valve does not interfere with ventricular wall tissue.
- The ventricular access site does not approximate the coronary vessel anatomy or transverse the right ventricle.
- The native anterior mitral leaflet is not at risk for SAM causing LVOT obstruction.

The risk of LVOT obstruction should be considered using the aforementioned measurements along with simulated virtual valve implantation with multiplanar reformatting.

4. What is the approach to Tendyne valve implantation, and what are the unique features?

After identifying the ideal location for transapical access on pre-operative imaging, a small left anterior thoracotomy is made, and the apex of the heart is visualized. The valve anchor to the apex should be orthogonal to the MV and not the true apex (Figure 40.3). Attention to the ideal placement of apical access is necessary to ensure alignment of the apical tether. The Tendyne system has a specific access point that is mapped relative to the true apex and corresponds to the patient's mitral orthogonal plane, which is unique for each patient. This access should be precise to minimize the risk of a canted valve position, which may result in PVL or LVOT obstruction. Next, pledgeted purse-string sutures are placed at the orthogonal access site of the LV myocardium, and the device sheath is inserted after obtaining a (chord-free) left atrial and ventricular access. The Tendyne valve may then be inserted through the sheath into the left atrium. The valve is partially deployed and visualized by transesophageal echocardiography (TEE) to ensure correct orientation. It may then be deployed fully in an intra-annular position. The device tether is then secured to the apical epicardial pad with the pad positioning system, which prevents device migration and assists in hemostasis.

The Tendyne valve system does not require any fixation to the native MV leaflets or annulus, and a high degree of prosthesis over-sizing or radial force is not needed. This minimal interaction with the native valve apparatus makes Tendyne a versatile solution for treating different disease etiologies of the MV (i.e. mitral annular calcification, degenerative MR [flail prolapse], functional MR, prior mitral rings, etc.). While transapical implantation is the current method described, a transseptal approach is being investigated.

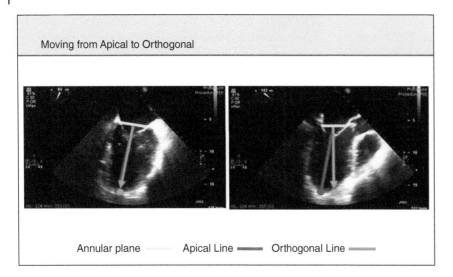

Figure 40.3 The Tendyne system has a specific axis point around the apex that corresponds to each patient's mitral orthogonal plane. This axis should be precise to minimize the risk of paravalvular leakage and left ventricular outflow tract obstruction.

5. What are specific challenges and potential complications of TMVR with the Tendyne system?

The rapid adoption and successes of transcatheter aortic valve replacement (TAVR) has provided a rationale for similar minimally invasive options to treat the MV. However, given the anatomic and physiologic complexity of the MV, unique challenges to system development and implementation exist.

Patients presenting with MR are generally younger than those with aortic stenosis but often significantly comorbid with advanced heart failure and cardio-renal syndrome. Ensuring valve durability and limiting structural valve deterioration is therefore imperative, although currently, no reported incidences of valve deterioration have been reported, with the longest follow-up now in a few patients over seven years. Additionally, while substantial advantages exist for patients undergoing TAVR for aortic stenosis, the benefit of TMVR in patients with secondary MR is less defined. The heterogeneity of MV pathology and the range of devices currently under investigation have implied that a "one-size fits all" strategy may not be appropriate for this disease process. However, early successes of the Tendyne system suggest this valve has the potential to challenge this paradigm and be a feasible solution to a wide range of mitral pathologies. Finally, the long-term durability and success of the Tendyne TMVR system have yet to be seen, although the upcoming SUMMIT (Clinical Trial to Evaluate the Safety and Effectiveness of Using the Tendyne Mitral Valve System for the Treatment of Symptomatic Mitral Regurgitation) trial and post-market clinical follow-up studies in Europe should address many of these questions.

Complications seen in early feasibility studies of the Tendyne system have included bleeding, access failure, LVOT obstruction, new conduction abnormalities, PVL, valve thrombosis, acute renal failure, and early and late cardiovascular rehospitalization. Challenges in the Tendyne global early feasibility trial by Muller and colleagues included a fall in mean LVEF from 47 to 41%, although this may be related to an increase in afterload and decrease in preload from the complete elimination of MR. However, provided the LVEF remains relatively stable or with only a minor reduction in LV function, the forward stroke volume will be substantially increased secondary to a reduction in post-capillary pulmonary artery pressures, providing for functional improvement of patients' heart failure symptomology.

Muller et al. reported one patient with valve thrombosis and another with significant hemolysis without evidence of PVL. Questions remain regarding the optimal anticoagulation strategy, rates of valve thrombosis or hemolysis, PVL, and conduction abnormalities requiring pacemaker implantation long-term. Pacemaker rates and new-onset atrial fibrillation at 30 days were very low – less than 5% in the first 100 patients as reported by Muller and colleagues – and this trend has persisted. The overall mortality risk is associated with advanced age and frailty, likely related to the surgical portion of the procedure. In the first 100 patients, incremental mortality was 6, 12, and 18% at one, two, and three months, respectively. Following the initial few months, the mortality curve flattens significantly, speaking to the importance of a patient's ability to tolerate the index procedure. Whether these adverse events seen in early trials represent isolated occurrences remains to be seen until larger trials are complete. The upcoming SUMMIT trial and post-market follow-up studies should provide more context in this cohort.

Conclusions

The Tendyne TMVR system is a promising transcatheter minimally invasive approach in the treatment of moderate-to-severe MR in select high-surgical risk patients. The system offers unique features, including a valve-tether pad that allows for valve repositioning, retrievability, and improved hemostasis. Excellent short-term results in early feasibility studies are promising; however, additional studies are ongoing. As minimally invasive approaches continue to advance, a paradigm shift in the available options for the treatment of mitral valve disease will unfold in the coming decade.

Acknowledgments

The authors would like to thank Thomas H. Vilkama, Abbott Medical Affairs, Minnesota, USA for his expert review, updates and images provided.

Bibliography

1 Alkhouli, M., Alqahtani, F., and Aljohani, S. (2017). Transcatheter mitral valve replacement: an evolution of a revolution. *J. Thorac. Dis.* 9 (Suppl 7): S668–S672.

2 Aoun, J., Reardon, M.J., and Goel, S.S. (2021). Transcatheter mitral valve replacement: an update. *Curr. Opin. Cardiol.* 36 (4): 384–389.

3 Bapat, V., Rajagopal, V., Meduri, C. et al. (2018). Early experience with new transcatheter mitral valve replacement. *J. Am. Coll. Cardiol.* 71 (1): 12–21.

4 Beller, J.P., Rogers, J.H., Thourani, V.H. et al. (2018). Early clinical results with the Tendyne transcatheter mitral valve replacement system. *Ann. Cardiothorac Surg.* 7 (6): 776–779.

5 Blanke, P., Dvir, D., Cheung, A. et al. (2014). A simplified D-shaped model of the mitral annulus to facilitate CT-based sizing before transcatheter mitral valve implantation. *J. Cardiovasc. Comput. Tomogr.* 8 (6): 459–467.

6 De Backer, O., Wong, I., Taramasso, M. et al. (2021). Transcatheter mitral valve repair: an overview of current and future devices. Open. *Heart* 8 (1).

7 Duncan, A. and Quarto, C. (2021). 6-year outcomes of first-in-man experience with Tendyne transcatheter mitral valve replacement: a single center experience. *JACC Cardiovasc. Interv.* 14 (20): 2304–2306.

8 Hensey, M., Brown, R.A., Lal, S. et al. (2021). Transcatheter mitral valve replacement: an update on current techniques, technologies, and future directions. *JACC Cardiovasc. Interv.* 14 (5): 489–500.

9 Lozonschi, L., Bombien, R., Osaki, S. et al. (2010). Transapical mitral valved stent implantation: a survival series in swine. *J. Thorac. Cardiovasc. Surg.* 140 (2): 422–426 e1.

10 Muller, D.W.M., Farivar, R.S., Jansz, P. et al. (2017). Transcatheter mitral valve replacement for patients with symptomatic mitral regurgitation: a global feasibility trial. *J. Am. Coll. Cardiol.* 69 (4): 381–391.

11 Quarto, C., Davier, S., Duncan, A. et al. (2016). Transcatheter mitral valve implantation: 30-day outcome of first-in-man experience with an apically tethered device. *Innovations (Phila)* 11 (3): 174–178.

12 Sorajja, P., Moat, N., Badhwar, V. et al. (2019). Initial feasibility study of a new transcatheter mitral prosthesis: the first 100 patients. *J. Am. Coll. Cardiol.* 73 (11): 1250–1260.

13 Lutter, G., Lozonschi, L., Ebner, A., et al. (2014). First-in-Human Off-Pump Transcatheter Mitral Valve Replacement. *JACC Cardiovasc. Interv.* 7 (9): 1077–1078.

41

Self-Expanding Transcatheter Mitral Valve Replacement Systems

Medtronic Intrepid Valve

Ignacio Inglessis-Azuaje

Structural Heart Disease Program, Massachusetts General Hospital, Boston, MA, USA
Harvard Medical School, Boston, MA, USA

1. What are the key features of the Medtronic Intrepid transcatheter mitral valve replacement (TMVR) valve?

The Intrepid bioprosthesis is a trileaflet bovine pericardial valve contained in a self-expanding Nitinol frame with a unique dual structure design consisting of a circular inner stent to house the valve and a conformable outer fixation ring to engage the mitral annular anatomy (Figure 41.1). The outer fixation ring is designed to accommodate the dynamic variability of the native mitral annulus while isolating the inner valve assembly throughout the cardiac cycle. A flexible brim attached to the atrial end of the fixation ring facilitates imaging during the procedure.

The bioprosthesis is built around a 27 mm inner valve structure with an effective orifice area (EOA) of 2.4 cm^2 and is being currently investigated in 42 and 48 mm outer diameters

2. How does the Medtronic Intrepid valve achieve fixation and sealing?

Fixation and sealing are achieved through a combination of design features: (i) the outer fixation ring is larger in circumference than the native mitral valve (MV) annulus with varying degrees of radial stiffness along its axial length; (ii) the atrial portion of the outer fixation ring is flexible where the frame and native annulus engage, allowing conformation to the native annulus – in contrast, the ventricular portion is stiffer and resists compression; and (iii) the flexible atrial portion deflects inward to allow annular alignment, while the stiff ventricular mid-section resists compression and maintains its shape, producing a final "champagne cork-like" conformation (narrow neck and wider body) to resist migration under systolic pressure. Three circumferential rings of frictional elements further help fixation. The prosthesis is designed to preserve the native leaflets and chordae and leverage them to seal around the device. The outer and inner stent frames are covered by a polyester fabric skirt to assist in preventing paraprosthetic leaks and facilitate tissue ingrowth for long-term fixation and sealing. The prosthesis has minimal protrusion downstream of the annulus to help maintain the patency of the left ventricular outflow tract.

3. How does the Medtronic Intrepid valve heal in the heart?

Healing of the atrial space between the stents follows a characteristic sequence of events that is common to virtually all cardiac devices (Figure 41.2). An initial layer of fibrin deposition (resulting from acute inflammation) resolves, leading to endothelial encapsulation as the surface thrombus organizes to provide a protective adherent coating. Ultimately, a pannus layer between the stents forms a new atrial floor.

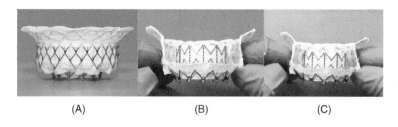

Figure 41.1 (a) The Intrepid transcatheter mitral valve replacement prosthesis (b) with cut-outs to demonstrate the innovative dual stent design and (c) overall flexibility, which allows the device to conform to the shape of the native mitral annulus. *Source:* Meredith et al. (2016), Europa Group.

4. What are the available delivery systems for the Medtronic Intrepid valve?

The Intrepid MV was first studied with transapical delivery, consisting of an apical introducer sheath (with dilator) and a hydraulically actuated delivery catheter. The prosthesis is compressed to 33 Fr before being loaded within the delivery capsule and then is advanced via the apical sheath into the left ventricle and across the MV.

A next-generation, 35-F transfemoral access system that enables transseptal delivery of the Intrepid valve is now under investigation.

5. How is the Medtronic Intrepid valve deployed via transapical delivery?

Under transesophageal echocardiographic guidance, the valve is advanced into the left atrium. Subsequently, the capsule is retracted hydraulically using a standard inflation device to gradually deploy and release the self-expanding prosthesis within the native MV. The hydraulic actuation system assists with the controlled expansion and deployment of the prosthesis. Importantly, the system does not require rotational alignment, tethering, or capture of native leaflets before or during device deployment (Figures 41.3 and 41.4).

6. What has been the experience with the Medtronic Intrepid transapical delivery system?

Patients with symptomatic mitral regurgitation (MR) who were deemed a high or extreme risk by the local heart teams were enrolled in a global pilot study evaluating the Intrepid transapical system at 14 sites in the United States, Australia, and Europe.

Fifty consecutively enrolled patients (mean age: 73 ± 9 years; 58.0% men; 84% secondary MR) underwent TMVR with the valve. The mean Society for Thoracic Surgery score was 6.4 ± 5.5; 86% of patients were New York Heart Association (NYHA) functional class III or IV, and the mean left ventricular ejection fraction was 43 ± 12%. The device implant was successful in 48 patients with a median deployment time of 14 minutes (interquartile range: 12–17 minutes). The 30-day mortality was 14%, with no disabling strokes or repeat interventions. The median follow-up was 173 days (interquartile

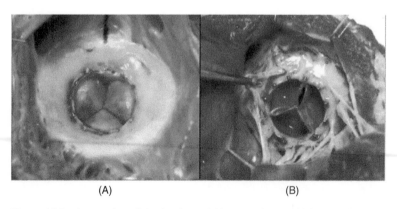

Figure 41.2 Integration of the implant within a porcine preclinical model. Healing response observed on the (a) atrial and (b) ventricular surfaces three months following Intrepid prosthesis implantation.

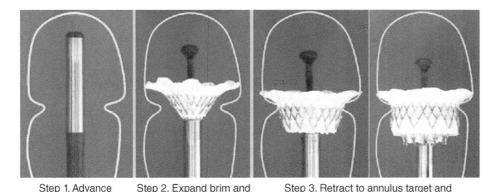

Step 1. Advance into left atrium.

Step 2. Expand brim and align with annulus target.

Step 3. Retract to annulus target and deploy the valve.

Figure 41.3 The delivery sequence for implantation of the Intrepid bioprosthesis.

range: 54–342 days). At the latest follow-up, echocardiography confirmed mild or no residual MR in all patients who received implants. Improvements in symptom class (79% in NYHA functional class I or II at follow-up; $p < 0.0001$ vs. baseline) and Minnesota Heart Failure Questionnaire scores (56.2 ± 26.8 vs. 31.7 ± 22.1; $p = 0.011$) were observed. This study confirmed that TMVR with the Intrepid transapical system with the valve was feasible in a study group at high or extreme risk for conventional MV replacement. The Intrepid valve is now undergoing evaluation in the APOLLO (Transcatheter Mitral Valve Replacement with the Medtronic Intrepid TMVR System in Patients with Severe Symptomatic Mitral Regurgitation) trial, a multicenter, global, prospective, nonrandomized trial enrolling patients with moderate to severe or severe mitral insufficiency who are not candidates for transcatheter mitral edge-to-edge repair. This trial includes a cohort with mitral annular calcification.

7. What has been the experience with the Medtronic Intrepid transseptal delivery system?

A prospective, multicenter, nonrandomized early feasibility study evaluated the safety and performance of the Intrepid valve using transfemoral access, enabling

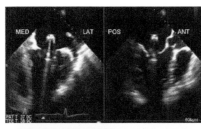

Step 1: Advance into the left atrium.

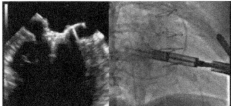

Step 2: Expand brim and align with annulus target.

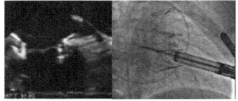

Step 3: Retract to annulus target and deploy the valve.

Figure 41.4 Deployment of the Intrepid valve via transapical delivery. Step 1: Advance into the left atrium, Step 2: Expand brim and align with the annulus target, Step 3: Retract to annulus target and deploy the valve.

transseptal delivery in patients with moderate to severe or severe symptomatic MR at high surgical risk.

Fifteen patients were enrolled at six sites from February 2020 to May 2021. The median age was 80 years, and the median Society of Thoracic Surgeons Predicted Risk of Mortality was 4.7%; 87% of patients were men, and 53% had undergone prior sternotomy. Fourteen implants were successful. One patient was converted to surgery during the index procedure. Patients stayed a median of five days postprocedure. There were 6 access site bleeds (40%) and 11 iatrogenic atrial septal defect closures (73%). At 30 days, there were no deaths, strokes, or reinterventions. All patients undergoing implantation had trace or no valvular or paravalvular MR, and the mean gradient was 4.7 mmHg (IQR: 3.0–6.7 mmHg).

Conclusions

Early experience has shown that the Medtronic Intrepid valve is a promising advance for the treatment of MV disease. The combination of a novel, straightforward delivery system and a uniquely designed bioprosthesis that does not require rotational alignment, tethering, or capture of the native mitral leaflets for fixation and the potential for transfemoral delivery lends itself as an attractive option.

Bibliography

1 Bapat, B., Rajagopal, V., Meduri, C. et al. (2018). Early experience with new transcatheter mitral valve replacement. *JACC* 72 (1): 12–21.

2 Zahr, F., Song, H., Chadderdon, S. et al. (2022). 30-day outcomes following transfemoral transseptal transcatheter mitral valve replacement. *JACC Interven.* 15: 80–89.

Part III

Structural Interventions for the Tricuspid Valve

42

Natural History and Hemodynamic Assessment of Tricuspid Valve Diseases

Nicholas Sturla[1] and Brian P. O'Neill[2]

[1] Department of Internal Medicine, Henry Ford Hospital, Detroit, MI, USA
[2] Division of Cardiology, Center for Structural Heart Disease, Henry Ford Hospital, Detroit, MI, USA

Epidemiology, Natural History, and Prognosis

1. How prevalent is tricuspid regurgitation?

It is estimated that at least 1.6 million Americans have moderate-to-severe tricuspid regurgitation (TR). The prevalence of TR significantly increases with age: 1.5% of men over the age of 70 have moderate-to-severe TR, and 5.6% of women.

2. What is the significance of TR?

Evidence suggests that severe TR is associated with increased mortality if left untreated. Moderate TR will worsen over time and cause permanent right ventricle (RV) dysfunction, leading to heart failure and death. Studies have shown an association with increased hospitalization rates, morbidity, and mortality. In the presence of TR in patients with left-sided heart disease, there was an increase in mortality.

Anatomy

3. What are the four components of the tricuspid valve?

The fibrous annulus. The annulus is a dynamic structure that varies with loading conditions. It is ovoid and saddle-shaped, with a normal diameter of 12 ± 1 cm and an area of 11 ± 2 cm^2. The annular area can increase to 29.6 cm^2 during atrial systole. The anatomy of the annulus is crucial to understand, given its significant role in the pathophysiology of secondary TR; it is the primary target of several interventions.

The three leaflets. The tricuspid valve consists of three leaflets: anterior, septal, and posterior. The anterior leaflet is the largest, with the most motion, and the septal is the shortest in the radial direction with the least movement. In the setting of functional dilation (i.e. secondary TR), the dilation primarily occurs on the septal and posterior leaflet attachments with relative sparing of the septal portion.

Papillary muscles and chordal attachments. Two papillary muscles are defined in the TV apparatus: anterior and posterior. The anterior papillary muscle lends chordal attachments to the anterior and posterior leaflets, while the posterior papillary muscle lends chordal attachments to the posterior and septal. Unlike the mitral valve, chordae may arise directly from the septum contributing to a more complicated trabecular meshwork. This is of particular significance when planning for interventions (Figure 42.1).

4. How do we classify TR, and what diseases fall into each category?

Tricuspid regurgitation is classified into primary, secondary, and isolated etiologies.

Primary disease is defined as an organic valvular disease and represents 10% of all cases of TR in adults. The abnormality occurs in one of the four components of the tricuspid valve. We can further classify the disease into congenital, acquired, and isolated. Congenital causes include Ebstein's disease, atrioventricular defects, and myxomatous prolapse. Acquired primary conditions include endocarditis, rheumatic disease, systemic lupus erythematosus, sarcoidosis,

(A) **View from Above**   (B) **View from Front**

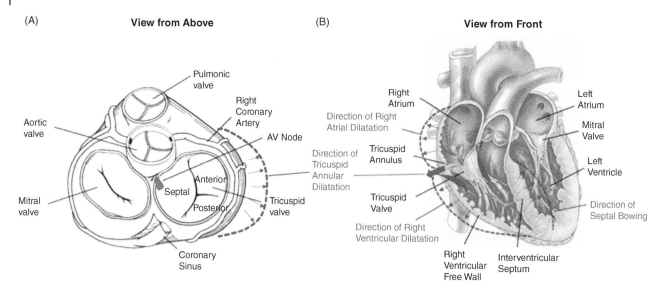

Figure 42.1 (a) The anatomy of the tricuspid valve and adjacent structures from a surgical view. (b) The relevant anatomy from the front view. The dotted lines show the direction of dilation of various structures in the setting of secondary tricuspid regurgitation. *Source:* Dahou, A., et al., 2019 / with permission of Elsevier.

iatrogenic injury from endomyocardial biopsy, transvenous pacing or defibrillator leads, carcinoid syndrome, and trauma.

Secondary valvular disease is the absence of organic valvular disease, and the primary mechanism results from annular dilation and leaflet tethering. Causes of secondary disease can arise from left-heart disease causing RV remodeling or RV dilation caused by dilated cardiomyopathies, RV infarct, and arrhythmogenic RV dysplasia. Chronic volume overload from high output states or intracardiac shunts is another cause.

Isolated TR has been described as a form of secondary disease. However, it is becoming recognized as a separate entity in the absence of pulmonary hypertension or left-sided heart disease. It is mostly found in elderly patients with atrial fibrillation.

5. What are the signs and symptoms of TR?

TR is mostly asymptomatic. Severe TR may present with stand-alone symptoms, including palpitations, edema, fatigue, dyspnea, abdominal bloating, and anorexia. Congestive hepatopathy is another finding, making liver function testing a helpful tool in patients with severe TR.

Physical exam findings suggestive of severe TR include a systolic murmur heard best at the left lower sternal border with increasing intensity on inspiration. A palpable right ventricular precordial thrust may be present with right ventricular hypertrophy. Prominent jugular V waves, jugular venous distention, and hepatic pulsations may also be present.

Evaluation/Diagnosis

6. What are the major imaging modalities used to assess the tricuspid valve?

Transthoracic and transesophageal echocardiogram, Cardiac magnetic resonance imaging (MRI), and multi-detector computed tomography (MDCT) all have valuable and unique utilities in assessing TR.

7. What are the advantages of each of these imaging modalities?

Echocardiography has a central role given its cost, safety, portability, and accessibility. It can provide information regarding RV function and examination of other heart valves. It can also to be performed during surgical or transcatheter interventions.

Cardiac magnetic resonance imaging (MRI) is the gold standard, given its spatial resolution and ability to provide volumetric quantification of the valve. The routine use of cardiac MRI may be challenging as many patients with TR have pacemakers or defibrillators.

Multidetector CT (MDCT) provides accurate measurements and assessments of the tricuspid valve itself in addition to surrounding structures. These features are useful during pre-procedural planning of transcatheter tricuspid valve intervention (TTVI).

8. How is the tricuspid valve evaluated with echocardiography?

TR is classically staged A–D, with stage A being at risk for TR, B representing progressive TR, C representing asymptomatic severe TR, and D representing symptomatic TR. Transthoracic echocardiography (TTE) is used to evaluate the etiology and severity of disease and assess for the presence of left-sided heart disease. This is done by using specific parameters to individually assess valve anatomy, valve hemodynamics, and hemodynamic consequences.

Valve anatomy differentiates primary from functional TR. Intrinsic leaflet and chordal abnormalities are seen in primary disease, while annular dilation and leaflet tethering are seen in functional disease.

Valve hemodynamic parameters comprise the central jet area, continuous-wave jet density and contour, vena contracta, and hepatic vein flow. The central jet area of regurgitant flow is measured by color Doppler, and the regurgitant jet area is associated with TR severity. Continuous-wave Doppler can measure the shape and density of the jet. The shape of a TR jet is normally symmetrically parabolic, indicating the equality of changes in acceleration. A severe TR jet will show an early peaked, asymmetric waveform due to the large regurgitant volume equalizing the right atrium (RA) and RV pressures earlier than normal. Jet density progressively darkens as TR severity increases. Vena contracta is a more quantitative assessment that measures the cross-sectional area of the blood column as it leaves the regurgitant valve, resulting in a surrogate for the regurgitant orifice area. Hepatic vein flow in mild cases of TR shows a systolic dominant pattern of flow contrasted with the systolic flow reversal seen in severe TR (Figure 42.2).

Hemodynamic consequences refer to changes seen in the RV, RA, and interior vena cava (IVC). These modalities are measured by 2D echocardiography. Hemodynamically significant TR will show dilation of the RV, RA, and IVC with changes in the variability pattern seen with respiration.

9. What are the characteristics of severe TR?

Valve hemodynamics consistent with severe TR are a central jet area $>10\,cm^2$, vena contracta width $>7\,mm$, dense and triangular continuous-wave jets with early peak, and reversal of hepatic vein flow. Hemodynamic effects are RA, RV, and IVC dilation with decreased respiratory variation, the presence of a c-V wave, and diastolic interventricular septal wall flattening.

Parameters	Mild	Moderate	Severe
Qualitative	Normal/mildly abnormal leaflets	Moderately abnormal leaflets	Flail leaflet, ruptured papillary muscle, large perforation or vegetation
	Flow convergence zone not visible, transient, or small	Flow convergence zone is moderate and central	Flow convergence zone is large and throughout systole
		Intermediate size and duration of CW signal TR jet	Dense, triangular with early peaking CW signal TR jet
			IVC dilated
	Faint/partial/parabolic CW signal TR jet	IVC normal or mildly dilated	Usually dilated RA/RV
	IVC normal in size	Normal or mildly dilated RA/RV	
	Normal RA and RV size		
Semi-quantitative	Color flow jet area not defined	Color flow jet area not defined	Color flow jet area $>10\,cm^2$
	Tricuspid inflow is A-wave dominant	Tricuspid inflow E-wave is variable	Tricuspid inflow E-wave $\geq 1\,m/sec$
	VC $<0.3\,cm$	VC $0.3–0.69\,cm$	VC $\geq 0.7\,cm$
	PISA radius $\leq 0.5\,cm$	PISA radius $0.6–0.9\,cm$	PISA radius $>0.9\,cm$
	Systolic dominance in hepatic vein flow	Systolic blunting in hepatic vein flow	Systolic flow reversal in hepatic vein flow
Quantitative	EROA by PISA $<20\,mm^2$	EROA by PISA $20–39\,mm^2$	EROA by PISA $\geq 40\,mm^2$
	RVol by PISA $<30\,mL$	RVol PISA $30–44\,m$	RVol by PISA $\geq 45\,mL$

IVC, inferior vena cava; RA, right atrium; RV, right ventricle; CW, continuous wave; TR, tricuspid regurgitation; VC, vena contracta; PISA, proximal isovelocity surface area; EROA, effective regurgitant orifice area; RVol, regurgitant volume; 3D, three-dimensional.

Figure 42.2 Criteria for grading tricuspid regurgitation based on qualitative, semi-quantitative, and quantitative measurements. *Source:* Zoghbi et al., 2017 / with permission of Elsevier.

Management

10. What are the broad categories of TR management?

The management of TR consists of medical therapy, surgical management, and TTVI. **Medical therapy** commonly includes diuretics and mineralocorticoid receptor antagonists. Studies demonstrating improvement in survival for patients with severe TR and medical therapy alone are lacking. Hence the current gold standard remains surgical tricuspid valve repair or replacement.

11. When is surgery considered the preferred option?

Surgery remains the gold standard for the treatment of symptomatic TR even though rates of surgical correction remain low and surgery is primarily performed in the setting of concomitant left-sided surgical repair.

12. What are the surgical methods for TR management?

Surgical management can be divided into three categories: annuloplasty, adjunctive repair techniques, and tricuspid valve replacement.

Tricuspid annuloplasty reduces annular dilation and thereby improves leaflet coaptation. It can be accomplished in one of two ways: ring annuloplasty or suture annuloplasty. Ring annuloplasty is the more commonly done procedure due to its relative ease and lower recurrence of TR. Numerous studies have demonstrated better outcomes with ring annuloplasty over suture annuloplasty.

Adjunctive repair techniques used in RV remodeling, leaflet tethering, and residual TR persist despite prior ring annuloplasty. The techniques for adjunctive repair include anterior leaflet augmentation, double orifice valve technique, and anterior leaflet augmentation.

Valve replacement carries a higher risk than valve repair and is pursued if valve repair cannot be performed or is not expected to have a durable outcome. Given the lack of data on valve repair on primary TR, valve replacement is often performed in complex cases of primary TR, including infective endocarditis, carcinoid heart disease, Ebstein's anomaly, and rheumatic heart disease.

13. Which patients are considered for TTVI?

Patients who are considered poor surgical candidates are the population for TTVI. As previously mentioned, many patients with significant TR have delayed presentation with significant comorbidities, and this large population of patients requires a less invasive means of repair.

14. What challenges are associated with TTVI?

Several factors make TTVI a complicated endeavor. First, the anatomy of the valve is difficult. As with surgical repair, the primary focus is the annulus, which lies in close proximity to the right coronary artery, lending itself to iatrogenic injury of the artery during the procedure. The structure of the annulus makes it difficult to anchor devices, given its mixed composition of muscular and fatty tissue with interspersed fibrous support.

Patients who are the typical candidates for TTVI also may have significant dilation of the annulus, which causes challenges in designing expandable valves that can be deployed through the femoral vein using current catheters and sheaths.

15. What are the major categories of TTVI?

Percutaneous techniques include annuloplasty systems, direct leaflet repair, transcatheter tricuspid value implantation, and caval aortic valve implantation (CAVI). These techniques will be discussed in detail in later chapters.

Bibliography

1 Alqahtani, F., Berzingi, C.O., Aljohani, S. et al. (2017). Contemporary trends in the use and outcomes of surgical treatment of tricuspid regurgitation. *J. Am. Heart Assoc.* 6 (12): e007597.

2 Badano, L.P., Muraru, D., and Enriquez-Sarano, M. (2013). Assessment of functional tricuspid regurgitation. *Eur. Heart J.* 34 (25): 1875–1885.

3 Dahou, A., Levin, D., Reisman, M. et al. (2019). Anatomy and physiology of the tricuspid valve. *JACC Cardiovasc. Imaging* 12 (3): 458–468.

4 Fender, E.A., Zack, C.J., and Nishimura, R.A. (2018). Isolated tricuspid regurgitation: outcomes and therapeutic interventions. *Heart* 104 (10): 798–806.

5 Hahn, R.T. (2016). State-of-the-art review of echocardiographic imaging in the evaluation and treatment of functional tricuspid regurgitation. *Circ. Cardiovasc. Imaging* 9 (12).

6 Mangieri, A., Montalto, C., Pagnesi, M. et al. (2017). Mechanism and implications of the tricuspid regurgitation: from the pathophysiology to the current and future therapeutic options. *Circ. Cardiovasc. Interv.* 10 (7).

7 Nishimura, R.A., Otto, C.M., Bonow, R.O. et al. (2014). 2014 AHA/ACC guideline for the Management of Patients with Valvular Heart Disease: executive summary: a report of the American College of Cardiology/American Heart Association Task Force on Practice Guidelines. *Circulation* 129 (23): 2440–2492.

8 Prihadi, E.A., Delgado, V., Leon, M.B. et al. (2019). Morphologic types of tricuspid regurgitation: characteristics and prognostic implications. *JACC Cardiovasc. Imaging* 12 (3): 491–499.

9 Sudhakar, B.G.K. (2020). Evaluation and management of primary tricuspid regurgitation. *Indian J. Clin. Cardiol.* 1 (3–4): 174–185.

10 Zoghbi, W.A., Adams, D., Bonow, R.O. et al. (2017). Recommendations for Noninvasive Evaluation of Native Valvular Regurgitation: A Report from the American Society of Echocardiography Developed in Collaboration with the Society for Cardiovascular Magnetic Resonance. *J. Am. Soc. Echocardiogr.* 30: 303.

43

Indications and Outcomes for Surgical Tricuspid Valve Repair

Ali Ghodsizad[1], Matthias Loebe[1] and Tomas Salerno[2]

[1] *Miami Transplant Institute, University of Miami Miller School of Medicine, Miami, FL, USA*
[2] *Cardiothoracic Surgery, University of Miami Miller School of Medicine, Miami, FL, USA*

Tricuspid Regurgitation (Tricuspid Valve Insufficiency)

Tricuspid regurgitation (TR) is a functional dynamic clinical picture caused by enlargement of the tricuspid annulus with right ventricular dilation. Right-heart failure secondary to left-sided valvular disease is often seen. Jerome Kay introduced repair techniques for functional TR repair in 1965 followed by Norberto DeVega in 1972. Kay and colleagues describe shortening the posterior tricuspid leaflet by placing several sutures across the posterior segment of the tricuspid valve annulus. The DeVega technique involves annular plication by placing two semicircular purse-string sutures on the tricuspid valve annulus. Both techniques were more or less replaced by ring annuloplasty after the introduction of the remodeling annuloplasty concept by Alain Carpentier. The development of transcatheter strategies for TR is in the early stages, but various approaches, including edge-to-edge repair and annuloplasty, have been reported in the literature.

The tricuspid valve functions in a dynamic relationship with the right ventricle (RV) with the anterior and posterior leaflet arising from the anterior papillary muscle.

1. What are known etiologies associated with TR?

Different etiologies are associated with TR. So-called severe primary TR is an indication for surgery but involves fewer than 10% of TR cases. More clinically relevant is functional TR, which is diagnosed on echocardiography (> 50%); an indication for surgical treatment is given when a concomitant indication for left-heart surgery is present. As reported by Nath and colleagues in a retrospective analysis including 5223 patients, moderate to severe TR was associated with worse survival despite adjustment for pulmonary artery systolic pressure (PASP), left ventricular ejection fraction (LVEF), RV size, and function. There is no clear evidence showing that surgical repair of isolated TR improves survival or symptoms. Based on a few observational studies, international guidelines recommend surgical annuloplasty of non-severe TR with annulus dilatation $\geq 40\,mm$ or $21\,mm/m^2$ by 2D echocardiography and valve repair or replacement for severe TR.

2. What is the reported mortality rate for surgical repair of TR?

High surgical short-term mortality, between 5 and 15%, is usually reported from small cohorts. A recent study by Axtell and colleagues showed no survival benefit when comparing surgery to medical treatment in a large cohort of 3276 patients. In addition, no difference could be shown between surgical repair and replacement.

3. Are there better clinical results using transcatheter tricuspid valve intervention (TTVI)?

Several new interventional devices are used for TTVI. The surgically established Alfieri-styled edge-to-edge procedure was proposed for the tricuspid valve as well as the mitral valve. But given the tricuspid valve anatomy, clipping only the anterior and posterior leaflets was shown not to be the best interventional step.

Mastering Structural Heart Disease, First Edition. Edited by Eduardo J. de Marchena and Camilo A. Gomez.
© 2023 John Wiley & Sons Ltd. Published 2023 by John Wiley & Sons Ltd.
Companion website: www.wiley.com/go/deMarchena/Mastering-Structural-Heart-Disease

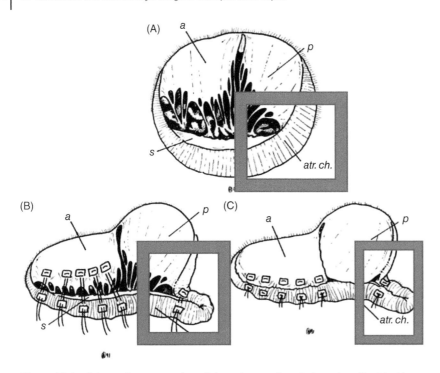

Figure 43.1 Schematic presentation of the valve repair technique described by Hetzer and colleagues. The technique was modified for bicuspidalization of the tricuspid valve and described by Loebe and Ghodsizad et al.: modification includes using two 2-3 pledgeted 3-0 Polypropylene mattress sutures at the posterior-septal commissure (blue labeled portion). *Source:* Roland Hetzer et al. 1998 / With permission of Elsevier.

The TriClip (Abbott) can be seen as a modification of the MitraClip percutaneous delivery system and was under investigation in the TRILUMINATE study (Trial to Evaluate Treatment with Abbott Transcatheter Clip Repair System in Patients with Moderate or Greater Tricuspid Regurgitation). Another device used was PASCAL (Edwards Lifesciences), successfully adapted from mitral to tricuspid use. Edwards Lifesciences has presented its FORMA device, which was used to reduce TR by creating a new surface for coaptation for tricuspid leaflets. The FORMA device consists of a foam-filled spacer that can be implanted using the subclavian or axillary vein, placed in the regurgitant orifice, and further anchored in the right ventricular apex. In a feasibility study with up to 20 patients, it has been shown to reduce TR. The SPACER (Repair of Tricuspid Valve Regurgitation Using the Edwards TricuSPid TrAnsCatheter REpaiR System) study will report further results.

4. Describe a surgical assessment and repair technique to repair a tricuspid valve

A saline test can reveal the loss of coaptation between all three leaflets due to annular dilation focused on TR

between the posterior and septal leaflets. Repair of a tricuspid valve using the DeVega technique can be assessed as follows: the surgeon should be able to pass two fingers through the valves, so two fingers can enter the RV without major challenge.

Different repair techniques have been described in the literature. Kay and colleagues described plication of the posterior leaflet by placing several sutures across the posterior leaflet of the tricuspid valve annulus. The repair is started by performing the first arm of support suture (3-0 Prolene) along the posterior annulus. The second arm of the support suture is completed using two pledgeted mattress sutures. The DeVega technique involves annular plication with the first arm starting at the anterior-septal commissure and ending at the posterior-septal commissure; the second arm strengthens the circumferential force and helps to plicate the annulus to correct annular dilation. The triangle of Koch is an important anatomic landmark visualized by imaginary lines between the coronary sinus and septal commissures.

A further technique was developed by Hetzer and colleagues and published as a modified repair technique for tricuspid valve insufficiency in patients with Ebstein anomaly. Loebe and colleagues modified the technique to repair severe TR in left ventricular assist device (LVAD) candidates: 2 × 3-0 polypropylene pledgeted sutures are used to plicate the posterior-septal commissure for a closer approximation of the anterior annulus toward the septum.

5. Which transcatheter annuloplasty technique resembles the surgical DeVega and Kay techniques?

The Trialign (Mitralign) and TriCinch (4Tech) devices are interventional devices that function similarly to surgical annuloplasty techniques. The Trialign device is a transcatheter suture annuloplasty technique that can be implanted using transjugular access. A wire is positioned in the RV and retrogradely crossed into the tricuspid annulus. Two pledgets are placed at the postero-septal and anteroposterior commissures. The goal is to obliterate the posterior tricuspid leaflet, leading to bicuspidization of the tricuspid valve. The TriCinch device requires femoral access. The myocardium is crossed, and an epicardial coil with two hemostasis seal devices is implanted in the mid-anterior part of the tricuspid annulus. Next, a Nitinol stent connected to the coil through a Dacron band is placed in the inferior vena cava (IVC). The device is used to maintain tension applied to the annulus as described in a small case series.

6. What are some of the most frequently described surgical annuloplasty systems in the literature?

Various flexible ring systems are available in the literature. The Carpentier surgical ring annuloplasty system is widely used. A sizing device (delivered as part of the system) allows measurement of the anterior and posterior leaflet surfaces and inter-commissural distance. The Carpentier-Edwards Classic is a widely used semi-rigid ring system. Its flexibility allows the surgical ring system to be shaped before implantation, with the septal portion slightly bent inward to match the anatomic annular structure.

7. What is the outcome of TR repair and LVAD implantation in patients not responding to advanced medical heart failure therapy?

There is no clear evidence for improved survival as a result of correcting TR at the time of the LVAD implantation. Biventricular heart failure patients often present with advanced pulmonary hypertension secondary to chronic high left atrial pressures. Some previous publications have shown that concomitant TR repair and LVAD insertion improves survival. Further research and scientific evidence are needed to establish guidelines.

Bibliography

1 Axtell, A.L., Bhambhani, V., Moonsamy, P. et al. (2019). Surgery is not associated with improved survival compared to medical therapy in isolated severe tricuspid regurgitation. *J. Am. Coll. Cardiol.* .

2 Barac, Y.D., Nicoara, A., Bishawi, M. et al. (2020). Durability and efficacy of tricuspid valve repair in patients undergoing left ventricular assist device implantation. *JACC Heart Fail.* 8 (2): 141–150. Epub 2019 Dec 11.

3 Baumgartner, H., Falk, V., Bax, J.J. et al. (2017). 2017 ESC/EACTS guidelines for the management of valvular heart disease. *Eur. Heart J.* 38 (36): 2739–2791.

4 Calen, C., Taramasso, M., Guidotti, A. et al. (2017). Successful TriCinch-in-TriCinch transcatheter tricuspid valve repair. *JACC Cardiovasc. Interv.* 10 (8).

5 Carpentier, A., Deloche, A., Dauptain, J. et al. (1971). A new reconstructive operation for correction of mitral and tricuspid insufficiency. *J. Thorac Cardiovasc. Surg. JANV* 61 (1): 1–13.

6 Carpentier, A., Deloche, A., Hanania, G. et al. (1974). Surgical management of acquired tricuspid valve disease. *J. Thorac. Cardiovasc. Surg.* 67: 53–55.

7 DeVega, N.F. (1972). La anuloplastia selectiva, regulable y permanente. *Rev. Esp. Cardiol.* 25: 555–556.

8 Dreyfus, G.D., Corbi, P.J., Chan, K.M.J., and Bahrami, T. (2005). Secondary tricuspid regurgitation or dilatation: which should be the criteria for surgical repair? *Ann. Thorac. Surg. Janv.* 79 (1): 127–132.

9 Dreyfus, G.D., Martin, R.P., Chan, K.M. et al. (2015). Functional tricuspid regurgitation: a need to revise our understanding. *J. Am. Coll. Cardiol.* 65: 2331–2336.

10 Fam, N.P., Ho, E.C., Zahrani, M. et al. (2018). Transcatheter tricuspid valve repair with the PASCAL system. *JACC Cardiovasc. Interv.* 11 (4): 407–408.

11 Gheorghe, L., Swaans, M., Denti, P. et al. (2018). Transcatheter tricuspid valve repair with a novel cinching system. *JACC Cardiovasc. Interv.* 11 (24): e199–e201.

12 Ghodsizad, A., Badiye, A., Loebe, M. et al. (2018). Modified Hetzer's technique for concomitant TK valve repair and LVAD implantation. Orlando ISHLT.

13 Hetzer, R., Nagdyman, N., Ewert, P. et al. (1998). 3-year outcomes of transcatheter mitral valve repair in patients with heart failure. *J. Thorac. Cardiovasc. Surg.* 115 (4): 857–868. http://dx.doi.org/10.1016/S0022 5223(98)70367-8.

14 Imamura, T., Narang, N., and Nnanabu, J. (2019). Hemodynamics of concomitant tricuspid valve procedures at LVAD implantation. 34 (12): 1511–1518. Epub 2019 Nov 6. J Cardiac Surgery.

15 Kay, J.H., Maselli-Campagna, G., and Tsuji, H.K. (1965). Surgical treatment of tricuspid insufficiency. *Ann. Surg.* 162: 53–58.

16 Lai, Y.-Q., Meng, X., Bai, T. et al. (2006). Edge-to-edge tricuspid valve repair: an adjuvant technique for residual tricuspid regurgitation. *Ann. Thorac. Surg. Juin.* 81 (6): 2179–2182.

17 Lavie, C.J., Hebert, K., and Cassidy, M. (1993). Prevalence and severity of Doppler-detected valvular regurgitation and estimation of right-sided cardiac pressures in patients with Normal two-dimensional echocardiograms. *Chest* 103 (1): 226–231.

18 Lindenfeld, J., Abraham, W.T., Grayburn, P.A. et al. (2021). Cardiovascular outcomes assessment of the MitraClip percutaneous therapy for heart failure patients with functional mitral regurgitation (COAPT) investigators. *JAMA Cardiol.* 6 (4): 427–436.

19 Mack, M.J. and Lindenfeld, J. (2021). Abraham WT et a al; 3-year outcomes of transcatheter mitral valve repair in patients with heart failure. COAPT Investigators. *J. Am. Coll. Cardiol.* 77 (8): 1029–1040.

20 McElhinney, D.B., Cabalka, A.K., Aboulhosn, J.A. et al. (2016). Transcatheter tricuspid valve-in-valve implantation for the treatment of dysfunctional surgical bioprosthetic valves: an international, multicenter registry study. *Circulation* 133 (16): 1582–1593.

21 Nath, J., Foster, E., and Heidenreich, P.A. (2004). Impact of tricuspid regurgitation on long-term survival. *J. Am. Coll. Cardiol.* 43 (3): 405–409.

22 Overtchouk, P., Piazza, N., Granada, J. et al. (2020). Advances in transcatheter mitral and tricuspid therapies. *BMC Cardiovasc. Disord.* 20: 1.

23 Puri, R. and Rodés-Cabau, J. (2016). Transcatheter interventions for tricuspid regurgitation: the FORMA repair system. *EuroIntervention J. Eur. Collab. Work Group Interv. Cardiol. Eur. Soc. Cardiol.* 12 (Y): Y113–Y115.

24 Rosser, B.A., Taramasso, M., and Maisano, F. (2016). Transcatheter interventions for tricuspid regurgitation: TriCinch (4Tech). *EuroIntervention* 12: Y110–Y112.

25 Schofer, J., Bijuklic, K., Tiburtius, C. et al. (2015). First-in-human transcatheter tricuspid valve repair in a patient with severely regurgitant tricuspid valve. *J. Am. Coll. Cardiol.* 65 (12): 1190–1195.

26 Singh, J.P., Evans, J.C., Levy, D. et al. (1999). Prevalence and clinical determinants of mitral, tricuspid, and aortic regurgitation (the Framingham heart study). *Am. J. Cardiol.* 83 (6): 897–902.

27 Song, H.K., Gelow, J.M., Mudd, J. et al. (2016). Limited utility of tricuspid valve repair at the time of left ventricular assist device implantation. *Ann. Thorac. Surg.* 101: 2168–2174.

28 Topilsky, Y., Khanna, A.D., Oh, J.K. et al. (2011). Preoperative factors associated with adverse outcome after tricuspid valve replacement. *Circulation* 123 (18): 1929–1939.

29 Wahlers, T., Wittwer, T., and Adams, D.H. (2018). *Cardiac Surgical Operative Atlas Atlas of Ccardiac Surgery*. Lehmanns Media GmbH.

44

Intra-Procedural Imaging of Tricuspid Valve Edge-to-Edge Interventions

Brijeshwar Maini[1,2,3] Hamza Lodhi[1,2] Adithya Mathews[1,2] and Houman Khalili[1,2]

[1] Department of Cardiovascular Diseases, Florida Atlantic University, Boca Raton, FL, USA
[2] Cardiology, Delray Medical Center, Delray Beach, FL, USA
[3] Tenet Healthcare Corporation, Delray Beach, FL, USA

Introduction

The tricuspid valve (TV) has remained the forgotten valve until recently, when there has been burgeoning interest in transcatheter solutions for tricuspid regurgitation (TR), especially given the associated poor survival. This has happened after success with catheter-based technologies for mitral regurgitation, which are becoming mainstream not only with edge-to-edge repair but also with transcatheter mitral valve replacement, as exemplified by multiple ongoing recent studies.

Advanced imaging to guide these procedures is critical to achieve technical success. This includes appropriate preoperative assessment of the patient with multi-modality imaging. Intra-procedural imaging is coming of age with both two-dimensional and three-dimensional transesophageal echocardiography (TEE) as well as intracardiac echocardiography imaging, which may complement the imaging endeavor.

Several devices are being developed to address this unmet need in a patient population in which there is high in-hospital mortality associated with isolated TV surgery as well as a significant impact on mortality and morbidity in patients with secondary TR. One such device is the Cardioband (Edwards Lifesciences), which received the CE mark award in April 2018. Transcatheter TV devices currently under investigation or development can be divided into those treating annular dilatation (i.e. Trialign [Mitralign], Cardioband, TriCinch [4Tech], Millipede [Boston Scientific], and Cardiac Implants), those approaching leaflet malcoaptation (i.e. MitraClip [Abbott Vascular],

PASCAL [Edwards Lifesciences], and FORMA [Edwards Lifesciences]), heterotopic valve implantation (i.e. caval valve implants [CAVIs; Tricentro]), and transcatheter TV replacements (i.e. GATE [NaviGate Cardiac Structures], Trisol, and valve-in-valve [ViV]). These devices use different access sites to reach the TV: the superior vena cava (SVC), inferior vena cava (IVC), and transatrial access. Other devices in development may access the pericardial space. This list is not exhaustive because there is ongoing development of new devices.

A comprehensive understanding of the TV anatomy is essential for intra-procedural imaging of transcatheter devices. It is inherently important to understand that while the TV is usually tricuspid, it may have up to six leaflets and may have clefts or folds, and therefore it is difficult to discriminate the differences. The tricuspid leaflets are also very thin and translucent. It is important to note that the anterior leaflet is generally the largest and has the greatest excursion, while the septal leaflet is the least mobile and shortest. Similarly, the anterior papillary muscle is the largest and supports the anterior and posterior leaflets, while the septal leaflet chordae insert directly into the septum and have multiple small papillary muscles. The tricuspid annulus is D-shaped and flat with a dynamic motion that is larger in diastole; the average perimeter is 12 ± 1 cm, and the average area is 11 ± 2 cm^2. It should also be noted that the right atrium (RA) is markedly dilated; in advanced disease, the SVC and IVC are also dilated. Also of note is that the coronary sinus enters the RA at the commissure between the septal and posterior leaflets. The atrioventricular (AV) node and bundle of His cross the septal leaflet attachment 3–5 mm posterior to the anteroseptal commissure, and the noncoronary sinus of Valsalva borders the anterior/superior annulus.

1. Is it important to understand the structures adjacent to the tricuspid valve?

The size of the RA is important because maneuvering these large-bore devices may be challenging in the small right atrial space, and if the RA is very large, imaging will be difficult. Understanding the size of the SVC and IVC is an important consideration for device implantation. The inflow of the coronary sinus is a good anatomic marker for the commissure between the septal and posterior leaflets. There is a risk of heart block with devices in the region of the AV node. Understanding the correlation of the TV to the coronary sinus decreases the risk of perforation with devices in the region, and the sinus of Valsalva can also be used as a marker for the septal anterior commissure. It is important to understand that tethering or tenting of the leaflets is a common etiology of secondary TR resulting in wider coaptation gaps and dilatation of the right ventricle and displacement of the papillary muscles. Understanding the chordal apparatus is important to prevent the interaction of the catheters and devices.

2. What should the transesophageal imaging protocol be?

Tricuspid valve imaging: Focused views of the TV (rightward rotation of the probe) should be obtained from the mid-esophageal and gastric views. Single-plane (preferred) with simultaneous multiplane image views should be performed from different rotational angles, as shown in Figure 44.1.

1) **Mid-esophageal view:**
   a. 0°: TV-focused view starting from the four-chamber view (RV apex seen) imaging the septal and typically anterior leaflets.
   b. 30°: Retroflexion may begin to image +/− anterior/posterior leaflets.
   c. 60–70°: Inflow-outflow view (may image all three leaflets (commissural view). The anteroseptal and posteroseptal commissures can be imaged using a biplane.
   d. 90–100°: Anterior and posterior leaflets can be seen; a biplane can be used to image either of them with a septal leaflet. Typically this is a bicaval view with the TV en face but out of plane. Retroflexion may bring the TV into view.

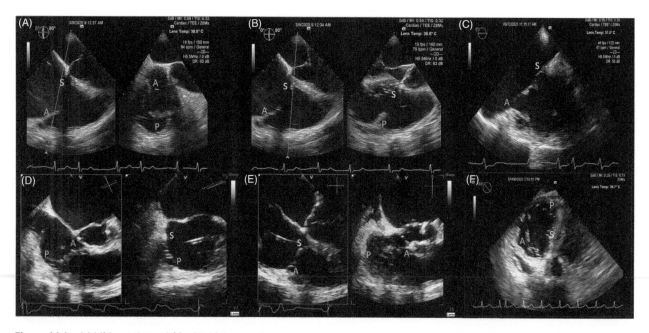

Figure 44.1 (a) Mid-esophageal 0° with biplane at the anterior leaflet showing the A, S, and P leaflets. (b) Mid-esophageal 0° with biplane at the septal leaflet showing A, S, and P leaflets. (c) Deep-esophageal 0° view without visualization of the left-sided heart structures. (d) 60–70° commissural view with biplane at the P leaflet, showing the P and S leaflets. (e) 60–70° commissural view with biplane at the A leaflet, showing the A and S leaflets. (f) Transgastric 0–40° view showing the A, S, and P leaflets. A, anterior; S, septal; P, posterior.

2) **Deep-esophageal view:** Similar to the mid-esophageal views, this view typically eliminates imaging of the left-sided structures and allows unobstructed views of the TV.

3) **Transgastric view:** 0–40°: From a SAX LV view, the right rotation of the probe should result in the SAX of the RV (and the TV).

4) **Deep transgastric view:** 0°: similar to an apical 4Ch view.

Doppler assessment:

1) At each of the previous views, with the TV imaged, record the color Doppler of the TV using the appropriate sector size to image the entire jet (the Nyquist limit should be between 0.5 and 0.6 m/s for the vena contracta and ~0.3 m/s for the proximal isovelocity surface area) (Figure 44.2).

2) Continuous wave Doppler of the TR jet to obtain a complete spectral profile of the jet. From multiple views, pulsed wave Doppler of the TV for TV Inflow (at the level of the annulus): Be sure to adjust the level of the PW sample volume so that it bisects the tricuspid annular plane in mid-diastole

3) TV inflow at the leaflet tips.

4) Record at least 5 beats (10 beats if there is atrial fibrillation).

3. Why is Tricuspid valve imaging challenging?

Tricuspid edge-to-edge repair is possible with the use of the MitraClip device off-label, or within the context of clinical trials in the United States. Both Abbott Triclip and Edwards Pascal have CE mark indication for tricuspid valve repair in Europe. The currently available edge-to-edge repair device requires perpendicular access to the TV. Intra-procedural echocardiographic imaging is more challenging than mitral valve imaging because of the following factors:

- The esophageal location of the transesophageal echocardiogram probe leads to shallow angles of insonation.
- Far-field, shadowing secondary to other cardiac structures, especially when there are calcified structures or a prosthesis present.
- Presence of multiple leaflets.
- Severe tethering.
- Annular dilatation.
- Wide coaptation gaps.

4. What are the steps in TV imaging?

Very thorough pre-procedural TEE imaging in a supine position is of paramount importance.

1) The basic imaging recommendations for tricuspid edge-to-edge repair start with a bicaval view with biplane imaging. This prevents tissue damage and can navigate the tricuspid edge-to-edge repair device to the tricuspid annular plane.

2) The second view is used to adjust the trajectory of the tricuspid clip, which should be done in the mid/deep esophageal view with the angle from 60° to 80° with biplane imaging to help identify the septal/anterior and septal/posterior leaflets and the secondary view (Figure 44.3.)

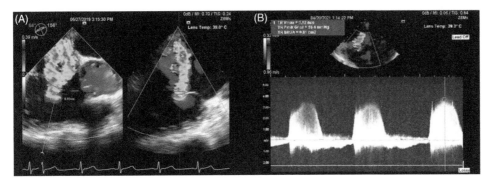

Figure 44.2 (a) Proximal isovelocity surface area (PISA) radius (green line), and biplane vena contracta (VC) (red lines). (b) Continuous-wave (CW) Doppler through the tricuspid valve evaluates the gradient across the tricuspid valve, maximum velocity (Vmax) helps to calculate the effective regurgitant orifice area (EROA), and the velocity time integral (VTI) helps to calculate regurgitant volume.

3) The final positioning of the clip should be performed in a deep transgastric view whereby all three leaflets are visualized. Biplane imaging may be used in the transgastric view as well to identify the septal/anterior and septal/posterior leaflets. The transgastric view is best obtained at 10° to 40° (Figure 44.3).

4) The grasping views are again performed with the mid/deep esophageal commercial views at 60° to 80° with biplane imaging.

5) The septal and anterior leaflets are generally intervened first, followed by moving posteriorly and intervening upon the septal and posterior leaflets. It is best to interrogate the three leaflets in the mid/deep esophageal view by interrogating the anterior and posterior leaflets with and without color Doppler to evaluate the color jet's location as well as reduction in the regurgitant flow.

6) Appropriate attention must be paid to the length of the leaflet incorporated within the clip arms.

7) Appropriate assessment of TR should be performed before the edge-to-edge repair using objective evaluation of the TV including proximal isovelocity surface area (PISA), effective regurgitant orifice, and regurgitant volumes along with the vena contractor and hepatic venous flow reversal. These should be compared after the edge-to-edge repair has been performed to evaluate reduction in TR.

8) It is also important to ensure that the gradient across the TV does not increase significantly. A gradient of <4 mmHg is considered acceptable

5. How is TR graded?

According to the American Society of Echocardiography, the severity parameters for TR are as shown in Figure 44.4. To better characterize the severity of TR currently being treated with various transcatheter devices, there has been a proposal to increase the grades to include very severe (or massive) as well as torrential. This requires further validation (see Table 44.1).

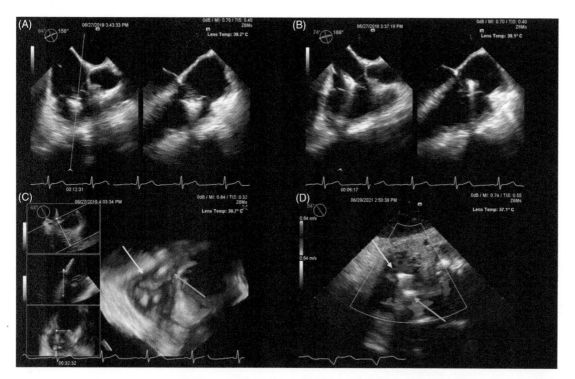

Figure 44.3 Intra-procedural TEE. (a) Commissural (grasping view) showing biplane at the anterior leaflet on the left and anterior and septal leaflets on the right. (b) Commissural (grasping view) showing biplane at the posterior leaflet on the left and the posterior and septal leaflets on the right. (c) 3D transesophageal echocardiography showing the MitraClip device (yellow arrow) and shaft (green arrow) approaching the anterior leaflet. (d) Final result with two deployed clips anterior and septal (green arrow) and posterior and septal (yellow arrow).

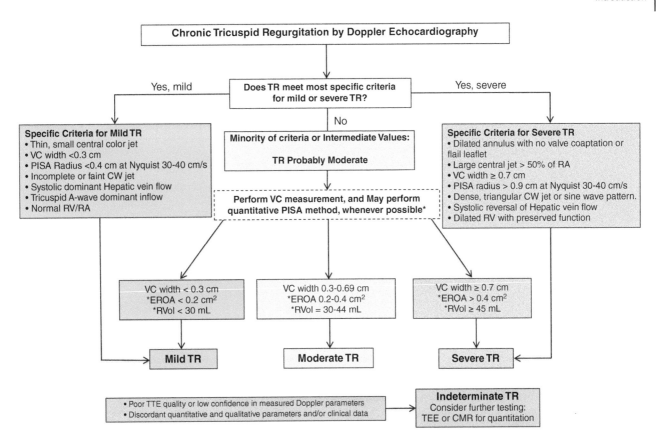

Figure 44.4 Algorithm for evaluating chronic tricuspid regurgitation by Doppler echocardiography. *Source:* Zoghbi et al. 2017/ with permission of Elsevier.

Table 44.1 Proposed expansion of the "severe grade" by Hahn et al.

Variable	Severe	Massive	Torrential
Vena contracta (biplane)	7–13 mm	14–20 mm	≥21 mm
Effective regurgitant orifice area (proximal isovelocity surface area)	40–59 mm²	60–79 mm²	≥80 mm²
3D VCA or quantitative effective regurgitant orifice area	75–94 mm²	95–114 mm²	≥115 mm²

6. How should post-procedural imaging be graded?

There is minimal data on how to evaluate residual TR after tricuspid valve interventions. In the registry of tricuspid edge-to-edge repair, several methods were used to assess regurgitation. These methods require further validation.

The guidelines for the evaluation of valvular regurgitation after percutaneous repair or replacement suggest the grading system in Table 44.2.

Table 44.2 Proposed grading of the severity of residual tricuspid regurgitation by echocardiography after tricuspid valve interventions.

Parameters	Mild	Moderate	Severe
Qualitative			
Color jet area[d]	Small, narrow, central	Moderate central	Large central jet or eccentric wall-impinging jet(s) of variable size swirling in the RA
Flow-convergence zone[a]	Not visible or small	Intermediate in size	Large
TR CW Doppler velocity waveform	Faint/partial/parabolic	Dense, parabolic, or triangular	Dense, often triangular
Tricuspid inflow	A-wave dominant	Variable	E-wave dominant[b, c]
Semi-quantitative			
VC width (cm)[d]	<0.3	0.3–0.69	0.7 or 2 moderate jets[c]
PISA radius (cm)[a]	0.5	0.6–0.9	>0.9
Hepatic vein flow[b]	Systolic dominance	Systolic blunting	Systolic flow reversal
Quantitative			
EROA (cm^2)[e]	<0.20	0.20–0.39	0.40[c]
RVol (ml)[e]	<30	30–44	45[c]

CW, continuous-wave; EROA, effective regurgitant orifice area; RA, right atrium; RVol, regurgitant volume; TR, tricuspid regurgitation; VC, vena contracta.

a) Not well-validated for quantitation; best used after interventions that leave the valve intact; baseline Nyquist limit shift to 25–35 cm/s.
b) Non-specific, influenced by other factors (RV diastolic function, atrial fibrillation, RA pressure).
c) Not suitable in procedures intervening with valve leaflets (e.g. edge-to-edge repair).
d) With Nyquist limit >50–60 cm/s.
e) EROA from 2D PISA is not suitable in patients with edge-to-edge valve repair because of a multiplicity of jets and non-hemispheric shape of flow convergence. Needs further validation of cut-offs by either the PISA or volumetric method.

Bibliography

1 Goode, D., Dhaliwal, R., and Mohammadi, H. (2020). Transcatheter mitral valve replacement: state of the art. *Cardiovasc. Eng. Technol.* 11: 229–253.

2 Hahn, R.T. and Zamorano, J.L. (2017). The need for a new tricuspid regurgitation grading scheme. *Eur. Heart J. Cardiovasc. Imaging* 18: 1342–1343.

3 Nath, J., Foster, E., and Heidenreich, P.A. (2004). Impact of tricuspid regurgitation on long-term survival. *J. Am. Coll. Cardiol.* 43: 405–409.

4 Nickenig, G., Kowalski, M., Hausleiter, J. et al. (2017). Transcatheter treatment of severe tricuspid regurgitation with the edge-to-edge MitraClip technique. *Circulation* 135: 1802–1814.

5 Ohno, Y., Attizzani, G.F., Capodanno, D. et al. (2014). Association of tricuspid regurgitation with clinical and echocardiographic outcomes after percutaneous mitral valve repair with the MitraClip system: 30-day and 12-month follow-up from the GRASP registry. *Eur. Heart J. Cardiovasc. Imaging* 15: 1246–1255.

6 Patel, J.S. and Kapadia, S.R. (2019). The Tendyne transcatheter mitral valve replacement system for the treatment of mitral regurgitation. *Future Cardiol.* 15: 139–143.

7 Zoghbi, W.A., Adams, D., Bonow, R.O. et al. (2017). Recommendations for noninvasive evaluation of native valvular regurgitation: a report from the American Society of Echocardiography developed in collaboration with the Society for Cardiovascular Magnetic Resonance. *J. Am. Soc. Echocardiogr.* 30: 303–371.

8 Zoghbi, W.A., Asch, F.M., Bruce, C. et al. (2019). Guidelines for the evaluation of valvular regurgitation after percutaneous valve repair or replacement: a report from the American Society of Echocardiography developed in collaboration with the Society for Cardiovascular Angiography and Interventions, Japanese Society of Echocardiography, and Society for Cardiovascular Magnetic Resonance. *J. Am. Soc. Echocardiogr.* 32: 431–475.

45

Transcatheter Tricuspid Valve Device Landscape

Sharon Bruoha, Andrea Scotti, Edwin Ho and Azeem Latib

Montefiore-Einstein Center for Heart and Vascular Care, Montefiore Medical Center, Albert Einstein College of Medicine, Bronx, NY, USA

1. What is the magnitude of tricuspid regurgitation disease and its impact on patient outcomes?

Tricuspid regurgitation (TR) is an exceedingly prevalent valve disease: approximately 1.6 million individuals across the United States alone have significant TR. Numerous studies have highlighted the adverse prognosis that patients with severe TR experience, independent of other comorbidities, including increased mortality, a greater number of hospital admissions, and prolonged hospitalizations. Currently, no effective medical treatment exists, and surgery for isolated TR is associated with in-hospital mortality of 8.8%. Delayed referrals, often associated with the presence of end organ damage, may account, at least in part, for these poor results. In addition, a high operative risk may preclude a significant number of patients from surgical treatment.

2. What is the pathophysiology of TR?

Functional TR (FTR), the most prevalent form of TR, is seen in approximately 80–90% of cases and is a consequence of right ventricular (RV) remodeling secondary to excessive pulmonary pressure loads (pressure overload) or long-standing volume overload, as seen in systemic-to-pulmonary shunts. RV deformation with subsequent annular dilation and leaflet tethering ultimately leads to FTR. Annular dilatation, typically the dominant mechanism involved in FTR, occurs predominantly along the anteroposterior valve plane, corresponding to the low resistant free wall of the RV. Alternatively, in "atrial" FTR (isolated TR), the right atrium (RA) undergoes progressive dilatation with subsequent annular expansion and leaflet malcoaptation in the absence of pulmonary hypertension (PH). In FTR, the valve leaflets and sub-valvular apparatus are anatomically normal. Less commonly, primary TR results from abnormalities of the valve leaflets themselves, such as prolapse, flail, perforation, fibrosis, retraction, or congenital abnormalities. Iatrogenic TR, frequently associated with cardiovascular implantable electronic device (CIED) leads, is an increasingly recognized form of primary TR, and the presence of device wires across the tricuspid valve (TV) may interfere with procedural imaging and device deployment during transcatheter procedures.

3. What are the current medical and surgical recommendations for managing TR?

Available drug therapy specific for TR is highly limited and mainly based on diuretics. Treating the underlying etiologies associated with secondary TR is strongly recommended (e.g. guideline-directed medical therapy for left-sided heart failure and PH). Surgical ring annuloplasty is currently considered the preferred repair procedure, especially during left-sided valve surgery. Surgical repair of isolated secondary TR in high-risk patients with evidence of end-organ damage is associated with poor outcomes and is rarely performed. Ideally, treatment should be pursued early, before the onset of severe PH and\or severe RV failure. However, if there is significant valve and ventricular remodeling, effective TR elimination can only be achieved with surgical valve replacement.

Mastering Structural Heart Disease, First Edition. Edited by Eduardo J. de Marchena and Camilo A. Gomez.

4. What are the main surgical TV repair techniques?

TV annuloplasty techniques target the pathophysiological hallmark of functional TR, anterolateral annular dilatation with consequent abnormal leaflet coaptation, by reducing the annular dimensions.

Annular reconstruction is the main approach utilized in surgical TV repair and is associated with significantly lower in-hospital mortality than valve replacement. Surgical annular reshaping can be achieved by suture-based or ring-assisted techniques. Suture bicuspidization (Kay procedure) is performed by applying pledget-protected sutures to the posterior annulus with subsequent plication and obliteration of the posterior leaflet. Alternatively, surgical annular reduction is performed by implanting an undersized (typically, incomplete) prosthetic ring, thereby reducing the annular perimeter.

5. What are the main challenges associated with transcatheter TV interventions?

The unique features of the TV apparatus, with its many anatomical variants – it has four functional leaflets in approximately 40% of individuals – combined with close proximity to the heart conduction system and the right coronary artery (RCA) and the heavy impact of loading conditions on its dimensions, render the process of patient selection and procedural planning challenging. Furthermore, the TV is positioned anteriorly and thus may be subjected to suboptimal imaging.

The D-shaped tricuspid annulus (TA) is a non-planar structure; it has a saddle-shaped, three-dimensional conformation and is devoid of a well-defined annulus fibrosus. The RV free wall attaches to the anterolateral portion of the TA, and the interventricular septum attaches to the relatively shorter septal aspect of the annulus. Histologically, the RV free wall contains small amounts of supportive connective tissue, while the septal segment is in close proximity to the fibrous skeleton of the heart and is more robust. Consequently, annular remodeling is especially pronounced along the axis with less resistance to dilation, along the lateral RV free wall, corresponding to the anteroposterior annulus.

An effective transcatheter tricuspid repair depends on meticulous imaging-based patient selection and the need to overcome multiple potential anatomic obstacles:

- The TV and TA area are dynamic in response to variable loading conditions (volume status), positive pressure ventilation, respiratory phase, and cardiac cycle. Thus, the anatomical details obtained during baseline evaluation using transesophageal echocardiography (TEE) or cardiac gated computed tomography (CT) may differ at the time of intervention. Ideally, baseline evaluation should be performed after a period of diuresis, when the patient is euvolemic.
- The TV proximity to the RCA and conduction system can potentially increase the procedure-related risk of iatrogenic injury, causing myocardial ischemia or conduction disturbances. The anatomic relationship of the TV to the RCA can be evaluated by CT angiography.
- The thin RV free wall is delicate and can easily be perforated during device manipulation.
- The thin TV leaflets and dense sub-valvular chordae are prone to injury and risk of device entrapment, respectively.
- There are often multiple mechanisms involved in FTR that can rarely be fully addressed using a single repair device. Even if annular dilatation is the predominant mechanism of FTR, associated leaflet coaptation defects, fibrosis, and tethering may result in residual TR despite successful percutaneous annuloplasty. The presence of CIED wires across the TV may also physically restrict leaflet mobility and reduce the efficacy of annular-directed therapies.

6. What transcatheter repair and replacement options are available?

Both transcatheter valve replacement and valve repair have emerged as feasible and effective interventions for severe TR (Table 45.1, Figure 45.1). Transcatheter valve repair techniques can broadly be grouped into two categories: leaflet-directed therapies and annulus-reshaping therapies. Leaflet-directed therapies are based on edge-to-edge leaflet approximation and currently constitute the majority of the outcomes data available. Alternatively, annular-reshaping therapies aim to reduce the TA diameter. Small case series with short- and intermediate-term outcomes with annular-reshaping devices have also been published.

TV replacement is an extensively investigated area with several potential advantages compared to valve repair. Valve replacement allows for complete elimination of TR, while repair often yields significant reduction but not complete elimination of regurgitant blood flow. Furthermore, valve replacement can be performed relatively independent of TA morphology, while repair techniques are limited by the degree of annular dilation, the severity of leaflet malcoaptation (large coaptation gap), and the complexity

Table 45.1 Transcatheter tricuspid valve devices landscape.

Coaptation Devices	Forma device
	TriClip
	PASCAL
Annuloplasty Devices	
Ring annuloplasty	
Direct	Cardioband
	Millipede IRIS
Indirect	TRAIPTA Transatrial intrapericardial tricuspid annuloplasty
Direct suture	Trialign
	TriCinch
	DaVingi TR system
	MIA-T
Heterotopic caval valve implantation (CAVI)	Balloon expandable valve
	Tricvalve

of the underlying sub-valvular apparatus. However, the utilization of some bulky transcatheter TV implants may be limited in the presence of small RV dimensions.

Registry data pooling outcomes following valve repair and valve replacement have demonstrated high rates of procedural success, significant reduction in TR severity, and substantial improvement in clinical symptoms at short and mid-term follow-up. The fundamental role of imaging in patient selection and procedural guidance for optimal results cannot be overestimated.

Leaflet-Directed Therapies

Leaflet-directed therapies target the TV leaflets to reduce the effective regurgitant orifice area (EROA) and are the most widely used modality for transcatheter TV repair. Currently, three devices have outcome data available following repair: MitraClip/TriClip (Abbot), PASCAL (Edwards Lifesciences), and FORMA Spacer (Edwards Lifesciences). However, only the MitraClip/TriClip and PASCAL systems are still available to operators. The ideal anatomical candidates for edge-to-edge repair are summarized in Table 45.2.

MitraClip/TriClip. The TriClip system (Abbot) uses the same clip-based device for leaflet approximation as the MitraClip but has a differentiated delivery system specifically designed to optimally approach the TV. The newest fourth-generation (4G) of the TriClip is a polyester-covered, V-shaped clip with four available device sizes for tailored repair: wide-arm (6 mm) clips available in arm lengths of 15 mm (NTW) or 18 mm (XTW) and narrow-arm (4 mm) clips available in 15 mm (NT) and 18 mm (XT) arm lengths. The wider-arm devices are designed to address wider regurgitant jets and larger baseline valve areas and are believed to reduce tissue stress due to the expanded distribution of tension. A new leaflet grasping technology, Controlled Gripper Actuation, also allows simultaneous or independent leaflet grasping to confirm

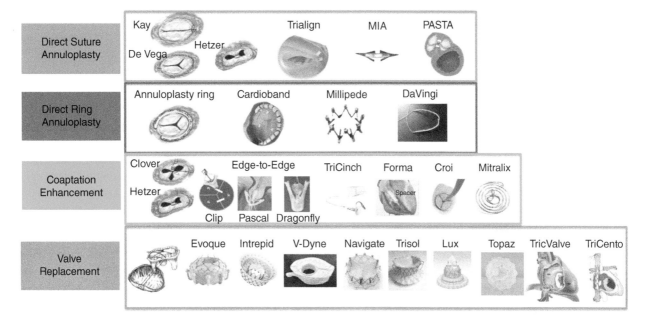

Figure 45.1 The transcatheter tricuspid landscape. *Source:* Adapted from Latib (2021).

Table 45.2 Eligibility criteria for tricuspid edge-to-edge repair.

Ideal TR for edge-to-edge repair	Edge-to-edge repair to be considered	Edge-to-edge repair not recommended or only in exceptional cases
Secondary TR with structurally normal-appearing leaflets	Secondary TR with normal-appearing leaflets or primary TR with leaflet prolapse[a]	Severe leaflet (rheumatic) thickening or shortening or destruction or very large leaflet prolapse
Small coaptation defect (<3–4 mm[b]) and good leaflet mobility	Moderate coaptation defect (4–7 mm[b]), reduced leaflet mobility	Large coaptation defect (>7 mm[b]) or severe leaflet tethering
Central TR jet extending in the anteroseptal commissure	Central TR jet extending in the posteroseptal or anteroposterior commissure	Non-central or very eccentric jets or jets originating from anteroposterior commissure
Good echocardiographic windows[c] for leaflet visualization	Sufficient echocardiographic windows[c] for leaflet visualization	Insufficient echocardiographic windows[c] for leaflet visualization
No PM/ICD lead	Presence of PM/ICD lead, no significant leaflet interaction, and no interaction with clip	PM/ICD lead-induced TR
Normal to moderately reduced RV function, normal to moderate RV dilatation	Moderately reduced RV function, moderate RV dilatation	Severely reduced RV function or severe RV dilatation
Normal sPAP	sPAP <60–65 mmHg and pulmonary capillary resistance <4 WU	sPAP >60–65 mmHg and/or pulmonary capillary resistance >4 WU

ICD, implantable cardioverter-defibrillator; PM, pacemaker; RV, right ventricular; sPAP, systolic pulmonary artery pressure; TR, tricuspid regurgitation.

In addition to the displayed suitability criteria for tricuspid edge-to-edge (E2E) repair, all patients should (i) be symptomatic with right-sided heart failure symptoms, (ii) be at high or prohibitive surgical risk, and (iii) have severe TR.

a) Leaflet prolapse width <10–12 mm and flail gap <10 mm.
b) Size of the coaptation defect must be assessed at the location of the planned clip placement orthogonally to the commissural plane.
c) Echocardiographic image quality must be assessed in a grasping view at the location of the planned clip placement.

and optimize leaflet insertion without releasing both leaflets. Multiple clips can be used depending on the size of the coaptation defect. The procedure is conducted via fluoroscopic and TEE guidance under general anesthesia.

The TRILUMINATE (Trial to Evaluate Treatment with Abbott Transcatheter Clip Repair System in Patients with Moderate or Greater Tricuspid Regurgitation) trial prospectively evaluated outcomes in 85 patients after TV repair with the TriClip. At 30-day follow-up, 87% of patients in the study had a reduction in TR severity by at least one grade. Additionally, most patients in the study had significant improvements in New York Heart Association (NYHA) class and six-minute walk distance on short-term follow-up. The six-month, one-year, and two-year outcomes, presented at the 2021 EuroPCR Valves Annual Meeting, showed excellent safety and efficacy of the TriClip system. TR reduction and improvement in patient functional capacity and quality of life achieved at 30 days post-procedure were sustained at two years. Furthermore, an overall reduction in hospitalizations was observed after the procedure compared to rates prior to the repair. The reported all-cause mortality was 18.7% at two years. The clinical benefits of edge-to-edge TR reduction with the TriClip have also

been shown in real-world settings and reconfirmed in interim data from post-marketing, real-world studies.

Of note, recruitment for the TRILUMINATE Pivotal IDE trial is currently ongoing with the aim to include approximately 700 patients with severe TR and to randomize them to medical therapy or TriClip repair. Long term follow-up of five years will be assessed in this trial.

PASCAL. The PASCAL system (Edwards Lifesciences), which is CE mark certified for the treatment of severe mitral regurgitation (MR) and TR, was originally developed for transcatheter mitral valve repair and subsequently repurposed for the percutaneous correction of TR. The implant consists of a central spacer (10 mm wide), two broad contoured paddles (about 25 mm wide in grasping position), and two clasps (10 mm long) that can be lowered independently to facilitate leaflet grasping in challenging anatomy. The larger clasps and contoured paddles are designed to place less tension on the leaflets during capture and closure and may be less traumatic. The central spacer fills in large coaptation gaps, prevents backflow after device delivery, and possibly further reduces leaflet load. These unique features potentially give PASCAL an advantage in treating valves with large coaptation gaps. Finally, the implant collapses into an elongated form, which reduces implant system length and helps minimize the risk of device retraction in the event of entanglement within dense sub-valvular chordae.

The early clinical experience in 28 patients undergoing repair with the PASCAL system showed promising results. The majority of patients (86%) had successful device implantation with a post-procedure TR grade of moderate or less. At follow-up of 30 days, 85% of patients had a TR grade of moderate or less, and 88% of patients were NYHA class I or II.

The six-month results of the CLASP TR (Edwards PASCAL Transcatheter Valve Repair System Pivotal Clinical Trial) early feasibility study, aiming to determine the safety and effectiveness of the Edwards PASCAL Transcatheter Valve Repair System in patients with severe, symptomatic functional or degenerative TR, despite medical therapy, was recently published. A total of 63 patients were enrolled. Massive or torrential TR was present in 69% of patients, and 70% had NYHA functional class III/IV. Successful implantation was reported in all treated subjects, and 98% experienced at least one grade of TR reduction. At six months, a TR grade reduction of ≥ 1 and ≥ 2 was seen in 89 and 70% of patients, respectively, with sustained improvement in NYHA class, six-minute walking test, and Kansas City Cardiomyopathy Questionnaire (KCCQ) score. The cardiovascular mortality rate (3.2%) and stroke rate (3.2%) at six months were unrelated to the study device or procedure. Five cases (7.9%) of severe bleeding were reported, and one patient required surgical explant of the study device. The randomized CLASP II TR pivotal trial is underway.

Annular-Reshaping Therapies

Annular-reshaping devices treat TR by directly or indirectly reshaping the TA without altering the valve leaflets. Direct transcatheter annuloplasty devices are designed to directly engage the TV annulus with sutures or rings. After securing the implant, tension is delivered to cinch the annulus. Alternatively, indirect annuloplasty devices are installed and secured in adjacent structures to the valve orifice, and subsequent tension exerted on the implant induces tissue approximation to achieve indirect annular contraction. A major advantage of annular-reshaping therapies is that they are "leaflet independent," thus allowing for operators to perform an additional edge-to-edge repair in the future if needed. Annular-reshaping devices have been shown to be efficacious in decreasing TR and improving functional status in the majority of patients with severe TR; however, the utility of these devices in the setting of extreme annular dilation is limited. The three annular-reshaping devices that have been implanted in humans are the Cardioband (Edwards Lifesciences), and TriCinch (4Tech), and Trialign (Mitralign). However, the Trialign and TriCinch are no longer available.

Direct Ring Annuloplasty Therapies

Cardioband. The Cardioband system for TV repair was the first CE mark approved transcatheter therapy for TR. It consists of a sutureless polyester sleeved contraction band that is fixed directly on the annulus using a series of helical anchors along the anterior, lateral, and posterior segments of the TA. A size-adjustment tool facilitates device contraction with a resultant reduction in annular septo-lateral diameter and improved leaflet coaptation. This is performed under real-time three-dimensional TEE and fluoroscopic guidance to evaluate the immediate effect of cinching on TR severity. Meticulous procedure planning is key to mitigating RCA injury during device anchoring and subsequent contraction.

Initial data reporting short-term outcomes following repair with the Cardioband system demonstrated high rates of procedural success and TR improvement. In a prospective multicenter study of 22 patients with severe TR at baseline, repair with the Cardioband system yielded a 96% technical success rate and no mortality at 30-day follow-up. In this cohort, patients had a 38% reduction in their EROA at 30 days. Additionally, the number of NYHA class I or II patients increased from 27% at baseline to 71% at 30-days post-procedure. Recently, results for the prospective TRI-REPAIR (TrIcuspid Regurgitation RePAIr with CaRdioband Transcatheter System) study were published, further highlighting the technical feasibility and long-term durability of TV repair with the Cardioband system. In the TRI-REPAIR study, 30 patients with at least moderate TR and unacceptably high surgical risk underwent TR repair with the Cardioband. Technical success was achieved in 100% of cases. At two-year follow-up, 82% of patients were NYHA class I or II compared to 17% at baseline, and 72% had a TR grade of moderate or less. Significant improvements in the six-minute walk distance and KCCQ score were also seen at follow-up.

The European, multicenter, post-market clinical follow-up study, TriBAND (Transcatheter Repair of Tricuspid Regurgitation With Edwards Cardioband TR System Post Market Study), is currently recruiting patients with severe TR treated with the Cardioband. Preliminary 30-day data show favorable results with device implantation success rate of 97%, mean reduction of septo-lateral diameter of 20%, TR reduction of at least one grade in 85% of patients, and all-cause mortality of 1.6%. A significant improvement in RV remodeling parameters was also documented.

Millipede IRIS. The Millipede IRIS device (Boston Scientific) is a complete Nitinol ring that is attached to the atrial aspect of the TA with helical anchors localized at the base of the implant. It functions as a direct annuloplasty device. The upper portion of the device has eight sliding collars, which, when advanced, shorten the distance between two adjacent anchoring elements. Each ring segment (consisting of one sliding collar and two anchors) can be adjusted independently, allowing selective remodeling of the most dilated portions of the annulus. The ring is completely retrievable for optimal repositioning prior to final deployment.

The Millipede IRIS has been implanted during open heart surgery as a proof-of-concept in two patients during a combined procedure to treat both TR and MR. After placement and anchoring, the collars were advanced to reduce the size of the device and attached annulus until leaflet coaptation was achieved and there was no TR by surgical "bulb" testing.

Significant reduction in TR to trace was noted, with an average TA septo-lateral diameter reduction of 36% that was stable at 6- and 12-month follow-up. A dedicated delivery catheter for transcatheter deployment to the TA is under development.

Other transcatheter tricuspid annuloplasty systems. Currently, several transcatheter devices that aim to replicate complete or incomplete surgical tricuspid annuloplasty are in the pre-clinical or clinical investigational phase of development (Table 45.1).

Indirect Ring Annuloplasty Therapies

TRAIPTA The TRAnsatrial IntraPericardial Tricuspid Annuloplasty (TRAIPTA; National Institutes of Health and Cook Medical) is an indirect annuloplasty system delivered through the pericardial space and across the atrioventricular groove. The system is introduced in the pericardium through the right atrial appendage to externally reduce the anterolateral portion of the TA. The system has been tested successfully in 16 Yorkshire swine. Implantation resulted in a reduction of annular dimensions, annular perimeter, and TV area. In four animal models with baseline TR, TRAIPTA achieved a significant and stable reduction of insufficiency. First-in-human implantation is pending.

Direct Suture Annuloplasty Therapies

Trialign. The Trialign percutaneous TV annuloplasty system is a transcatheter incomplete direct annuloplasty system designed to mimic the Kay surgical procedure. Using a transjugular approach, two pledgets are placed at the anteroposterior and postero-septal commissures, followed by cinching using a plication lock device to eliminate the posterior leaflet to bicuspidize the valve. The performance of the device has been tested in the SCOUT I (Symptomatic Chronic Functional Tricuspid Regurgitation) and SCOUT II trials. Device development has since been interrupted due to financial reasons.

TriCinch. The TriCinch Coil System is an indirect annuloplasty device in its second generation. Unlike the first-generation device, which was anchored directly to the hinge point of the lateral TA using a corkscrew-shaped anchor, the second-generation device is secured in the pericardial space using a Nitinol coil with a hemostasis seal anchor. This anchor is connected to a Nitinol stent placed in the inferior vein cava through a tensioning band that pulls the lateral annulus toward the septum. These modifications to the second-generation device were designed to overcome the main limitation of the previous TriCinch system, i.e. dehiscence and loss of efficacy.

In the PREVENT (Percutaneous Treatment of TV Regurgitation with the TriCinch System) trial, implantation of the first-generation TriCinch was successful in 18 cases, and a reduction of TR by at least one grade occurred in 94% of the cases. Two patients had hemopericardium after the procedure, and late detachment of the corkscrew-shaped anchor was observed in four patients.

After two successful procedures in the United States and many in Europe, the TriCinch coil system was under investigation in the Early Feasibility Study of the Percutaneous 4Tech TriCinch Coil Tricuspid Valve Repair System. However, device development has since been interrupted for financial reasons.

DaVingi. The DaVingi TR system (Cardiac Implants) is a transcatheter tricuspid annuloplasty system consisting of a fabric-coated ring, a set of anchoring elements, and an adjustment cord. The device is implanted in a two-step procedure. First the device is delivered through a 22 Fr catheter from the jugular vein and anchored on the atrial aspect of the TA. The presence of a prosthesis ring stimulates the healing process with new tissue growth around the implant. In the second step, performed approximately three months later, the encapsulated ring is cinched by the adjustment cord and fixed to the jugular vein to reduce the annular size. The multicenter first in-human study of the DaVingi TR system for functional TR is currently recruiting patients.

MIA-T. The MIA-T system (Micro Interventional Devices) consists of a series of low-mass, polymeric, self-tensioning PolyCor anchors and a thermoplastic elastomer, MyoLast, for tensioning of the anchors, including annular plication. A dedicated 12 Fr delivery catheter is used for anchor deployment. Once delivered, the anchors are linked using a connection band, which is then tightened to bicuspidize the valve by obliterating the posterior leaflet. A total of 31 patients have supposedly been enrolled thus far in the percutaneous arm of the STTAR (Study of Transcatheter Tricuspid Annular Repair) trial. The company has reported significant reductions in annular dimensions and TR with MIA-T system and durable results at one-year follow-up. However, there are no published data on these patients. Based on these data, the company has recently submitted the required technical documentation for CE mark approval.

Heterotopic Caval Valve Implantation (CAVI)

A transcatheter heterotopic ("hetero-" meaning "other" and "topos" meaning "place") caval valve implantation (CAVI) consists of implanting, via femoral venous access, bioprosthetic valves in the inferior vena cava (IVC) or, less commonly, in the superior vena cava (SVC; biCAVI), thereby reducing regurgitant blood flow into the central venous system and thus secondary organ congestion. The main conceptual advantage of this strategy is the complete independence of the underlying mechanism of TR and the TV remodeling pattern. On the other hand, CAVI does not treat TR and only addresses the repercussions of blood regurgitation on the venous system to reduce organ blood stasis.

The bioprosthetic valves used in CAVI are balloon-expandable valves (BEVs; Edwards SAPIEN XT and SAPIEN 3) and the self-expandable TricValve (P&F).

In BEV CAVI, the complex anatomy of the IVC-RA junction (large diameter and high compliance of the IVC and proximity of the hepatic veins) precludes direct implantation of a BEV and requires the preparation of a landing zone by implanting a self-expandable stent to facilitate BEV fixation. Thus, a self-expandable stent is first deployed in the IVC at the level of the diaphragm with a slight protrusion in the RA. Then a 29 mm BEV is deployed inside the stent, proximal to the hepatic vein-IVC confluence. A guidewire is used to mark the proximal hepatic vein trajectory and thus avoid it during valve implantation. The same procedural sequence can be repeated in the SVC (biCAVI) in selected cases.

The TricValve is a set of two separate self-expandable valves designed to be implanted in the IVC and SVC. The IVC implant is tapered, while the SVC implant has a central bulbar configuration for anchoring.

The safety and efficacy of CAVI with either a BEV (SAPIEN XT/3; n = 18) or TricValve (n = 6) were evaluated in the setting of compassionate use in patients with massive functional TR. All patients had debilitating heart failure symptoms despite medical therapy. Patients with severe RV dysfunction or systolic pulmonary artery pressure >60 mmhg were excluded. Most patients were treated with CAVI (IVC only; 76%) and only a minority with biCAVI and were followed for up to 12 months. Procedural success was achieved in the vast majority of cases. Two events (8%) of device migration (one from the IVC and the second from the SVC) were reported and required open heart surgery for device removal. No intra-procedural deaths occurred. In-hospital mortality was 24%, mainly due to multiorgan failure and septic complications. All patients experienced a reduction in IVC backflow, and 84% of patients discharged from the hospital had symptomatic improvement in heart failure symptoms.

Bibliography

1 Asmarats, L., Puri, R., Latib, A. et al. (2018). Transcatheter tricuspid valve interventions: landscape, challenges, and future directions. *J. Am. Coll. Cardiol.* 71 (25): 2935–2956. https://doi.org/10.1016/j.jacc.2018.04.031.

2 Belluschi, I., Del Forno, B., Lapenna, E. et al. (2018). Surgical techniques for tricuspid valve disease. *Front. Cardiovasc. Med.* 5: 118. https://doi.org/10.3389/fcvm.2018.00118.

3 Besler, C., Orban, M., Rommel, K.P. et al. (2018). Predictors of procedural and clinical outcomes in patients with symptomatic tricuspid regurgitation undergoing transcatheter edge-to-edge repair. *JACC Cardiovasc. Interv.* 11 (12): 1119–1128. https://doi.org/10.1016/j.jcin.2018.05.002.

4 Curio, J., Demir, O.M., Pagnesi, M. et al. (2019). Update on the current landscape of transcatheter options for tricuspid regurgitation treatment. *Interv. Cardiol.* 14 (2): 54–61. https://doi.org/10.15420/icr.2019.5.1.

5 Dahou, A., Levin, D., Reisman, M., and Hahn, R.T. (2019). Anatomy and physiology of the tricuspid valve. *JACC Cardiovasc. Imaging* 12 (3): 458–468. https://doi.org/10.1016/j.jcmg.2018.07.032.

6 Davidson, C.J., Lim, D.S., Smith, R.L. et al. (2021). Early feasibility study of cardioband tricuspid system for functional tricuspid regurgitation: 30-day outcomes. *JACC Cardiovasc. Interv.* 14 (1): 41–50. https://doi.org/10.1016/j.jcin.2020.10.017.

7 Dreyfus, G.D., Martin, R.P., Chan, K.M. et al. (2015). Functional tricuspid regurgitation: a need to revise our understanding. *J. Am. Coll. Cardiol.* 65 (21): 2331–2336. https://doi.org/10.1016/j.jacc.2015.04.011.

8 Dreyfus, J., Ghalem, N., Garbarz, E. et al. (2018). Timing of referral of patients with severe isolated tricuspid valve regurgitation to surgeons (from a French Nationwide Database). *Am. J. Cardiol.* 122 (2): 323–326. https://doi.org/10.1016/j.amjcard.2018.04.003.

9 Fam, N.P., Braun, D., von Bardeleben, R.S. et al. (2019). Compassionate use of the PASCAL transcatheter valve repair system for severe tricuspid regurgitation: a multicenter, observational, first-in-human experience. *JACC Cardiovasc. Interv.* 12 (24): 2488–2495. https://doi.org/10.1016/j.jcin.2019.09.046.

10 Fender, E.A., Zack, C.J., and Nishimura, R.A. (2018). Isolated tricuspid regurgitation: outcomes and therapeutic interventions. *Heart* 104 (10): 798–806. https://doi.org/10.1136/heartjnl-2017-311586.

11 Hahn, R.T., Meduri, C.U., Davidson, C.J. et al. (2017). Early feasibility study of a transcatheter tricuspid valve annuloplasty: SCOUT trial 30-day results. *J. Am. Coll. Cardiol.* 69 (14): 1795–1806. https://doi.org/10.1016/j.jacc.2017.01.054.

12 Hausleiter, J., Braun, D., Orban, M. et al. (2018). Patient selection, echocardiographic screening and treatment strategies for interventional tricuspid repair using the edge-to-edge repair technique. *EuroIntervention* 14 (6): 645–653. https://doi.org/10.4244/EIJ-D-17-01136.

13 Hołda, M.K., Zhingre Sanchez, J.D., Bateman, M.G., and Iaizzo, P.A. (2019). Right atrioventricular valve leaflet morphology redefined: implications for transcatheter repair procedures. *JACC Cardiovasc. Interv.* 12 (2): 169–178. https://doi.org/10.1016/j.jcin.2018.09.029.

14 Lauten, A., Figulla, H.R., Unbehaun, A. et al. (2018). Interventional treatment of severe tricuspid regurgitation: early clinical experience in a multicenter, observational, first-in-man study. *Circ. Cardiovasc. Interv.* 11 (2): e006061. https://doi.org/10.1161/CIRCINTERVENTIONS.117.006061.

15 Mehr, M., Taramasso, M., Besler, C. et al. (2019). 1-year outcomes after edge-to-edge valve repair for symptomatic tricuspid regurgitation: results from the TriValve registry. *JACC Cardiovasc. Interv.* 12 (15): 1451–1461. https://doi.org/10.1016/j.jcin.2019.04.019.

16 Nath, J., Foster, E., and Heidenreich, P.A. (2004). Impact of tricuspid regurgitation on long-term survival. *J. Am. Coll. Cardiol.* 43 (3): 405–409. https://doi.org/10.1016/j.jacc.2003.09.036.

17 Nickenig, G., Friedrichs, K.P., Baldus, S. et al. (2021). Thirty-day outcomes of the Cardioband tricuspid system for patients with symptomatic functional tricuspid regurgitation: the TriBAND study. *EuroIntervention* https://doi.org/10.4244/EIJ-D-21-00300.

18 Nickenig, G., Kowalski, M., Hausleiter, J. et al. (2017). Transcatheter treatment of severe tricuspid regurgitation with the edge-to-edge MitraClip technique. *Circulation* 135 (19): 1802–1814. https://doi.org/10.1161/CIRCULATIONAHA.116.024848.

19 Nickenig, G., Weber, M., Lurz, P. et al. (2019). Transcatheter edge-to-edge repair for reduction of tricuspid regurgitation: 6-month outcomes of the TRILUMINATE single-arm study. *Lancet* 394 (10213): 2002–2011. https://doi.org/10.1016/S0140-6736(19)32600-5.

20 Nickenig, G., Weber, M., Schüler, R. et al. (2020). Two-year outcomes with the cardioband tricuspid system from the multicentre, prospective TRI-REPAIR study. *EuroIntervention* https://doi.org/10.4244/EIJ-D-20-01107.

21 Otto, C.M., Nishimura, R.A., Bonow, R.O. et al. (2021). 2020 ACC/AHA Guideline for the Management of Patients with Valvular Heart Disease: a report of the American College of Cardiology/American Heart Association Joint Committee on Clinical Practice Guidelines. *Circulation* 143 (5): e72–e227. https://doi.org/10.1161/CIR.0000000000000923.

22 Rodés-Cabau, J., Taramasso, M., and O'Gara, P.T. (2016). Diagnosis and treatment of tricuspid valve disease: current and future perspectives. *Lancet* 388 (10058): 2431–2442. https://doi.org/10.1016/S0140-6736(16)00740-6.

23 Rogers, J.H., Boyd, W.D., and Bolling, S.F. (2019). Tricuspid annuloplasty with the millipede ring. *Prog. Cardiovasc. Dis.* 62 (6): 486–487. https://doi.org/10.1016/j.pcad.2019.11.008.

24 Rogers, T., Ratnayaka, K., Sonmez, M. et al. (2015). Transatrial intrapericardial tricuspid annuloplasty. *JACC Cardiovasc. Interv.* 8 (3): 483–491. https://doi.org/10.1016/j.jcin.2014.10.013.

25 Sadeghpour, A., Hassanzadeh, M., Kyavar, M. et al. (2013). Impact of severe tricuspid regurgitation on long term survival. *Res. Cardiovasc. Med.* 2 (3): 121–126. https://doi.org/10.5812/cardiovascmed.10686.

26 Santaló-Corcoy, M., Asmarats, L., Li, C.H., and Arzamendi, D. (2020). Catheter-based treatment of tricuspid regurgitation: state of the art. *Ann. Transl. Med.* 8 (15): 964. https://doi.org/10.21037/atm.2020.03.219.

27 Sanz, J., Sánchez-Quintana, D., Bossone, E. et al. (2019). Anatomy, function, and dysfunction of the right ventricle: JACC state-of-the-art review. *J. Am. Coll. Cardiol.* 73 (12): 1463–1482. https://doi.org/10.1016/j.jacc.2018.12.076.

28 Taramasso, M., Benfari, G., van der Bijl, P. et al. (2019). Transcatheter versus medical treatment of patients with symptomatic severe tricuspid regurgitation. *J. Am. Coll. Cardiol.* 74 (24): 2998, 10.1016/j.jacc.2019.09.028–3008.

29 Topilsky, Y., Khanna, A.D., Oh, J.K. et al. (2011). Preoperative factors associated with adverse outcome after tricuspid valve replacement. *Circulation* 123 (18): 1929–1939. https://doi.org/10.1161/CIRCULATIONAHA.110.991018.

30 Zack, C.J., Fender, E.A., Chandrashekar, P. et al. (2017). National trends and outcomes in isolated tricuspid valve surgery. *J. Am. Coll. Cardiol.* 70 (24): 2953–2960. https://doi.org/10.1016/j.jacc.2017.10.039.

46

Progress in Transcatheter Tricuspid Valve Repair and Replacement

Ankit Agrawal, Vinayak Nagaraja, Toshiaki Isogai and Samir R. Kapadia

Department of Cardiovascular Medicine, Heart Vascular and Thoracic Institute, Cleveland Clinic, Cleveland, OH, USA

1. Describe the anatomy of the tricuspid valve.

The tricuspid valve (TV) is the largest of the four cardiac valves. The apparatus is a complex structure made of three leaflets (anterior, posterior, and septal). These leaflets are inserted into the tricuspid annulus (TA) and attached to the papillary muscle of the right ventricle (RV) via chordae tendinae. The anterior leaflet is the largest and the longest in the radial direction with the greatest motion. The posterior leaflet is the shortest. The septal leaflet is the least mobile and shortest in the radial direction. Although the typical TV has three leaflets (anterior, posterior, and septal), there is a huge variation in the number and size of leaflets, as has been recognized in patients referred for percutaneous tricuspid therapies. The TV can be bicuspid or quadricuspid. Four leaflets are seen in 40% of the cases, and as many as seven leaflets have also been observed.

Several structures are adjacent to the apparatus. The right coronary artery (RCA) surrounds the parietal attachment of the valve. The non-coronary sinus of Valsalva is next to the commissure between the anterior and septal leaflets, and the atrioventricular node and bundle of His cross the septal leaflet attachment 3–5 mm posterior to the anteroseptal commissure. The gross and illustrated anatomy are shown in Figure 46.1.

2. What are the causes and pathophysiology of tricuspid regurgitation?

Tricuspid regurgitation (TR) is the most frequently encountered disease of the TV. Even though it is common, the TV was considered the "forgotten valve" until recently. Lack of

technology to evaluate the right-heart structure and function in the past, minimal effect of TR on prognosis, and greater mortality rate during TV surgery resulted in the notion of the neglected valve. Although mild TR is usually benign and is not considered pathological in the presence of anatomically normal valves, moderate or severe TR is reportedly associated with increased mortality rates in patients undergoing cardiac surgery or transcatheter valve interventions for aortic or mitral valves. TR is usually an incidental finding in routine echocardiography (echo). The Framingham Heart Study demonstrated that the presence of any severity of TR (trace to more than moderate) was 82% and 85.7% in men and women, respectively. The prevalence of significant TR increases with increasing age. In men and women aged >70 years, the prevalence of moderate to severe TR is estimated to be up to 1.5% and 5.6%, respectively. The prevalence of moderate and severe TR in the United States is estimated to be 1 600 000.

There are primary and secondary etiologies of TR. Secondary TR is more common and is caused mostly by TA and RV dilation. It can be classified under four different types depending upon the underlying pathology; the etiologies are summarized in Table 46.1.

Device-induced TR (caused by transvenous pacemaker or defibrillator leads) occurs very frequently. The incidence is documented to be as high as 45%, although a clear causal relationship to TR may exist in a far fewer patients. Bulky leads and apical lead placement have been associated with more TR. The potential mechanism could be related to lead-induced valve dysfunction leading to perforation, impingement, adherence to the leaflets, or lead entrapment in the subvalvular apparatus of the TV. There is neo-endocardium formation as early as 12 hours after device implantation, resulting in the development of fibrous sheaths surrounding the electrode. Consequently, multiple endocardial attachments, fibrosis, and adhesion can

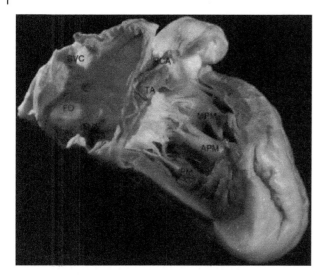

Figure 46.1 Anatomy of the TV and valvular apparatus. The anterolateral walls of the RA and RV are removed to demonstrate the TV attachment to the ventricle. The relation of the tricuspid annulus to the right coronary artery is visualized. Interatrial septal relations with the SVC, IVC, and coronary sinus are clearly visualized. IVC, inferior vena cava; RA, right atrium; RV, right ventricle; SVC, superior vena cava; TV, tricuspid valve. *Source:* Reproduced with permission from Agarwal et al. (2009) / American Heart Association, Inc.

Table 46.1 Etiologies of tricuspid regurgitation.

Primary tricuspid regurgitation	Secondary tricuspid regurgitation
• Ebstein anomaly • Tricuspid valve dysplasia, hypoplasia, or cleft • Congenital isolated right atrial enlargement with annular remodeling • Endomyocardial fibrosis • Infective endocarditis • Carcinoid disease • Serotonin active drugs • Tricuspid valve prolapse, flail • Myxomatous changes • Radiation • Chest wall trauma • Rheumatic (with left-sided disease) • Iatrogenic (from RV biopsy, pacemaker, or defibrillator leads)	• Due to left-sided valve disease or left ventricular dysfunction • Secondary to pulmonary arterial hypertension, which could be multifactorial like pulmonary thromboembolism, chronic lung diseases, left to right shunt, or systolic pulmonary artery pressure of >50 mm Hg estimated via Doppler without any other identifiable cause • Due to RV dysfunction (RV ischemia or infarction) • Idiopathic

compromise TV functions. Al-Bawardy et al. conducted a retrospective study that reflected a small but significant increase in the prevalence of moderate and severe TR both acutely and chronically after cardiac device implantation. It also revealed that pre-implantation TR was associated with early mortality and post-implantation TR with late mortality despite relatively steady right ventricular systolic pressure (RVSP). Leads can also alter the RV geometry, which can cause TR. With the increase in the pacemaker-requiring population, the prevalence of TR is also expected to grow. Höke et al. conducted a retrospective cohort study that showed significant TR (38%) after lead placement. This subgroup also had a poor long-term prognosis (hazard ratio [HR] = 1.687, p-value = 0.040) and more heart failure–related events (HR = 1.641, p-value = 0.019). Lead-induced TR was also independently associated with all-cause mortality.

Left-sided valvular involvement, ischemic or non-ischemic RV or left ventricle (LV) dilation, and cor pulmonale are the most common causes of secondary TR. Left-sided cardiac pathologies like mitral regurgitation or stenosis and left-sided congestive heart failure result in elevated left atrial filling pressure, causing pulmonary venous hypertension or heightened pulmonary vascular resistance with pulmonary arterial hypertension. Subsequently, RV dilation occurs with or without RV dysfunction and dilation of the tricuspid annulus and right atrium (RA), causing TR.

Primary RV involvement in cases of ischemia/infarction can also result in RV and TA dilation. Mid-RV dilation causes tethering of the TV leaflets with malcoaptation, which further worsens the TR.

3. What are the signs and symptoms of TR?

The signs and symptoms of TR can indicate the type and help us understand the stage of presentation. TR can remain asymptomatic for an extended period, leading to it being called the "forgotten valve." In such scenarios of advanced TR with minimal or no symptoms, precise assessment of TV and RV function becomes challenging, and the optimal timing of intervention remains unclear. The pathophysiology behind these signs and symptoms is due to pulmonary and central venous congestion. Patients with secondary TR in the early stages can have exertional dyspnea, orthopnea, and paroxysmal nocturnal dyspnea due to pulmonary venous congestion from left-sided heart disease. Primary TR and the late stages of secondary TR present with central venous congestion. Clinical features include peripheral edema, third heart sound, epigastric fullness, right upper quadrant discomfort, hepatomegaly, and ascites.

Early in the disease, TR can activate compensatory remodeling of the RV due to central venous congestion. This compensatory remodeling is short-lasting as compared to LV remodeling due to RV anatomic characteristics. Therefore, in the severe stages of TR, symptoms of low cardiac output can take over the clinical presentation, such as fatigue, poor appetite from gut edema, asthenia, and overall poor functional capacity. Severe TR can also result in elevated right atrial pressure, which in turn is channeled to the hepatic veins. It causes congestive hepatopathy and liver dysfunction and, if left untreated, can lead to cardiac cirrhosis. Central venous congestion can similarly result in poor perfusion to the kidneys, resulting in renal dysfunction.

4. What are the indications of treatment of TR in the current guidelines?

The current guidelines recommend concomitant surgical correction of TR while undergoing surgery for left-sided lesions in patients with severe TR or significant annular dilation (end-diastolic ≥ 40 mm or >21 mm/m^2 in the four-chamber transthoracic view, even in cases of mild or moderate TR. Due to the increasing burden and poor effect on the overall prognosis of progressive TR, timely optimal management is vital. The American Heart Association and American College of Cardiology (AHA/ACC) 2020 recommendations for managing TR are summarized in Table 46.2.

5. What constitutes the pre-procedural planning for tricuspid valve intervention?

To accurately plan an intervention, a multi-modality imaging approach is needed.

Echocardiography

Transthoracic echocardiography (TTE) and three-dimensional transesophageal echocardiography (3D TEE) are the cornerstone imaging modalities. They are used to scan the severity of TR and the anatomy of the TV. Simultaneous evaluation of all the TV leaflets can be difficult, and different views like long-axis RV inflow, short axis at the aortic valve, apical four-chamber view, and subcostal views are used. To overcome this difficulty, real-time 3D TTE can see all the leaflet dynamics simultaneously during the cardiac cycle in a short-axis view. Visualizing the commissures and attachment to the TA and assessing RV volumes is also possible with 3D TTE.

Table 46.2 American Heart Association and American College of Cardiology (AHA/ACC) 2020 guidelines: recommendations for management of tricuspid regurgitation.

Class of recommendation	Recommendation
Ia	Presence of severe primary or secondary TR in patients undergoing left heart surgery.
IIa	TR repair for progressive TR during left left-sided surgery with tricuspid annular dilation or prior right-heart failure.
	Symptomatic patients with primary severe TR and signs and symptoms of right-sided heart failure.
	Isolated TV surgery is also considered in patients with signs or symptoms of right-sided heart failure with severe secondary TR from annular dilation in the absence of pulmonary hypertension or left-sided heart disease.
IIb	Asymptomatic patients with severe primary TR and progressive RV dilation or systolic dysfunction.
	Re-surgery for isolated TV repair/ replacement can be considered for continued symptoms of severe TR in patients who underwent prior left-sided valvular surgery in the absence of pulmonary hypertension or considerable RV systolic dysfunction.

RV, right ventricle; TR, tricuspid regurgitation; TV, tricuspid valve.

The following echo parameters can be used to assess the severity of TR:

- *Color Doppler jet area:* A prior study reported that a jet area of >10 cm^2 is an independent predictor of survival free from TV reoperation, heart transplantation, and readmission for heart failure among patients undergoing TV repair or bioprosthetic valve replacement even after adjustment was done for pre-operative risk factors (p-value = 0.036) (Figure 46.2).

- *Vena contracta (VC):* Measuring the width of the color jet where it is the narrowest while passing through the VC is another way to assess TR severity. American Society of Echocardiography (2017) valve regurgitation guidelines recommended that a VC width of <3 mm suggests mild TR and a width of ≥ 7 mm denotes severe TR. Numerous studies have shown the adequacy of 3D color Doppler to quantify TR. Velaudhan et al. conducted one of the pioneer studies that correlated Doppler methods of quantifying TR with planimetry of the 3D VC area (VCA). A 3D VCA of 0.75 cm^2 was the most sensitive cutoff value (sensitivity 85.2% and specificity 82.1%), using a right atrial

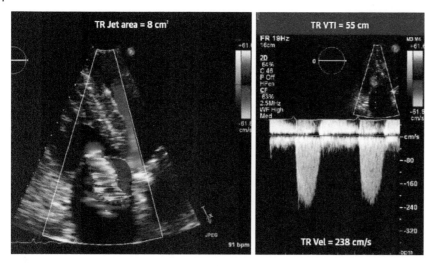

Figure 46.2 Color flow jet area in tricuspid regurgitation. *Source:* Reproduced with permission from Nagaraja et al. (2020) / Elsevier.

or regurgitant jet area of >34% and regurgitant jet area of >10 cm^2 to define severe TR. In contrast, Chen et al. showed that a 3D VCA of 0.36 cm^2 was a significant cut-off value to define severe TR (sensitivity 89% and specificity 84%). This variability can be explained by the lack of a gold standard to compare the findings with and different criteria used to define severe TR.

- *Continuous-wave velocity profile:* The shape and density of continuous-wave spectral tracing of TR provide qualitative information about the TR severity. Most TR tracing is parabolic in shape, but in cases of severe TR, dense triangular continuous-wave spectral tracing is noticed due to an early systolic rise in RA pressure (Figure 46.2). In such cases of severe wide-open TR, the peak jet velocity is low (<2.5 m/s).

- *Systolic flow reversal in hepatic veins:* Severe TR is associated with systolic flow reversal in hepatic veins identified by pulse wave spectral Doppler from a subcoastal view. The flow reversal is harmonized by the size and compliance of RA and RV functions. A small amount of TR is enough to reverse the flow in cases with small RA, high systemic pressure, or poor RV function.

- *Volumetric quantification:* This method compares the stroke volume (SV) across the regurgitant valve with the SV from a cardiac area where there is no regurgitation or shunting. For example, the diastolic SV across the regurgitant TV can be compared with the LV outflow tract stroke volume.

- *Proximal convergence analysis:* The flow convergence zone is transient or small in cases of mild TR and large throughout the systole in severe TR.

- *RV function:* Echocardiographic assessment of RV dilation and dysfunction constitutes an integral part of the pre-procedural assessment. The presence of significant secondary TR is related to larger TA, end-systolic tethering area, and RV eccentricity index on 2D echo. Global RV function can be assessed by systolic peak tissue Doppler imaging, percentage of fractional area change, 3D RV ejection fraction, 2D longitudinal strain, and tricuspid annulus plane systolic excursion. In cases of severe TR, volume overload causes greater RV dysfunction and dilation, furthering the malcoaptation of the TV leaflets. RV end-systolic area ≥20 cm^2 predicts poor event-free survival in the population undergoing TV surgery. With increasing RV dilation, there is a high degree of loss of coaptation, pseudo-normal TR gradients, and elevated central venous pressure. The grading of severity of TR via echo is summarized in Table 46.3.

Hahn et al. have proposed a new grading system for the severity of TR. The parameters of severe TR fail to include the patient population who present with late-stage disease. These end-stage patients were thus categorized under massive TR, which again fails to define the patient population with extreme disease who were treated in early feasibility trials of transcatheter devices. The SCOUT (Percutaneous Tricuspid Valve Annuloplasty System for Symptomatic Chronic Functional Tricuspid Regurgitation) trial demonstrated an average reduction in quantitative effective regurgitant orifice area (EROA) of -0.22 ± 0.29 mm^2, which is the comparable to a full grade. But the baseline and resulting quantitative EROA were 0.85 ± 0.22 and 0.63 ± 0.29 mm^2, respectively. Hence, the grade of torrential TR is introduced. This grading system is designed to better study the relationship between the evolution of severity of TR and long-term outcomes after percutaneous transcatheter TV intervention. The new classification system is summarized in Table 46.4.

Table 46.3 Severity of tricuspid regurgitation by echocardiogram.

TR severity	Mild	Moderate	Severe
Structural			
TV morphology	Normal or mildly abnormal leaflets	Moderately abnormal leaflets	Severe valve lesions (e.g. flail leaflets, severe retraction, large perforation)
RV and RA size	Usually normal	Normal or mild dilation	Usually dilated[a]
IVC diameter	Normal <2 cm	Normal or mildly dilated 2.1–2.5 cm	Dilated > 2.5 cm
Qualitative Doppler			
Color flow jet area[b]	Small, narrow, central	Moderate central	Large central jet or eccentric wall-impinging of jet variable size
Flow convergence zone	Not visible, transient, or small	Intermediate in size and duration	Large throughout systole
Continuous-wave Doppler jet	Faint/partial/parabolic	Dense, parabolic, or triangular	Dense, often triangular
Semiquantitative			
Color flow jet area $(cm^2)^b$	Not defined	Not defined	>10
Vena contracta width $(cm^2)^b$	<0.3	0.3–0.69	≥0.7
Proximal isovelocity surface area (PISA) radius $(cm)^c$	≤0.5	0.6–0.9	>0.9
Hepatic vein flow[d]	Systolic dominance	Systolic blunting	Systolic flow reversal
Tricuspid inflow[d]	A-wave dominant	Variable	E-wave > 1.0 m/s
Quantitative			
Effective regurgitant orifice area (cm^2)	<0.20	$0.2–0.39^e$	≥0.40
Regurgitant volume (mL/beat)	<30	$30–44^e$	≥45

IVC, inferior vena cava; RA, right atrium; RV, right ventricle; TV, tricuspid valve.
a)   RV and RA size can be within the "normal" range in patients with acute severe TR.
b)   With Nyquist limit > 50–70 cm/s.
c)   With baseline Nyquist limit shift of 28 cm/s.
d)   Signs are non-specific and are influenced by many other factors (RV diastolic function, atrial fibrillation, RA pressure).
e)   There are few data to support further separation of these values.
Source: Asmarats et al. (2018) / with permission of Elsevier.

Table 46.4 Proposed expansion of the "Severe" grade.

Variable	Mild	Moderate	Severe	Massive	Torrential
VC in mm (biplane)	<3	3–6.9	7–13	14–20	≥21
EROA in mm^2 (PISA)	<20	20–39	40–59	60–79	≥80
3D VCA or quantitative EROA $(mm^2)^a$			75–94	95–114	≥115

EROA, effective regurgitant orifice area; VC, vena contracta; VCA, vena contracta area.
a)   3D VCA and quantitative Doppler EROA cutoffs may be larger than PISA EROA.
Source: Hahn and Zamorano (2017) / with permission of Oxford University Press.

Multi-detector Computed Tomography

Multi-detector computed tomography (MDCT) is another imaging modality that provides fine details regarding tricuspid annulus measurements and adjacent structures, yields high-quality motion-free images of the right ventricular outflow tract, and helps identify access routes for percutaneous intervention (Figure 46.3). MDCT gives a variety of necessary information:

- MDCT provides optimal measurements of the TA (maximal anteroposterior and septolateral diameter,

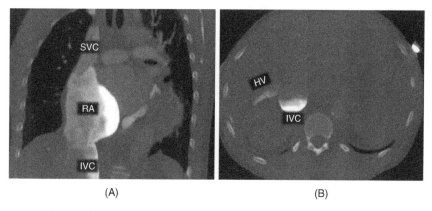

Figure 46.3 (a) Coronal projection showing intravenous contrast arriving from the SVC, passing through the RA, and being directed toward the IVC due to severe TR. (b) Axial imaging shows intravenous contrast arriving in the IVC and reaching the HV, which is a specific finding for severe TR. HV, hepatic vein; IVC, inferior vena cava; RA, right atrium; SVC, superior vena cava; TR, tricuspid regurgitation. *Source:* Reproduced with permission from Nagaraja et al. (2020) / Elsevier.

perimeter, and RV measurements). It can also help assess the maximal distance from the tricuspid annulus to the RV apex.

- MDCT becomes necessary to evaluate the target anchoring site for some replacement devices. For example, when using coaptation devices, an anchoring site can be selected by making a perpendicular line connecting the annular plane with RV septal free wall on a sagittal reconstruction. It also evaluates the safety of the landing zone of the device and confirms the optimal annular tissue and shelf for annuloplasty devices.

- MDCT is crucial for evaluating adjacent anatomic structures like the RCA course relative to the TA and the distance between the RCA and anterior and posterior tricuspid leaflet insertion. The RCA course via the right atrioventricular groove and distance from the TA varies, and MDCT helps delineate the spatial distribution to prevent RCA impingement during transcatheter TV intervention. A distance of ≤2 mm from the RCA to the TA is considered unfavorable and has been reported in 40% of patients with severe TR. MDCT also screens for anatomic structures like large papillary muscles, prominent moderate bands, or trabeculations that would prevent device navigation.

- MDCT helps assess the status of the various venous access sites (jugular, axillary, or subclavian veins). It also evaluates the size of the inferior vena cava (IVC) at the cavoatrial junction and the level of the first hepatic vein. The distance between the cavoatrial junction and the first hepatic vein can also be calculated. This is important for heterotopic caval valve implantation.

- MDCT provides coplanar fluoroscopic projections assisting coaxial device deployment.

Cardiac magnetic resonance (CMR) is another imaging modality that is the gold standard for estimating right ventricular volumes and physiology. CMR complements 3D echo for functional and anatomic evaluation of TV and TA and is an integral constituent of pre-procedural planning.

The advantages and disadvantages of all of these imaging modalities are summarized in Table 46.5.

6. What are the indications of transcatheter tricuspid valve replacement?

Isolated TV surgery carries a high mortality rate. Although surgical TV repair is performed more commonly, return of TR post-repair occurs in 42% by 5 years, and there is 14% recurrence of moderate to severe TR on one-week follow-up. In patients in whom transcatheter TV repair is indicated, the valve anatomy sometimes is not favorable due to large coaptation gaps (>6–8 mm), tethered septal leaflets, or complex anatomy including four or more leaflets. This suggests that transcatheter TV repair could be suboptimal, demanding an alternative approach to valve replacement. Transcatheter TV replacement can also be considered in patients with fibrotic leaflets (as seen in carcinoid syndrome or rheumatic valve involvement) or large leaflet prolapse. Patient populations with extremely dilated annuli or extreme leaflet tethering are considered primarily for TV replacement over repair. If residual TR is expected to be moderate or worse after the repair, replacement is also preferred in those cases. Certain conditions such as endocarditis, iatrogenic or inflammatory diseases, and Ebstein

Table 46.5 Advantages and disadvantages of each imaging modality used for the assessment of tricuspid valve function.

Modality	Advantages	Disadvantages
Echocardiography	Readily available and portable Transthoracic and transesophageal approaches Multiplane 2D and 3D real-time imaging No iodinated intravenous contrast No radiation Excellent temporal resolution and good spatial resolution Functional and hemodynamic information Automated post-processing tools (becoming more available)	3D acquisition and interpretation require more skill. Transesophageal echocardiography is semi-invasive, and sedation is typically required. Limitations of ultrasonography physics (i.e. acoustic shadowing, lateral resolution, far-field imaging, 3D volume rates, and so forth). Incomplete vascular assessment.
Cardiac magnetic resonance	Good temporal and spatial resolution Minimal effect of body habitus Gold standard for ventricular volumes, mass, and ejection fraction (no contrast required) Excellent for valvular regurgitation (no contrast) Excellent myocardial tissue characterization No radiation and non-invasive Can assess anatomy without intravenous gadolinium Vascular assessment Hemodynamic information	Spatial resolution is inferior to computed tomography angiography and echocardiography (thick slices). Lower temporal resolution than echocardiography. Requires adequate training for comprehensive examination acquisition and interpretation. Longer examination (free breathing examination is possible). Claustrophobia. Incompatible with certain intracardiac devices (e.g. intracardiac cardioverter-defibrillator, cardiac resynchronization therapy, older permanent pacemakers). Suboptimal quantification can occur with fast and irregular cardiac rhythms (unless newer pulse sequences are available). Cannot visualize calcification as well. Peak velocities may be underestimated.
Computed tomography angiography	Excellent spatial resolution (gold standard for anatomical information and structural planning) Noninvasive and fast Extensive training not required Automated post-processing tools are available with comprehensive vascular assessment.	Frequently requires iodinated intravenous contrast (elevated risk in patients with chronic kidney dysfunction). Radiation dose has improved but is high in 4D (functional) imaging. Poor temporal resolution (better with dual-source imaging). Suboptimal with fast and irregular cardiac rhythms. Not portable. Blooming artifacts can occur with calcium, valve stent frames, intracardiac leads, and others.

Source: Hahn et al. (2019) / with permission of Elsevier.

anomaly require replacement. The first-in-human percutaneous TV replacement was performed by Navia et al. using a NaviGate valved stent in a patient who presented with refractory right heart failure, severe TR secondary to annular dilation, severe RV dysfunction, and severe pulmonary hypertension.

7. What are different types, outcomes, and complications of transcatheter tricuspid valve replacement devices?

These devices can be categorized as orthotopic or heterotopic (Figures 46.4 and 46.5). Orthotopic devices include NaviGate, TRiCares, LuX (Ningbo Jenscare), Trisol, Cardiovalve (Boston Medical), Intrepid (Medtronic) and EVOQUE (Edwards Lifesciences). Heterotopic devices include SAPIEN (Edwards Lifesciences), TricValve (P&F), and Tricento (NVT).

Coaptation Devices

FORMA. The FORMA Repair System (Edwards Lifesciences) is a coaptation transcatheter device system that occupies the regurgitant orifice area, thereby increasing the native leaflet coaptation surface. It can be introduced using the left axillary or subclavian vein through a 20–24- F sheath introducer. It is positioned within the TA over a rail anchored at the RV apex septal segment. It is available in three sizes: 12, 15, and 18 mm. It is fully retrievable during any step of the procedure. A total of 18 patients were treated on compassionate grounds, and successful device implantation was seen in 16 patients with no in-hospital mortality. A complete one-year follow-up was successful in 15 patients. Among the 14 patients with successful device implantation and a one-year follow-up period, 86% had improvement in New York Heart Association (NYHA) functional class, six-minute walking distance (6-MWD), and overall quality of life (QoL). Device-related thrombosis was seen in one patient (due to sub-therapeutic international normalized ratio [INR]),

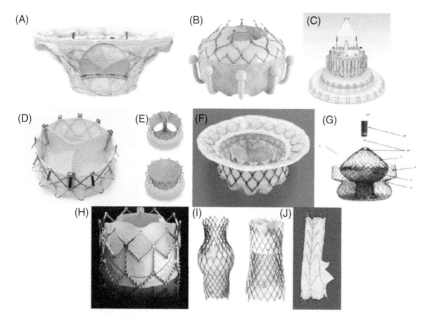

Figure 46.4 Transcatheter tricuspid valve replacement devices. *Source:* Reproduced with permission from Goldberg et al. (2021) / Frontiers Media S.A. / CC BY 4.0.

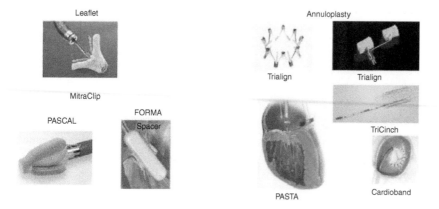

Figure 46.5 Transcatheter tricuspid valve repair devices. *Source:* Reproduced with permission from Bapat (2017) / Taylor & Francis Group.

and there was one re-hospitalization due to congestive heart failure. At the end of one year, severe TR in 96% was reduced to moderate to severe or less in 46% of cases. The 30-day outcomes of the US Early Feasibility Study reported RV perforation in two patients; nine patients had at least one 30-day adverse event, including death in two, vascular injury in one, major or life-threatening bleeding in six, device-related surgery in three, and acute kidney injury in three. On compassionate grounds, improvement in NYHA, 6-MWD, and QoL was seen at 30-day follow-up. However, the development of this device has been halted due to business decisions.

TriClip and MitraClip. The MitraClip system (Abbott Vascular) has an off-label use for treating high-risk patients with functional TR. More than 650 procedures using the MitraClip have been conducted worldwide. Nickenig et al. reported procedural success in 97% of the patients with the TriClip: 64 high-risk patients with moderate to severe TR underwent TV clipping, of which 22 patients underwent simultaneous mitral repair. No serious intra-procedural complications were seen, and three in-hospital deaths were reported. Most patients showed significant improvement in NYHA class and exercise capacity at 30-day follow-up. Orban et al. reported six-month outcomes of 50 patients treated with transcatheter edge-to-edge TV repair, of which 36 patients underwent parallel mitral valve repair. Procedural success was reported in 46 patients. At six-month follow-up, improvement in NYHA functional class and TR grade was seen in 79% and 90% of patients, respectively, with a 16% mortality rate. Recently, the international multicenter TRILUMINATE (Trial to Evaluate Treatment with Abbott Transcatheter Clip Repair System in Patients with Moderate or Greater Tricuspid Regurgitation) single-arm trial ($n = 85$) reported that TR was decreased to moderate or less at one year after TriClip therapy in 71% of cases, along with RV remodeling and improvements in NYHA functional class, 6-MWD, and Kansas City Cardiomyopathy Questionnaire (KCCQ) Score. No peri-procedural deaths, myocardial infarction (MI), or stroke were witnessed. At six-month follow-up, all-cause mortality was seen in 5% of patients, and the rate of major bleeding was 11%. Single leaflet device attachment and TV stenosis were reported in 7% and 9% of the patients, respectively. More recently, two-year outcomes of the TRILUMINATE trial were presented, which showed a sustained reduction in TR grading to moderate or less (60%), sustained improvement in NYHA class, 6-MWD, and KCCQ score, and a significant reduction in the rate of hospitalization (49%). There were no safety issues or peri-procedural mortality. The bRIGHT (An Observational Real-world Study Evaluating Severe Tricuspid Regurgitation Patients Treated with the Abbott TriClip Device) study also showed a 100% implant and procedural

success rate with a short procedural time. It enrolled 75 patients. Most patients ($n = 41$) had two clips, and most clips (78%) were implanted in the anterior-septal coaptation line. All patients had TR reduced by at least one grade, with 84% reduced to moderate or less. A pivotal trial is ongoing at this time comparing TriClip to medical management.

PASCAL. The Edwards Lifesciences PASCAL transcatheter mitral valve repair system combines the technicalities of the MitraClip and FORMA device systems by integrating a 10 mm central spacer, two paddles approximately 25 mm wide, and clasps 10 mm long. These attach the device to the valve leaflets. The device is repositionable and retrievable. The system has a 2-F steerable guide sheath, and an implantation catheter. The first successful case using the PASCAL device system to treat severe TR was reported by Fam et al.. The patient was an 82-year-old woman with advanced right-sided heart failure and secondary TR. Two devices were implanted, and on one-month follow-up, the dose of diuretics was lowered, resolution of ascites was seen, and improvement in QoL and 6-MWD was witnessed. Fam et al. also conducted a multicenter observational study that investigated the feasibility and safety of the PASCAL device system and short-term clinical outcomes in 28 patients with severe TR. Procedural success was 86% without any intra-procedural complications. At 30-day follow-up, mortality was 7.1%, and 88% of patients were in NYHA class I or II with a TR grade of ≤2+ in 85% of cases. There was improvement in 6-MWD and single leaflet device attachments treated conservatively. The CLASP TR (Edwards PASCAL Transcatheter Valve Repair System Pivotal Clinical Trial) trial using the PASCAL device for transcatheter edge-to-edge repair showed that 70% of 64 enrolled patients had NYHA class III–IV, and 69% were categorized as massive or torrential TR at baseline. At six-month follow-up, 84% were NYHA class I–II, the massive or torrential group of patients dropped to 8%, 89% improved by at least one TR grade, and 70% showed at least a two-TR-grade reduction along with significant improvement in QoL and KCCQ score. Two patients died of cardiovascular causes or developed stroke, but there was no MI. Severe bleeding was seen in 7.9% of cases. A pivotal trial is ongoing comparing medical management and PASCAL.

Suture Annuloplasty Systems

Trialign (Mitralign). This is a transcatheter annuloplasty system that simulates the modified Kay surgical procedure. A catheter is established via a transjugular approach to further an insulated radiofrequency wire across the TA. Two pledgets are anchored at the posteroseptal and anteroposterior commissures. They are cinched together using a plication lock device, resulting in posterior leaflet plication and bicuspid TV. The first multicenter study conducted by Yzeiraj et al. demonstrated a significant post-procedural reduction in TR severity with a single procedural complication of arrhythmia. Hahn et al. conducted a prospective, multicenter, single-arm, early feasibility study from November 2015 to June 2016, SCOUT I, which showed implantation success in all 15 patients with 93% procedural success (one patient required RCA stenting due to extrinsic compression) and 80% technical success (there were three events of single-pledget dehiscence without the need for re-intervention). No major adverse events occurred at 30-day follow-up, with improvement in NYHA functional class. At one-year follow-up, one patient needed elective re-intervention, and one had a non-device-related death. There was continued improvement in NYHA functional class and QoL.

TriCinch System (4Tech). This is also a Kay-like annuloplasty system that decreases the septolateral diameter of the TA. It does so by cinching the anteroposterior commissure. An 18-F delivery system is advanced using a 24-F femoral vein sheath introducer into the RA. Next, a corkscrew anchor is positioned near the anteroposterior commissure. Post-right coronary angiography, a self-expanding stent connected to the anchor via a Dacron band is situated in the subhepatic region of the IVC. Data from the TriCinch device in the PREVENT Percutaneous Treatment of Tricuspid Valve Regurgitation with the TriCinch System) trial showed that 18 of 24 patients had successful device placement with a significant acute reduction in TR severity in 94% of cases. Hemopericardium was noticed in two patients, and late annular anchor detachment was noticed in five patients. Improvement in functional status and QoL was seen at six-month follow-up. First-in-human implantation of the second-generation TriCinch device has been performed without any procedural complications. There was 30-day improvement in QoL and TR severity.

Ring Annuloplasty Systems

Cardioband. This is a direct, sutureless ring annuloplasty system. The transfemoral approach is used to introduce the device using a 24-F access sheath. Up to 17 anchors are established on the atrial side of the anteroposterior TA to position the device. A size-adjustment tool is advanced over the wire, and the band is cinched. For the Cardioband Tricuspid Repair System, 30-day outcomes among 30 patients showed procedural success in all, with a 17% average reduction in septolateral diameter. RV failure and non-device-related life-threatening bleeding were seen in two patients and led to death; one stroke and three major bleeding cases were reported. These were the outcomes of

the first-in-human TRI-REPAIR (TrIcuspid Regurgitation RePAIr with CaRdioband Transcatheter System) trial. Nickenig et al. reported the results of the TriBAND (Transcatheter Repair of Tricuspid Regurgitation with Edwards Cardioband TR System Post Market Study) study, which involved 61 patients with severe symptomatic functional TR who failed diuretic therapy. At 30-day follow-up, there was one MI and one all-cause death but no cardiovascular mortality or stroke. Severe bleeding was seen in seven patients, a new need for renal replacement therapy in two patients, major access site/vascular complications in four patients, and coronary artery injury needing reintervention in four patients. NYHA class I-II was witnessed in 74% of patients, with an overall improvement in KCCQ score.

Millipede IRIS (Boston Scientific). This is an adjustable, semi-rigid annuloplasty ring that is fully retrievable. It has been surgically implanted in two patients who underwent simultaneous mitral valve repair. No TR was reported on 12-month follow-up. This device system does not require anticoagulation and preserves the native valve anatomy.

MIA-T (Micro Interventional Devices). The minimally invasive annuloplasty (MIA) technology is a sutureless, transcatheter annuloplasty system. It has a thermoplastic elastomer and low-mass polymeric, compliant, self-tensioning anchor, which allows reduction of the TV annulus. The device is surgically implanted via a 16-F steerable dispatching system that allows the delivery of the device in a 270° partial ring pattern. The STTAR (Study of Transcatheter Tricuspid Annular Repair) trial will assess the safety and efficacy of the MIA-T device system.

PASTA. Pledget-assisted suture tricuspid annuloplasty (PASTA) is a "percutaneous surgical" technique that replicates the Hetzer double-orifice suture technique. Two sutures and one pledget are consecutively placed in the posteroseptal and midanterior TA, after which each suture is secured using a Cor-Knot device. The procedure can be conducted through the internal jugular or apical right ventricular access. It has been used in humans once so far under compassionate grounds.

DaVingi TR system (Cardiac Implants). This is a two-step annuloplasty device that commences with the delivery of a flexible, barbed ring around the TA. A chronic healing process fixes the implant and cinches the neo-annulus. It is delivered using a highly maneuverable 22-F delivery system. The first-in-human study is currently ongoing.

Transatrial Intrapericardial Tricuspid Annuloplasty (TRAIPTA). This device consists of an adjustable Nitinol loop that is inserted in the pericardial space via right atrial puncture. Later, the device is adjusted as per the TA dimensions, resulting in external compression of the TA along the AV groove. Pre-clinical data showed acute feasibility in swine, and the latest versions are under development for in-human use.

Heterotopic Devices

SAPIEN and TricValve. SAPIEN is a balloon-expandable, heterotopic 29 mm caval implantation valve system whose first off-label use was reported by Laule et al. TricValve is another self-expandable pericardial valve whose implantation can be safely conducted using a single- or dual-valve approach. It is available in 38 and 43 mm sizes for the superior vena cava (SVC) and IVC, respectively. Compassionate use of the SAPIEN valve or TricValve has been reported in 25 patients. Single IVC valve implantation was done in 19 patients. Balloon-expandable valves were used in single-valve procedures, and self-expandable valves were used in double-valve procedures. Procedural success was witnessed in 92% of the cases, and two device embolizations required surgical removal. There was 12% 30-day mortality and 63% one-year mortality because of high comorbidities. TricValve is planning a pivotal trial in the United States with the breakthrough device exemption.

Tricento. The Tricento device is composed of a 13.5 cm covered stent with the SVC and IVC as landing zones and a low intra-atrial porcine bicuspid valve segment. It also has a non-covered segment for hepatic vein outflow. Transfemoral access via a 24-F sheath is used. The first successful in-human implantation of Tricento was reported in 2017; since then, 31 Tricento valve systems have been implanted in Europe.

Orthotopic Devices

NaviGate. This was the first orthotopic device in the literature and was used for transcatheter TV replacement with transjugular access in one patient and mini-thoracotomy for transatrial access in another patient. It is composed of a self-expanding atrioventricular valved stent and a delivery system. It is available in five sizes: 36, 40, 44, 48, and 52 mm. A transjugular or transatrial approach is used to introduce the delivery catheter through a 42-F introducer sheath. In a single-site experience study on transcatheter TV replacement using the NaviGate system conducted by Hahn et al., 30-day follow-up showed improvement in NYHA functional class in all patients, RV remodeling, and improved cardiac output on echo. In another study conducted by Hahn et al., there was significant improvement in TR and improvement in symptoms, with admissible in-hospital mortality of 10%. At a median follow-up of 127 days, there

were no device-related late adverse events among live patients. NaviGate is currently planning an outside the US (OUS) trial for approval outside of the United States.

LuX. This is also a self-expanding bovine pericardial tissue valve that is mounted on a covered Nitinol stent. There are varied sizes for the annulus (50, 60, and 70 mm) and the inner valve (26 and 28 mm). A minimally invasive right thoracotomy approach is used to place the 32-F system in the RA. It has been used on compassionate grounds in China, and an early feasibility study in Canada will soon be underway.

Intrepid. This is a dual-stent system with a bovine pericardial valve (29 mm), available in three sizes: 43, 46, and 50 mm. A transfemoral approach is used via a 35-F delivery system, and a 29-F delivery system is under production. The use of Intrepid has been successful in three cases on compassionate grounds, and an early feasibility trial begin soon in the United States.

EVOQUE. This device is composed of bovine pericardial leaflets with an intra-annular sealing skirt and anchors. It is available in two sizes: 44 and 48 mm. A transfemoral access is used to introduce the 28 F delivery system. The first transfemoral TV replacement was performed using the EVOQUE system. Fam et al. reported data on 25 compassionate cases that showed a significant success rate of 92% with no procedural deaths and excellent safety profile; 8% of patients needed a permanent pacemaker. The conduct of this valve was studied during the TRISCEND (Edwards EVOQUE Tricuspid Valve Replacement) trial. It enrolled 56 patients, 84% of whom were NYHA class III–IV; 92% had at least severe TR, 68% had functional etiology, 11% had degenerative TR, and the rest had mixed etiologies. The baseline TR grade was reported to be 46% severe, 29% massive, and 15% torrential. At 30-day follow-up, 98% had mild or no/trace TR. All patients showed a reduction of at least one TR grade, 95% had a decrease of ≥2 grades, three-quarters were NYHA class I-II, and there was significant improvement in 6-MWD and KCCQ score.

Trisol. The Trisol valve system comprises a single bovine pericardial dome-shaped leaflet and a self-expandable conical Nitinol stent. Access is obtained through a 30-F transjugular delivery system. The valve is retrievable and repositionable.

Cardiovalve. The Cardiovalve comprises bovine pericardial leaflets mounted on a Nitinol frame. It is available in three sizes: 45, 50, and 55 mm. A 60 mm valve is under production. Transfemoral access is obtained with a 28-F delivery system.

TRiCares. This is also a bovine pericardial self-expandable valve arranged on a Nitinol frame. It is extremely early in its development.

Complications

Transcatheter TV intervention has complications that should be kept in mind. Improper anchoring of the valve can lead to post-procedural device malfunction and paravalvular leakage. Pressure on the bundle of His from the transcatheter valve can lead to conduction disturbance. Lower blood velocity on the right side of the heart imposes a risk of valve thrombosis. Lifelong anticoagulation is recommended after the procedure, but if there is no concomitant indication for long-term anticoagulation, switching to dual antiplatelet therapy six months post-procedure has been suggested. There is also a risk of post-procedural RV failure, for which patients should be monitored.

Future Development of Devices

An early feasibility study of the Cardiovalve system is underway in the US. The primary endpoints of the trial are intra-procedural technical success and significant device-related adverse events at 30-day follow-up.

The TRICAVAL (Treatment of Severe Secondary TRIcuspid Regurgitation in Patients With Advance Heart Failure With CAval Vein Implantation of the Edwards Sapien XT VALve) study for the SAPIEN XT valve was prematurely stopped due to high rates of valve dislodgements, and the HOVER (Heterotopic Implantation Of the Edwards-Sapien Transcatheter Aortic Valve in the Inferior VEna Cava for the Treatment of Severe Tricuspid Regurgitation) trial is underway to evaluate the safety and efficacy of the SAPIEN following IVC implantation.

Although the first successful in-human TricValve was reported, the early feasibility studies TRICUS (NCT03723239; Safety and Efficacy of the TricValve Device) and TRICUS Euro (NCT04141137) are ongoing in the United States and Europe, respectively. Some preliminary data from TRICUS have been reported. Of nine patients, technical and procedural success was seen in eight. There was zero in-hospital mortality, with one device embolization/migration event and one conversion to surgery. There was significant improvement in NYHA class, 6-MWD, and KCCQ score at six-month follow-up.

The TriCinch system is currently being studied in clinical trials (NCT03294200 and NCT03632967). The SCOUT II trial (NCT03225612) is studying patients with functional TR secondary to annular dilation for the Trialign system. The CLASP II TR pivotal trial is underway in the United States for PASCAL device systems. The first in-human data on Trisol, TRiCares, and Intrepid are awaited. Ongoing and future studies on transcatheter TV intervention are summarized in Table 46.6.

8. What are the limitations of transcatheter tricuspid valve replacement?

The devices utilized in replacement are new, and tricuspid anatomy presents challenges:

- The normally 3D saddle-shaped TA loses its shape and dilates because the RA and RV are stretched in the setting of TR. Therefore, TA in patients undergoing valve replacement may require large transcatheter valves with potentially large-bore venous access. More importantly, these large devices may impair the function of the RV, which may require some annular mobility. Acute right-heart failure with large devices has been reported.
- 3D curves of the annulus, a not-well-defined annulus, and variable subvalvular anatomy make anchoring the transcatheter valve challenging.
- The interaction of the valve with the conduction system is still undisclosed. It is also unknown whether the procedure will lead to indefinite conduction irregularities. Patients with devices pose a different challenge with regard to device interaction or reliability of pacing after valve placement.
- Data regarding optimal patient selection, appropriate device type, and timing of intervention are limited.
- Several risk scores have been validated to predict short-term mortality and morbidity post-cardiac surgeries. The European System for Cardiac Operative Risk Evaluation II Score and the Society of Thoracic Surgeons score are the most used and accepted for mitral and aortic valve interventions. Although these scores can be used for TV intervention, that use has not yet been validated.
- No long-term durability data exists for transcatheter TV interventions.

Table 46.6 Summary of ongoing and future studies on transcatheter therapies for tricuspid regurgitation.

Device	Study	Study design	Patients	Select inclusion criteria	Select exclusion criteria	Primary endpoint
FORMA	SPACER (NCT02787408)	Prospective registry	78	**Clinical:** • 18 yr of age or more • Functional TR as primary etiology • Clinically significant symptomatic TR • NYHA class II or more or signs of persistent right-heart failure despite optimal medical therapy	**Clinical:** • Moderate or more tricuspid stenosis • Clinically significant CAD requiring immediate revascularization • MI within 30 d of procedure • Stroke within 3 mo of procedure • Life expectancy <12 mo **Echocardiographic:** • PASP > 70 mm Hg • LVEF <25% within 90 d of procedure	Safety: cardiac mortality at 30 d, compared with a research-derived performance goal based on high-risk surgical outcomes for tricuspid repair/replacement
	Early Feasibility Study of the Edwards Forma Tricuspid Transcatheter Repair System (NCT02471807)	Prospective registry	30	**Clinical:** • 18 yr or older • Clinically significant, symptomatic, and functional TR	**Clinical and imaging:** • Moderate or more tricuspid stenosis • Severe RV dysfunction • Tricuspid valve anatomy not suitable for intervention	Procedural success defined as device success and freedom from device- or procedure-related SAEs at 30 d
MitraClip	TRILUMINATE (NCT03227757)	Prospective registry	75	**Clinical:** • Increased risk for cardiac surgery • Moderate TR with NYHA class III-IV • Severe TR with NYHA class II, III, IV • No indication of other valve therapy **Echocardiographic:** • Moderate or more (≥2+) TR • Moderate TR with TV annulus ≥40 mm	**Clinical:** • Prior TV procedure • Life expectancy <12 mo **Echocardiographic:** • Tricuspid stenosis • Pacemaker leads that would hinder clipping • LVEF <20% • Significant MR • PASP > 60 mm Hg	Echocardiographic tricuspid regurgitation reduction at least 1 grade (30 d) Composite of MAE (6 mo)
	MitraClip for Severe TR (NCT02863549)	Prospective registry	100	**Clinical:** • Moderate to severe TR • Patients not suitable for surgery	**Echocardiographic:** • Poor quality of echo images	Tricuspid regurgitation grade and incidence of major adverse cerebrovascular events (1–12 mo)

(Continued)

Table 46.6 (Continued)

Device	Study	Study design	Patients	Select inclusion criteria	Select exclusion criteria	Primary endpoint
	SCOUT II (NCT03225612)	Prospective registry	60	**Clinical:** • NYHA II, III, or ambulatory IV • High-risk cardiac surgery • LVEF ≥35% • Symptomatic moderate or more TR **Echocardiographic:** TV annulus ≤55mm (or 29mm/m²)	**Clinical:** • Severe CAD • Previous procedure of TV • MI or any PCI <30d • Life expectancy <12mo	All-cause mortality at 30d
Trialign	Early feasibility of the Mitralign PTVAS, also known as Trialign (NCT02574650)	Prospective registry	30	**Clinical:** • NYHA II, III, or ambulatory IV • High-risk cardiac surgery • LVEF ≥35% • Symptomatic moderate or more TR **Echocardiographic:** TV annulus ≤55mm (or 29mm/m²)	**Clinical:** • Severe CAD • Previous TV procedure • MI or any PCI <30d • Life expectancy <12mo	Technical success at 30d, defined as freedom from death with successful access, delivery, and retrieval of the device delivery system, and deployment and correct positioning of the intended device, and no need for additional unplanned or emergency surgery or reintervention related to the device or access procedure
	PREVENT (NCT02098200)	Prospective registry	24	**Clinical:** • Moderate or more functional TR **Echocardiographic:** TV annulus ≥ 40mm	**Clinical:** • Cardiac procedure planned up to 3 mo before or after TV repair • Life expectancy <12mo • TV or MV endocarditis within 1yr	Safety: participants with MAE[a] within 30d of the procedure Efficacy: reduction of tricuspid regurgitation by at least one degree immediately after the procedure and at discharge
TriCinch	Clinical Trial Evaluation of the Percutaneous 4Tech TriCinch Coil Tricuspid Valve Repair System (NCT03294200)	Prospective registry	90	**Clinical:** • NYHA class ≥II • Symptomatic moderate or more TR **Echocardiographic:** • LVEF ≥30% • TV annulus ≥ 40mm	**Clinical:** • Stroke within 6 mo • Severe renal impairment or on dialysis • Recent percutaneous, cardiac, or surgical intervention • TV tethering >10mm • Previous TV procedure • CIED leads across the TV **Echocardiographic:** • Systolic PAP >60mmHg • Moderate aortic, mitral, and/or pulmonic valve stenosis and/or regurgitation Moderate or severe TS	All-cause mortality of the per protocol cohort at 30d post-procedure

(Continued)

Device	Study	Study design	Patients	Select inclusion criteria	Select exclusion criteria	Primary endpoint
MIA	STTAR (not registered)	Prospective registry	40	**Clinical:** • Symptomatic functional TR • NYHA class II, III, IVa **Echocardiographic:** • LVEF ≥30% • TV annulus ≥40 mm and ≤55 mm (or 29 mm/m²)	**Clinical:** • Prior TV procedure • Life expectancy <12 mo **Echocardiographic:** • Severe RV dysfunction • Pulmonary hypertension with PAP mean 2/3rd MAP	Safety: rate of MAEs at 30 d follow-up Performance: technical success rate of MIA implant and reduction in the valve area
	TRI-REPAIR (NCT02981953)	Prospective registry	30	**Clinical:** • Symptomatic functional TR • NYHA class II, III, IVa **Echocardiographic:** • TV annulus ≥40 mm • Systolic PAP ≤60 mm Hg • LVEF ≥ 30	**Clinical:** • Previous TV procedure • Cardiac cachexia • Recent MI/PCI or severe untreated CAD • CIED/permanent pacemaker leads across TV • Moderate aortic, mitral, and/or pulmonic valve stenosis and/or regurgitation **Echocardiographic:** • Severe RV dysfunction	Overall rate of major SAEs and serious adverse device effects at 30 d Intra-procedural successful access, deployment, and positioning of the Cardioband device and septolateral diameter reduction
Cardioband			15			Change in septolateral dimension at 30 d
	Edwards Cardioband Tricuspid Valve Reconstruction System Early Feasibility Study (NCT03382457)	Prospective registry		**Clinical:** Symptomatic functional TR	**Clinical:** • Previous TV procedure • Primary TV disease	Freedom from device or procedure-related adverse events (30 d)

(Continued)

Table 46.6 (Continued)

Device	Study	Study design	Patients	Select inclusion criteria	Select exclusion criteria	Primary endpoint
	HOVER (NCT02339974)	Prospective registry	15	**Clinical:** • 21 yr or older • Severe, symptomatic TR	**Clinical:** • MI within 30 d of procedure • Upper GI bleed within 30 mo of procedure • Stroke or TIA within 6 mo of procedure **Echocardiographic:** • Mean PAP ≥ 40 mm Hg • LVEF <40% • Echo evidence of intracardiac mass, vegetation, or thrombus	Procedural success at 30 d, defined as device success and no SAE[b] Individual success at 30 d, defined by device success and positive clinical outcomes[c]
Heterotopic CAVI	TRICAVAL (NCT02387697)	Randomized open label	40	**Clinical:** • Optimal medical therapy • NYHA class II at least • High risk for cardiac surgery • Severe symptomatic TR with significant regurgitation to the hepatic and caval veins	**Clinical:** • Stroke or TIA within 180 d of the procedure • Acute MI within 1 mo of the procedure • Life expectancy <12 mo **Echocardiographic:** • LVEF <30% • Severe mitral insufficiency • Echo evidence of intracardiac mass, thrombus, or vegetation	Maximum relative VO₂ at 3 mo (difference of means in maximum relative VO₂ at 3 mo compared with control group)

CAD, coronary artery disease; CIED, Cardiovascular implantable electronic device; GI, Gastrointestinal; HOVER, Heterotopic Implantation of the Edwards-SAPIEN Transcatheter Aortic Valve in the IVC for the Treatment of Severe Tricuspid Regurgitation; KCCQ, Kansas City Cardiomyopathy Questionnaire; LVEF, left ventricular ejection fraction; MAE, major adverse event; MAP, Mean arterial pressure; MI, myocardial infarction; MIA, minimally invasive annuloplasty; NYHA, New York Heart Association; PAP, pulmonary artery pressure; PASP, pulmonary artery systolic pressure; PCI, percutaneous coronary intervention; PREVENT, Percutaneous Treatment of Tricuspid Valve Regurgitation with the TriCinch System; PTVAS, percutaneous tricuspid valve annuloplasty system; RV, right ventricle; SAE, serious adverse event; SCOUT, Safety and Performance of the Trialign Percutaneous Tricuspid Valve Annuloplasty System; SPACER, Repair of Tricuspid Valve Regurgitation Using the Edwards Tricuspid Transcatheter Repair System; STTAR, Study of Transcatheter Tricuspid Annular Repair; TIA, Transient ischemic attack; TR, tricuspid regurgitation; TRICAVAL, Treatment of Severe Secondary Tricuspid Regurgitation in Patients With Advanced Heart Failure With Caval Vein Implantation of the Edwards SAPIEN XT Valve; TRILUMINATE, Evaluation of Treatment With Abbott Transcatheter Clip Repair System in Patients With Moderate or Greater Tricuspid Regurgitation; TRI-REPAIR, Tricuspid Regurgitation Repair With Cardioband Transcatheter System; TV, tricuspid valve; VAD, ventricular assist device; VO₂, oxygen consumption.

a) Including death, Q-wave myocardial infarction, cardiac tamponade, cardiac surgery for failed TriCinch implantation, stroke, and septicemia.

b) Including all death, all stroke, myocardial infarction, acute kidney injury grade 3, life-threatening bleeding, major vascular complications, pericardial effusion or tamponade requiring drainage, and vena cava syndrome.

c) Positive clinical outcomes defined as no readmissions to hospital for right-sided heart failure or right-sided heart failure equivalents including drainage of ascites or pleural effusions, new listing for heart transplantation, VAD, or other mechanical support; improvement in 1 of 3 variables: KCCQ improvement >15 versus baseline and 6MWT improvement >70 m versus baseline, or VO₂ peak improvement >6% versus baseline. *Sources:* Asmarats et al. (2018) and Nagaraja et al. (2020).

Bibliography

1 Addetia, K., Harb, S.C., Hahn, R.T. et al. (2019). Cardiac implantable electronic device lead-induced tricuspid regurgitation. *JACC: Cardiovasc. Imaging* 12 (4): 622–636. https://doi.org/10.1016/j.jcmg.2018.09.028.

2 Agarwal, S., Tuzcu, E.M., Rodriguez, E.M. et al. (2009). Interventional cardiology perspective of functional tricuspid regurgitation. *Circ. Cardiovasc. Interv.* 2 (6): 565–573. https://doi.org/10.1161/CIRCINTERVENTIONS.109.878983.

3 Al-Bawardy, R., Krishnaswamy, A., Brargava, M. et al. (2015). Tricuspid regurgitation and implantable devices. *PACE – Pacing Clin. Electrophysiol.* 38 (2): 259–266. https://doi.org/10.1111/PACE.12530.

4 Al-Bawardy, R. et al. (2013). Tricuspid regurgitation in patients with pacemakers and implantable cardiac defibrillators: a comprehensive review. *Clin. Cardiol.* 36 (5): 249. https://doi.org/10.1002/CLC.22104.

5 Arsalan, M., Walther, T., Smith, R.L. et al. (2017). Tricuspid regurgitation diagnosis and treatment. *Eur. Heart J.* 38 (9): 634–638. https://doi.org/10.1093/eurheartj/ehv487.

6 Asmarats, L., Puri, R., Latib, A. et al. (2018). Transcatheter tricuspid valve interventions: landscape, challenges, and future directions. *J. Am. Coll. Cardiol.* 71 (25): 2935–2956. https://doi.org/10.1016/j.jacc.2018.04.031.

7 Bapat, V. (2017). New percutaneous tricuspid valve repair system. Transcatheter Cardiovascular Therapeutics; October 30, 2017; Denver, CO.

8 Bapat, V. N. and Cth, F. (2020) 'The INTREPID valve for severe tricuspid regurgitation : first-in-man case experience. Cardiovascular Research Technologies Conference, National Harbor, MD.

9 Boudoulas, K.D., Barbetseas, J., Pitsis, A.A. et al. (2019). Tricuspid valve disease: the "Forgotten Valve". *Cardiology (Switzerland)* 142 (4): 235–238. https://doi.org/10.1159/000497816.

10 Cao P. (2019). *A new, non-radial force transcatheter tricuspid valve replacement (LuX Medical)*. https://www.tctmd.com/slide/new-non-radial-force-transcatheter-tricuspid-valve-replacement-lux-medical.

11 Chen, T.E., Kwon, S.H., Enriquez-Sarano, M. et al. (2013). Three-dimensional color Doppler echocardiographic quantification of tricuspid regurgitation orifice area: comparison with conventional two-dimensional measures. *J. Am. Soc. Echocardiogr.* 26 (10): 1143–1152. https://doi.org/10.1016/j.echo.2013.07.020.

12 Cox, C.E. (2021). *Tricuspid Trio: TRISCEND, CLASP TR, and TriBAND studies show advances* https://www.tctmd.com/news/tricuspid-trio-triscend-clasp-tr-and-triband-studies-show-advances.

13 Dahou, A., Levin, D., Reisman, M. et al. (2019). Anatomy and physiology of the tricuspid valve. *JACC: Cardiovasc. Imaging* 12 (3): 458–468. https://doi.org/10.1016/j.jcmg.2018.07.032.

14 Demir, O.M., Regazzoli, D., Magieri, A. et al. (2018). Transcatheter tricuspid valve replacement: principles and design. *Front. Cardiovasc. Med.* 5 (September): 1–10. https://doi.org/10.3389/fcvm.2018.00129.

15 Denti, P. (2017). 4Tech—clinical outcomes and current challenges. PCR London Valves; September 26, 2017; Paris, France.

16 Eleid, M., Gavazzoni, M., Kodali, S. et al. (2021). *EuroPCR 2021 Hotlines/late-breaking trials: TRILUMINATE, CLASP TR, bRIGHT, TRISCEND, TriBAND, and more!*. https://www.pcronline.com/Cases-resources-images/Resources/Course-videos-slides/2021/EuroPCR-2021-Hotlines-Late-Breaking-Trials-TRILUMINATE-CLASP-TR-bRIGHT-TRISCEND-TriBAND-and-more?auth=true.

17 Fam, N.P., Ho, E.C., Zahrani, M. et al. (2018). Transcatheter tricuspid valve repair with the PASCAL system. *JACC: Cardiovasc. Interv.* 11 (4): 407–408. https://doi.org/10.1016/j.jcin.2017.12.004.

18 Fam, N.P., Braun, D., von Bardeleben, R.S. et al. (2019). Compassionate use of the PASCAL transcatheter valve repair system for severe tricuspid regurgitation: a multicenter, observational, first-in-human experience. *JACC: Cardiovasc. Interv.* 12 (24): 2488–2495. https://doi.org/10.1016/j.jcin.2019.09.046.

19 Fam, N.P., von Bardeleben, S., Hensey, M. et al. (2021). Transfemoral transcatheter tricuspid valve replacement with the EVOQUE system: a multicenter, observational, first-in-human experience. *JACC: Cardiovasc. Interv.* 14 (5): 501–511. https://doi.org/10.1016/j.jcin.2020.11.045.

20 Goldberg, Y.H., Ho, E., Latib, A. et al. (2021). Update on transcatheter tricuspid valve replacement therapies. *Front. Cardiovasc. Med.* 8619558 (February): https://doi.org/10.3389/fcvm.2021.619558.

21 Greenbaum, A.B., Khan, J.M., Rogers, T. et al. (2021). First-in-human transcatheter pledget-assisted suture tricuspid annuloplasty for severe tricuspid insufficiency. *Catheter. Cardiovasc. Interv.* 97 (1): E130. https://doi.org/10.1002/CCD.28955.

22 Hahn, R.T., George, I., Kodali, S.K. et al. (2019). Early single-site experience with transcatheter tricuspid valve replacement. *JACC: Cardiovasc. Imaging* 12 (3): 416–429. https://doi.org/10.1016/j.jcmg.2018.08.034.

23 Hahn, R.T., Kodali, S., Fam, N. et al. (2020). Early multinational experience of transcatheter tricuspid valve replacement for treating severe tricuspid regurgitation. *JACC: Cardiovasc. Interv.* 13 (21): 2482–2493. https://doi.org/10.1016/j.jcin.2020.07.008.

24 Hahn, R.T., Meduri, C.U., Davidson, C.J. et al. (2017). Early feasibility study of a transcatheter tricuspid valve annuloplasty: SCOUT trial 30-day results. *J. Am. Coll. Cardiol.* 69 (14): 1795–1806. https://doi.org/10.1016/j.jacc.2017.01.054.

25 Hahn, R.T.. (2017). SCOUT I 12-month data. Transcatheter Cardiovascular Therapeutics; November 1, 2017; Denver, CO.

26 Hahn, R.T. and Zamorano, J.L. (2017). The need for a new tricuspid regurgitation grading scheme. *Eur. Heart J. Cardiovasc. Imaging* 18 (12): 1342–1343. https://doi.org/10.1093/ehjci/jex139.

27 Hahn, R.T., Thomas, J.D., Khalique, O.K. et al. (2019). Imaging assessment of tricuspid regurgitation severity. *JACC: Cardiovasc. Imaging* 12 (3): 469–490. https://doi.org/10.1016/j.jcmg.2018.07.033.

28 Harb, S.C. and Kapadia, S.R. (2019). Patients' selection for transcatheter tricuspid valve interventions: who will benefit? *Prog. Cardiovasc. Dis.* 62 (6): 467–472. https://doi.org/10.1016/j.pcad.2019.09.002.

29 Höke, U., Auger, D., Thijssen, J. et al. (2014). Significant lead-induced tricuspid regurgitation is associated with poor prognosis at long-term follow-up. *Heart* 100 (12): 960–968. https://doi.org/10.1136/heartjnl-2013-304673.

30 Holda, M.K., Zhingre Sanchez, J.D., Bateman, M. et al. (2019). Right atrioventricular valve leaflet morphology redefined: implications for transcatheter repair procedures. *JACC: Cardiovasc. Interv.* 12 (2): 169–178. https://doi.org/10.1016/J.JCIN.2018.09.029.

31 Kefer, J., Sluysmans, T., and Vanoverschelde, J.L. (2014). Transcatheter sapien valve implantation in a native tricuspid valve after failed surgical repair. *Catheter. Cardiovasc. Interv.* 83 (5): 841–845. https://doi.org/10.1002/ccd.25330.

32 Kelly, B.J., Luxford, J.M.H., Goldberg Butler, C. et al. (2018). Severity of tricuspid regurgitation is associated with long-term mortality. *J. Thorac. Cardiovasc. Surg.* 155 (3): 1032.e2–1038.e2. https://doi.org/10.1016/j.jtcvs.2017.09.141.

33 Kim, J.B., Jung, S.H., Choo, S.J. et al. (2013). Clinical and echocardiographic outcomes after surgery for severe isolated tricuspid regurgitation. *J. Thorac. Cardiovasc. Surg.* 146 (2): 278–284. https://doi.org/10.1016/j.jtcvs.2012.04.019.

34 Kocak, A., Govsa, F., and Aktas, E.O. (2004). Structure of the human tricuspid valve leaflets and its chordae tendineae in unexpected death. A forensic autopsy study of 400 cases. *Saudi Med J.* 25 (8): 1051–1059.

35 Lama, P., Tamang, B.K., and Kulkarni, J. (2016). Morphometry and aberrant morphology of the adult human tricuspid valve leaflets. *Anat. Sci. Int.* 91 (2): 143–150. https://doi.org/10.1007/S12565-015-0275-0.

36 Lauten, A., Doenst, T., Hamadanchi, A. et al. (2014). Percutaneous bicaval valve implantation for transcatheter treatment of tricuspid regurgitation clinical observations and 12-month follow-up. *Circ. Cardiovasc. Interv.* 268–272. https://doi.org/10.1161/CIRCINTERVENTIONS.113.001033.

37 Lauten, A., Figulla, H.R., Unbehaun, A. et al. (2018). Interventional treatment of severe tricuspid regurgitation. *Circ. Cardiovasc. Interv.* 11 (2): e006061. https://doi.org/10.1161/CIRCINTERVENTIONS.117.006061.

38 Leon, M. (2019). *Cardiac implants Da Vingi. . . proof of concept – technology and clinical updates.* https://www.tctmd.com/slide/cardiac-implants-da-vingi-proof-concept-technology-and-clinical-updates.

39 Lu, F.L., Ma, Y., An, Z. et al. (2020). First-in-man experience of transcatheter tricuspid valve replacement with LuX-valve in high-risk tricuspid regurgitation patients. *JACC: Cardiovasc. Interv.* 13: 1614–1616. https://doi.org/10.1016/j.jcin.2020.03.026.

40 Montorfano, M., Beneduce, A., Ancona, M.B. et al. (2019). Tricento transcatheter heart valve for severe tricuspid regurgitation: procedural planning and technical aspects. *JACC: Cardiovasc. Interv.* 12 (21): e189–e191. https://doi.org/10.1016/j.jcin.2019.07.010.

41 Muntané-Carol, G., Alperi, A., Faroux, L. et al. (2021). Transcatheter interventions for tricuspid valve disease: what to do and who to do it on. *Can. J. Cardiol.* https://doi.org/10.1016/j.cjca.2020.12.029.

42 Nagaraja, V., Kapadia, S.R., Miyasaka, R. et al. (2020). Contemporary review of percutaneous therapy for tricuspid valve regurgitation. *Expert Rev. Cardiovasc. Ther.* 18 (4): 209–218. https://doi.org/10.1080/14779072.2020.1750370.

43 Nagaraja, V., Mohananey, D., Navia, J. et al. (2020). Functional tricuspid regurgitation: feasibility of transcatheter interventions. *Clevel. Clin. J. Med.* 22 (11): 4–14. https://doi.org/10.3949/ccjm.87.s1.01.

44 Navia, J.L., Kapadia, S., Elgharably, H. et al. (2017). First-in-human implantations of the NaviGate bioprosthesis in a severely dilated tricuspid annulus and in a failed tricuspid annuloplasty ring. *Circ. Cardiovasc.*

Interv. 10 (12): e005840. https://doi.org/10.1161/CIRCINT ERVENTIONS.117.005840.

45 Nickenig, G. (2017). TRI-REPAIR: 30-day outcomes of transcatheter tricuspid valve repair in patients with severe secondary tricuspid regurgitation. Transcatheter Cardiovascular Therapeutics; November 2, 2017; Denver, CO.

46 Nickenig, G., Kowalski, M., Hausleiter, J. et al. (2017). Transcatheter treatment of severe tricuspid regurgitation with the edge-to-edge mitraclip technique. *Circulation* 135 (19): 1802–1814. https://doi.org/10.1161/ CIRCULATIONAHA.116.024848.

47 Nickenig, G., Weber, M., Lurz, P. et al. (2011). Transcatheter edge-to-edge repair for reduction of tricuspid regurgitation: 6-month outcomes of the TRILUMINATE single-arm study. *The Lancet* 394 (10213): 2002–2011. https://doi.org/10.1016/ S0140-6736(19)32600-5.

48 Orban, M., Besler, C., Braun, D. et al. (2018). Six-month outcome after transcatheter edge-to-edge repair of severe tricuspid regurgitation in patients with heart failure. *Eur. J. Heart Fail.* 20 (6): 1055–1062. https://doi.org/10.1002/ ejhf.1147.

49 Otto, C.M., Nishimura, R.A., Bonow, R.O. et al. (2021). 2020 ACC/AHA guideline for the management of patients with valvular heart disease. *J. Am. Coll. Cardiol.* 77 (4): e25–e197. https://doi.org/10.1016/j. jacc.2020.11.018.

50 Prihadi, E.A., Delgado, V., Leon, M.B. et al. (2019). Morphologic types of tricuspid regurgitation: characteristics and prognostic implications. *JACC: Cardiovasc. Imaging* 12 (3): 491–499. https://doi .org/10.1016/j.jcmg.2018.09.027.

51 Rogers, T., Ratnayaka, K., Sonmez, M. et al. (2015). Transatrial intrapericardial tricuspid annuloplasty. *JACC. Cardiovasc. interv.* 8 (3): –483. https://doi.org/ 10.1016/J.JCIN.2014.10.013.

52 Schaefer, U. (2020).*The updated experience of the Tricento bioprosthesis for tricuspid regurgitation.* https://www .tctmd.com/slide/updated-experience-tricento-bioprosthesis-tricuspid-regurgitation.

53 Singh, J.P., Evans, J.C., Levy, D. et al. (1999). Prevalence and clinical determinants of mitral, tricuspid, and aortic regurgitation (The Framingham Heart Study). *Am. J. Cardiol.* 83 (6): 897–902. https://doi.org/10.1016/ S0002-9149(98)01064-9.

54 Stuge, O. and Liddicoat, J. (2006). Emerging opportunities for cardiac surgeons within structural heart disease. *J. Thorac. Cardiovasc. Surg.* 132: 1258–1261. https://doi .org/10.1016/j.jtcvs.2006.08.049.

55 Taramasso, M., Gavazzoni, M., Pozzoli, A. et al. (2019). Tricuspid regurgitation: predicting the need for intervention, procedural success, and recurrence of disease. *JACC: Cardiovasc. Imaging* 12 (4): 605–621. https://doi.org/10.1016/j.jcmg.2018.11.034.

56 Toggweiler, S., De Boeck, B., Brinkert, M. et al. (2018). First-in-man implantation of the tricento transcatheter heart valve for the treatment of severe tricuspid regurgitation. *EuroIntervention* 14 (7): 758–761. https:// doi.org/10.4244/EIJ-D-18-00440.

57 Van Rosendael, P.J., Kamperidis, V., Kong, W.K.F. et al. (2017). Computed tomography for planning transcatheter tricuspid valve therapy. *Eur. Heart J.* 38 (9): 665–674. https://doi.org/10.1093/eurheartj/ehw499.

58 Velayudhan, D.E., Brown, T.M., Nanda, N.C. et al. (2006). Quantification of tricuspid regurgitation by live three-dimensional transthoracic echocardiographic measurements of vena contracta area. *Echocardiography* 23 (9): 793–800. https://doi. org/10.1111/j.1540-8175.2006.00314.x.

59 Yzeiraj, E. (2016). *TCT 86: early experience with the trialign system for transcatheter tricuspid valve repair: A multicenter experience.* https://www.tctmd.com/slide/ tct-86-early-experience-trialign-system-transcatheter-tricuspid-valve-repair-multicenter.

47

Tricuspid Valve-in-Valve and Valve-in-Ring

Antonio Mangieri[1,2], Sharon Bruoha[3], Kuno Toshiki[3], Andrea Scotti[3] and Azeem Latib[3]

[1] *Department of Biomedical Sciences, Humanitas University, Milan, Italy*
[2] *Humanitas Research Hospital IRCCS, Rozzano, Milan, Italy*
[3] *Montefiore-Einstein Center for Heart and Vascular Care, Montefiore Medical Center, Albert Einstein College of Medicine, Bronx, NY, USA*

Tricuspid Regurgitation

1. How is tricuspid regurgitation classified?

Moderate to severe tricuspid regurgitation (TR) affects 1 in every 25 patients above 75 years of age, with a significant impact on the patient's prognosis and quality of life. TR can be primary (organic) or secondary (functional) in etiology. Organic TR, the less prevalent form, results from damage to one or more components of the tricuspid valve (TV) apparatus and can be either congenital or acquired. Conversely, in functional TR, the valve components are anatomically normal, and valve dysfunction is usually secondary to the combination of left-sided heart disease, pulmonary hypertension, and right ventricular (RV) remodeling that leads to distorted annular geometry with loss of its saddle shape configuration and leaflet tethering.

2. When should TR be treated?

For years, it was believed that correction of the concurrent left-sided valvulopathies would reduce or eliminate the associated secondary TR. However, more recent evidence has shown that uncorrected TR may deteriorate, especially when the mitral and/or aortic valve disease are not completely resolved or when high pulmonary pressure is persistent. Accordingly, recent guidelines recommend a low threshold for concomitant TV repair at the time of mitral valve surgery in patients with tricuspid annular dilation (end diastolic diameter ≥ 40 mm or area > 21 mm/m^2; Class IIa; evidence C), regardless of the grade of regurgitation.

For functional TR, surgical repair strategies based on annular reduction represent the gold standard of treatment; conversely, valve replacement is considered only in those rare cases of TR associated with a severely diseased valve. However, despite the satisfactory short-term results of surgical repair, the recurrence of significant regurgitation during long-term follow-up is not uncommon. This chapter describes the valve-in-valve and valve-in-ring procedures to manage failure of surgical tricuspid annuloplasties and replacements with bioprostheses.

Surgical TV Annuloplasty

3. What is the rationale behind TV annuloplasty?

As opposed to the mitral annulus, which has robust structural support due to its anatomical relationship with the fibrous trigone, the TV annulus is constituted of less resistant fibro-fatty tissue, in particular in its anterolateral aspect. It is thus more prone to dilatation along the free wall of the RV. Annular dilatation is the first anatomical alteration seen in secondary TR, while defects of leaflet coaptation and tethering typically appear later in the course of RV remodeling as a consequence of progressive chamber dilatation and dysfunction.

Suture-based or prosthetic ring-based annuloplasty techniques target the anterolateral and posterior portions of the annulus, while the septal portion is usually spared due to its minor contribution to annular dilatation and its proximity to the conduction system.

Mastering Structural Heart Disease, First Edition. Edited by Eduardo J. de Marchena and Camilo A. Gomez.
© 2023 John Wiley & Sons Ltd. Published 2023 by John Wiley & Sons Ltd.
Companion website: www.wiley.com/go/deMarchena/Mastering-Structural-Heart-Disease

4. What are the most common suture-based annuloplasty techniques?

Suture-based techniques are generally simple, rapid, and cost-effective, and include the following:

- The **Kay procedure** aims to achieve tricuspid competency by plication and exclusion of the posterior leaflet, thus obtaining a functionally bicuspid valve (suture bicuspidization). The original "figure -eight" technique has been replaced by the double pledget-supported suture running from the anteroposterior to the posteroseptal commissure.

- The **De Vega** procedure reduces the annular dimensions by placing two parallel running sutures (with 5–6 mm bites) along the annulus perimeter, from the posteroseptal to the anteroseptal commissure, where they are tied together. The interposition of Teflon pledgets between each bite of the suture or the use of interrupted pledget-supported sutures has been used to reinforce the result.

5. What are the properties of prosthetic rings?

Prosthetic ring-based techniques are currently the surgical annuloplasty treatment of choice.

Ring annuloplasty techniques are designed to reinforce and restore the 3D shape of the tricuspid annulus to achieve leaflet coaptation and valve competency. The incomplete C-shaped prosthetic rings are fixed along the anterolateral portion of the tricuspid annulus in correspondence with the RV free wall. The numerous commercially available prosthetic rings can be classified according to three main parameters: size, 3D shape, and stiffness. Undersized rings are frequently chosen to favor annular contraction, RV geometry restoration, and leaflet coaptation. Device conformation may be denoted as "flat" (2D) or "remodeling/contoured" (3D), whereas the stiffness scale includes three ring consistencies: "flexible", "semi-rigid", and "rigid".

Flexible bands (such as the Cosgrove-Edwards annuloplasty system [Edwards Lifesciences]) adapt to the contour of the annulus and preserve its dynamic ability during the cardiac cycle. However, due to their elastic properties, flexible rings may not completely restore the optimal nonplanar spatial configuration of the annulus.

Conversely, **semi-rigid or rigid rings** (such as the Edwards MC3 annuloplasty system [Edwards Lifesciences] and the Contour 3D annuloplasty ring [Medtronic]) may

be preconfigured to reproduce the physiologic saddle shape of the annulus thus providing a more physiological plasty. However, their stiffness limits the full range of dynamic annular excursion in the beating heart. Contemporary evidence suggests that compared to the flexible band, overall and long-term (five years) freedom from significant TR are better following rigid ring annuloplasty. Tricuspid plasty using the Contour 3D has excellent early valve function and a low rate of residual regurgitation that is maintained up to two years after implantation.

6. What are the outcomes of TV annuloplasty?

Approximately 8000 tricuspid annuloplasties are performed each year in the United States. However, the volume of surgical TV repairs is expected to increase in the near future due to the increased prevalence of functional TR in the population and the rise in awareness of its clinical repercussions on prognosis if left untreated. Furthermore, the absence of added operative risk (including mortality risk, increased bleeding due to right atriotomy and the risk of atrioventricular block requiring pacemaker implantation) along with the positive impact on RV remodeling of concomitant tricuspid annuloplasty at the time of mitral valve surgery would lead to more liberal TV annuloplasties during left-side valve surgery, when indicated.

Nevertheless, long-term outcomes of surgical tricuspid annuloplasty are far from optimal, with residual TR of at least moderate severity recorded in 13% of patients at hospital discharge and clinically relevant recurrent TR reported in up to 14% of patients five years after surgical annuloplasty.

7. How can the results of TV annuloplasty be predicted?

Predictors of early and late TR recurrence include higher degrees of pre-operative TR, reduced left ventricular ejection fraction (LVEF), presence of pacemaker leads across the TV, and the use of non-ring annuloplasty. Treatment of TR at earlier stages of disease and the avoidance of suture-based annuloplasties are useful strategies to improve acute outcomes after surgery and reduce the rate of TR recurrence at follow-up. In addition, prosthetic ring annuloplasty is the preferred approach in patients with an enlarged tricuspid annulus and risk factors for TR recurrence; in cases of concomitant leaflet tethering, the addition of a leaflet plasty using the clover technique or leaflet augmentation techniques may be useful to achieve durable results. Conversely, when TR arises in a background of complex anatomical scenarios, concomitant RV dilatation, and/or compromised leaflets, TV replacement may offer a better long-term outcome.

8. What is the role of imaging after a failed surgical TV annuloplasty?

Multi-modality imaging plays a key role in evaluating patients with recurrent TR after surgery and should be performed and interpreted by properly trained personnel. Accurate and comprehensive assessment of the various anatomic and functional aspects of the failing valve and its surroundings are indispensable for optimal patient selection and procedural planning.

In particular, echocardiography is fundamental to confirm the diagnosis of TR, quantify its severity, and determine the mechanism of failure. Real-time echocardiography is also essential for procedural guidance. Both transthoracic and transesophageal echocardiography (TEE) are utilized for TR quantification. Since no specific recommendations exist regarding TR grading in the setting of tricuspid annuloplasties, the general consensus is to use a multiparametric approach similar to the grading of native valve regurgitation. Nevertheless, the echocardiographic assessment of a surgically reconstructed valve may have significant limitations. For instance, the presence of the prosthetic material may affect the imaging quality due to shadowing and reverberations, leading to suboptimal evaluation.

Accurate echocardiographic assessment of RV function is also challenging. Not uncommonly, a post-operative reduction of RV contraction is appreciated when Doppler and bidimensional-based measurements are utilized to assess RV performance; the RV fractional area change (FAC) can be used, but foreshortening of the RV on 2D echo views may lead to significant underestimation of function. However, when the post-surgical RV ejection fraction (RVEF) is evaluated by 3D echocardiography, preserved RV function can be seen despite a decrease in the tricuspid annular plane systolic excursion (TAPSE), suggesting geometrical rather than functional changes in RV performance. A post-operative RVEF <45% assessed on 3D echocardiography is consistent with dysfunction. Cardiac magnetic resonance imaging (CMR) is considered the reference standard for evaluating RV function, giving important data on both function and anatomy; the 3D evaluation (with either CMR or echocardiography) is also useful for the assessing the RV longitudinal dimension and characterizing the trabeculated apex, which are

extremely relevant for the safe navigation of transcatheter devices in the ventricle.

9. What information can be obtained from computed tomography?

When planning a valve-in-ring procedure, knowledge of the surgical ring type and dimensions is essential for transcatheter heart valve (THV) sizing. Direct measurements of ring dimensions can be best achieved with ECG-gated computed tomography (CT). Multiplanar reconstructions (MPRs) can precisely delineate the actual 3D conformation of the ring, which is often oval rather than circular, and thus can potentially predict the risk of embolization and residual paravalvular leak (PVL) after implantation of a cylindrical valve platform.

However, the CT scan does not account for the presence of valvular tissue inside the ring that may alter the true dimensions of the available space for implantation; it also does not account for potential, even if rare, dynamic changes in ring geometry during valve deployment. For this purpose, intra-procedural balloon sizing prior to valve implantation should also be considered in addition to the pre-procedural CT scan. Balloon sizing can also anticipate the persistence of residual TR and better understand the mobility and predict the final positioning of pacemaker leads across the prosthetic ring once the THV is implanted. Furthermore, the CT scan provides invaluable information regarding the subclavian, axillary, and femoral vein dimensions and course; in addition, the ECG-gated CT scan is highly useful for evaluating the cavotricuspid angle and the distance between the tricuspid annulus and the apex of the RV, which are fundamental to appreciate before the procedure to facilitate the steering of the delivery system. Despite its fundamental role in procedural planning, the use of contrast-enhanced ECG-gated CT may be limited in patients with kidney dysfunction or poorly controlled atrial fibrillation or in the presence of prosthetic devices that can impair imaging quality.

10. How do you manage a failed tricuspid annuloplasty?

TR recurrence after annuloplasty is associated with high morbidity and frequent rehospitalizations due to progressive right-heart failure. Persistent volume overload triggers a vicious cycle that promotes RV dilatation and dysfunction. Diuretics are often used to mitigate right-heart failure symptoms by attenuating hypervolemia. However, medical therapy does not interrupt disease progression and has no favorable impact on RV reverse remodeling; moreover, there is a lack of solid evidence of the benefit of renin-angiotensin-aldosterone blockers in the setting of right-heart failure. Surgical redo can effectively restore the continency of the TV, but the associated high rate of in-hospital morbidity and mortality limits its practical use. Therefore, innovative transcatheter approaches are rapidly evolving as low-risk therapeutic alternatives for residual or recurrent TR. Specifically, standardized transcatheter tricuspid valve-in-valve (TTViV) and valve-in-ring (TTViR) procedures demonstrate satisfactory results and a good safety profile. However, patient selection is key for procedural success; and multiple factors, as briefly mentioned – especially prosthetic ring type and dimensions – must be taken into consideration during procedural planning to ensure optimal and reproducible results.

Transcatheter Tricuspid Valve-in-Ring Procedure

11. Can you always perform a TTViR?

TTViR, unlike TTViV, has some unique challenges that limit its wide applicability. In most cases, tricuspid prosthetic annuli are incomplete in the area of the interventricular septum, thus creating a non-circumferential landing zone that increases the risk of valve embolization and predisposes to incomplete sealing and PVL. In addition, certain implanted rings have a tridimensional contour that may hamper the precise alignment and final positioning of the THV. Finally, larger prosthetic annuli cannot accommodate the commercially available bioprosthetic valves (Figure 47.1).

12. What does the literature say about TTViR procedures?

An international experience describing the use of THV for the treatment of residual or recurrent TR after surgical repair reported the outcome of 22 patients treated with the SAPIEN (Edwards Lifescience) or Melody (Medtronic). The procedure was aborted in two cases due to the persistence of a regurgitant jet in correspondence with the open portion of the prosthetic ring during balloon sizing.

All procedures were performed under general anesthesia with TEE guidance. The femoral vein was the preferred access site (73%). Rapid pacing, necessary to reduce heart motion and balloon movement during valve deployment, was utilized in 56% of cases, via either an existing pacing system (n = 9) or a temporary transvenous atrial pacing wire (n = 2). In four cases, a permanent pacemaker lead was present across the prosthetic ring and was entrapped upon valve implantation. In one case, the RV lead was dislodged, although that patient did not require ventricular

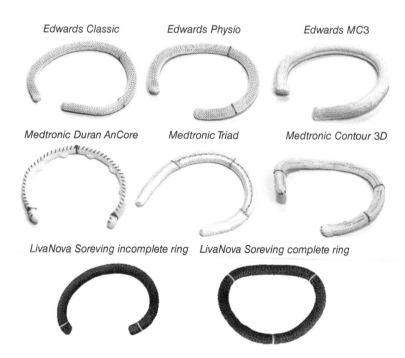

Edwards Classic   Edwards Physio   Edwards MC3

Medtronic Duran AnCore   Medtronic Triad   Medtronic Contour 3D

LivaNova Soreving incomplete ring   LivaNova Soreving complete ring

Figure 47.1 Surgical annuloplasty rings for tricuspid valve repair.

pacing. One case of valve embolization into the RV was reported and was managed with its surgical retrieval followed by the placement of a new valve. Significant PVL that required treatment occurred in six patients (30%). THV malposition was responsible for one case of severe PVL and was managed with a second THV implant. In the remaining patients, the PVL was treated with an Amplatzer Vascular Plug II (St. Jude Medical) or an Amplatzer Muscular Ventricular Septal Occluder. However, surgical treatment was eventually necessary for two patients to eliminate the PVL.

To date, only one case report describes the outcome of a dedicated transcatheter TV implanted in a failed surgical annuloplasty. Navia et al. reported the transjugular implantation of the NaviGate valved stent (36 mm) in a failed 34 mm annuloplasty ring. The procedure, performed under fluoroscopic monitoring and TEE guidance, was successful with final mild PVL and improved RV function. In the future, the development of new transcatheter valves will expand the armamentarium of percutaneous bioprostheses suitable for treating failed tricuspid annuloplasties.

Transcatheter Tricuspid Valve-In-Valve Procedure

13. What is the rate of bioprosthetic TV failure?

Despite the demonstrated excellent performance of mechanical valves in tricuspid position with low freedom from reintervention at 10-year follow-up, the use of bioprostheses for treating TV pathology is increasing. Recent data show freedom from reoperation at 1, 5, and 10 years of 100, 86, and 81%, respectively, and freedom from prosthesis dysfunction detected by echocardiography at 1, 5, and 10 years of 89, 66, and 58%, respectively. Younger age at implantation is the main predictor for early bioprosthetic failure, whereas the mechanism responsible for most cases of implant dysfunction is valve insufficiency.

14. What does the literature say about TTViV procedures?

TTViV procedures for treating failed surgical bioprostheses are rapidly gaining importance, with remarkable data supporting their efficacy and safety. The first successful TTViV for treating degenerated bioprostheses was performed in 2010 using the Melody valve in a patient who received a 27 mm Medtronic Mosaic valve eight years before for endocarditis. One year later, the first SAPIEN THV was implanted via the jugular venous approach entirely percutaneously. The introduction of steerable delivery systems paved the way for the transfemoral approach, now considered the standard access site for TTViV; in addition, similarly to mitral ViV procedures, TTViV procedures can be safely performed without rapid pacing due to the attenuated pressure gradients on the right heart, which make the delivery and deployment of the THV more predictable (Figure 47.2).

The largest TTViV series published to date, the tricuspid VIV International Data (VIVID) registry, included 152 patients. As many as 30% of patients experienced surgical bioprosthesis failure within five years of implantation, highlighting the accelerated degeneration process observed in tricuspid bioprostheses. Procedural success was high (99%), with one procedural death and one patient who required an acute conversion to open-heart surgery. Two cases of valve embolization were managed percutaneously. The echocardiographic results were optimal, with significant improvement of the gradients and abolition of the regurgitation; 76% of patients experienced a sustained functional improvement, and 85% of the whole cohort had freedom from reintervention at one-year follow-up. All-cause mortality was low, with a reported incidence of 3% at 30 days and a total of 22 deaths (15%) during a median follow-up period of 13 months.

Conclusions

Surgical annuloplasty and bioprosthetic valve failures in the tricuspid position are relatively infrequent events. Conservative medical management can be adopted in patients with multiple comorbidities and limited life expectancy; however, in patients with reasonable anticipated longevity and functional status and an acceptable procedural risk profile, TTViV and TTViR are attractive alternatives to redo surgery with good results in terms of safety and efficacy. Longer follow-up periods and accumulating procedural experience are needed to clarify whether these new percutaneous solutions can be considered the gold standard for treating failed tricuspid annuloplasty and replacement in the appropriate context.

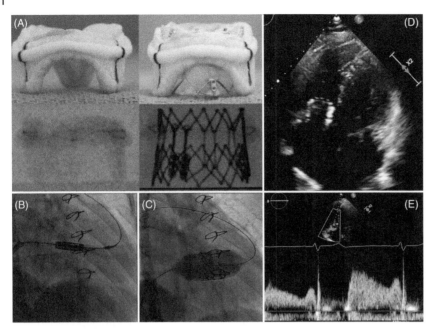

Figure 47.2 Transcatheter tricuspid valve-in-valve (TTViV) using a minimalistic approach: the patient presented with symptomatic degenerated biological 33 mm Epic valve (Abbott) and refused a surgical replacement. The patient underwent successful implantation of a 29 mm SAPIEN via the right femoral vein without pacing. Upon completion of the procedure, the patient had no perivalvular leaks and a mean transprosthetic gradient of 1 mmHg. (a) Illustration of a Biocor Epic valve before and after the implantation of a SAPIEN TTViV with corresponding angiographic views. (b) Valve positioning and (c) and deployment during TTViV. Final echocardiographic assessment: (d) four-chamber view and (e) mean transprosthetic gradient.

Bibliography

1 Aboulhosn, J., Cabalka, A.K., Levi, D.S. et al. (2017). Transcatheter valve-in-ring implantation for the treatment of residual or recurrent tricuspid valve dysfunction after prior surgical repair. *JACC Cardiovasc. Interv.* 10 (1): 53–63. https://doi.org/10.1016/j.jcin.2016.10.036.

2 Asmarats, L., Puri, R., Latib, A. et al. (2018). Transcatheter tricuspid valve interventions: landscape, challenges, and future directions. *J. Am. Coll. Cardiol.* 71 (25): 2935–2956. https://doi.org/10.1016/j.jacc.2018.04.031.

3 Baumgartner, H., Falk, V., Bax, J.J. et al. (2017). 2017 ESC/EACTS guidelines for the management of valvular heart disease. *Eur. Heart J.* 38 (36): 2739–2791. https://doi.org/10.1093/eurheartj/ehx391.

4 Belluschi, I., Del Forno, B., Lapenna, E. et al. (2018). Surgical techniques for tricuspid valve disease. *Front Cardiovasc. Med.* 28 (5): 118. https://doi.org/10.3389/fcvm.2018.00118.

5 Braunwald, N.S., Ross, J. Jr., and Morrow, A.G. (1967). Conservative management of tricuspid regurgitation in patients undergoing mitral valve replacement. *Circulation* 35 (4 Suppl): I63–I69. https://doi.org/10.1161/01.cir.35.4s1.i-63.

6 Burri, M., Vogt, M.O., Hörer, J. et al. (2016). Durability of bioprostheses for the tricuspid valve in patients with congenital heart disease. *Eur. J. Cardiothorac. Surg.* 50 (5): 988–993. https://doi.org/10.1093/ejcts/ezw094.

7 Calafiore, A.M., Bartoloni, G., Al Amri, H. et al. (2012). Functional tricuspid regurgitation and the right ventricle: what we do not know is more than we know. *Expert Rev. Cardiovasc. Ther.* 10 (11): 1351–1366. https://doi.org/10.1586/erc.12.114.

8 Calafiore, A.M., Lorusso, R., Kheirallah, H. et al. (2020). Late tricuspid regurgitation and right ventricular remodeling after tricuspid annuloplasty. *J. Card. Surg.* 35 (8): 1891–1900. https://doi.org/10.1111/jocs.14840.

9 Chikwe, J. and Fischer, G. (2013). Tricuspid valvular disease. In: *Perioperative Transesophageal Echocardiography: A Companion to Kaplan's Cardiac Anesthesia*, 156–162. Elsevier Inc.

10 Dreyfus, G.D., Corbi, P.J., Chan, K.M., and Bahrami, T. (2005). Secondary tricuspid regurgitation or dilatation: which should be the criteria for surgical repair? *Ann. Thorac. Surg.* 79 (1): 127–132. https://doi.org/10.1016/j.athoracsur.2004.06.057.

11 Filsoufi, F., Salzberg, S.P., Coutu, M., and Adams, D.H. (2006). A three-dimensional ring annuloplasty for

the treatment of tricuspid regurgitation. *Ann. Thorac. Surg.* 81 (6): 2273–2277. https://doi.org/10.1016/j.athoracsur.2005.12.044.

12 Fukuda, S., Gillinov, A.M., McCarthy, P.M. et al. (2006). Determinants of recurrent or residual functional tricuspid regurgitation after tricuspid annuloplasty. *Circulation* 114 (1 Suppl): I582–I587. https://doi.org/10.1161/CIRCULATIONAHA.105.001305.

13 Fukuda, S., Song, J.M., Gillinov, A.M. et al. (2005). Tricuspid valve tethering predicts residual tricuspid regurgitation after tricuspid annuloplasty. *Circulation* 111 (8): 975–979. https://doi.org/10.1161/01.CIR.0000156449.49998.51.

14 Guenther, T., Mazzitelli, D., Noebauer, C. et al. (2013). Tricuspid valve repair: is ring annuloplasty superior? *Eur. J. Cardiothorac. Surg.* 43 (1): 58–65. discussion 65. https://doi.org/10.1093/ejcts/ezs266.

15 Hahn, R.T., Meduri, C.U., Davidson, C.J. et al. (2017). Early feasibility study of a transcatheter tricuspid valve annuloplasty: SCOUT trial 30-day results. *J. Am. Coll. Cardiol.* 69 (14): 1795–1806. https://doi.org/10.1016/j.jacc.2017.01.054.

16 Kay, J.H. (1992). Surgical treatment of tricuspid regurgitation. *Ann. Thorac. Surg.* 53 (6): 1132–1133. https://doi.org/10.1016/0003-4975(92)90411-v.

17 Kochav, J., Simprini, L., and Weinsaft, J.W. (2015). Imaging of the right heart - CT and CMR. *echocardiography* 32 (S1): 53–68.

18 Lang, R.M., Badano, L.P., Mor-Avi, V. et al. (2015). Recommendations for cardiac chamber quantification by echocardiography in adults: an update from the American Society of Echocardiography and the European Association of Cardiovascular Imaging. *J. Am. Soc. Echocardiogr.* 28 (1): 1.e14–39.e14. https://doi.org/10.1016/j.echo.2014.10.003.

19 Mangieri, A., Lim, S., Rogers, J.H., and Latib, A. (2018). Percutaneous tricuspid annuloplasty. *Interv. Cardiol. Clin.* 7 (1): 31–36. https://doi.org/10.1016/j.iccl.2017.08.006.

20 Mangieri, A., Montalto, C., Pagnesi, M. et al. (2017). Mechanism and implications of the tricuspid regurgitation: from the pathophysiology to the current and future therapeutic options. *Circ. Cardiovasc. Interv.* 10 (7): e005043. https://doi.org/10.1161/CIRCINTERVENTIONS.117.005043.

21 Mathur, M., Malinowski, M., Timek, T.A., and Rausch, M.K. (2020). Tricuspid annuloplasty rings: a quantitative comparison of size, nonplanar shape, and stiffness. *Ann. Thorac. Surg.* 110 (5): 1605–1614. https://doi.org/10.1016/j.athoracsur.2020.02.064.

22 McCarthy, P.M., Bhudia, S.K., Rajeswaran, J. et al. (2004). Tricuspid valve repair: durability and risk factors for

failure. *J. Thorac. Cardiovasc. Surg.* 127 (3): 674–685. https://doi.org/10.1016/j.jtcvs.2003.11.019.

23 Navia, J.L., Kapadia, S., Elgharably, H. et al. (2017). First-in-human implantations of the NaviGate bioprosthesis in a severely dilated tricuspid annulus and in a failed tricuspid annuloplasty ring. *Circ. Cardiovasc. Interv.* 10 (12): e005840. https://doi.org/10.1161/CIRCINTERVENTIONS.117.005840.

24 Prihadi, E.A., Delgado, V., Hahn, R.T. et al. (2018). Imaging needs in novel transcatheter tricuspid valve interventions. *JACC Cardiovasc. Imaging* 11 (5): 736–754. https://doi.org/10.1016/j.jcmg.2017.10.029.

25 Rabago, G., De Vega, N.G., Castillon, L. et al. (1980). The new De Vega technique in tricuspid annuloplasty (results in 150 patients). *J. Cardiovasc. Surg. (Torino)* 21 (2): 231–238.

26 Raja, S.G. and Dreyfus, G.D. (2009). Surgery for functional tricuspid regurgitation: current techniques, outcomes and emerging concepts. *Expert Rev. Cardiovasc. Ther.* 7 (1): 73–84. https://doi.org/10.1586/14779072.7.1.73.

27 Ratschiller, T., Guenther, T., Guenzinger, R. et al. (2014). Early experiences with a new three-dimensional annuloplasty ring for the treatment of functional tricuspid regurgitation. *Ann. Thorac. Surg.* 98 (6): 2039–2044. https://doi.org/10.1016/j.athoracsur.2014.07.023.

28 Roberts, P., Spina, R., Vallely, M. et al. (2010). Percutaneous tricuspid valve replacement for a stenosed bioprosthesis. *Circ. Cardiovasc. Interv.* 3 (4): e14–e15. https://doi.org/10.1161/CIRCINTERVENTIONS.110.957555.

29 Stuge, O. and Liddicoat, J. (2006). Emerging opportunities for cardiac surgeons within structural heart disease. *J. Thorac. Cardiovasc. Surg.* 132 (6): 1258–1261. https://doi.org/10.1016/j.jtcvs.2006.08.049.

30 Tamborini, G., Muratori, M., Brusoni, D. et al. (2009). Is right ventricular systolic function reduced after cardiac surgery? A two- and three-dimensional echocardiographic study. *Eur. J. Echocardiogr.* 10 (5): 630–634. https://doi.org/10.1093/ejechocard/jep015.

31 Taramasso, M., Calen, C., Guidotti, A. et al. (2017). Management of Tricuspid Regurgitation: the role of transcatheter therapies. *Interv. Cardiol.* 12 (1): 51–55. https://doi.org/10.15420/icr.2017:3:2. Erratum in: Interv Cardiol. 2020 Jul 29;15:e12.

32 Topilsky, Y., Maltais, S., Medina Inojosa, J. et al. (2019). Burden of tricuspid regurgitation in patients diagnosed in the community setting. *JACC Cardiovasc. Imaging* 12 (3): 433–442. https://doi.org/10.1016/j.jcmg.2018.06.014.

33 Topilsky, Y., Nkomo, V.T., Vatury, O. et al. (2014). Clinical outcome of isolated tricuspid regurgitation. *JACC*

Cardiovasc. Imaging 7 (12): 1185–1194. https://doi .org/10.1016/j.jcmg.2014.07.018.

34 Van Garsse, L.A., Ter Bekke, R.M., and van Ommen, V.G. (2011). Percutaneous transcatheter valve-in-valve implantation in stenosed tricuspid valve bioprosthesis. *Circulation* 123 (5): e219–e221. https://doi.org/10.1161/ CIRCULATIONAHA.110.972836.

35 Van Praet, K.M., Stamm, C., Starck, C.T. et al. (2018). An overview of surgical treatment modalities and emerging transcatheter interventions in the management of tricuspid valve regurgitation. *Expert Rev. Cardiovasc. Ther.* 16 (2): 75–89. https://doi.org/10.1080/14779072.201 8.1421068.

36 Wang, N., Phan, S., Tian, D.H. et al. (2017). Flexible band versus rigid ring annuloplasty for tricuspid regurgitation: a systematic review and meta-analysis. *Ann. Cardiothorac. Surg.* 6 (3): 194–203. https://doi.org/10.21037/acs.2017.05.05.

48

Caval Valve Implantation (CAVI) for the Treatment of Severe Tricuspid Regurgitation
Brian P. O'Neill[1]

[1] *Division of Cardiology, Center for Structural Heart Disease, Henry Ford Hospital, Detroit, MI, USA*

1. What is the concept behind caval valve implantation (CAVI)?

Severe tricuspid regurgitation (TR) causes a large amount of the total blood volume of the heart to be ejected retrograde into the right atrium (RA) and inferior vena cava (IVC). By inserting a one-way valve into this circuit, this volume is thereby contained within the RA and superior vena cava (SVC), where it may be better tolerated.

2. What is the initial data to support CAVI as a treatment for TR?

Lauten et al. showed that when acute TR was created, IVC pressure increased. This pressure was decreased with the implantation of a valve within the IVC. In addition, cardiac output, which initially decreased, subsequently increased when a valve was implanted. The elevated central venous pressures that occur with TR may contribute to renal dysfunction, which may in turn lead to progressive insensitivity to diuretics. In theory, this reduction in IVC pressure may increase the trans-renal gradient to the kidneys, helping to relieve this diuretic resistance (Figure 48.1). The initial human case series of CAVI showed improvement in peripheral edema, ascites, and New York Heart Association (NYHA) functional class.

3. Who is a candidate for CAVI?

First, patients should have severe TR with evidence of congestion despite diuretics. Second, patients should have evidence of reverse caval flow. This is most readily determined using hepatic vein flow reversal by echocardiogram. Finally, right atrial pressure should be elevated to allow a gradient that will open and close the heterotopic caval valve leaflets. This is based on data from the US Caval Valve Registry, where patients had a baseline mean right atrial pressure of 15 mmHg.

4. What information is needed to perform CAVI?

The evaluation of anatomical suitability for CAVI begins with a gated cardiac computed tomography (CT). The first measurement is the size of the IVC at the superior hepatic vein (SHV) of the IVC and right atrial caval junction. This diameter, in our experience, should be no greater than a mean diameter of 30.5 mm. This is because of the limitations of valve sizes with the SAPIEN valve (Edwards Lifesciences), which is the main valve used in the United States. The valve may be placed at a point within the IVC that meets this criterion; however, the valve skirt must be located above the SHV so that the vein is protected by the regurgitant volume of the right heart (Figure 48.2).

5. What are the steps in CAVI?

A detailed description of the procedural steps has previously been published. Briefly, venous access is obtained in the femoral vein and internal jugular vein to create a rail. A radiolucent marking tape is placed on the chest to help define previously established distances of the venous structures by CT. A right atrial angiogram is performed to document reverse caval flow, and an intravascular ultrasound

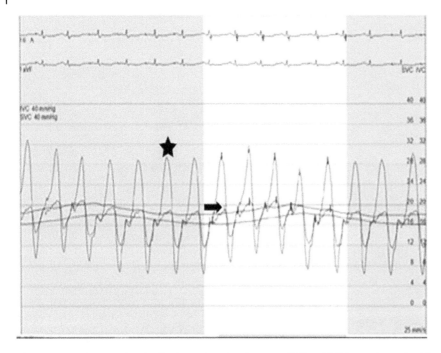

Figure 48.1 Post-caval valve implantation simultaneous SVC and IVC hemodynamics. The star shows the persistent v-wave present in the SVC. The arrow shows the blunted v-wave in the IVC. The mean pressure lines are also shown, demonstrating a slightly higher mean pressure in the SVC than the IVC. IVC, inferior vena cava; SVC, superior vena cava.

(IVUS) catheter may be used to verify identified landmarks for implantation (SHV and RA/IVC junction (Figure 48.2a.) Pre-stenting is performed to avoid interaction with the SAPIEN valve, a 24×65 Gore DrySeal sheath may be advanced over the wire across the stents to allow implantation of the valve (Figure 48.2b).

6. What are the current data with CAVI?

The current data surrounding CAVI are primarily in the form of registries. Lauten et al. studied 25 patients who underwent CAVI with several different valves, as well as

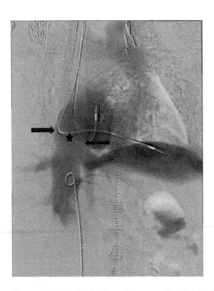
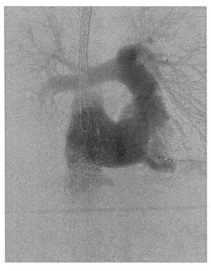

Figure 48.2 (a) IVC angiogram. The RA/IVC junction is shown near where the ventricular lead passes through into the right ventricle. The RA/hepatic vein diameter is shown at the bottom of the right atrial lead. The skirt of the valve is deployed here to prevent reflux into the hepatic vein. The greater the distance between these two measurements, the less of the valve that will protrude into the RA or across the hepatic vein. (b) Final placement of the SAPIEN valve showing improvement in reverse caval flow in IVC. IVC, inferior vena cava; RA, right atrium.

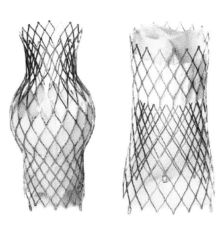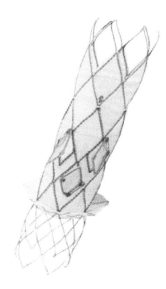

Figure 48.3 (a) The TricValve is composed of two separate valves that are anchored in the SVC and IVC with a self-expanding stent. (b) The Trillium system has a stent graft that anchors in the SVC and IVC. At the level of the tricuspid valve, there are valve leaflets allowing blood to return to the right atrium but isolating the right atrium during ventricular systole and preventing venous backflow. IVC, inferior vena cava; SVC, superior vena cava.

some patients who underwent both IVC and SVC implantation. Procedural success in this cohort of patients was 96%. NYHA class symptoms improved by ≥1 class in 84.2% of patients. In the US Caval Valve Registry, 24 patients underwent CAVI with an IVC approach only with primarily a SAPIEN valve. All procedures were acutely successful, and in patients in whom follow-up data were available, 72.7% improved at least one NYHA class.

recently received a CE mark designation in Europe and in January 2021 received a breakthrough device designation from the Food and Drug Administration (FDA). The Trillium device (Innoventric) (Figure 48.3b) is composed of a long, covered, bare-metal stent that anchors in the IVC and SVC with a series of valves that allow blood inflow and a sealing skirt at the bottom to prevent reflux into the IVC. The valve is currently only available in clinical trials.

7. What is the future of CAVI?

The current challenges with CAVI are primarily related to the size of the vena cava. Two dedicated devices are in development to help address these shortcomings. The first is the TricValve (P+F), a bi-caval implantation system composed of two self-expanding stents and valves that prevent blood reflux into the IVC and SVC (Figure 48.3a). The device has

8. What are the unknowns of CAVI?

The long-term impact of CAVI on indices of right ventricular (RV) size and function is currently unknown and requires further study. Additional data are needed to determine whether these patients require indefinite anticoagulation. As many patients are referred late, the relationship of baseline RV function to outcome in CAVI will need to be established.

Bibliography

1 Laule, M., Stangl, V., Sanad, W. et al. (2013). Percutaneous transfemoral management of severe secondary tricuspid regurgitation with Edwards Sapien XT bioprosthesis: first-in-man experience. *J. Am. Coll. Cardiol.* 61 (18): 1929–1931.

2 Lauten, A., Figulla, H.R., Unbehaun, A. et al. (2018). Interventional treatment of severe tricuspid regurgitation: early clinical experience in a multicenter, observational, first-in-man study. *Circ. Cardiovasc. Interv.* 11 (2): e006061.

3 Lauten, A., Figulla, H.R., Willich, C. et al. (2010). Percutaneous caval stent valve implantation: investigation of an interventional approach for treatment of tricuspid regurgitation. *Eur. Heart J.* 31 (10): 1274–1281.

4 Maeder, M.T., Holst, D.P., and Kaye, D.M. (2008). Tricuspid regurgitation contributes to renal dysfunction in patients with heart failure. *J. Card. Fail.* 14 (10): 824–830.

5 O'Neill, B., Wang, D.D., Pantelic, M. et al. (2015). Transcatheter caval valve implantation using multimodality imaging: roles of TEE, CT, and 3D printing. *JACC Cardiovasc. Imaging* 8 (2): 221–225.

6 O'Neill, B.P., Negrotto, S., Yu, D. et al. (2020). Caval valve implantation for tricuspid regurgitation: insights from the United States caval valve registry. *J. Invasive Cardiol.* 32 (12): 470–475.

7 O'Neill, B.P., Wheatley, G., Bashir, R. et al. (2016). Study design and rationale of the heterotopic implantation of the Edwards-Sapien XT transcatheter valve in the inferior vena cava for the treatment of severe tricuspid regurgitation (HOVER) trial. *Catheter. Cardiovasc. Interv.* 88 (2): 287–293.

Part IV

Structural Interventions for Management of Paravalvular Leaks

49

Aortic Paravalvular Leak Closure

Techniques and Devices for Surgical and Transcatheter Prostheses

Chak-yu So[1] and Pedro A. Villablanca[2]

[1] *Division of Cardiology, Department of Medicine and Therapeutics, Prince of Wales Hospital, Chinese University of Hong Kong, HKSAR, China*
[2] *Division of Cardiology, Center for Structural Heart Disease, Henry Ford Hospital, Detroit, MI, USA*

1. What are the indications for percutaneous aortic paravalvular leak (PVL) closure?

Indications for PVL closure includes moderate to severe PVL with heart failure symptoms or clinically significant hemolytic anemia.

2. What are the contraindications for percutaneous aortic PVL closure?

Contraindications for percutaneous PVL closure include (i) active endocarditis; (ii) regurgitation involving more than one-third of the circumference of the prosthetic annulus or an unstable or rocking prosthesis; and (iii) the presence of intracardiac thrombus with risk of distal embolism.

3. How do you plan an aortic PVL closure procedure?

If available, multimodality imaging should be used to plan aortic PVL closure to reduce the procedure time, increase the success rate, and optimize the repair result. The number, location(s), and size of PVL defects are assessed using transthoracic echocardiography (TTE) and transesophageal echocardiography (TEE) (Figure 49.1a). Electrocardiogram-gated computed tomography (CT) is used to measure the dimensions and identify the path of the PVL, measure the distance from the defect to the coronary ostium, and identify the optimal fluoroscopic projection to cross the defect (Figure 49.1b). A personalized 3D printed model can also be used for device simulation in selected cases (Figure 49.1c). The procedure can be performed under fluoroscopic guidance alone with TTE or TEE guidance.

4. How do you cross the aortic PVL defect?

A baseline aortogram using a pigtail catheter can be obtained to isolate the PVL to guide defect crossing. The optimal projection to isolate the leak can be obtained from pre-procedural CT. The PVL is usually crossed with a 0.035-in. stiff angled Glidewire (Terumo) through a telescoped 125 cm, 5-Fr multipurpose (MP) catheter and a 6- or 7-Fr multipurpose guiding catheter (Cordis), respectively (Figure 49.2a). Other outer catheter choices includes 6- or 7-Fr Amplatzer-left 1 or 2 guiding catheters.

5. What are the techniques to deliver occluder devices?

Three common techniques are used to deliver occluder devices: (i) catheter only, (ii) anchor or safety wire, and (iii) simultaneous deployment. The catheter-only technique is the simplest and is useful for a small or circular defect with a leak that is likely to be sealed with one device. After crossing the defect with a Glidewire, the 5-Fr MP catheter is delivered across the defect and then the 6- or 7-Fr guiding catheters is railed across the defect for device delivery. If a bigger profile device is needed, the Glidewire is exchanged for a pre-shaped left ventricle (LV) stiff wire (e.g. Confida [Medtronic] or Safari2 [Boston Scientific]). Then, a 6- or 7-Fr Shuttle sheath

Mastering Structural Heart Disease, First Edition. Edited by Eduardo J. de Marchena and Camilo A. Gomez.
© 2023 John Wiley & Sons Ltd. Published 2023 by John Wiley & Sons Ltd.
Companion website: www.wiley.com/go/deMarchena/Mastering-Structural-Heart-Disease

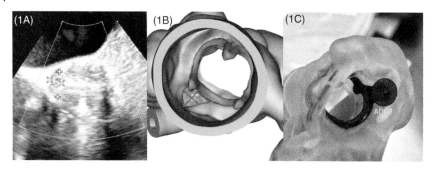

Figure 49.1 Pre-procedural planning. (a) Paravalvular leak (PVL) sizing by transesophageal echocardiogram. (b) PVL sizing by 3D computed tomography reconstruction. (c) Device simulation on a patient-specific 3D printed model.

(Cook Medical) is inserted for device delivery. The disadvantage of the catheter-only technique is that it gives up guidewire access across the leak after device deployment.

The anchor wire technique preserves access across the leak and allows sequential deployment of multiple devices if necessary. In this method, after crossing the leak, the Glidewire is exchanged for a stiff wire. Then the telescoping system is exchanged for a 6-8Fr Shuttle sheath. The closure device is advanced alongside the anchor wire and deployed across the defect but not released. If an additional device is needed, the delivery catheter is removed and placed back on the anchor wire, leaving the device cable outside the delivery catheter. The disadvantage of this technique is that the anchor wire might interact with the device deployment and affect the angulation of device deployment. If this happens, you may consider replacing the Glidewire with two stiff

wires after crossing the defect and then remove the telescoping system and inserting a delivery sheath over one of the stiff wires, leaving a second stiff wire as a safety wire (Figure 49.2b). If the anchor/safety wire technique is planned, a Gore DrySeal sheath can be used to reduce bleeding from the access site.

The simultaneous deployment technique can be considered if the leak is long and crescent shaped and multiple devices are expected. If a large sheath (e.g. Gore DrySeal sheath) is used for single access, the Glidewire is exchanged for two stiff wires after crossing the leak. Then, two small delivery sheaths are inserted over the stiff wires to allow simultaneous insertion and deployment of two devices (Figure 49.2c). If two small arterial accesses are used, the defect needs to be crossed from each arterial access, respectively. The advantage of the simultaneous deployment

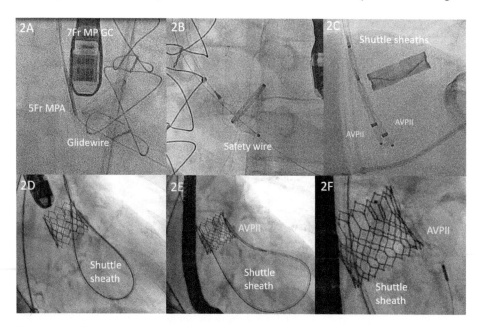

Figure 49.2 Procedural techniques for percutaneous aortic paravalvular leak (PVL) closure. (a) The aortic PVL is crossed using a telescoping system (5-Fr MPA diagnostic catheter, 7-Fr MP Guiding Catheter, Terumo Glidewire). (b) To maintain access across the PVL, a safety wire can be kept outside the delivery sheath for device deployment. (c) In the simultaneous deployment technique, two delivery sheaths were used to allow simultaneous deployment of two Amplatzer Vascular Plugs (AVPs). (d–f) In the retro-antegrade deployment, the Shuttle sheath was delivered retrograde across the transcatheter heart valve and then antegrade across the PVL via an established arterio-arterial rail to allow delivery and deployment of the device (AVP II).

technique is that it allows the two devices to be deployed at the same time, so adjustment of the devices is feasible if interaction happens during deployment.

6. How to negotiate an uncrossable defect?

Small PVL or PVL with a tortuous course can be difficult to cross. After passing the Glidewire through the defect, a few tricks can be used to get the MP catheter or device delivery system across. First, a 4-Fr catheter (e.g. NaviCross microcatheter [Terumo] or Glidecath [Terumo]) can be used to negotiate through the defect; then exchange the Glidewire for a stiff wire to rail the delivery system across. Second, an arterio-arterial rail can be established for better support if it is a bioprosthetic aortic valve. After crossing the defect, the Glidewire is sent antegrade across the bioprosthesis to the descending aorta. The Glidewire is snared and externalized from a second arterial access to establish an arterio-arterial access. Then the delivery system is railed across the defect through the additional support from the arterio-arterial rail. In the presence of a mechanical aortic valve, an arterio-arterial rail is not recommended due to the risk of mechanical leaflet interference and acute aortic regurgitation. Instead, an arterio-apical rail via an apical access or an arterio-venous rail via transseptal access can be built. Third, on rare occasions, the defect is still difficult to cross despite a rail support; a small coronary or peripheral balloon can be used to modify the PVL size and geometry and facilitate the passage of a delivery system.

7. What are the device choices for aortic PVL closure?

A number of devices have been used to close aortic PVL. The Amplatzer Vascular Plug II (AVP II, Abbott) is the most commonly used device. It is circular and suitable for round PVLs. AVP III devices (Abbott) are rectangular and can be used to occlude more crescent-shaped PVLs. Other Amplatzer devices like the Muscular Ventricular Septal Defect Occluder (Abbott) and Duct Occluder II (Abbott) are occasionally used too.

8. What are the mechanisms and treatments for post-transcatheter aortic valve replacement (TAVR) PVL?

PVL after TAVR is becoming less common with the addition of sealing skirts in new valve designs, better and standardized CT sizing, and better operator experience. Three different mechanisms cause PVL: (i) undersized prosthesis relative to the annulus, (ii) prosthesis mal-positioning (too high to too low relative to the annulus), and (iii) mal-apposition of the valve to the annulus due to a protruding annulus or LV outflow tract calcium. An undersized prosthesis can be prevented by better pre-op CT sizing or intra-procedurally with post-dilatation or valve-in-valve TAVR. Prosthesis mal-positioning should be managed with valve-in-valve TAVR. Mal-apposition of the TAVR valve to the annulus can be managed with balloon post-dilatation or plug device closure. Aggressive balloon post-dilatation risks annulus rupture due to significant protruding annular calcium; therefore, it should be performed cautiously.

9. What are the specific anatomical challenges to close post-transcatheter aortic valve PVLs?

In TAVR, PVLs are classically due to protruding annulus calcification. Together with the unresected native calcified aortic leaflet, the path to cross the PVL is typically more tortuous. In the case of the CoreValve system (Medtronic), the long valve stent makes the crossing more challenging as the wire delivery system needs to go through the valve stent frame and across the native aortic valve and then the PVL defect.

10. What are some tips and tricks while closing post-TAVR PVLs?

When closing post-CoreValve PVLs, it is advised to cross the valve stent frame at a higher level before negotiating the PVL. This allows more room for catheter manipulation as higher valve stent frames are bigger and catheter manipulation is easier when going from the top down the PVL. Techniques to negotiate PVLs can be used, as stated earlier. In addition, if the device size is suitable, you can consider using a small-profile Amplatzer Vascular Plug 4 (AVP 4) device (Abbott) sized up to 8 mm, which can be delivered through a 0.038 catheter. Finally, the retro-antegrade approach to the delivery of the catheter can be considered. In the retro-antegrade approach, after crossing the PVL from the aortic side, a snare is placed across the center of the TAVR valve from contralateral femoral access to snare the Glidewire. Then the wire is externalized to build an arterio-arterial rail. Through the antegrade limb of the arterio-arterial rail, the delivery system is passed across the center of the TAVR valve retrograde and across the PVL antegrade with the rail support (Figure 49.2d–f). This technique allows the delivery system to bypass the need to cross the TAVR valve frame and calcified native leaflets and potentially allows easier passage of the delivery system.

11. What are the potential complications of aortic PVL closure?

Important and specific complications of aortic PVL closure include device embolization (<1%), coronary impingement (<1%), and prosthetic leaflet impingement (4%). Device embolization is rare and usually is due to inadequate device compression (Figure 49.3a). Careful assessment of device compression and a tug test should be performed to reduce the risk of device embolization after device release. When performing PVL closure, it is also important to prepare essential equipment for percutaneous device retrieval in the cath lab, e.g. different sizes and types of snares, bioptome, and large-size access sheaths (Figure 49.3b). Coronary impingement is rare and can be prevented by pre-operative planning. If there is any concern of coronary impingement by the occluder device, a semi-selective or selective angiogram should be performed before device release (Figure 49.3c,d). Prosthetic leaflet impingement can be assessed by cine for mechanical prosthesis, ensuring complete leaflet opening and closing (Figure 49.3e–g) and by TEE for bioprostheses. This might be successfully managed by changing the occlusion device size of deployment orientation.

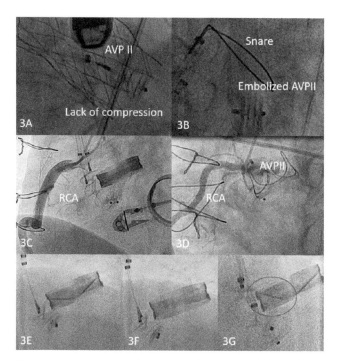

Figure 49.3 Potential complication of percutaneous aortic paravalvular leak closure. (a, b) Embolized Amplatzer Vascular Plug II (AVP II) to descending aorta due to lack of compression, which required endovascular snaring. (c) A selective angiogram of the right coronary artery (RCA) showed no impingement by the deployed occluder devices. (d) A selective angiogram showed possible impingement to ostial RCA by the AVP II device after its release. (e, f) High-resolution cine showed normal mechanical leaflet closing and opening after occluder device deployment. (g) Impingement of mechanical aortic leaflet by the occluder device, leading to incomplete closure (red circle).

Bibliography

1 Athappan, G., Patvardhan, E., Tuzcu, E.M. et al. (2013). Incidence, predictors, and outcomes of aortic regurgitation after transcatheter aortic valve replacement: meta-analysis and systematic review of literature. *J. Am. Coll. Cardiol.* 61: 1585–1595.

2 Cruz-Gonzalez, I., Rama-Merchan, J.C., Rodríguez-Collado, J. et al. (2017). Transcatheter closure of paravalvular leaks: state of the art. *Neth. Heart J.* 25: 116–124.

3 Eleid, M.F., Cabalka, A.K., Malouf, J.F. et al. (2015). Techniques and outcomes for the treatment of paravalvular leak. *Circ. Cardiovasc. Interv.* 8: e001945.

4 Feldman, T., Salinger, M.H., Levisay, J.P., and Smart, S. (2014). Low profile vascular plugs for paravalvular leaks after TAVR. *Catheter. Cardiovasc. Interv.* 83: 280–288.

5 Gafoor, S., Franke, J., Piayda, K. et al. (2014). Paravalvular leak closure after transcatheter aortic valve replacement with a self-expanding prosthesis. *Catheter. Cardiovasc. Interv.* 84: 147–154.

6 Mohamad, A., Mohammad, S., Elad, M. et al. (2016). Techniques and outcomes of percutaneous aortic paravalvular leak closure. *JACC Cardiovasc. Interv.* 9 (23): 2416–2426. https://doi.org/10.1016/j.jcin.2016.08.038.

7 Okuyama, K., Jilaihawi, H., Kashif, M. et al. (2015). Percutaneous paravalvular leak closure for balloon-expandable transcatheter aortic valve replacement: a comparison with surgical aortic valve replacement paravalvular leak closure. *J. Invasive Cardiol.* 27: 284–290.

8 Ruiz, C.E., Jelnin, V., Kronzon, I. et al. (2011). Clinical outcomes in patients undergoing percutaneous closure of periprosthetic paravalvular leaks. *J. Am. Coll. Cardiol.* 58: 2210–2217.

9 Smolka, G., Pysz, P., Jasinski, M. et al. (2016). Multiplug paravalvular leak closure using Amplatzer vascular plugs III: a prospective registry. *Catheter. Cardiovasc. Interv.* 87: 478–487.

10 So, C.Y., Kang, G., Lee, J.C., and Eng, M.H. (2020). The retro-antegrade approach to paravalvular leak closure after transcatheter aortic valve replacement. *EuroIntervention* 16 (9): e763–e764. https://doi.org/10.4244/EIJ-D-19-01122.

11 Sorajja, P., Cabalka, A.K., Hagler, D.J., and Rihal, C.S. (2011). Long-term follow-up of percutaneous repair of paravalvular prosthetic regurgitation. *J. Am. Coll. Cardiol.* 58: 2218–2224.

12 Sorajja, P., Cabalka, A.K., Hagler, D.J., and Rihal, C.S. (2011). Percutaneous repair of paravalvular prosthetic regurgitation: acute and 30-day outcomes in 115 patients. *Circ. Cardiovasc. Interv.* 4: 314–321.

13 Wells, J.A. 4th, Condado, J.F., Kamioka, N. et al. (2017). Outcomes after paravalvular leak closure: transcatheter versus surgical approaches. *JACC Cardiovasc. Interv.* 10 (5): 500–507. https://doi.org/10.1016/j.jcin.2016.11.043. PMID: 28279317.

14 Yildirim, A., Goktekin, O., Gorgulu, S. et al. (2016). A new specific device in transcatheter prosthetic paravalvular leak closure: a prospective two-center trial. *Catheter. Cardiovasc. Interv.* 88: 618–624.

50

Mitral Paravalvular Leak: Imaging and Interventional Approaches

Matthew S. Wu[1], Sankalp P. Patel[2], Creighton W. Don[3] and Robert J. Cubeddu[4]

[1] University of Washington, Seattle, WA, USA
[2] Naples Community Hospital, Naples, FL, USA
[3] Department of Interventional Cardiology at University of Washington, Seattle, WA, USA
[4] Department of Interventional Cardiology, Naples Heart Institute, Naples, FL, USA

Imaging

Echocardiography is the mainstay option for paravalvular leak (PVL) diagnosis, evaluation, procedural guidance, and surveillance; however, imaging modalities such as cardiac computed tomography (CT), cardiac magnetic resonance imaging (MRI), intracardiac echocardiography (ICE), and angiography can provide important adjunctive information. Quantifying the severity of mitral PVL should be a process in which multiple imaging modalities are considered. In fact, the American Society of Echocardiography recommends against using any single imaging modality when evaluating mitral PVL.

Echocardiography

1. What imaging modality should be considered first with suspicion of mitral PVL following repair?

Transthoracic echocardiogram (TTE) should be the first imaging modality used for PVL evaluation. Clinical presentation of heart failure symptoms or evidence of hemolysis should prompt further workup. PVLs may also be found incidentally on screening TTE during the surveillance period (6–12 months) following mitral repair.

TTE with color Doppler provides good visualization of both paravalvular and intravalvular regurgitation. Paravalvular jets are pathologic and characterized as turbulent, eccentric, high-velocity jets. The irregular nature of these regurgitant jets often leads to underestimation of mitral regurgitation (MR) severity. These are best seen with a parasternal short-axis view of the mitral valve (MV).

Mechanical valves have built-in regurgitant functions to decrease clotting risk. These intravalvular regurgitant flows are narrow, symmetric jets that are short in duration. These should be differentiated from paravalvular regurgitant jets, as these do not require intervention.

2. What are the limitations of TTE in assessing mitral PVL? What are adjunctive quantitative measures used to ascertain mitral PVL?

TTE is limited in accurately grading PVLs due to the acoustic shadowing effect of the prosthetic ring or mechanical leaflets, which underestimates PVL. Additionally, PVLs may be inadequately visualized, even with off-axis views. Many quantitative/qualitative parameters help define prosthetic valve regurgitation (Table 50.1). Quantitative measures can include flow convergence in the left ventricle (LV) during systole, increased mitral peak E wave velocity ($>2\,\text{m/s}$), mean gradient $>6\,\text{mmHg}$, and DVI greater than 2.2. Qualitative evidence of occult MR includes the presence of unexplained pulmonary arterial hypertension, a hyperkinetic LV, and pulmonary vein flow reversal.

3. What is the next study considered after screening TTE for better visualization of the MV?

If PVL is suspected on screening TTE, direct evaluation with transesophageal echocardiogram (TEE) is recommended,

Table 50.1 Echocardiographic parameters to assess the degree of paravalvular leak for mitral valve prosthesis.

Parameters	Mild	Moderate	Severe
LV size	Normal	Normal to moderately dilated	Moderately to severely dilated
Prosthetic valve	Normal	Abnormal	Abnormal
RV size and function	Normal	Normal to moderately dilated	Moderately to severely dilated
Color flow jet area	Small, central jet (usually <4cm^2 or <20% of LA area)	Variable	Large, central jet (usually >8cm^2 or >40% LA area)
Proximal flow convergence	None or minimal	Intermediate	Large
Jet density	Incomplete/faint	Dense	Dense
Jet contour	Parabolic	Variable	Early peaking, triangular, holosystolic
Pulmonary venous flow	Normal	Systolic blunting	Systolic flow reversal
Mean gradient	Normal	Increased	>5 mmHg
Diastolic PHT	Normal (<130 ms)	Normal (<130 ms)	Normal (<130 ms)
PASP	Normal	Variable, usually increased	Increased (TR velocity ≥3 m/s, PASP ≥50 mmHg at rest or with exercise)
Vena contracta width (mm)	<3	3–6.9	≥7
Circumferential extent of PVL, %	<10	10–29	≥30
MVPR; LVOT flow	Approximately 1	Intermediate	≥2.5
RVol, ml/beat	<30	30–59	≥60
RF, %	<30	30–49	>50
EROA, mm^2	<20	20–39	>40

EROA, effective regurgitant orifice area; LA, left atrium; LV, left ventricle; LVOT, left ventricular outflow tract; PASP, pulmonary artery systolic pressure; PVL, paravalvular leak; RF, regurgitant fraction; RV, right ventricle. *Source:* Gursoy (2020).

as it offers improved visualization of the MV and annular ring. TEE is useful in characterizing the size and shape of the PVL, determining if there are multiple convergent or separate defects, and identifying the mechanism such as insufficiency in the surgical repair sites, annular tearing, ring dehiscence, calcification, or aorto-atrial fistulae (Figure 50.1).

Although TEE can be limited by acoustic shadowing, combining both echocardiography techniques typically is sufficient in evaluating mitral PVLs and determining the feasibility of closure.

4. What nomenclature is used to anatomically define the PVL location? Where are severe mitral PVLs most often found?

The anatomic location of PVLs is based on the clock-face nomenclature from the left atrial, or "surgeon's" view (Figure 50.2b). Severe mitral PVLs are mostly found around the anterolateral segments (from the left atrial appendage [LAA] and aorto-atrial curtain at 12 o'clock) and postero-medial around 5–6 o'clock. However, it is important to

remember that TEE views are based on the sonographer's view as a mirror image of the clock face (Figure 50.2a). Multiple TEE views, including the use of biplane imaging using a 3D TEE probe, should be used to pinpoint the PVL location. The shape and size of the PVL should also be determined, as regurgitant jets can be wide/thin, crescent-shaped, oval/round, linear, slit-like, or serpiginous tunnels. The width/length of the PVL should also be evaluated in multiple views, measuring the narrowest width of color Doppler flow with a Nyquist limit of 50–60 cm/s to avoid overestimating the PVL size if set too low or underestimating it if set too high.

5. What echocardiographic parameters exist for grading the severity of mitral PVLs?

With caution, echocardiographic parameters that are validated for intravalvular regurgitation can be used to grade mitral PVLs (Table 50.1). For example, the American Society of Echocardiography recommends using the effective regurgitant orifice area (EROA) as the standard

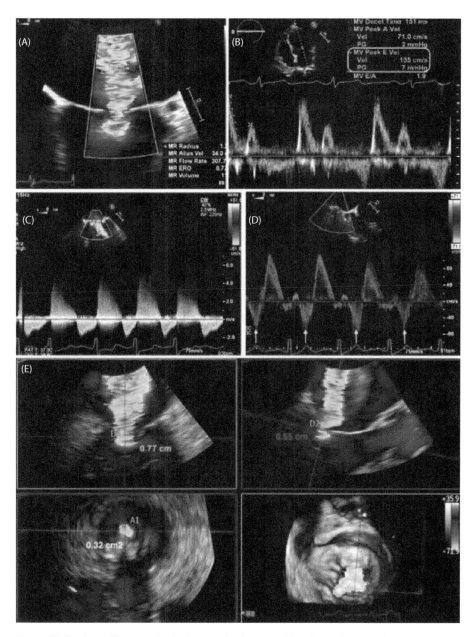

Figure 50.1 Quantification of mitral regurgitation with 2D echocardiogram views. (a) Effective regurgitant orifice area using the proximal isovelocity surface area (PISA) method. (b) CW Doppler signal. (c) Systolic reversal of pulmonary vein flow. (d) Systolic flow reversal of pulmonary vein flow. (e) Mitral regurgitation flow by 2D echocardiogram. *Source:* Garcia-Sayan E, et al. (2021) / Frontiers Media S.A. / CC BY 4.0.

measurement for quantifying MR. Common approaches to estimating EROA use single-frame measurements such as jet area, vena contracta width, or the proximal isovelocity surface area method (PISA). In intravalvular MR, these parameters are well-validated in determining EROA and regurgitant volume.

Nonetheless, it is important to keep in mind that these methods assume flows to be circular, as in traditional MR. The PISA method relies on the assumption that flow approaching a circular orifice forms a concentric, hemispheric shape. Color Doppler is then used to find the

area of flow convergence and measure the radius proximal to the orifice for estimation. PISA is less accurate when applied to non-hemispheric flow shapes and underestimates EROA in the elliptical and crescentic orifices encountered in PVLs. Furthermore, the color Doppler signal must properly align with the regurgitant jet for accurate measurement. The eccentric regurgitation of mitral PVLs can lead to incorrect alignment of the Doppler signal, underestimating the velocity and overestimating the EROA. Additionally, significant acoustic shadowing from the sewing ring or valve frames further complicates the

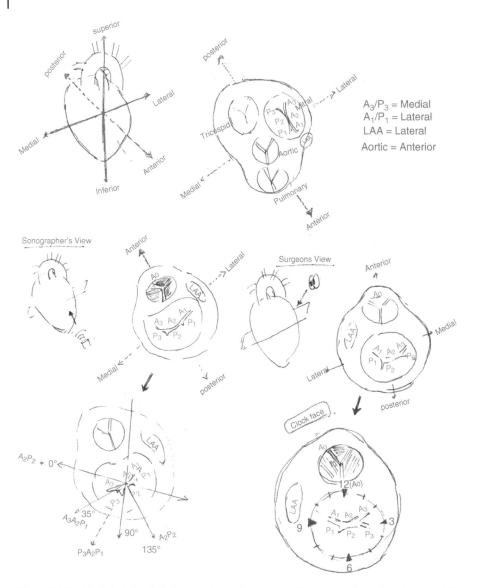

A_3/P_3 = Medial
A_1/P_1 = Lateral
LAA = Lateral
Aortic = Anterior

Figure 50.2 The "clock face" of the mitral annulus seen on fluoroscopy is a mirror image of the en face mitral valve shown on 3D transesophageal echocardiography (TEE). The anterior and posterior remain the same, but medial leaks appear at 3 o'clock on TEE and 9 o'clock on fluoroscopy; conversely, lateral leaks appear at 9 o'clock on TEE and 3 o'clock on fluoroscopy.

quantification of EROA using single-frame measurements. Finally, these techniques only apply when evaluating a single regurgitant jet, while patients may have multiple PVLs.

6. What role does 3D TEE play in evaluating mitral PVLs?

The advent of 3D TEE has been pivotal for diagnosing and treating PVL (Figure 50.3). 3D TEE provides greater accuracy than 2D TEE and avoids the PISA method, as EROA can be directly measured. EROA multiplied by MR jet velocity-time integral on color Doppler gives the regurgitant volume. 3D TEE also measures the anatomic regurgitant orifice (ARO),

although using EROA has been shown to better correlate with paravalvular regurgitant severity. Furthermore, 3D TEE elucidates the defect anatomy, entry/exit points, tunnel length, and spatial relationship with valve and ring and distinguishes multiple PVLs. The use of biplane TEE imaging using a 3D echo probe localizes the defects as well.

7. What role does cardiac MRI play in evaluating mitral PVLs?

Cardiac magnetic resonance imaging (CMRI) is a novel technology enabling excellent visualization of cardiac chambers for volume, function, and mass. However,

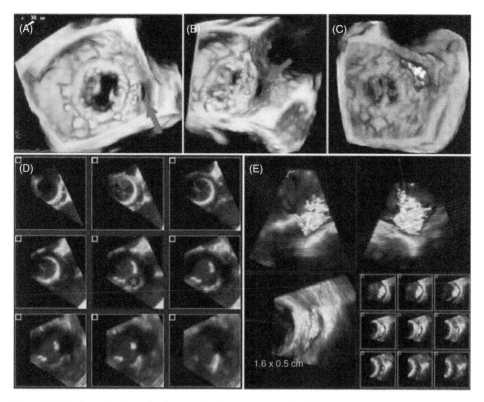

Figure 50.3 Paravalvular mitral regurgitation assessment by 3D transesophageal echocardiography (TEE). (a) En face surgeon's view with posteromedial defect around 5 o'clock (arrow). (b) Rotated view of a posteromedial defect on 3D TEE. (c) Color Doppler added to characterize regurgitant jets and rule out other defects. (d, e). *Source:* Garcia-Sayan E, et al (2021) / Frontiers Media S.A. / CC BY 4.0.

quantitative evaluation of mitral PVLs by CMRI has not yet been validated as studies are limited to native valves. PVLs are characterized on MRI as dark jets, or "negative contrast," due to dephasing on SSFP sequencing. Regurgitation can be quantified with phase-contrast MRI. Indirect methods of quantification have been described, such as using the difference between LV stroke volume and forward stroke volume (SV) flow in the ascending aorta. However, using this method assumes no co-existing transvalvular MR. CMRI parameters can also be implemented as markers of severity, including regurgitant fraction (RF) and PVL volume.

artifacts that can confound diagnosis. A slice thickness of 0.5–0.6 mm is used for maximal spatial resolution. True axial double-oblique reconstruction should be obtained, as crescent-shaped contrast columns can be lost in a coronal/sagittal single plane. Mitral PVL can be visualized on CT by a contrast column spanning from the left atrium (LA)-LV lumina. Additionally, 4D CT can be used to record multiple images in video form to assess paravalvular flow throughout the cardiac cycle.

Cardiac CT has its own limitations. Thin surgical material appears as ill-defined triangular high-attenuation, mimicking PVL. Additionally, shadowing from the annular ring may obscure PVLs. Nevertheless, in patients with complex anatomy, including those with periannular calcification/fibrosis, CT helps localize and understand the mechanism for PVL.

8. What role does cardiac CT play in evaluating mitral PVLs? What are some of its limitations?

Cardiac CT assists in locating PVLs in those with complex anatomy or significant acoustic shadowing prohibiting echocardiographic evaluation. CT imaging should be performed with contrast. ECG-gated (prospective/retrospective) techniques are used to obtain images during diastole in which cardiac motion is minimum. This reduces motion

9. What are the potential benefits of using intracardiac echocardiography in percutaneous leak closure?

Interest has grown in using ICE in percutaneous PVL closure. ICE offers benefits over TEE. Since ICE can be performed by the primary operator under conscious sedation, it precludes general anesthesia and endotracheal intubation, eliminating the risk of esophageal trauma by TEE. For high-risk surgical populations, many with severe lung disease or esophageal varices, ICE offers an attractive solution for patient safety. Additionally, ICE reduces fluoroscopy exposure to both the patient and operator. While ICE is also gaining traction in mitral valvuloplasty procedures, it has not been well-studied in mitral PVL closure. 2D ICE provides limited views of the mitral annulus even when imaging from the LA, and 3D ICE currently only provides a 70° field of view. Nevertheless, in straightforward cases, ICE could be used as the sole imaging modality to guide PVL closure.

10. What combination imaging modalities are useful when evaluating and intervening in mitral PVLs?

Technologies combining imaging modalities have emerged in recent years to improve structural cardiac views for pre- and intra-procedural imaging. Echocardiography-fluoroscopic fusion (EFF) technologies have made the different spatial frames of echocardiography and fluoroscopy compatible with visualizing 3D spatial anatomy in real-time. The ability to overlay 3D echocardiography projection on the fluoroscopic image in real-time improves transseptal sheath position, maneuvering, defect crossing, and device deployment in mitral PVL closure. Additionally, combining CCTA and fluoroscopy provides enhanced pre-procedural mapping, facilitating transapical puncture and PVL identification and crossing. However, the fidelity of the mapped image and the fluoroscopic image, along with challenges in gating to overlay a real-time moving image, have limited the utility of these technologies. As these techniques improve, the use of these modalities should increase.

Transcatheter Closure of Mitral PVLs

Percutaneous mitral PVL closure is difficult and requires a thorough understanding of the patient's anatomy, the techniques for a transseptal puncture, PVL crossing and closure, and the numerous catheters, wires, and devices utilized. Anatomical diversity combined with complexity multimodality imaging guiding the procedure makes mitral PVL closure very challenging.

No universally accepted techniques for mitral PVL closure exist, and several nuanced differences in approaches and devices used have been described. Nonetheless, basic principles of PVL closure are generally well accepted and are described in this chapter. Most commonly, an anterograde transseptal approach is used, although retrograde PVL crossing from a catheter placed in the LV across the aortic valve is used when anterograde crossing cannot be achieved. The procedure is relatively safe, with few short-term complications reported and significantly fewer complications than cardiac surgery.

11. What is the most common approach to mitral PVL closure?

Anterograde Transseptal Approach

Mitral PVL closure most commonly occurs through the anterograde transseptal approach with anterograde defect crossing (Figure 50.4a). For simple defects, a single 8F or 9F femoral venous sheath may suffice; but with multiple defects, using multiple devices simultaneously or keeping a safety wire across the defect to maintain access while deploying a large device with a larger 12F or greater sheath is preferable. The Agilis or Direx steerable catheters are 8.5F with an 11F outer diameter. The usual delivery sheaths are the Flexor Shuttle Sheath (Cook Medical) and Pinnacle Destination Sheath (Terumo), ranging in size from 5F to 9F. The French size of a sheath or guide catheter refers to its internal diameter, although the actual internal diameter can vary slightly by manufacturer. Knowing the minimal delivery catheter requirements for each device is critical for preprocedural planning in ensuring the compatibility of delivery sheaths with required devices (Table 50.2).

Transseptal Puncture

12. Describe the approach an interventionalist should take with transseptal puncture. How does this change with (a) posterior defects, (b) anterior defects, and (c) medial defects?

PVL location is important in determining the site of transseptal puncture to optimize maneuverability in the LA. Typically, a more posterior puncture will position the catheter farther away from the MV (more height), allowing more room to maneuver in the LA. However, given the relationship of PVL to the ring and atrial size, too much height affects the trajectory from the catheter to the leak,

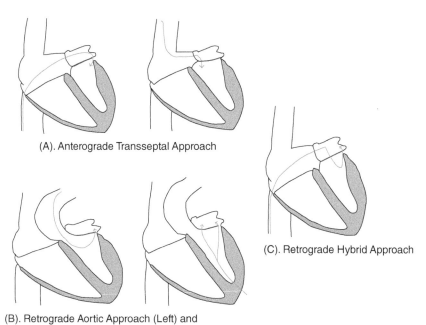

(A). Anterograde Transseptal Approach

(C). Retrograde Hybrid Approach

(B). Retrograde Aortic Approach (Left) and
Transapical Approach (Right)

Figure 50.4 Approaches to mitral paravalvular leak closure. (a) Anterograde transseptal approach. (b) Retrograde aortic approach (left) and transapical approach (right). (c) Retrograde hybrid approach. *Source:* Sankalp Patel.

making PVL crossing difficult. In most patients, a mid-septal puncture is reasonable, but if maneuvering the steerable guide to the PVL and crossing prove difficult, the operator should consider performing a new transseptal puncture. Additionally, if a patient has a PVL in a challenging location (e.g. medial), a more specific transseptal puncture could be tried up front.

Generally, difficulty crossing PVLs is due to a lack of coaxial alignment of the steerable guide with the puncture site in a different position spatially from the PVL. In considering optimizing the transseptal puncture, the location of the transseptal puncture should generally be at the same level on the superior–inferior axis as the defect to avoid an acute angle between the trajectory of the catheter and the path of the leak. This can be observed on fluoroscopy or 3D TEE, noting the tip of the transseptal needle and mitral annular ring. A posterior leak may require a slightly inferior puncture to avoid an acute angle of trajectory toward the leak. Likewise, an anterior leak is sometimes better approached with a slightly more superior "aorta hugger" puncture. In medial defects, a more midline or slightly anterior puncture places the catheter closer to the leak allowing for an easier crossing of the defect and a more coaxial orientation to the leak. A posterior puncture often places the catheter too far away from the medial annulus. Lateral leaks are typically the easiest to cross with any transseptal puncture.

13. In what position should the fluoroscopic gantries be oriented for transseptal puncture? What techniques or equipment should be considered when performing transseptal puncture?

Transseptal puncture is traditionally performed in the left anterior oblique (LAO) position on fluoroscopy. Right anterior oblique (RAO) views should be used to ensure that the catheter position is directed toward the area of the mitral annulus of interest. ICE or TEE can be used to help direct the precise localization of the puncture site and document the crossing of the wire or needle into the LA. Pressure tracings can confirm access to the LA. A dilator is then advanced, followed by a transseptal sheath into the LA. The needle and dilator should be removed. Patients should be anticoagulated immediately after the transseptal puncture is performed to avoid LA thrombus formation.

Transseptal puncture can be difficult in this population due to distorted cardiac anatomy post-surgery and atrial septal fibrosis, scarring, or patch repair. Radiofrequency ablation and electrocautery can be helpful adjunctive tools to facilitate precise transseptal puncture. The VersaCross wire (Baylis Medical) is stiff enough to puncture the septum and is equipped with a j-tip or pigtail tip allowing for

Table 50.2 Devices used for occlusion of mitral paravalvular leaks (Amplatzer portfolio and Gore portfolio 2016, 2021).

Device	Company	Device Diam. (mm) – middle waist	Retention disc diameter	Delivery catheter requirement	Minimal internal diameter requirements (mm/in.)	Max length of delivery system (cm)	
AVP 2	Abbott	8	8	6F guide catheter	1.42/0.056	125	
		10	10	6F guide catheter	1.78/0.070	125	
		12	12	6F guide catheter	1.78/0.070	125	
AVP 4	Abbott	6	6	5F diagnostic catheter	0.038	125	
		7	7	5F diagnostic catheter	0.038	125	
		8	8	5F diagnostic catheter	0.038	125	
ADOII	Abbott	5	11	5F guide catheter	1.50/0.059	125	
		6	12	5F guide catheter	1.50/0.059	125	
Amplatzer Duct Occluder	Abbott	8/6	12	6F sheath	2.11/0.08	110	
		10/8	16	6F sheath	2.11/0.08	110	
		12/10	18	7F sheath	2.44/0.10	110	
Amplatzer Ventricular Septal Duct Occluder	Abbott	8	16	6F sheath	2.11/0.08	110	
		10	18	6F sheath	2.11/0.08	110	
		12	20	7F sheath	2.44/0.10	110	
Non-Fenestrated Cardio-form Septal Occluder	Gore	20, 25, 30	8	10Fr or 12Fr with Guidewire	3.45/0.136	75	

Sources: Matthew Wu and Sankalp Patel.

looping to prevent atrial wall trauma. A SafeSept Transseptal Guidewire (Pressure Products Medical Supplies) can also be used. Balloon septostomy can be used for dilation if sheath crossing is difficult or it is anticipated that multiple large sheaths will be used.

14. Describe the retrograde transapical approach to mitral PVL closure

A transapical approach (Figure 50.4b) may be used for mitral PVLs if there is difficulty crossing the leak due to extreme tortuosity or the leak location is difficult to access from a transseptal left atrial or retrograde aortic valve approach. A medial PVL posing a difficult acute angle for access between the atrial septum and mitral annulus occasionally warrants a transapical approach. For the transapical approach, echocardiographic-guided puncture can be made in the left fifth intercostal space. CTA-fluoroscopy fusion can be used to identify appropriate landmarks and ideal pre-procedural insertion site, with the CT overlay on the fluoroscopy guiding puncture.

Alternatively, a hybrid surgical/transcatheter approach has been studied for the transapical approach. The procedure is performed by teams of cardiothoracic surgeons and interventional cardiologists. The surgeon performs a small thoracotomy at the left fifth intercostal space exposing the cardiac apex. A needle is used with direct visualization to puncture the LV and exchange it for a sheath. Similar techniques with telescoping are used by the interventionalist to cross the defect into the LA. Retrograde delivery of the device is executed.

15. Describe the retrograde femoral approach to mitral PVL closure

Retrograde Femoral Approach

A retrograde femoral approach may be used to access difficult-to-cross medial PVLs (Figure 50.4b). Access is obtained through the common femoral artery, across the aortic valve into the LV. A curved catheter, such as an EBU guide, is advanced into the LV with the catheter elbow looped in the apex and the catheter tip directed toward the mitral annulus. This is typically done in RAO cranial view to provide clear visualization of the mitral annulus and facilitate crossing the PVL; however, the LAO view may be needed to direct the catheter toward the medial or lateral aspects of the annulus. This approach can be challenging because the steerable guides are not long enough to direct the wires across the defect, and once across the PVL, advancing a delivery sheath and device over the aortic arch, around the LV apex, and through the leak is not trivial.

Hybrid Anterograde-Retrograde Approach

Often, if the PVL can only be crossed from a retrograde approach, an operator will snare and externalize a wire from a transseptal sheath in the LA and then deliver the closure device from an antegrade approach. This approach has been described in cases where high-velocity regurgitant flows and serpiginous defects posed difficulty crossing the defect using the anterograde LA-LV approach.

The PVL is typically crossed retrograde from the arterial side across the aortic valve, but a novel hybrid anterograde transseptal-retrograde transmitral approach has also been described (Figure 50.4c). In this approach, dual transseptal access is obtained with a steerable guide catheter and a JR-4 catheter. A 5-Fr left internal mammary artery (LIMA) catheter can be inserted through the steerable guide and is maneuvered through the bioprosthetic MV into the LV. The LIMA catheter is positioned in the subvalvular space near the PVL and crossed retrograde. The Guidewire is then snared in the LA with a large snare inserted through the transseptal JR-4 catheter. The device delivery sheath can then be advanced retrograde using the snared wire for stability, or the wire can be externalized, and the delivery sheath advanced retrograde.

Defect Crossing and Telescoping Catheters

16. Describe the steps required to cross a mitral PVL

Fluoroscopy gantries are oriented to show the mitral annulus en face. Often a RAO cranial or LAO caudal view can achieve this, but this can be variable for each patient. The deflectable catheter is then aimed toward the defect using fluoroscopic and TEE guidance. It should be noted that the "clock face" of the mitral annulus seen on fluoroscopy is a mirror image of the en-face MV shown on 3D TEE (Figure 50.2). Anterior and posterior will remain the same, but medial leaks will appear at 3 o'clock on TEE and 9 o'clock on fluoroscopy, and conversely, lateral leaks at 9 o'clock on TEE and 3 o'clock on fluoroscopy.

Using a combination of TEE and fluoroscopic imaging, or EFF imaging if available, the catheters can be positioned just above the PVL. Often color Doppler is used to confirm that the catheter is in the correct position. A straight hydrophilic wire such as a straight Glidewire (Terumo) is used to probe the mitral annulus, attempting to cross through the leak. One challenge is that the wire will often cross through the MV rather than the leak, but careful interrogation on fluoroscopy or echocardiography is needed to determine if the wire is inside or outside the annular ring.

Many small vascular devices can be advanced through a 5-6F guide catheter, but if a larger device/larger delivery sheath is required, a stiff exchange length wire is used to deliver the larger sheath (e.g. an Abbott Trevisio, Flexor Shuttle, or Destination sheath). The stiff wire can be looped in the LV or externalized after crossing the aortic valve and snared from an arterial access site, which may be required if a large stiff sheath is needed.

If a safety wire to maintain access across the defect is needed, or multiple devices will be deployed in the defect, two 0.032-in. Amplatzer Extra-Stiff wires (Abbott) are placed, or a combination of a stiff exchange length 0.014-/0.018-in. wire and a 0.032-/0.035-in. wire is placed across the PVL. The delivery sheath is then advanced over the larger wire, and the smaller wire is left in place during device deployment. Alternatively, the smaller wire can be left across the defect while the device is advanced in the same sheath. This requires a sheath to be sized larger than the nominal size needed for the device itself.

17. Describe the concept of telescoping catheters for mitral PVL closure

Telescoping catheters are an important technique for mitral PVL closure. The concept is to use a deflectable catheter to help maneuver toward the leak and provide backup support, through which a smaller, longer, lower-profile catheter is inserted to cross the leak.

If the transseptal puncture is performed using a dedicated transseptal catheter, it is exchanged for a deflectable catheter such as an Agilis NTX Steerable Introducer (Abbott) or a Direx Steerable Sheath (Boston Scientific), which are 8.5F sheaths with a dial used to deflect the catheter tip toward the PVL. These catheters typically have a 70 cm usable length with 10 cm for the handle, so the catheter telescoped within the deflectable sheath should be >100 cm in length. The catheter curve size depends on LA size and PVL location. A 5-6F multipurpose guide/diagnostic catheter, or a sheath such as a Cook Flexor Shuttle Sheath or Pinnacle Destination Sheath, is often used to cross through the PVL (Table 50.3). A Judkins Right catheter can also be used, which has the advantage of providing extra angle maneuvering and directing a wire across the PVL, often required for leaks originating at an off angle from the annulus or medial leaks. If the PVL is very small or has a tortuous tunnel preventing crossing with a 5F catheter, a third 120 cm 4F catheter can be telescoped within the 5-6F guide, such as a Terumo Glidecath. The soft, hydrophilic catheter is more easily advanced through small, tortuous leaks, using the telescoped 8.5F and 6F catheters for pushability and backup. This low-profile catheter can then be exchanged over a stiff wire for the device delivery sheath such as a Flexor Shuttle Sheath.

Device Selection

18. What are common devices used for mitral PVL closure?

Several devices have been used to occlude the space between the annular ring and the prosthetic valve (Table 50.2). While there are no devices in the United States with FDA approval for this indication, the most-used devices are the Amplatzer Vascular Plug (AVP) II and IV (Abbott). These are made with expandable Nitinol mesh delivered through 5-8F catheters. The size/type of the occluder should be determined by the diameter, length, and shape of the PVL via TEE. The type of device chosen also determines the sheath size required. The AVP III has been designed specifically for PVL closure, with smaller pore sizes, improved surface contact, and a design shaped for crescentic PVLs. This explains why the AVP III is the most commonly used device for PVL closure in Europe; however, the device is not yet available in the United States.

Other off-label devices for PVL closure include the Amplatzer Septal Occluder, Amplatzer Muscular Occluder, Amplatzer Duct Occluder, and Gore CARDIOFORM Septal Occluder (CSO). The Amplatzer Duct Occluder II is a low-profile device effective for small leaks delivered through a small 5F sheath. A round, circular defect can be occluded with a single AVPII, while larger, crescentic leaks might be suitable for multiple smaller devices or larger atrial or

Table 50.3 Sheaths employed for the delivery of closure devices (Cook Medical and Terumo 2021).

Device	Company	Diameter	Internal diameter		Wire diameter
Flexor shuttle sheath	Cooks Medical Inc.	5F	0.074 (1.9 mm)		0.038 down
		6F	0.087″ (2.2 mm)		
		7F	0.100″ (2.5 mm)		
		8F	0.113″ (2.9 mm)		
Pinnacle Destination Sheath	Terumo	5F	0.076″ (1.92 mm)		
		6F	0.087″ (2.21 mm)		
		7F	0.101″ (2.57 mm)		
		8F	0.115″ (2.92 mm)		

Source: Matthew Wu.

ventricular septal occluders. The nonfenestrated Gore CSO has been reported to amend rather large PVLs without residual hemolysis or valve dysfunction. Nevertheless, its reduced flexibility and larger sheath requirement limit its transseptal delivery, necessitating an invasive transapical approach. In general, the operator should choose slightly oversized devices that maintain tissue apposition and device anchoring, conforming to the leak. There are ongoing efforts to design a specific PVL plug by Occlutech.

Device Deployment

19. What technique should be used for single-device deployment?

In single-device deployment, the delivery sheath is slowly withdrawn, and the device is partially deployed on the LV side of the annulus. For the AVP II, the first disc is fully deployed, but the body of the device remains sheathed. The device and sheath are then withdrawn so that the distal part of the device gently apposes the ventricular aspect of the annulus; the operator must be careful not to withdraw too quickly or forcefully such that the device is pulled through the defect. The device is then unsheathed within the defect so the body fills the PVL. Counterclockwise turns of the delivery cable release the device.

20. What techniques should be considered with multiple-device deployment?

Simultaneous Deployment Technique (Double Wire)

A double-wire technique can be used for deploying multiple devices. Use a >16F transvenous sheath for venous access. After the defect is crossed with a 6F catheter, two 0.032-in. Amplatzer Extra-Stiff Guidewires are inserted through the 6F catheter across the defect. The 6F is withdrawn, leaving only the two guidewires in the LV. Two 6F or smaller delivery systems are advanced over the guidewires into the LV. The guidewires are removed, and the devices can be deployed through the 6F catheters simultaneously. This technique typically requires a 12F venous access sheath.

Sequential Deployment Technique (Anchor Wire)

When the PVL size/shape requires multiple devices for defect occlusion and simultaneous deployment is not possible, sequential deployment techniques can be used. After

catheter crossing of the defect, two wires are placed into the LV. The catheter is removed, and a sheath is advanced over one wire across the defect, with the second wire parallel to the sheath, across the defect. Once the initial device is deployed, the sheath is removed and reloaded onto the second guidewire, leaving the first device on its delivery cable outside the sheath. The sheath is advanced across the second wire alongside the first device, and a second device is deployed. If the closure is sufficient, both devices are deployed. The anchor wire technique offers the advantage in maintaining LV position if devices must be exchanged.

21. What technique can be used to increase stability for catheter passage across a serpiginous defect that is difficult to cross?

Sequential Deployment Technique Using Arteriovenous or Transapical Rail

Due to the serpiginous nature of PVLs, the passage of a delivery catheter across a defect can be difficult. Using a transcatheter rail provides improved stability for catheter passage. In concept, a transcatheter rail uses snaring of a guidewire that will be exteriorized to allow the operator to have control of both ends of the wire. A second operator is required to hold both ends of the wire to manipulate wire tension. For a mitral PVL, the wire route can be left atrial-ventricular-aortic, left atrial-ventricular-apical, or left atrial-ventricular-left atrial. Once the rail is secured, the deployment technique is similar to sequential deployment methods as described earlier. A sheath is typically advanced over an antegrade guidewire. The first device is advanced through the shuttle sheath alongside the guidewire. Once deployed, the sheath is removed and placed over the rail again, allowing the subsequent devices to be deployed in a similar sequence.

While the rail can be extremely useful for facilitating catheter passage and device deployment, the risks of a transapical puncture are not trivial, and damage to the aortic valve or annulus or mitral chords can occur when a wire is externalized across the aortic valve. Additionally, severe bradycardia can result from nodal impingement from the externalized wire.

Conclusion

Although often technically challenging, with a detailed assessment of patient anatomy, high-quality imaging, and a thorough understanding of the techniques and devices, percutaneous mitral PVL can be successfully performed and be highly effective in addressing patients' heart failure symptoms.

Bibliography

1 Alkhouli, M., Rihal, C.S., Zack, C. et al. (2017). Transcatheter and surgical management of mitral paravalvular leak: long-term outcomes. *JACC Cardiovasc. Interv.* 10 (19): 1946–1956.

2 Cubeddu, R.J., Crespo, H., Novaro, G.M. et al. (2018). Retrograde transmitral paravalvular leak closure through an antegrade transseptal approach: a novel technique. *Catheter. Cardiovasc. Interv.* 92 (6): 1196–1200.

3 Cubeddu, R.J., Sancehz, A.M., Perez, E. et al. (2020). First experience using a nonfenestrated cardioform septal occluder for closure of giant mitral paravalvular leak. *J. Am. Coll. Cardiol. Case Rep.* 2: 468–472.

4 Eleid, M.F., Cabalka, A.K., Malouf, J.F. et al. (2015). Techniques and outcomes for the treatment of paravalvular leak. *Circ. Cardiovasc. Interv.* 8 (8): 1945.

5 Franco, E., Almeria, C., de Agustin, J.A. et al. (2014). Three-dimensional color Doppler transesophageal echocardiography for mitral paravalvular leak quantification and evaluation of percutaneous closure success. *J. Am. Soc. Echocardiogr.* 27 (11): 1153–1163.

6 Garcia-Sayan, E., Chen, T., Khalique, O.K. et al. (2021). Multimodality cardiac imaging for procedural planning and guidance of transcatheter mitral valve replacement and mitral paravalvular leak closure. *Front. Cardiovasc. Med.* 8: 44.

7 Grayburn, P.A., Carabello, B., Hung, J. et al. (2014). Defining "severe" secondary mitral regurgitation: emphasizing an integrated approach. *J. Am. Coll. Cardiol.* 64 (25): 2792–2801.

8 Grayburn, P.A., Weissman, N.J., Zamorano, J.L. et al. (2012). Quantitation of mitral regurgitation. *Circulation* 126 (16): 2005–2017.

9 Gursoy, M.O., Guner, A., and Kalcik, M. (2020). A comprehensive review of the diagnosis and management of mitral paravalvular leakage. *Anatol. J. Cardiol.* 24 (6): 350.

10 Haberka, M., Pysz, P., Kozlowski, M. et al. (2021). Cardiovascular magnetic resonance and transesophageal echocardiography in patients with prosthetic valve paravalvular leaks: towards an accurate quantification and stratification. *J. Cardiovasc. Magn. Reson.* 23 (1): 1–10.

11 Jone, P., Haak, A., Petri, N. et al. (2019). Echocardiography-fluoroscopy fusion imaging for guidance of congenital and structural heart disease interventions. *JACC Cardiovasc. Imaging* 12 (7): 1279–1282.

12 Krishnaswamy, A., Kapadia, S.R., Tuzcu, E.M. et al. (2012). Percutaneous paravalvular leak closure–imaging, techniques and outcomes. *Circ. J.* 77: 19-27.

13 Rajiah, P., Moore, A., Saboo, S. et al. (2019). Multimodality imaging of complications of cardiac valve surgeries. *Radiographics* 39 (4): 932–956.

14 Ruparelia, N., Cao, J., Newton, J.D. et al. (2018). Paravalvular leak closure under intracardiac echocardiographic guidance. *Catheter. Cardiovasc. Interv.* 91 (5): 958–965.

15 Sorajja, P. (2015). Mitral paravalvular leak closure. *Interv. Cardiol. Clin.* 5 (1): 45–54.

16 Sorajja, P., Bae, R., Lesser, J.A. et al. (2015). Percutaneous repair of paravalvular prosthetic regurgitation: patient selection, techniques and outcomes. *Heart* 101 (9): 665–673.

17 Yamama, H. and Sanghvi, K. (2021). Use of railway™ dilator as a novel technique to cross prosthetic aortic and mitral paravalvular leak. *Cardiovasc. Revasc. Med.* 28: 109–113.

18 Zoghbi, W.A., Asch, F.M., and Bruce, C. (2019). Guidelines for the evaluation of valvular regurgitation after percutaneous valve repair or replacement: report from the American Society of Echocardiography developed in collaboration with the Society for Cardiovascular Angiography and Interventions, Japanese Society of Echocardiography, and Society for Cardiovascular Magnetic Resonance. *J. Am. Soc. Echocardiogr.* 32 (4): 431–475.

19 Zoghbi, W.A., Enriquez-Sarano, M., Foster, E. et al. (2003). Recommendations for evaluation of the severity of native valvular regurgitation with two-dimensional and Doppler echocardiography. *J. Am. Soc. Echocardiogr.* 16 (7): 777–802.

Part V

Left Atrial Appendage Closure

51

Current Indications for Percutaneous Left Atrial Appendage Occlusion

Ryan M. Smith[1] and Giselle A. Baquero[1,2]

[1] *Hawaii Heart Associates, Kaneohe, HI, USA*
[2] *John Burns School of Medicine, University of Hawaii, Honolulu, HI, USA*

1. Is there a rationale for left atrial appendage occlusion (LAAO)?

Stroke risk reduction in patients with nonrheumatic atrial fibrillation (AF) has been the center of extensive clinical investigation due to the increasing prevalence of this condition, the well-documented relationship between increasing age and concomitant comorbidities with the development of cardioembolic events and the resulting morbidity/mortality and economic burden from consequential stroke. The left atrial appendage (LAA) has been implicated as the most common source of cardioembolic thrombi in nonrheumatic AF. Oral anticoagulation (OAC) with vitamin K antagonist (VKAs) and, most recently, direct-acting oral anticoagulants (DOACs), have been the mainstay of treatment for cardioembolic stroke risk reduction in AF. Although effective, VKAs are limited by their narrow therapeutic profile, multiple medication and food interactions, and the need for lifelong coagulation monitoring. Also, substantial data show that fewer than 60% of patients adhere to VKAs. More worrisome is that even when patients are adherent, a time in therapeutic range (TTR) has consistently shown to be below target (TTR of ≥65% is commonly accepted as the definition of international normalized ratio [INR] stability), with values ranging within 20–40%, even with the rigorous monitoring involving modern-day randomized controlled trials (RCTs), translating into unfavorable clinical outcomes including development of thromboembolic or hemorrhagic events, higher level of medication nonadherence with discontinuation, increased utilization of healthcare resources, and higher costs.

Consequently, the DOACs seemed to be the long-expected redeemers for stroke risk reduction with their fastest onset of action, lower potential for food and drug interactions, reduced need for routine therapeutic monitoring, greater predictability, and patient convenience. These advantages rapidly conferred popular favoritism over VKAs and their fast adoption into society treatment guidelines and clinical practice. With time, some of their initial disadvantages have been overcome with the development of reversal agents and cost-effective analysis studies. However, recent data involving more than 570 000 patients with AF also showed troubling suboptimal adherence to DOACs of 69%. This was associated with poor clinical outcomes, with a 39% higher hazard of stroke and increased risk of thromboembolic events and all-cause mortality in the nonadherent patients. The DOACs' praised shorter half-lives may result in more rapid elimination of anticoagulation effect in nonadherent DOAC patients, inheriting potentially greater harm from poor DOAC adherence compared to nonadherence with VKAs. Another interesting point of view the authors raised regarding perceived DOAC advantages was their ease of use and lack of required routine monitoring, perhaps predisposing patients to nonadherence due to diminished clinician oversight of therapeutic regimens. In addition, among other challenges, many patients with AF have relative or absolute contraindications to long-term OAC, resulting in nearly 40% of eligible patients not receiving OAC and being at substantial risk for stroke. As an alternative, a mechanical approach to exclude the LAA has become an attractive and recently proven effective stroke-risk reduction strategy for high-risk AF patients intolerant to OAC.

2. Left atrial appendage occlusion: why percutaneous?

The wide diversity in existing surgical techniques, lack of large or powered randomized trials, and controversial results from retrospective cohorts are some obstacles to supporting routine surgical LAAO. Surgical LAAO is more commonly performed concomitant to other cardiac surgeries, although it may also be performed as a pure stand-alone procedure. The latter continues to hold little attraction, not even being considered within the cardiothoracic surgery guidelines. Results of surgical LAAO remain suboptimal, with echocardiographic follow-up suggesting incomplete occlusion in >50% of patients, regardless of the used technique, with thrombus being identified in ≥25% of patients with unsuccessful occlusion. Retrospective analyses continue to demonstrate a strong association between incomplete LAAO and the occurrence of thromboembolic events. Additionally, following successful LAA exclusion, life-long anticoagulation remains recommended by the 2016 the European Society of Cardiology (ESC)/European Society for Cardio-Thoracic Surgery (EACTS) Guidelines (Class I, level of evidence B). All this has led to fast advancement in the development of catheter-based techniques for LAAO, providing patients with AF and no other associated valvular heart disease an alternative option to long-term OAC.

3. What is the level of evidence supporting percutaneous LAAO?

RCTs for Percutaneous LAAO

Since 2005, numerous devices have been approved for this purpose outside the United States. In 2015, the US Food and Drug Administration (FDA) approved the WATCHMAN (Boston Scientific) LAAO device for patients deemed suitable for long-term oral anticoagulation. Approval was based on the findings of the PROTECT AF (WATCHMAN Left Atrial Appendage System for Embolic PROTECTion in Patients With Atrial Fibrillation) and PREVAIL (WATCHMAN Left Atrial Appendage System for Embolic PROTECTion in Patients With Atrial Fibrillation) RCTs. In PROTECT AF, 707 patients with nonvalvular atrial fibrillation and at least one additional stroke risk factor (CHADS2 score ≥1) were randomized (2 : 1) to percutaneous LAAO vs. VKA. The LAAO arm demonstrated both noninferiority and superiority for preventing the combined outcome of stroke, systemic embolism, and cardiovascular death, as well as superiority for cardiovascular and all-cause mortality, but at the expense of a small percentage of serious complications. The PREVAIL trial followed and included 461 patients with higher CHA2DS2-VASc score, randomized into LAAO vs. VKA. The study demonstrated that LAAO was noninferior to VKA in preventing ischemic stroke or systemic embolism, with significant improvement in procedural safety and device-related complications. The FDA approval of the WATCHMAN device was restricted to patients deemed suitable for long-term VKA, keeping true to the enrollment indications in the clinical trials (Table 51.1). A year later, the Centers for Medicare & Medicaid (CMS) approved the utilization of the WATCHMAN device as an alternative option for patients not suitable for long-term anticoagulation but able to tolerate short-term VKA. The approval was accompanied by specific criteria for device implantation in patients with non-valvular AF (Table 51.2) (https://www.cms.gov/medicare-coverage-database/details/nca-decision-memo.aspx?NCAId=281&bc=ACAAAAAAgAAAA%3d%3d&).

Registries for Percutaneous Left Atrial Occlusion

Following the FDA and CMS approval, the American College of Cardiology (ACC), Heart Rhythm Society (HRS), and Society for Cardiovascular Angiography and Interventions society (SCAI) recommended the development of prospective registries of LAAO, with an emphasis on patient selection and outcomes. The Continued Access to PROTECT-AF (CAP) and Continued Access to PREVAIL

Table 51.1 FDA indications for percutaneous left atrial appendage occlusion.

1. Age 18 years and older
2. Paroxysmal, persistent, or permanent nonvalvular atrial fibrillation
3. CHADS2 ≥ 2, CHA2DS2-VASc ≥ 2
4. Eligibility for long-term anticoagulation with VKA

Post-procedural Antithrombotic Regimen: VKA (INR goal, 2–3) plus aspirin for 45 d, followed by DAPT with clopidogrel and aspirin through 6 mo and then aspirin indefinitely

TEE was performed at 45 d and 12 mo

CHA2DS2-VASc, congestive heart failure, hypertension, 65 years of age and older, diabetes mellitus, previous stroke or transient ischemic attack, vascular disease, 65–74 years of age, female; VKA, vitamin K antagonist; TEE, transesophageal echocardiography.

Table 51.2 CMS indications for percutaneous left atrial appendage occlusion.

1. CHA2DS2-VASc of ≥ 3 or CHADS2 ≥ 2

2. Formal shared decision utilizing an independent, non-interventional physician whose opinion must be written in the medical record

3. Suitability for short-term warfarin, but deemed unable to take long-term anticoagulation

4. Procedure must be performed in a hospital with an established structural heart disease or electrophysiology program.

5. Procedure must be performed by an interventional cardiologist, electrophysiologist or cardiovascular surgeon, who must have received formal training by the manufacturer, have performed ≥ 25 transseptal procedures, and continue to perform ≥ 25 transseptal procedures, including 12 of which are LAA occlusion, over a two-year period.

6. Patient is enrolled, and physicians and hospital participate in, a prospective, national, audited registry for at least four years from the time of implantation.

CHA2DS2-VASc, congestive heart failure, hypertension, 65 years of age and older, diabetes mellitus, previous stroke or transient ischemic attack, vascular disease, 65–74 years of age, female; LAA, left atrial appendage.

(CAP2) registries have continued to demonstrate that the WATCHMAN device remains noninferior to VKAs for prevention of stroke/systemic thromboembolism, with proven lower rates of hemorrhagic stroke, nonprocedural related major bleeding, and mortality at five-year follow-up. The registries included 566 and 578 patients, respectively, meeting the inclusion/exclusion criteria from the original RCTs. The registries also compared the observed rate of ischemic stroke with the predicted rate based on CHA2DS2-VASc scores and showed that the WATCHMAN device reduced the relative risk of ischemic stroke by 78% in CAP and by 69% in CAP2. Most recently, the National Cardiovascular Data Registry (NCDR) LAAO Registry, the result of extensive collaboration between the ACC, SCAI, FDA, CMS, and Boston Scientific to help provide real-world procedural utilization and outcomes, presented its analyzed data. From 2016 to 2018, a total of 38 158 procedures from 495 hospitals in the United States were performed by 1318 physicians. In the registry, the average patient age was 76 ± 8.1, the average CHA2DS2-VASc was 4.6 ± 1.5, and the average HAS-BLED score was 3.0 ± 1.1. Implant success was 98.1%. Major in-hospital adverse events occurred in 2.16% of patients; the most common reported complications were pericardial effusion requiring intervention (1.39%) and major bleeding (1.25%).

Stroke and death were rare, below 0.20%. By the first quarter of 2019, a total of 44 950 procedures from 597 hospitals had been performed by over 1300 physicians in the United States.

In contrast to the FDA/CMS indications in the United States, the European Society of Cardiology (ESC) guidelines recommend the use of percutaneous LAAO in AF patients with a history of prior life-threatening bleeding or contraindications to long-term OAC, using dual antiplatelet therapy in the post-procedural period. The recommendation is largely based on multicenter prospective observational registries. The ASAP study included 150 patients with a mean CHA2DS2-VASc score of 4.4 ± 1.7 and contraindications to OAC who underwent LAAO with WATCHMAN. Post-procedural antithrombotic therapy consisted of six months of dual antiplatelet therapy (DAPT), with an observed ischemic stroke rate of 1.7%, representing a 77% event reduction compared to aspirin alone, based on the CHA2DS2-VASc score of the patient cohort. The EVOLUTION registry included 1020 patients with contraindication to OAC from 47 centers in the European Union who received the WATCHMAN device. The patients had mean CHA2DS2-VASc and HAS-BLED scores of 4.5 ± 1.6 and 2.3 ± 1.2, respectively, higher than patients included in previous RCTs. Device implantation was successful in 98.5% of the patients. Peri-procedural anticoagulation included VKA in 16%, no VKA in 11%, dual antiplatelet therapy in 60%, single antiplatelet therapy in 7%, and no anticoagulation in 6%. At one year, device-related thrombus (DRT) was observed in 3.7% of the patients, irrespective of the type of perioperative antithrombotic regimen (P = 0.14). The ischemic stroke rate was 1.1% (84% fewer events than expected for untreated patients). The major bleeding rate was 2.6% and was predominantly (2.3%) non-procedural-related. At two years, 85% of patients were treated with single antiplatelet or no antithrombotic therapy. The observed annual stroke rate was only 1.3%, and the combined annual endpoint of ischemic stroke and systemic embolism was 2% (83 and 80% fewer events, respectively, than expected for untreated patients). These are similar to the annualized rates of all strokes/systemic thromboembolism (1.7%) and ischemic strokes (1.6%) in the combined data from the PROTECT AF and PREVAIL RCTs (https://www.cms.gov/medicare-coverage-database/details/nca-decision-memo.aspx?NCAId=281&bc=ACAAAAAAgAAAA%3d%3d&). The rate of DRT at two years was 4.1%, with 91% of the cases identified in the first 90 days. This was comparable to the 3.7% observed in the combined analysis of PROTECT AF, PREVAIL, CAP, and CAP-2, in which the VKA/DAPT regimen was used, and the 4% reported in the ASAP study. Interestingly, the risk of stroke/systemic embolism in patients with DRT was low and not significantly different between those with and without DRT (1.7% vs. 2.2%; P = 0.8). It remains unknown if DRT is a cause or manifestation of an increased prothrombotic state, as the majority of patients with DRT do not suffer ischemic events, and the majority of patients that suffer ischemic events following LAAO do not have DRT.

Until this date, WATCHMAN is the only device approved by the FDA and CMS for LAAO. Multiple other devices are in varying stages of development/investigation. In July 2020, based on the data from the single-arm Pinnacle FLX US Investigational Device Exemption (IDE) trial, the FDA approved the newer generation WATCHMAN FLX device (https://www.fda.gov/medical-devices/recently-approved-devices/watchman-left-atrial-appendage-closure-device-delivery-system-and-watchman-flx-left-atrial-appendage). The trial enrolled 400 patients in 29 US sites, with mean CHA2DS2-VASc and HAS-BLED scores of 4.2 and 2.0, respectively. About 33% of patients had a prior major bleed or predisposition to bleeding, and 22% had a history of stroke/TIA or thromboembolism. The post-procedural antithrombotic regimen included a DOAC plus aspirin for 45 days, followed by clopidogrel plus aspirin for six months and then aspirin indefinitely. TEE was performed at 45 days and 12 months. The primary safety endpoint was the occurrence of all-cause death, ischemic stroke, systemic embolism, or device/procedure-related events requiring open cardiac surgery or major endovascular intervention between implantation and either seven days or discharge (whichever came later). The incidence of the primary safety endpoint was 0.5%, with a one-sided 95% upper confidence interval (CI) of 1.6%, meeting the performance goal of 4.2% (P < 0.0001). The newer device was successfully deployed in 98.8% of cases, with an average of 1.2 devices required per case. The rate of effective LAAO at one year was 100%, significantly above the 97% performance goal derived from the first-generation device studies (P < 0.0001). There were no cases of device embolization. The rate of DRT was 1.8%; 0.45% (two patients) developed ischemic stroke or systemic embolism, including one who died. The newer device approval indications by CMS are summarized in Table 51.3, as well as the professional societies recommended list to describe the patient population with contraindications to long-term OAC (https://www.acc.org/-/media/Non-Clinical/Files-PDFs-Excel-MS-Word-etc/Latest-in-Cardiology/Advocacy-and-Policy/advocacy_ pdf_LAA_NCD_2015_12_10.pdf?la=en&hash=81604 9C427250AC5184502AAE9EF702415485102).

4.   What are the current US society recommendations for percutaneous LAAO?

Among the most noticeable changes in the 2019 ACC/AHA Task Force on Clinical Practice Guidelines updates for the management of patients with AF, percutaneous LAAO was included as a Class IIb recommendation to be considered as a treatment option for those AF patients at an increased risk of stroke who have contraindications to long-term anticoagulation and who are at high risk of thromboembolic events.

5.   Are there additional considerations related to LAAO?

Chronic kidney disease is a well-known prothrombotic and pro-hemorrhagic condition. Worsening creatinine clearance (CrCl) is a better independent predictor of ischemic stroke/systemic embolism and bleeding than renal impairment per se. Patients with CrCl 15–29 ml/min, end-stage kidney disease with CrCl ≤ 15 ml/min, or on dialysis were excluded from the RCTs. The evidence of the benefits of OAC in these patients is limited or controversial. Data from observational studies suggest possible bleeding risk reduction by taking a DOAC compared with VKA, but there is no solid evidence for a reduction in embolic events with either new oral anticoagulants (NOACs) or VKAs, as demonstrated in a systematic review and meta-analysis. The RENAL-AF (Trial to Evaluate Anticoagulation Therapy in Hemodialysis Patients with Atrial Fibrillation) trial, investigating apixaban vs. VKA in AF patients on hemodialysis, was terminated early with inconclusive data on relative stroke and bleeding rates. Conspicuously, DOACs have not been approved in Europe for patients with CrCl ≤ 15 ml/min or on dialysis.

In contrast, our guidelines state that it may be reasonable (Class IIb) to use VKAs or apixaban for OAC in these patients. These patients, particularly if they have associated chronic anemia or thrombocytopenia, may benefit from LAAO. Routine LAAO is not necessarily being advocated, and more data are required, but it is definitely an option worth considering.

Table 51.3 Current indications for percutaneous left atrial appendage occlusion with the WATCHMAN device in the United States.

FDA WATCHMAN FLX IDE

1. Patients with AF who are at increased risk for stroke and systemic embolism based on CHADS2 or CHA2DS2-VASc scores and are recommended for anticoagulation therapy
2. Patients deemed by their physicians to be suitable for anticoagulation therapy
3. Patients who have an appropriate rationale to seek a non-pharmacologic alternative to anticoagulation therapy, taking into account the safety and effectiveness of the device compared to anticoagulation therapy

CMS National Coverage Determination

1. CHADS2 ≥2 or a CHA2DS2-VASc ≥3
2. Patients must be suitable for short-term warfarin but deemed unable to take long-term oral anticoagulation.
3. Documented evidence of a formal shared decision interaction between the patient and an independent, non-interventional physician

ACC/HRS/SCAI: Recommendations on appropriate contraindications to anticoagulation

1. History of intracranial bleeding (intracerebral or subdural) where benefits of LAAO outweigh risks
2. History of spontaneous bleeding other than intracranial (e.g. retroperitoneal bleeding)
3. Documented poor compliance with anticoagulant therapy
4. Inability or significant difficulty with maintaining patients in the therapeutic anticoagulation range
5. Intolerance of warfarin and DOACs
6. High risk of recurrent falls
7. Cognitive impairment
8. Severe renal failure
9. Occupation-related high bleeding risk
10. Need for prolonged dual antiplatelet therapy
11. Increased bleeding risk not reflected by the HAS-BLED score (e.g. thrombocytopenia, cancer, or risk of tumor-associated bleeding in case of systemic anticoagulation)
12. Other situations for which anticoagulation is inappropriate

CHA2DS2-VASc, congestive heart failure, hypertension, 65 years of age and older, diabetes mellitus, previous stroke or transient ischemic attack, vascular disease, 65–74 years of age, female; FDA, Food and Drug Administration; CMS, Center for Medicare and Medicaid Services; ACC, American College of Cardiology; HRS, Heart Rhythm Society; SCAI, Society for Cardiovascular Angiography and Interventions; LAAO, left atrial appendage occlusion; DOACs, direct-acting oral anticoagulants; HAS-BLED, hypertension, abnormal renal/liver function, stroke, bleeding history or predisposition, labile international normalized ratio, elderly, drugs/alcohol concomitantly.

Bibliography

1 Adcock, D.M. and Gosselin, R. (2015). Direct Oral Anticoagulants (DOACs) in the laboratory: 2015 review. *Thromb. Res.* 136: 7–12.

2 Benussi, S., Mazzone, P., Maccabelli, G. et al. (2011). Thoracoscopic appendage exclusion with an atriclip device as a solo treatment for focal atrial tachycardia. *Circulation* 123: 1575–1578.

3 Birman-Deych, E., Radford, M.J., Nilasena, D.S. et al. (2006). Use and effectiveness of warfarin in Medicare beneficiaries with atrial fibrillation. *Stroke* 37 (4): 1070–1074.

4 Blackshear, J.L. and Odell, J.A. (1996). Appendage obliteration to reduce stroke in cardiac surgical patients with atrial fibrillation. *Ann. Thorac. Surg.* 61 (2): 755–759.

5 Boersma, L.V., Ince, H., Kische, S. et al. (2017). EWOLUTION Investigators. Efficacy and safety of left atrial appendage closure with WATCHMAN in patients with or without contraindication to oral anticoagulation: 1-year follow-up outcome data of the EWOLUTION trial. *Heart Rhythm.* 14: 1302–1308.

6 Boersma, L.V., Schmidt, B., Betts, T.R. et al. (2016). EWOLUTION Investigators. Implant success and safety of left atrial appendage closure with the WATCHMAN device: periprocedural outcomes from the EWOLUTION registry. *Eur. Heart J.* 37: 2465–2474.

7 Bungard, T.J., Ghali, W.A., Teo, K.K. et al. (2000). Why do patients with atrial fibrillation not receive warfarin? *Arch. Intern. Med.* 160 (1): 41–46.

8 Chatterjee, S., Alexander, J.C., Pearson, P.J. et al. (2011). Left atrial appendage occlusion: lessons learned from surgical and transcatheter experiences. *Ann. Thorac. Surg.* 92: 2283–2292.

9 Coleman, C.I., Kreutz, R., Sood, N.A. et al. (2019). Rivaroxaban versus warfarin in patients with nonvalvular atrial fibrillation and severe kidney disease or undergoing hemodialysis. *Am. J. Med.* 132: 1078–1083.

10 Dukkipati, S.R., Kar, S., Holmes, D.R. et al. (2018). Device-related thrombus after left atrial appendage closure. *Circulation* 138: 874–885.

11 Fauchier, L., Bisson, A., Clementy, N. et al. (2018). Changes in glomerular filtration rate and outcomes in patients with atrial fibrillation. *Am. Heart J.* 198: 39–45.

12 Freeman, J.V., Varosy, P., Price, M.J. et al. (2020). The NCDR left atrial appendage occlusion registry. *J. Am. Coll. Cardiol.* 75 (13): 1503–1518.

13 Girotra, T., Lekoubou, A., Bishu, K.G., and Ovbiagele, B. (2020). A contemporary and comprehensive analysis of the costs of stroke in the United States. *J. Neurol. Sci.* 410: 116643.

14 Ha, J.T., Neuen, B.L., Cheng, L.P. et al. (2019). Benefits and harms of oral anticoagulant therapy in chronic kidney disease: a systematic review and metaanalysis. *Ann. Intern. Med.* 171: 181–189.

15 Hart, R.G., Pearce, L.A., and Aguilar, M.I. (2007). Metanalysis: antithrombotic therapy to prevent stroke in patients who have nonvalvular atrial fibrillation. *Ann. Intern. Med.* 146 (12): 857–867.

16 Healey, J.S., Crystal, E., Lamy, A. et al. (2005). Left Atrial Appendage Occlusion Study (LAAOS): results of a randomized controlled pilot study of left atrial appendage occlusion during coronary bypass surgery in patients at risk for stroke. *Am. Heart J.* 150: 288–293.

17 Holmes, D.R. Jr., Kar, S., Price, M.J. et al. (2014). Prospective randomized evaluation of the Watchman Left Atrial Appendage Closure device in patients with atrial fibrillation versus long-term warfarin therapy: the PREVAIL trial. *J. Am. Coll. Cardiol.* 64 (1): 1–12.

18 January, C.T., Wann, L.S., Alpert, J.S. et al. (2014). ACC/AHA Task Force Members. 2014 AHA/ACC/HRS guideline for the management of patients with atrial fibrillation: a report of the American College of Cardiology/American Heart Association Task Force on practice guidelines and the Heart Rhythm Society. *Circulation* 130 (23): e199–e267.

19 January, C.T., Wann, L.S., Calkins, H. et al. (2019). 2019 AHA/ACC/HRS focused update of the 2014 AHA/ACC/HRS guideline for the management of patients with atrial fibrillation: a report of the American College of Cardiology/American Heart Association task force on clinical practice guidelines and the Heart Rhythm Society

in collaboration with the Society of Thoracic Surgeons. *Circulation* 140 (2): e125–e151.

20 Kanderian, A.S., Gillinov, A.M., Pettersson, G.B. et al. (2008). Success of surgical left atrial appendage closure: assessment by transesophageal echocardiography. *J. Am. Coll. Cardiol.* 52: 924–929.

21 Kar, S., Doshi, S.K., Sadhu, A. et al. (2021). PINNACLE FLX Investigators. Primary outcome evaluation of a next-generation left atrial appendage closure device: results from the PINNACLE FLX trial. *Circulation* 143 (18): 1754–1762.

22 Kimmel, S.E., Chen, Z., Price, M. et al. (2007). The influence of patient adherence on anticoagulation control with warfarin: results from the Inter- national Normalized Ratio Adherence and Genetics (IN-RANGE) Study. *Arch. Intern. Med.* 167: 229–235.

23 Lin, H.J., Wolf, P.A., Kelly-Hayes, M. et al. (1996). Stroke severity in atrial fibrillation. The Framingham Study. *Stroke* 27: 1760–1764.

24 Lloyd-Jones, D.M., Wang, T.J., Leip, E.P. et al. (2004). Life- time risk for development of atrial fibrillation: the Framingham Heart Study. *Circulation* 110: 1042–1046.

25 López-López, J.A., Sterne, J.A.C., Thom, H.H.Z. et al. (2017). Oral anticoagulants for prevention of stroke in atrial fibrillation: systematic review, network metaanalysis, and cost effectiveness analysis. *BMJ* 359: j5058.

26 Masoudi, F.A., Calkins, H., Kavinsky, C.J. et al. (2015). 2015 ACC/HRS/SCAI left atrial appendage occlusion device societal overview. *Heart Rhythm* 12: e122–e136.

27 Meier, B., Blaauw, Y., Khattab, A.A. et al. (2014). Document Reviewers. EHRA/EAPCI expert consensus statement on catheter-based left atrial appendage occlusion. *Europace* 16 (10): 1397–1416.

28 Olesen, J.B., Lip, G.Y., Kamper, A.L. et al. (2012). Stroke and bleeding in atrial fibrillation with chronic kidney disease. *N. Engl. J. Med.* 367: 625–635.

29 Ozaki, A.F., Choi, A.S., Le, Q.T. et al. (2020). Real-world adherence and persistence to direct oral anticoagulants in patients with atrial fibrillation: a systematic review and metaanalysis. *Circ. Cardiovasc. Qual. Outcomes.* 13 (3): e005969.

30 Price, M. (2019). *Transcatheter LAA Occlusion in the United States - Update from the NCDR LAAO Registry*. San Francisco, CA, USA: TCT.

31 Randhawa, M.S., Vishwanath, R., Rai, M.P. et al. (2020). Association between use of warfarin for atrial fibrillation and outcomes among patients with end-stage renal disease: a systematic review and metaanalysis. *JAMA Netw. Open.* 3 (4): e202175.

32 Reddy, V.Y., Doshi, S.K., Kar, S. et al. (2017). PREVAIL and PROTECT AF Investigators. 5-year outcomes after left atrial appendage closure: from the PREVAIL and PROTECT AF trials. *J. Am. Coll. Cardiol.* 70: 2964–2975.

33 Reddy, V.Y., Möbius-Winkler, S., Miller, M.A. et al. (2013). Left atrial appendage closure with the Watchman de-vice in patients with a contraindication for oral anticoagulation: the ASAP study (ASA Plavix Feasibility Study With Watchman Left Atrial Appendage Closure Technology). *J. Am. Coll. Cardiol.* 61: 2551–2556.

34 Reddy, V.Y., Sievert, H., Halperin, J. et al. (2014). Percutaneous left atrial appendage closure vs warfarin for atrial fibrillation. A randomized clinical trial. *JAMA* 312 (19): 1988–1998.

35 Schein, J.R., White, C.M., Nelson, W.W. et al. (2016). Vitamin K antagonist use: evidence of the difficulty of achieving and maintaining target INR range and subsequent consequences. *Thromb. J.* 14: 14.

36 Siontis, K.C., Zhang, X., Eckard, A. et al. (2018). Outcomes associated with apixaban use in patients with end-stage kidney dis- ease and atrial fibrillation in the United States. *Circulation* 138: 1519–1529.

37 Stroke Risk in Atrial Fibrillation Working Group (2007). Independent predictors of stroke in patients with atrial fibrillation: a systematic review. *Neurology* 69 (6): 546–554.

38 Weimar, T., Vosseler, M., Czesla, M. et al. (2012). Approaching a paradigm shift: endoscopic ablation of lone atrial fibrilla- tion on the beating heart. *Ann. Thorac. Surg.* 94: 1886–1892.

52

Imaging for LAA Interventions

Ignacio Cruz- Gonzalez, Ana E. Laffond and Manuel Barreiro-Perez[1]

[1] University Hospital of Salamanca, Salamanca, Spain

Cardiac CT Pre-procedural Planning

1. What are the main objectives of pre-procedural cardiac tomography in left atrium appendage occlusion?

Cardiac tomography (CT) is a noninvasive technique with high spatial resolution, which allows 3D and multiplanar imaging acquisition. When performed in candidates for left atrial appendage occlusion (LAAO), it should focus on determining the feasibility of the procedure, providing accurate sizing of left atrial appendage (LAA) dimensions, LAA morphology, exclusion of LAA thrombus and peri-procedural planning (Table 52.1).

2. How should the patient be prepared before CT?

The patient should receive a comprehensive and understandable explanation of the procedure and provide written informed consent. The last glomerular filtration rate (GFR) should be reviewed. When inferior to 30 ml/min/1.73 m^2, 3D transesophageal echocardiogram (TEE) should be considered as an alternative. A venous line should be obtained, ideally located in the antecubital fossa and at least 18 gauge.

As LAA dimensions are influenced by loading conditions, the scan should be performed with patients in the non-fasting state. A further oral intake of 250 ml of water might be considered upon arrival. If the patient is in the fasting state for other reasons, an intravenous 5–10 ml/kg fluid infusion may be administered. In subjects on chronic hemodialysis, the scan shall be performed before the dialysis session. Caffeinated drinks before the procedure should be avoided. Routine use of beta-blockers or sublingual nitroglycerine is not recommended, although it may be considered to improve the study's quality or when the evaluation of the coronary anatomy is required.

3. What is the technical protocol for imaging acquisition?

The study should be acquired with ECG gating. To reduce radiation exposure, a prospective electrocardiographically gated acquisition is preferred. Images should be obtained in a phase corresponding to 30–60% of the cardiac cycle when the LAA dimension is the largest and with the narrowest predefined R-R interval possible. Tube potential and current should be set depending on body mass index (BMI), vendor specifications, and local protocols. A topogram is necessary to guarantee coverage of the LAAO area, and the complete inclusion of the cardiac silhouette is recommended. Contrast should be injected with a biphasic protocol at 5–7 ml/s, followed by a saline chaser of 50 ml. To ensure adequate synchronization of scan sequence, a bolus-tracking technique with a region of interest in the ascending aorta should be used. After obtaining ECG-gated images of the heart and the LAA, it is highly advisable to perform delayed imaging acquisition to exclude the presence of thrombus. Images are acquired 60–90 seconds from the initial scan (the arterial phase), enabling contrast distribution and preventing low-flow artifacts. The delayed acquisition does not require further contrast administration and is performed at low tube voltage (80–100 kV) and covering the LAA area.

Mastering Structural Heart Disease, First Edition. Edited by Eduardo J. de Marchena and Camilo A. Gomez.
© 2023 John Wiley & Sons Ltd. Published 2023 by John Wiley & Sons Ltd.
Companion website: www.wiley.com/go/deMarchena/Mastering-Structural-Heart-Disease

Table 52.1 Key elements to be described in a cardiac tomography scan report before the left atrial appendage occlusion procedure.

Thrombus

- Report the presence/absence of contrast repletion in both phases (early and delayed).
- In the event of a repletion defect, describe its shape and attenuation value compared with descending aorta.

Morphology and measurement of the landing zone

- Describe morphology (chicken wing, cactus, cauliflower, windsock, whale-tail, cone-shaped) and the presence of additional proximal lobes. In chicken-wing-shaped left atrial appendage (LAA), the distance from the ostium and first curvature should be reported.
- Measure the LAA depth and length.
- Measure the landing zone as specified by the device manufacturer. The shape of the landing zone should be described.
- Define the optimal fluoroscopic projection angle.

Relevant anatomical aspects

- Report the presence of interatrial septal aneurysm, patent foramen ovale, interatrial communication, lipomatous hypertrophy of the interatrial septum, or other anatomical anomalies.
- Describe the left atrium absolute and indexed sizing.
- Describe pulmonary veins anatomy.
- Report the presence of pericardial effusion.

Optional aspects

- Describe the coronary anatomy and presence of coronary artery disease.
- Valvular anatomy and calcification.
- Distance from the landing zone to the pulmonary artery.

---

4. Explain how to exclude the presence of thrombus in the LAA with CT

To exclude the presence of thrombus, images in the arterial and delayed phase should be acquired. The absence of contrast repletion in the arterial but not in the venous phase is interpreted as low flow. Lack of repletion in both phases is highly suggestive of the presence of thrombus and should be confirmed with other imaging techniques (i.e. TEE) (Figure 52.1).

5. How is anatomic feasibility of LAAO assessed by CT?

The CT report should reflect LAA morphology and dimensions to allow optimal device selection and procedure planning:

LAA morphology. The morphological classification is based on compared anatomy (chicken wing, cactus, cauliflower, windsock, whale tail, cone-shaped). It is best assessed in the volume-rendered 3D reconstruction.

LAA sizing. LAA sizing is performed with multiplanar reconstruction. The definition of the landing zone is variable and depends on the type of device, which should be considered during interpretation. However, certain general principles should be followed in all cases. From the axial acquisition, a two-chamber long-axis oblique view is obtained. The crosshairs are positioned at the base of the LAA, with the axes aligned with the left upper pulmonary vein and the left circumflex coronary artery. Multiplanar

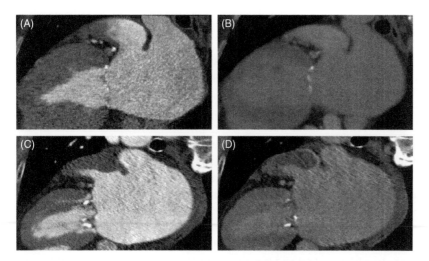

Figure 52.1 Differential diagnosis of left atrial appendage (LAA) thrombus and low flow. Arterial phase images (a, c) show a lack of repletion of the LAA in both cases. However, the defect is only visible in the venous phase in the second case. (b) LAA by CT. (d) Thrombus.

reconstruction generates an en face view of the landing zone, and measurements are obtained after polygon reduction. Usually, device size is based on the maximum diameter of the landing zone. LAA depth (perpendicular distance from the landing zone to the LAA wall) and length (distance from the landing zone to the dominant lobe end) should be reported. Spatial relationship and distance to neighboring structures, such as the left circumflex coronary artery, should also be assessed. Finally, to guarantee adequate transseptal crossing, a description of atrial septal anatomy, the spatial relationship to the LAA ostium, and the optimal C-arm angulation during the procedure is advisable.

TEE Pre-procedural Planning

6. What is the role of transthoracic echocardiography (TTE) before LAA closure procedure?

TTE is used to assess LA dimensions and volumes and left ventricle (LV) function and to exclude contraindications for LA closure. However, the role of TTE in pre-procedural planning of LAAO is limited, as the LAA cannot be adequately evaluated with TTE alone.

7. What are the objectives of TEE in pre-procedural planning for LAAO?

As with pre-procedural CT, the objectives of TEE before an LAAO procedure are to evaluate the 3D geometry of LA/LAA and its relationship to major structures, exclude the presence of LA or LAA thrombus, and provide procedural guidance. TEE is the reference imaging technique for assessing LAA thrombus and should be used to support diagnosis when LAA thrombosis is suspected in a CT scan. The use of echocardiographic contrast can enhance its diagnostic performance, particularly in the presence of artifacts or sludge.

8. How should the measurements of the LAA be performed during pre-procedural TEE?

Measurements should be performed at ventricular telesystole and under normal LA filling conditions. Imaging of the LAA is best obtained with a multiplane approach, with long-axis and short-axis views and with the use of 3D TEE. The probe should be placed at the mid-esophagus, and interrogation of the LAA from 0° to 180° should be performed. At least four planes should be recorded (usually at 0°, 45°, 90°, and 135°), where measurements are made. Specific indications on how these measurements are performed should follow the manufacturer's instructions, as they depend on the type of the device. Landing zone and LAA orifice measurements, as well as LAA depth, should be reported. Additionally, the length of the anchoring lobe (in the expected axis of the device) should be indicated (Figure 52.2).

9. What is the advantage of using 3D TEE compared with 2D TEE?

Although 2D offers higher-resolution images, different studies have reported 3D TEE to provide more accurate diameters of the LAA and LAA orifice compared with 2D TEE. 3D TEE allows better differentiation between adjacent structures and provides a more thorough examination of the LAA. While TEE tends to underestimate LAA sizing in relation to CT, real-time 3D TEE is less biased and shows a higher correlation with CT for assessing the LAA orifice area.

10. Apart from LAA sizing, what other information is relevant during pre-procedural planning with TEE?

The angle between the ostium, neck, and main anchoring lobe should be reported, as transseptal puncture may be conditioned by these measurements. Furthermore, LAA morphology, the number and origin of additional LAA lobes, and the relationship of the LAA to other atrial structures should be assessed.

11. Which imaging technique is preferred for pre-procedural planning for LAAO?

Both TEE and CT are adequate techniques for pre-procedural imaging. CT is a noninvasive technique with higher spatial resolution, which provides better morphological assessment and sizing accuracy. Therefore, CT is the preferred imaging modality for pre-procedural planning. On the other hand, TEE is more widely available and prevents further radiation and iodinated contrast administration – it is preferable in patients with severe renal impairment. Furthermore, TEE is the gold standard to exclude the presence of thrombus, although CT with protocol adaptation can achieve high positive and negative predictive values (Table 52.2).

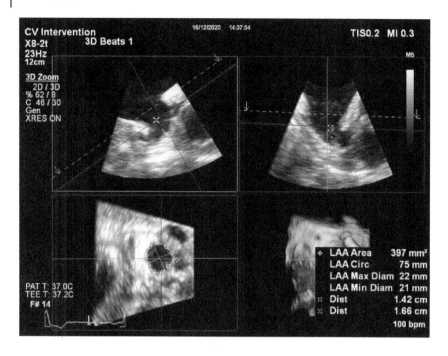

Figure 52.2 Left atrial appendage (LAA) sizing with multiplanar transesophageal echocardiography. LAA area, circumference, and maximum and minimum diameters are reported. Measurements have been performed with specific software that automatically provides the landing zone diameters without the need for user intervention.

Table 52.2 Comparison between transesophageal echocardiography (TEE) and computerized tomography (CT) in left atrial appendage occlusion (LAAO) pre-procedural planning.

	TEE	CT
Availability	+++	+
Noninvasive	No	Yes
Radiation	No	Yes
Iodinated contrast	No	Yes
3D imaging	Only on (3D-TEE)	Yes
Spatial resolution (mm)	0.5 × 1 mm (2D) 0.5 × 1.2 × 1.2 (3D)	0.3–0.6
Temporal resolution (ms)	20 (2D), 50 (3D)	50–100

Intra-procedural TEE and ICE Guided Intervention

12. Which imaging modalities can be used for intra-procedural guidance in LAA closure?

Multiplanar 2D TEE is the most commonly used imaging modality for intra-procedural guidance. However, real-time 3D TEE can provide a single-view composition of

LAA, wires, catheters, and devices, facilitating device alignment and deployment. Therefore, the optimal guidance of the procedure is performed using 2D and 3D TEE in combination. Transoral micro-TEE probes are a safe and effective alternative to conventional TEE and allow to perform the procedure under conscious sedation. Another alternative modality that may be used to guide the procedure is intracardiac echocardiography (ICE). This modality does not require general anesthesia but does not provide multiplanar views and implies the need for further vascular access to insert the probe (Table 52.3, Figure 52.3).

13. What are the main objectives of intra-procedural TEE during LAAO?

TEE is the gold standard imaging technique to guide LAAO. During the procedure, real-time echocardiographic guidance is crucial to guide the transseptal puncture, catheter position in LAA, and device delivery, as well as to verify LAA optimal sealing and identify immediate complications. Before transseptal puncture, the presence of thrombus in the LAA should be excluded once again, and LAA morphology and dimensions should be reassessed to guarantee optimal device type and size choice.

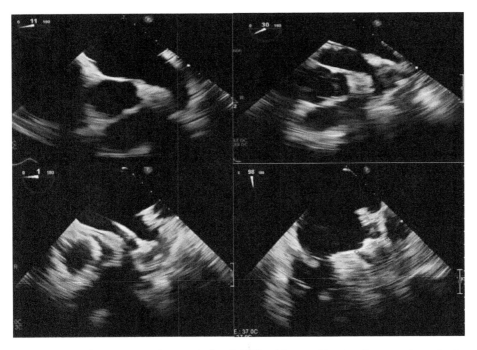

Figure 52.3 Left atrial appendage occlusion (LAAO) guidance with micro-transesophageal echocardiography: progression of catheter and sheath within the left atrium, device deployment, and final result.

Table 52.3 Comparison between conventional transesophageal echocardiography (TEE), transesophageal echocardiography with micro-probes (micro-TEE), and intracardiac echocardiography (ICE) for left atrial appendage occlusion (LAAO) intra-procedural guidance.

	2D and 3D TEE	Micro-TEE	ICE
Image quality	+++	++	++
Multiplanar view/3D	Yes	No	No/Yes with 4D ICE
General anesthesia	Usually needed	Not needed	Not needed
Additional vascular access	No	No	Yes
Procedure duration	Longer	Shorter	Longer
Experience	+++	++	+

14. What are the best perspectives for each of the steps of the procedure?

- *Transseptal crossing:* 2D TEE bicaval plane, 3D visualization of tenting of the atrial septum, and transseptal puncture from a lateral perspective.
- *Position of the catheter and sheath in the LA:* Acquire an en face view of the LAA orifice and then angulate to display the tip of the catheter. Obtain a long-axis view to

establish the relation of the catheter, LAA wall, and LAA lobes.
- *Expansion of the device:* In the same view as the previous, to simultaneously visualize the edges of the lobe and LAA orifice as the device is deployed.
- *Deployment control:* Obtain an overhead perspective of LAA to confirm complete occlusion of the LAA by the device. 2D TEE color Doppler is used to evaluate the presence and severity of peri-device leak (Figure 52.4).

15. Explain how transseptal puncture is guided with TEE

Although transseptal puncture may be performed with only fluoroscopy guidance by experienced operators, intra-procedural TEE use has demonstrated lower rates of complications. The safest point for transseptal crossing is the inferior region of the fossa ovalis. To locate the fossa ovalis, an en face view from the right atrial perspective may be particularly helpful, as it matches the fluoroscopic right anterior oblique projection. To determine whether the location of the catheter is optimal within the fossa ovalis, the point of "tenting" (deformation of the interatrial septum caused by the pressure of the tip of the catheter) should be identified. The interatrial septum is visualized in 2D TEE bicaval plane. When using 3D TEE, a lateral

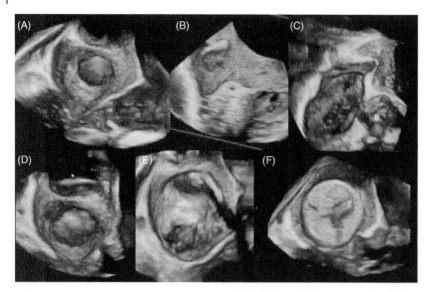

Figure 52.4 3D transesophageal echocardiography intra-procedural guidance: en face view of the left atrial appendage (LAA); transseptal puncture; sheath progression within the LAA; device deployment.

perspective should be obtained, rotating from left to right around the y-axis from the en-face view.

16. When is the device considered to be correctly placed within the LAA?

The occluder device should be centered within the LAA below the ostium or at the ostial plane. Definition of adequate device positioning depends on the type of device used:

- FLX: PASS criteria
  - **P**osition: Device is at the ostium of the LAA:
  - **A**nchor: Fixation anchors are engaged/device is stable
  - **S**ize: Device is compressed 10–30% of the original size.
  - **S**eal: Device spans the ostium, and all lobes of LAA are covered.
- Amulet: CLOSE criteria
  - **C**X: Two-thirds of the device lobe are distal to the left circumflex artery.
  - **L**obe compression.
  - **O**rientation of the device: axis of device lobe in line with the axis of the LAA neck.
  - **S**eparation between the device lobe and disc.
  - **E**lliptical: concave disc.
- Lambre: COST criteria
  - Umbrella deployed beyond **C**ircumflex artery
  - Umbrella was full **O**pen.
  - Peridevice optimal **S**ealing.
  - Device stability confirmed by **T**ug test.

17. When intracardiac echocardiography is used to guide TEE, where should the probe be placed?

Contrary to TEE, ICE probes are positioned at a fixed point and only provide a bidimensional view. Therefore, the choice of the positioning of the probe significantly influences the quality of the LAA view. The most frequent place for probe positioning is the left atrium (LA), which requires advancing the ICE probe through the interatrial septum. Although it provides a good LAA view, the position of the probe is unstable, and repositioning the probe might be necessary throughout the procedure. Furthermore, as the probe is placed inside the LA, it may interfere with manipulating the catheter and sheath system.

Alternative probe locations include the right atrium (RA), the pulmonary artery, and the upper left pulmonary vein. The RA prevents transseptal crossing of the probe, but the view of the LAA is unsatisfactory and therefore is not recommended as the standard positioning. Positioning the probe in the pulmonary artery does not require transseptal crossing, although placing the probe might be particularly challenging. Locating de probe in the upper pulmonary vein usually provides a good, stable LAA view and prevents interference with the delivery system. However, in certain cases, the upper pulmonary vein may be located distantly from the LAA, and the image quality may be suboptimal (Figure 52.5).

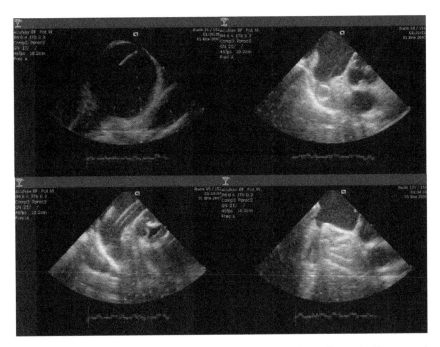

Figure 52.5 Intra-procedural guidance with intracardiac echocardiography. Transseptal puncture; device progression; device deployment; final result.

18. What are the advantages of double transseptal puncture for ICE probe transseptal crossing?

When using the single transseptal puncture approach, the subsequent atrial septal defect is usually larger. Furthermore, the probe's position is more unstable, and it interferes more frequently with the delivery system due to its closer positioning. On the other hand, when using a double transseptal approach, the probe position is more stable and provides complete LA and delivery system visualization. On the other hand, a second transseptal puncture can theoretically increase the risks inherent to the transseptal puncture, such as perforation, air embolism, and thromboembolism.

19. Is ICE a safe and effective alternative to TEE for intra-procedural LAAO guidance?

Several studies, including one metaanalysis of both prospective and retrospective studies, have reported similar success and complication rates for ICE and TEE for LAAO guidance. However, some groups have reported longer procedure duration and higher radiation doses with ICE. ICE probes are significantly more expensive, although the final cost might be reduced because the procedure does not require an additional operator to manipulate the probe or an anesthetist. The use of conscious sedation rather than general anesthesia has not been associated with lower complication rates or shorter length of stay in these patients (Figure 52.6).

Bibliography

1 Barreiro-Perez, M., Cruz-Gonzalez, I., Moreno-Samos, J.C. et al. (2019). Feasibility, safety, and utility of microtransesophageal echocardiography guidance for percutaneous LAAO under conscious sedation. *JACC: Cardiovasc. Interv.* 12 (11): 1091–1093.

2 Beigel, R., Wunderlich, N.C., Ho, S.Y. et al. (2014). The left atrial appendage: anatomy, function, and noninvasive evaluation. *JACC: Cardiovasc. Imaging* 7 (12): 1251–1265.

3 Faletra, F.F. (2014). 3D TEE during catheter-based interventions. *JACC: Cardiovasc. Imaging* 7 (3): 292–308.

4 Faletra, F.F., Pedrazzini, G., Pastti, E. et al. (2021). Imaging for patient's selection and guidance of LAA and ASD percutaneous and surgical closure. *JACC: Cardiovasc. Imaging* 14 (1): 3–21.

5 Korsholm, K., Berti, S., Iriart, X. et al. (2020). Expert recommendations on cardiac computed tomography for

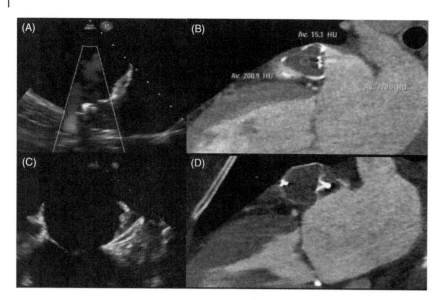

Figure 52.6 Post-procedural follow-up with cardiac tomography and transesophageal echocardiography. Imaging follow-up should assess the presence of (a, b) peridevice leaks and (c, d) thrombus formation.

planning transcatheter left atrial appendage occlusion. *JACC: Cardiovasc. Interv.* 13 (3): 277–292.

6 Mráz, T., Neuzil, P., Mandysova, E. et al. (2007). Role of echocardiography in percutaneous occlusion of the left atrial appendage. *Echocardiography* 24 (4): 401–404.

7 Nielsen-Kudsk, J.E., Berti, S., De Backer, O. et al. (2019). Use of intracardiac compared with transesophageal echocardiography for left atrial appendage occlusion in the amulet observational study. *JACC: Cardiovasc. Interv.* 12 (11): 1030–1039.

8 Nucifora, G., Faletra, F.F., Regoli, F. et al. (2011). Evaluation of the left atrial appendage with real-time 3-dimensional transesophageal echocardiography implications for catheter-based left atrial appendage closure. *Circ. Cardiovasc. Imaging* 4 (5): 514–523.

9 Pathan, F., Hecht, H., Narula, J. et al. (2018). Roles of transesophageal echocardiography and cardiac computed tomography for evaluation of left atrial thrombus and associated pathology: a review and critical analysis. *JACC: Cardiovasc. Imaging* 11 (4): 616–627.

10 Patti, G. (2019). Intracardiac versus transesophageal echocardiography for assisting percutaneous left atrial appendage occlusion?: "Veni, vidi, vICE"! *JACC: Cardiovasc. Interv.* 12 (11): 1040–1043.

11 Velagapudi, P., Turagam, M.K., Kolt, D. et al. (2019). Intracardiac vs transesophageal echocardiography for percutaneous left atrial appendage occlusion: a meta-analysis. *J. Cardiovasc. Electrophysiol.* 30 (4): 461–467.

12 Wunderlich, N.C., Beigel, R., Swaans, M.J. et al. (2015). Percutaneous interventions for left atrial appendage exclusion: Options, assessment, and imaging using 2D and 3D echocardiography. *JACC: Cardiovasc. Imaging* 8 (4): 472–488.

53

Devices for Left Atrial Appendage Closure

Pedro F. Gomes Nicz[1,4], Guilherme Bratz[1], Rogério Sarmento-Leite[2,3], and Fábio S. de Brito, Jr[1,4]

[1] *Structural Heart Disease Intervention, Interventional Cardiology Department at Heart Institute (InCor), University of São Paulo, São Paulo, São Paulo, Brazil*
[2] *Interventional Cardiology at Heart Institute, Fundação Universitária de Cardiologia (IC – FUC), Porto Alegre, Rio Grande do Sul, Brazil*
[3] *Interventional Cardiology at Hospital Moinhos de Vento, Porto Alegre, Rio Grande do Sul, Brazil*
[4] *Interventional Cardiology at Hospital Sírio Libanês, São Paulo, São Paulo, Brazil*

1. LAA occlusion: does one device fit all?

The left atrial appendage (LAA) is a finger-like heart structure coated with trabeculated pectinate muscle and located anterolaterally in the atrioventricular groove. This embryonic remnant is typically the smallest part of the left atrium (LA), but it is the most variable anatomically. Its wide variability in size and shape confers to the LAA a fingerprint-like characteristic.

The LAA anatomy is classically divided into two components: an ostium, which connects the lobar region of the LAA to the left atrial body, and the lobar region with its anatomical variability. An autopsy study found that 54% of LAAs had two lobs, 23% had three lobes, 20% had one lobe, and 3% had four lobes. Furthermore, there is significant variability within each of these groups, as many lobes are subdivided internally into progressively smaller parts. These characteristics were categorized in four recognizable patterns: chicken wing, cactus, windsock, and cauliflower (Figure 53.1); nevertheless, sometimes it is not easy to classify the anatomical shape as one of these types. In these cases, a careful anatomical assessment of the ostium and landing zone should be performed.

Considering this wide anatomic spectrum, noninvasive methods such as cardiac computed tomography angiography (CCTA) and transesophageal echocardiogram (TEE), especially three-dimensional echocardiography (3D echo), play an important role in procedural planning, helping either to choose the best device for each patient or to predict the risk of complications. So, anatomy matters, and one device does not fit all!

2. What are the main differences among LAA occlusion device designs?

Taking into account the risk of thrombus formation and unique LAA anatomical characteristics, many types of devices have been developed to close the LAA and mitigate the risk of stroke. Ideally, the device should have three important characteristics:

- *Ease of use:* The device should fit easily in a wide spectrum of LAA anatomies.
- *Safety:* Low rates of procedural complications and device thrombus formation.
- *Efficacy:* Complete exclusion of the LAA from circulation and reduction of stroke rate.

There are several methods of LAA occlusion (LAAO), including percutaneous or surgical approaches. Current catheter-based devices can be divided based on three principles:

- *Plug:* A device lobe or umbrella is used to occlude the neck of the LAA in order to prevent blood flow into the body of the LAA. LAA exclusion relies on sealing/endocardialization of the device. These devices include the WATCHMAN (Boston Scientific) and WaveCrest (Biosense Webster).
- *Lobe and disc:* A device lobe or umbrella with an additional disc is used to seal the ostium of the LAA from the left atrial side. LAA exclusion relies on sealing/endocardialization by the device lobe/umbrella and/or by the sealing disc. These devices include the Amplatzer

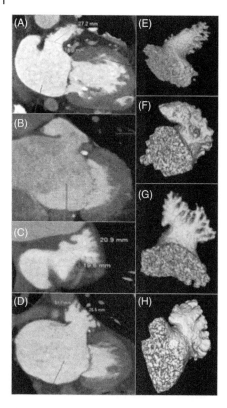

Figure 53.1 Cardiac computed tomography angiography illustration of left atrial appendage shapes. (a, e) Windsock; (b, f) retroflex chicken-wing; (c, g) cactus; (d, h) cauliflower. *Source:* Reprinted from Michael et al. (2020), European Society of Cardiology.

Cardiac Plug (ACP), Amulet (both Abbott Vascular), Ultraseal (Cardia), and LAmbre (Lifetech).

- *Ligation:* The Lariat (SentreHEART) is a snare is used to ligate the body of the LAA using an endocardial and epicardial approach. LAA exclusion relies on complete ligation of the neck of the LAA.

These devices are made with Nitinol, and their implantation is performed either by pushing the device out of a specific delivery sheath, retracting the sheath, or a combination of both maneuvers.

3. What are the characteristic of the WATCHMAN FLX device?

The WATCHMAN 2.5 LAAO device has demonstrated high procedural success rates and favorable clinical efficacy outcomes. However, in some challenging anatomies, such as a chicken-wing-shaped LAA with a short proximal segment associated with a broad landing zone, or some shallow LAAs, optimal implantation is not always possible.

WATCHMAN FLX, the new generation of WATCHMAN device, is a Nitinol-based device, fully recapturable, and repositionable. To overcome the limitations of the previous version of the device, the WATCHMAN FLX incorporates some novel features designed to simplify its implantation, reduce peri-procedural complications, and improve long-term device success. Its major improvements are as follows (Figure 53.2):

- 10–20% device length reduction, which facilitates device deployment in shallow anatomies. The minimum required LAA depth for safe implantation is 50% of the device size.
- Atraumatic closed distal end with a fluoroscopic mark (vs. an open end), which allows device advancement into the LAA in a "ball" configuration, reducing the likelihood of perforation.
- 18J-shaped anchors distributed in two rows to improve fixation.

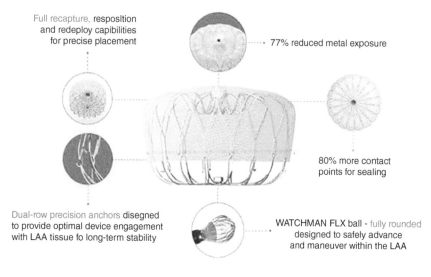

Full recapture, resposition and redeploy capibilities for precise placement

77% reduced metal exposure

80% more contact points for sealing

Dual-row precision anchors disegned to provide optimal device engagement with LAA tissue fo long-term stability

WATCHMAN FLX ball - fully rounded designed to safely advance and maneuver within the LAA

Figure 53.2 WATCHMAN FLX LAA closure device features. *Source:* Courtesy of Boston Scientific.

- Less metal exposure. The extended polyester fabric coverage reduces peri-device leak, and the delivery cable screw is recessed to reduce the risk of device-related thrombosis.
- The size range is broader (20–35 mm in five sizes: 20, 24, 27, 31, and 35 mm) than that of the previous version (21–33 mm), allowing implantation in a wider range of anatomies (LAA sizes ranging from 14 to 31.5 mm).

Pre-procedural planning can be done with either TEE or CCTA and is essential for understanding the LAA morphology and evaluating its dimensions. The WATCHMAN landing zone is located between the left circumflex coronary artery (LCx), at the inferior part of the ostial plane, at a point 1–2 cm distal to the left upper superior vein ridge. Sizing is performed using the maximal LAA landing zone dimension. The device should be selected to obtain a final compression between 10 and 30%, according to the manufacturer's instructions, but most operators prefer a compression rate of over 15%.

The first step of the procedure is the transseptal puncture (TSP). LAAO is advised to cross the atrial septum through an inferior and posterior position at the fossa ovalis, aiming to achieve a coaxial alignment between the delivery system and the LAA. Through a stiff guidewire placed within the left upper pulmonary vein, the delivery system is introduced into the LA and, assisted by a pigtail catheter, advanced into the LAA. At this moment, an angiogram is usually performed. The selected WATCHMAN FLX device should be placed at the tip of the delivery system and then unsheathed to form a ball. After achieving the device's final position, its deployment can be done by either unsheathing, pushing forward on the delivery cable, or a combination of both. Finally, device position, anchoring, size, and sealing (PASS criteria) should be checked using an echocardiogram and angiogram before full device release.

After a successful procedure, WATCHMAN trials usually suggest oral anticoagulation with warfarin and aspirin for 45 days. A TEE is advised at 45 days; in the absence of severe leaks (>5 mm), anticoagulation is stopped and dual antiplatelet therapy (DAPT) initiated and maintained for at least six months, with aspirin alone thereafter. This pharmacological scheme should be adjusted according to the patient's bleeding risk.

4. What are the characteristics of the Amulet device?

The Amulet, a second-generation Amplatzer LAAO device, is a self-expandable Nitinol-based LAA occluder that forms one lobe and a larger disc with polyester fabric and peripheral fixation hooks. This device, implanted through a 12- or 14-Fr delivery sheath, works by multiple mechanisms of occlusion with the lobe and disc, together with the polyester mesh, which is supposed to provide a superior seal of the LAA (Figure 53.3).

Although its design is similar to that of the ACP, the Amulet device has a wider lobe, a longer waist, a recessed proximal end screw, and more stabilizing wires. These adjustments were made to improve stability and reduce the risk of thrombus formation. The device comes in eight sizes covering a wide range of LAA landing zone sizes (from 12.6 mm to 32 mm). Its sizing is determined by the landing zone's widest diameter. The recommendation is to upsize this measure by 2–4 mm with the Amulet. The landing zone can be measured by TEE or CCTA, and it is located 12–15 mm from the LAA orifice (echocardiographic LAA ostium).

The procedure consists of an inferior and posterior TSP followed by placement of the specific delivery sheath at the LAA landing zone. After that, the planned device is advanced to the tip of the sheath. At this point, the first step of the deployment is unsheathing by pulling the delivery sheath. Once the ball is formed, the device can be moved (backward or forward) to achieve an optimal position. Then the entire lobe and disc are deployed, and imaging is used to confirm appropriate implantation. If there is any concern about the device's position or fixation, the device can be easily recaptured and repositioned.

Optimal deployment should achieve five criteria before the ACP/Amulet device is released:

1) A tire-shaped lobe ensures adequate compression of the lobe and engagement of stabilizing wire.
2) The distance between the lobe and disc ensures that the disc is pulled against the LAA orifice, providing a good seal.
3) The concavity of the disc indicates traction of the disc against the lobe, with a good seal.
4) The lobe axis is perpendicular to the neck axis at the landing zone with contact of the lobe and stabilizing wires against the LAA.
5) The lobe is ≥2/3 within the LCx, which ensures that the device is deep enough.

If any doubt remains about the device's stability, a gentle tug test can be performed. At the final position, echocardiographic assessment and fluoroscopy are important to detect and quantify any residual leaks and confirm the device's position and an absence of complications. The last step is to release the device from its cable and take the delivery sheath out of the LAA.

Despite the absence of randomized data regarding antithrombotic therapy after a successful ACP/Amulet

DISC

Designed to completely
seal the LAA at the orifice.

STABILIZING WIRES

Engage with the wall of the LAA
and help hold the device in place.

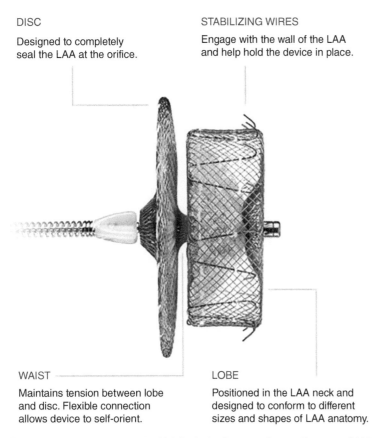

WAIST

Maintains tension between lobe
and disc. Flexible connection
allows device to self-orient.

LOBE

Positioned in the LAA neck and
designed to conform to different
sizes and shapes of LAA anatomy.

Figure 53.3 Amplatzer Amulet LAA Occluder features. *Source:* Courtesy of Abbott Vascular.

implantation, aspirin plus clopidogrel for one to six months followed by aspirin alone thereafter is suggested by the European Heart Rhythm Association (EHRA)/European Association of Percutaneous Cardiovascular Interventions (EAPCI) consensus statement on LAA occlusion.

5. What are the characteristic of the LAmbre device?

The LAmbre LAA occluder is a Nitinol device made up of two components: a left atrial cover and an umbrella, connected through a short central link. The cover is a flat disc made with Nitinol elastic mesh with a recessed hub connecting to the delivery cable. The umbrella is a framework with hooks to enhance adhesion to the LAA wall and mitigate the risk of device embolization. The hooks are recessed within the umbrella until it is in its final position. Both parts are covered by polyethylene terephthalate (PET) membrane to prevent blood entry (Figure 53.4).

This device is delivered through a single (45°) or double-curved (45 and 30°) 8–10F sheath. It is available in 17 sizes, and the disc can extend 4–16 mm from the umbrella. This characteristic allows it to be successfully implanted in a wide range of anatomies. Another exclusive attribute of this device is the articulating waist, which permits both parts of the device to be at different angles, maintaining the tension and assisting the cover to be self-oriented to its final position.

Pre-procedural planning and the procedure steps, from the vein puncture until the instrumentation of the LAA, are quite similar to those of the other devices discussed. After positioning the delivery system at the proximal LAA, the umbrella should be pushed out without moving the sheath. Then the umbrella and delivery system are gently advanced until they reach the landing zone. Finally, after umbrella deployment, the delivery sheath is retracted, exposing the disc. Before the full release of the device, angiography and TEE must be performed to confirm the position. In special cases, presented with thrombus within the LAA, a "no-touch" technique can be used to implant the device from the LA without advancing the delivery system inside the LAA.

6. Lobe and disc vs. plug: is one approach superior to the other?

A few small trials compared different types of LAAO devices prior to 2021. In 2013, two LAAO systems, ACP and

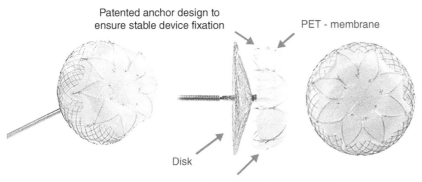

Patented anchor design to
ensure stable device fixation

PET - membrane

Disk

Umbrella - Suitable to various LAA anatomies

Figure 53.4 LAmbre LAA closure system features.

WATCHMAN, were prospectively assessed. Eighty patients treated in a single center were divided into two groups according to the device type used. Both groups presented high success rates (≥95%) without significant differences between them.

Six years later, Cheung et al. performed a single-center retrospective analysis of 161 patients, comparing three devices: 77 (47.5%) ACP/Amulet, 67 (41.4%) WATCHMAN, and 18 (11.1%) LAmbre, with 28.3 ± 24.4 months mean follow-up. In this small study, LAAO was a safe and effective treatment option for stroke prevention, and there was no significant difference among the three devices.

At the end of 2021, Amulet IDE (AMPLATZER Amulet LAA Occluder Trial), the first large-scale randomized, multicenter clinical trial comparing two types of devices, was published. This sponsor (Abbott) designed a trial to compare the Amulet with the WATCHMAN device with respect to safety and effectiveness. Safety was equivalent with both LAA occluders at 12 months (14.5 vs. 14.7%) despite nearly twice as high a rate of procedural complications with the Amulet device (4.5% vs. 2.5%), driven by pericardial effusion and device embolization. With respect to effectiveness at 18 months, the Amulet device was also noninferior. Procedural success rates were high with both devices (Amulet 96% vs. WATCHMAN 94.5%). Rates of LAAO (including residual jets ≤5 mm) were high with both devices, with the Amulet being statistically superior by TEE evaluation at 45 days (Amulet 98.9% vs. WATCHMAN 96.8%). It is important to note that this trial compared the Amulet with the first generation of the WATCHMAN device, not the last-generation WATCHMAN FLX.

The SWISS-APERO (Comparison of Amplatzer Amulet and Watchman Device in Patients Undergoing Left Atrial Appendage Closure) trial, a multicenter randomized clinical trial comparing Amulet with WATCHMAN (77.3% WATCHMAN FLX), has shown that only a minority of LAAs are totally sealed at 45 days based on multislice computed tomography (MSCT) evaluation (Amulet 32.3% vs.

WATCHMAN 30%; p = NS). Despite that, the impact of the type of LAA leaks remains uncertain; in this trial, the Amulet device has shown fewer side leaks (22.9% Amulet vs. 34% WATCHMAN) or mixed leaks (3.8% Amulet vs. 14% WATCHMAN) but more intra-device leak (44.8% Amulet vs. 23% WATCHMAN).

7. What is in the pipeline?

Several devices are being developed worldwide to reduce the risk of stroke by closing the LAA. Other devices with CE mark approval are the WaveCrest (plug; CE mark 2013), Ultraseal (lobe and disc; CE mark 2016) and Lariat (ligation; CE mark 2015) (Figure 53.5).

The WaveCrest is a Nitinol device designed to close the LAA based on a plug mechanism like the WATCHMAN device. It is made of three parts: occluder, anchors, and delivery system. The occluder is a sealing skirt made of polytetrafluoroethylene (PTFE) externally (toward the LA). It is connected to 20 anchors distal to the sealing skirt. There are three different sizes covering an LAA size from 14 to 32 mm. The advantage of this device is that the anchoring system and the occluder can be operated independently.

The Cardia Ultraseal LAAO device is constructed with a Nitinol frame, and its design combines a distal anchoring bulb with a proximal sail to close the LAA orifice. These parts are connected with a dual articulating joint allowing self-orientation of the disc at the LAA ostium. Sealing depends solely on a disc.

The Lariat is an LAAO ligation device that combines an epicardial and an endocardial approach. A magnet-tipped wire is inserted in the pericardial access, and a compliant occlusion balloon catheter with a second magnet-tipped wire is introduced through a TSP. After the two magnets are connected, the Lariat snare delivery system is advanced over the LAA. The snare is closed, and the suture is tightened to ligate LAA. This method has the theoretical

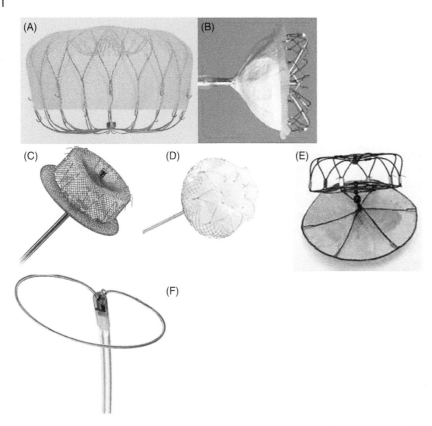

Figure 53.5 Percutaneous left atrial appendage occlusion devices. Plug devices: (a) WATCHMAN FLX; (b) WaveCrest. Lobe and disc devices: (c) Amulet; (d) LAmbre; (e) Cardia Ultraseal. Ligation device: (f) Lariat.

advantage that no foreign material is in contact with blood and potential electrical isolation of LAA. For this procedure, CCTA is mandatory to better understand the LAA anatomy.

There are other devices, such as the Sideris plug patch (a bioabsorbable device with polyurethane cover [Custom Medical Devices]) and the Prolipsis plug patch (a redesigned second-generation Sideris patch device [Occlutech]). Other investigational devices include the Lefort device (umbrella-shaped Nitinol device [Lepu Medical Technology]), the pfm device (Christmas tree-shaped pacifier device [pfm medical]), the SeaLA Occluder (umbrella-shaped Nitinol plug device [Hangzhou Valued Medtech]), the Sierra Ligation System (epicardial ligation device [Aegis Medical Innovations]), and the Conformal Left Atrial Appendage Seal (CLAAS; flexible Nitinol endoskeleton combined with a porous polyurethane-carbonate matrix foam cup [Conformal Medical]).

Bibliography

1 Al-Saady, N.M., Obel, O.A., and Camm, A.J. (1999). Left atrial appendage: structure, function, and role in thromboembolism. *Heart* 82: 547–554.

2 Bartus, K., Han, F.T., Bednarek, J. et al. (2013). Percutaneous left atrial appendage suture ligation using the Lariat device in patients with atrial fibrillation: initial clinical experience. *J. Am. Coll. Cardiol.* 62: 108–118.

3 Cheung, G.S., So, K.C., Chan, C.K. et al. (2019). Comparison of three left atrial appendage occlusion devices for stroke prevention in patients with non-valvular atrial fibrillation: a single-centre seven-year experience with Watchman, AMPLATZER Cardiac Plug/Amulet, LAmbre: comparison of three LAAO devices for stroke prevention. *AsiaIntervention* 5: 57–63.

4 Chun, K.R.J., Bordignon, S., Urban, V. et al. (2013). Left atrial appendage closure followed by 6 weeks of antithrombotic therapy: a prospective single-center experience. *Heart Rhythm* 10: 1792–1799.

5 Collado, F.M.S., Lama Von Buchwald, C.M., Anderson, C.K. et al. (2021). Left atrial appendage occlusion for stroke prevention in nonvalvular atrial fibrillation. *J. Am. Heart Assoc.* 10: e022274.

6 Cruz-González, I., Korsholm, K., Trejo-Velasco, B. et al. (2020). Procedural and short-term results with the new Watchman FLX left atrial appendage occlusion device. *J. Am. Coll. Cardiol. Intv.* 13: 2732–2741.

7 Ernst, G., Stöllberger, C., Abzieher, F. et al. (1995). Morphology of the left atrial appendage. *Anat. Rec.* 242: 553–561.

8 Galea, R., Marco, F.D., Meneveau, N. et al. Amulet or Watchman device for percutaneous left atrial appendage closure: primary results of the SWISS-APERO randomized clinical trial. *Circulation* 145: 724–738.

9 Glikson, M., Wolff, R., Hindricks, G. et al. (2020). EHRA/EAPCI expert consensus statement on catheter-based left atrial appendage occlusion – an update. *EuroIntervention* 15.

10 Gloekler, S., Shakir, S., Doblies, J. et al. (2015). Early results of first versus second generation Amplatzer occluders for left atrial appendage closure in patients with atrial fibrillation. *Clin. Res. Cardiol.* 104: 656–665.

11 Huang, H., Liu, Y., Xu, Y. et al. (2017). Percutaneous left atrial appendage closure with the LAmbre device for stroke prevention in atrial fibrillation: a prospective, multicenter clinical study. *J. Am. Coll. Cardiol. Intv.* 10: 2188–2194.

12 Kar, S., Price, M.J., and Saw, J. (2016). *Left Atrial Appendage Closure: Mechanical Approaches to Stroke Prevention in Atrial Fibrillation*. Humana Press.

13 Lakkireddy, D., Thaler, D., Ellis, C.R. et al. (2021). Amplatzer amulet left atrial appendage occluder versus Watchman device for stroke prophylaxis (amulet IDE): a randomized, controlled trial. *Circulation* 144: 1543–1552.

14 Price, M.J. (2018). The WATCHMAN left atrial appendage closure device: technical considerations and procedural approach. *Interv. Cardiol. Clin.* 7: 201–212.

15 Sabiniewicz, R., Hiczkiewicz, J., Wańczura, P. et al. (2016). First-in-human experience with the cardia ultraseal left atrial appendage closure device: the feasibility study. *Cardiol. J.* 23: 652–654.

16 Veinot, J.P., Harrity, P.J., Gentile, F. et al. (1997). Anatomy of the normal left atrial appendage. *Circulation* 96: 3112–3115.

17 Whisenant, B. and Weiss, P. (2014). Left atrial appendage closure with transcatheter-delivered devices. *Interv. Cardiol. Clin.* 3: 209–218.

18 Wunderlich, N.C., Beigel, R., Swaans, M.J. et al. (2015). Percutaneous interventions for left atrial appendage exclusion: options, assessment, and imaging using 2D and 3D echocardiography. *JACC Cardiovasc. Imaging* 8: 472–488.

54

LAA Occlusion Technique and Challenging Scenarios

Blanca Trejo Velasco and Ignacio Cruz-Gonzalez[1]

[1] University Hospital of Salamanca, Salamanca, Spain

1. What are the main prerequisites for left atrial appendage occlusion (LAAO)?

Pre-procedural imaging with either transesophageal echocardiography (TEE) or cardiac computed tomography angiography (CCTA) is highly recommended to rule out left atrial appendage (LAA) thrombus and ascertain a patient's suitability for LAAO based on the LAA's morphology and dimensions. With the current dedicated devices, LAAO can be performed in LAAs that measure between 11 mm at the level of the landing zone (LZ) and 40 mm at the ostium, although successful LAAO of larger LAAs has been reported employing a double-device technique. LAA thrombus has traditionally been considered an absolute contraindication. However, LAAO has recently proven feasible and safe in patients with resistant thrombus located in the distal LAA segments when performed by experienced operators with some procedural modifications.

2. What are the main imaging techniques employed to guide LAAO?

TEE is most commonly employed to guide LAAO, although the use of micro-TEE and intracardiac echocardiography (ICE) has increased substantially in the past few years to avoid the need for general anesthesia. The main limitations of these techniques are the need for an additional contralateral venous access, the high cost of the probe for ICE, and the lack of 3D images and simultaneous orthogonal views (X-plane) with micro-TEE. Also, most institutions require an additional examination with either 3D-TEE or CCTA before LAAO for more accurate device sizing.

Although LAAO guided by fluoroscopy alone has proven feasible in large-volume centers with significant experience, the general consensus is to employ additional imaging techniques to improve procedural outcomes.

3. What are the mains steps of LAAO?

1. Femoral venous access
2. Transseptal puncture (TSP)
3. Cannulation of the LAA with the delivery system
4. Device sizing
5. Device implantation
6. Stability test and device release

4. What features of femoral venous access are most relevant for LAAO?

The right femoral vein is preferred over the left as it enables a more linear trajectory of the transseptal and delivery sheaths toward the interatrial septum. If left femoral access is required, a transseptal needle with a sharper curve should be employed. In very obese patients, a larger-bore introducer sheath (16–18-French) may be considered to improve torque transmission to the delivery system.

5. What are the keys steps for TSP?

TSP in LAAO procedures is generally performed with the Brockenbrough (BRK)-0 (minor curve) or BRK-1 (larger curve) transseptal needle along with a SL-0

Swartz sheath (Abbott Vascular), which facilitates advancing a wire toward the left upper pulmonary vein (LUPV) (Figure 54.1a). The steerable Agilis NX-T (Abbott Vascular) or SureFlex sheaths (Baylis Medical) can also prove useful in more complex anatomies. In patients with a hypermobile, rigid, and/or thickened septum that hinders a straightforward puncture, employing an extra-sharp BRK-XS needle or advancing the stylet or the stiff end of an 0.014–0.018-in. guidewire through the trans-septal needle may be helpful. Other alternatives include applying radiofrequency to the proximal end of the BRK needle, using a dedicated radiofrequency catheter, or the SafeSept wire (Pressure Products Medical Supplies). After removal of the stylet, the Luer lock of the transseptal needle should be connected to a pressure line to allow continuous pressure monitoring (Figure 54.1d). Once the needle enters the left atrium (LA), the sheath and dilator are advanced over the needle into the LA. If resistance is met, applying mild forward tension and rotation maneuvers usually allows the sheath to cross. Alternatively, a pigtail-shaped 0.025-in. ProTrack wire (Baylis Medical) can be advanced to the LA to increase support, or the TSP site can be dilated with a 4 mm coronary balloon.

Use of TEE or ICE to guide the precise location of TSP that will enable coaxial alignment of the delivery system with the LAA is highly recommended, as this step largely determines procedural success. In general, TSP for LAAO

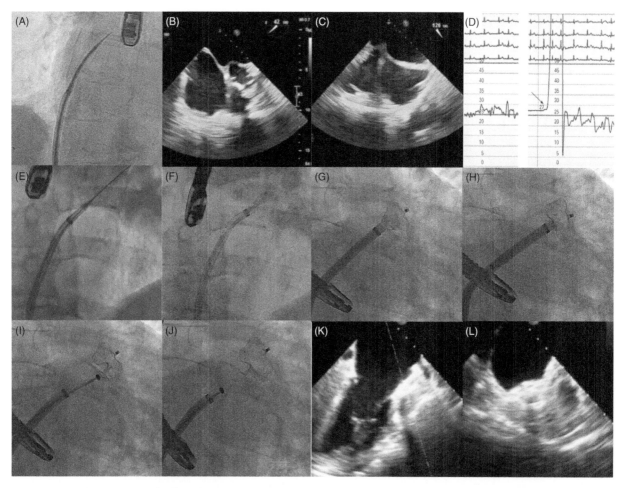

Figure 54.1 Transseptal puncture in the inferior posterior region of the fossa ovalis. (a–d) The Luer lock of the transseptal needle is connected to a pressure line to allow continuous pressure monitoring and confirm entry into the left atrium. (e–f) The transseptal sheath is exchanged for the delivery sheath by advancing a 0.035-in. guidewire to the left upper pulmonary vein, and the delivery sheath is advanced into the left atrial appendage with the protection of a pigtail catheter on its distal end. (g–h) For Amulet device deployment, the delivery sheath is withdrawn slightly until the device is partially deployed in the "ball" configuration. (i–j) Next, the delivery cable is advanced so that the device can unfold laterally into the triangle and subsequent tire conformations. (k–l) Before device release, device stability is tested by exerting traction tension to the delivery cable while the delivery sheath is retracted 2–4 cm from the device hub ("tug test"), and intra-procedural imaging with transesophageal echocardiography confirms adequate device positioning and rules out significant peri-device leak.

targets the infero-posterior region of the fossa ovalis, as most LAAs are oriented anterolaterally and superiorly (Figure 54.1b,c). However, in patients with extremely anterior LAAs, a more posterior puncture can be helpful, while TSP in the mid fossa ovalis may be considered if the LAA is laterally or posteriorly oriented.

The presence of pericardial effusions must be assessed before TSP so that new-onset or worsening effusions after TSP can be promptly identified and dealt with. Next, a 100UI/kg dose of non-fractioned heparin is administered to attain an activated clotting time (ACT) >250–300 seconds. Some operators recommend the administration of a 1000–2000 UI bolus after venous access cannulation, especially in more complex cases where TSP may be more time-consuming.

6. Can LAAO be performed through a patent foramen oval (PFO) or atrial septum defect (ASD)?

In patients with a preexistent PFO or ASD, performing a selective angiogram of the LAA through the defect may help determine if coaxial alignment of the delivery sheath and the LAA can be attained by crossing the septum through the defect. If this is the case, a TSP can be spared, and LAAO can be attempted through the defect, while a separate TPS is recommended for PFOs wih a long and tight tunnel.

7. What steps are required to position the delivery system at the LAA?

Once the transseptal sheath is located in the LA, it is exchanged for the delivery system. The safest location to perform this maneuver is in the LUPV. For this purpose, a 0.035-in. J-tipped stiff guidewire (Amplatz Extra-Stiff J-wire [Cook Medical] or a Backup wire [Boston Scientific]) is progressed into the LUPV, with the potential assistance of a Multipurpose or JR 5-French catheter (Figure 54.1e). Rotating the transseptal sheath (SL0) clockwise to attain a more posterior orientation further facilitates this step. If LUPV cannulation proves complex, another safe option is to advance a support guidewire with a pigtail curve (Safari wire [Boston Scientific]) into the LA. Sheath exchange can also be performed in the area contiguous to the LAA orifice by very experienced operators or in cases with a difficult LAA engagement, such as an upward LAA uptake, while carefully monitoring that the tip of the exchange wire does not progress into the LAA. The delivery sheath is advanced through the septum by exerting continuous light pressure

and small rotational movements under fluoroscopic and TEE guidance.

Next, a 5–6-French pigtail catheter is advanced through the delivery system to facilitate LAA engagement and progression of the delivery sheath inside the LAA without injuring its thin wall (Figure 54.1f).

In general, the best projection to engage the LAA and assess the pigtail's position within the LAA is the RAO/caudal, although this may be modified based on CCTA images. The pigtail catheter should be maintained in place until the occlusion device has been selected and prepared to avoid accidental advancement of the delivery sheath into the LAA and potential LAA injury. After removal of the pigtail, a certain degree of catheter torque is frequently required to maintain the sheath position.

8. How is device sizing performed?

The size of the device should be selected according to the recommended sizing chart, taking into account the mean LZ diameter for 3D imaging techniques (CCTA and 3D TEE) or the maximum LZ diameter for 2D techniques (2D TEE, including micro-TEE and fluoroscopy), with 2–6 mm of device oversizing, depending on the device selected. In general, CCTA measurements have proven slightly larger than those obtained with 3D-TEE and up to 2–3 mm greater than quantified by 2D-TEE. If sizes measured in the same view with different imaging modalities differ by >2 mm, sizing should rely on the largest measurement.

Intra-procedural angiographic measurements of the LZ and ostial diameters are generally performed in addition to other imaging techniques by means of a 5–6-French pigtail. Standard projections include the RAO 30°/cranial 10–20° view (Figure 54.2a), which displays the ostium and LZ of the LAA and the right anterior oblique (RAO) 30°/caudal 10–20° projection (Figure 54.2b), which assesses the mid to distal LAA segments. To integrate fluoroscopy and TEE images, it is important to remember that the RAO/cranial and RAO/caudal projections correspond to the mid-esophageal 45° (Figure 54.2c) and 135° views (Figure 54.2d), respectively.

Note that angiographic measurements should only be performed after confirming that LA pressure is >12 mmHg to avoid device undersizing. If baseline LA pressure is <12 mmHg, volume loading with 500–1000 ml of saline is recommended, as this can increase LAA diameters by ≈2 mm. Finally, measurements in patients with paroxysmal atrial fibrillation (AF) should ideally be performed during the same rhythm, as smaller diameters are generally observed during sinus rhythm than in AF.

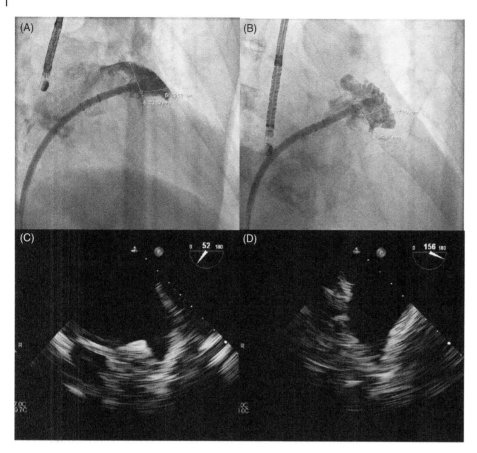

Figure 54.2 LAA angiogram in the RAO/CRA view (a) displays the ostium and LZ of the LAA and the RAO/CAU projection (b) that assesses the mid-distal LAA's segments. Transesophageal echocardiography images in the (c) 45° and (d) 135° mid-esophageal views corresponding to RAO/CRA and RAO/CAU projections, respectively. CAU, caudal; CRA, cranial; LAA, left atrial appendage; LZ, landing zone; RAO, right anterior oblique

9. What are the anatomical landmarks for LAAO device implantation?

For single-lobe devices such as the WATCHMAN (Boston Scientific) and WaveCrest (Biosense Webster), the LZ is measured from the inferior part of the LAA ostium at the level of the circumflex coronary to a point 1–2 cm distally to the tip of the rim to the LUPV. In addition, the LAA depth from ostium to apex is also determined.

In the case of lobe and disc devices such as the ACP/Amulet (Abbott Vascular), LAmbre (Lifetech Scientific), and Ultraseal (Cardia), the LZ is measured 10–12 mm distally from the ostial plane into the lobe.

Device Deployment

The device introducer and delivery sheath should be connected in a fluid-to-fluid manner to avoid air embolisms. This can be done by flushing with heparinized saline from the Y-connector side arm joined to the device introducer while blood backflow is obtained from the delivery sheath. Once the device is advanced to the tip of the delivery sheath, the first common step for all devices is to slightly withdraw the tip of the sheath while maintaining the device in place, to allow partial device unfolding. This measure reduces the risk of LAA perforation during subsequent device positioning maneuvers. Once placed in an optimal implant position and after assessing for peri-device leaks, the device is released by counterclockwise rotation of the delivery cable.

10. What specific considerations must be taken into account with each dedicated LAAO device?

WATCHMAN FLX

The WATCHMAN FLX has a significantly shorter length than its prior device iteration, the WATCHMAN 2.5, which enables LAAO of shallow LAAs. This new-generation device is implanted through the 14-Fr WATCHMAN TrueSeal Access sheath, available in three different shapes to facilitate coaxial LAA engagement (double curve for superior-anterior LAAs, single curve for mid-to-inferior LAAs and anterior curve for superior, rightward and posterior, "retroflex" LAAs). In addition, the sheath has three proximal radiopaque markers to ensure adequate sheath placement depending on the size of the device (Figure 54.3a).

The 12-Fr device introducer is advanced through the access sheath until the distal markers of both catheters align. The device is then deployed. This can be performed by unsheathing the device from the more distal LAA segments, as for the WATCHMAN 2.5 device, but the device can also be advanced in a ball configuration obtained by pulling the sheath back until the WATCHMAN FLX is partially unfolded and presents a width of ≈2 times that of the delivery sheath (Figure 54.3b–h).

Once the device is deployed in an optimal position, the four PASS device release criteria should be met before device release: (i) position (adequate LAA ostium coverage, shoulder protrusion <40–50%), (ii) anchor (tug test: confirmation of device stability by applying traction to the delivery cable ≈30 seconds), (iii) size (10–30% device compression), and (iv) seal (absence of peri-device leaks >5 mm).

Amulet

The Amulet is implanted through a 12–14-Fr TorqVue 45°×45° sheath. First the delivery sheath is partially withdrawn while maintaining the delivery cable fixed until the device is partially deployed in the ball configuration. In this way, the whole system can be advanced and retracted as a unit. Additional counterclockwise rotation may be needed to obtain a more coaxial orientation, especially in cases with a more superiorly oriented LAA. Alternatively, the recently approved 14Fr Amplatzer Steerable Delivery Sheath that allows for bidirectional deflection from 0º to 120º and a 1:1 torque response can be used in more complex anatomies to facilitate LAA engagement and co-axial alignment. Once an optimal position is achieved, the delivery cable is advanced so that the device can unfold laterally into the triangle and subsequent tire conformations (Figure 54.1g–h). It is important to keep in mind that this maneuver does not advance the device further into the LAA. After deploying the lobe, the sheath is retracted until the disc unfolds. Partial device recapture to the level of the lobe anchors enables device repositioning in a more proximal and also distal position.

After device deployment, a sustained ≈30 second traction test should be performed (Figure 54.1i–j) and the CLOSE criteria met, to ensure device stability: (i) Cx: at least two-thirds of the lobe should be distal to the circumflex artery,

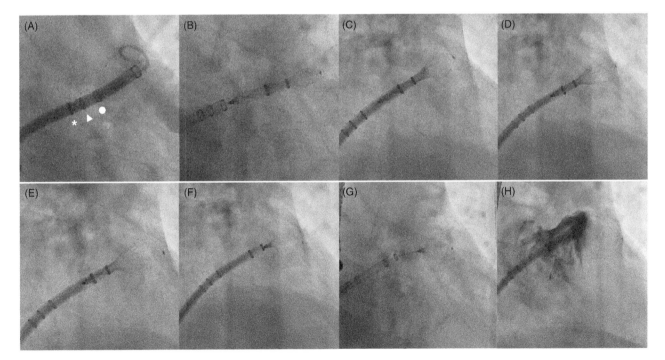

Figure 54.3 (a) The WATCHMAN TrueSeal access sheath has three proximal markers corresponding to the 35 mm (asterisk), 31 and 27 mm (arrowhead), and 24 and 20 mm (circle) devices. (b–h) Deployment steps of the WATCHMAN FLX device.

(ii) lobe: the lobe must be slightly compressed in the tire configuration, (iiii) orientation: the lobe must be aligned with the axis of the LAA neck, (iv) separation: there must be a separation between lobe and disc, and (v) elliptical: the disc should present a certain degree of concavity that reflects the attracting force exerted from the lobe.

LAmbre

The LAmbre is implanted through an 8–10-Fr delivery sheath, available in two shapes: double curve (45°×30°) and single curve (45°). Deployment of the LAmbre does not require deep intubation of the delivery sheath into the LAA and is not as dependent on optimal catheter alignment with the LAA as the device can be partially unsheathed outside the LAA. The partially unfolded umbrella is then advanced and anchored at the LZ, while subsequent device unsheathing releases the disc of the device at the level of the LAA ostia. This approach is particularly useful in the setting of dense spontaneous echo contrast or distal LAA thrombus. On the other hand, the unsheathing method can also be performed after advancing the device sheath distally into the LAA, which can be helpful in more intricate multilobe or shallow LAAs. Signs of optimal device placement include a concave-shaped cover and a rectangular-shaped, completely unfolded umbrella, which should be positioned beyond the left circumflex artery.

Ultraseal

In the case of the Ultraseal, the 10–12-Fr 45°×45° double-curve delivery sheath is advanced inside the LAA to the plane of the LZ. Once in this position, the delivery sheath is maintained in place while advancing the device until the bulb is completely deployed by pushing on the device forceps. Next, the sheath is pulled back until the sail is unfolded and deployed. Note that the Ultraseal allows for partial or total recapture up to five times. Before device release, it should be assessed that the anchor markers of the bulb have a non-symmetric shape, indicating bulb compression, and a tug test should confirm device stability.

11. What are the main steps to perform a "sandwich technique"?

In chicken-wing shaped LAAs with an early and severe (>90°) bend of the main lobe that determines a short LAA neck (<15–20 mm), a conventional LAAO technique may not be feasible, given the insufficient depth at

the LZ that hinders adequate device deployment and ostium coverage.

In this setting, the "sandwich technique" is a valuable option for LAAO employing lobe and disc devices such as the Amulet and LAmbre. Implantation of the occlusion device is performed in parallel to the distal LAA wall. The lobe is therefore inserted inside the chicken wing while the disc covers the LAA ostium, leaving the LAA ridge sandwiched between the lob and the disc of the device (Figure 54.4).

Device sizing is generally larger than would be needed for a conventional LAAO technique and should consider the following measurements: (i) ridge distance, (ii) height and (iii) width of the chicken wing, and (iv) maximal LAA ostial diameter.

The size of the device should be selected so that the lobe is ≥20–30% larger than the device ridge, without exceeding

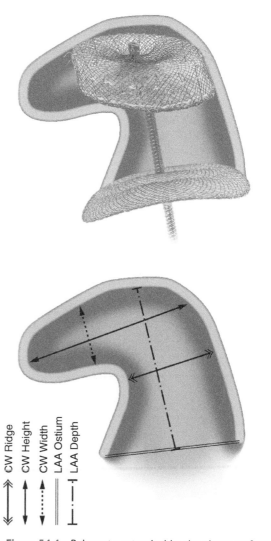

CW Ridge
CW Height
CW Width
LAA Ostium
LAA Depth

Figure 54.4 Relevant anatomical landmarks to perform left atrial appendage occlusion using the sandwich technique in chicken-wing left atrial appendages with an early and severe bend.

the chicken-wing height, while the disc seals the LAA ostium completely. The width of the chicken wing is critical, as the lobe is deployed inside it.

12. What other LAA anatomies can pose a challenge for LAAO?

Broad and shallow LAAs can also complicate LAAO. In this setting, using the LAmbre's special sizes that combine a smaller lobe with a 12–14 mm larger cover can be useful. Alternatively, LAAO closure using a double device technique has been reported with the ACP, WATCHMAN 2.5, and LAmbre devices with favorable safety and feasibility results in selected cases (Figure 54.5).

In addition, LAAs with a sharp upward uptake, as opposed to the conventional downward course, can challenge coaxial LAA engagement. In these cases, performing a more inferior and posterior TSP and/or marked counterclockwise sheath rotation can be helpful.

13. Can LAAO be performed in the presence of LAA thrombus?

Several publications have reported favorable safety and feasibility results of LAAO in the presence of distal LAA thrombus. Lobe and disc devices are preferred in this setting, as they enable a shallow deployment and do not require the engagement of the delivery catheter into the LAA. The WATCHMAN FLX is also useful in this scenario, as it features a shorter length and can also be advanced from the proximal to distal LAA segments in the ball configuration. Another important consideration is to avoid contrast injection inside the LAA. In addition, pre-procedural planning should be especially meticulous in determining the optimal device size and implant position and avoiding the need for device retrieval and repositioning, which may substantially increase the risk of thrombus embolization. Finally, the use of adjunctive cerebral embolic protection devices can be considered.

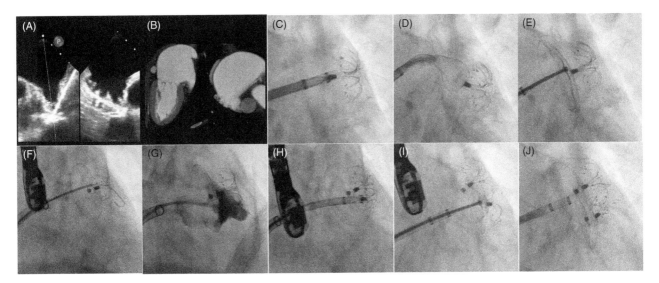

Figure 54.5 Procedural steps required for left atrial appendage occlusion of a very large left atrial appendage using double LAmbre device implantation. (Clinical case at the online companion website).

References

1 Cruz-González, I., Núñez, J.C., and Díaz-Peláez, E. (2020). Double LAmbre occlusion technique for extra-large and shallow left atrial appendage. *Rev. Esp. Cardiol.* 73 (12): 1061. https://doi.org/10.1016/j.recesp.2020.05.011.

2 Glikson, M., Wolff, R., Hindricks, G. et al. (2020). EHRA/EAPCI expert consensus statement on catheter-based left atrial appendage occlusion-an update. *EuroIntervention* 15 (13): 1133–1180. https://doi.org/10.4244/EIJY19M08_01.

3 Saw, J. and Lempereur, M. (2014). Percutaneous left atrial appendage closure: procedural techniques and outcomes. *JACC Cardiovasc. Interv.* 7 (11): 1205–1220. https://doi.org/10.1016/j.jcin.2014.05.026.

55

Preventing and Managing Complications of LAA Closure

Jean C. Núñez García and Ignacio Cruz- González[1]

[1] *University Hospital of Salamanca, Salamanca, Spain*

1. What is the relevance of this topic?

Percutaneous left atrial appendage closure (LAAC) has become an alternative to oral anticoagulation for the prevention of thromboembolic events related to nonvalvular atrial fibrillation (NVAF). The rate of complications in the initial studies penalized the procedure whose "preventive" nature requires a low percentage of complications. Device and technique improvements have reduced the rate of complications, with a current incidence <3%. The LAA's variable anatomy, its thin wall, the high-risk profile of patients, and the skills of the operators are factors that can influence the frequency of complications. Although some studies question the influence of the learning curve and experience with the technique, we consider that training is necessary and advise performing this procedure with special caution.

Pericardial Effusion (PE)

2. What is the current incidence of PE?

PE is the most frequent complication of LAAC, with a current incidence around 0.6–2% (considering those that require drainage). Most of these are detected in the first 24 hours.

3. What are the causes of PE, and how can they be prevented?

Transseptal puncture (TSP) is a critical point that can lead to perforation:

- Except in exceptional cases, LAACs should be performed guided by a transesophageal (TEE) or intracardiac echocardiogram (ICE).
- TSP should be performed in the inferior-posterior aspect of the fossa ovalis. TSP at other levels hinders the maneuverability of the sheaths, compromising the result and facilitating complications.
- Before puncturing, the tenting should be checked in two views.
- Thick or aneurysmal septa can make puncture challenging. Use a radiofrequency needle or maintain the tenting without additional pressure; using the back-end of a coronary wire or the stylet of the TSP sheath can help puncture. After the puncture, returning the sheath and needle to the 3 o'clock position can prevent the puncture of the posterior wall of the atrium.

Navigation of the guidewires or device delivery sheath (DDS). Improper handling of the material can lead to trauma or perforation of the LAA or pulmonary veins (PVs). The LAA wall is very thin, so all movements must be performed with caution and under fluoroscopic vision.

- Once TSP is done, the exchange for the DDS must be done over a stiff guidewire.
- Some operators do the exchange in the LAA; however, we consider it safer to do it in the PV.
- It is advisable to locate the LAA and advance the DDS with a pigtail in front, and once inside the LAA, advance the DDS over the pigtail.

Trauma due to LAAC devices. Devices and their hooks can perforate the LAA:

- Avoid pushing the devices out of the DDS. The correct way is to bring the delivery catheter to the tip and, maintaining the position, pull back the sheath.

- Device recaptures or repositioning increase the possibility of perforation. Good planning with CT or 3D-TEE can reduce the attempts or recaptures and avoid excessive oversizing.

Chronic oral anticoagulation (OAC). Management of peri-procedural OAC is a controversial issue. Some trials required an international normalized ratio (INR) <2.0 at the time of procedure, but in other studies it is not described; and some authors have reported the safety of keeping the patient on (or single-held dose) novel oral anticoagulants (NOACs) or warfarin before the procedure. Management of periprocedural OAC should be individualized based on thromboembolic and hemorrhagic risk.

It is important to exclude pericardial efussion (PE) before starting the procedure.

4.   How do you manage a LAAC-related PE?

- Mild PE without hemodynamic instability can be managed conservatively with monitoring.
- In the event of hemodynamic instability or significant rapid-onset PE, emergency pericardiocentesis should be performed at the same time as other general measures (volume expansion or vasopressor drugs) are taken.
- Once pericardiocentesis has been performed, some cases with abundant bleeding can benefit from autotransfusion.
- If pericardiocentesis has been performed and catheters have been removed, reversal of anticoagulation can be considered. Early reversal can lead to clotting of the PE and make it difficult to drain.
- If the perforation is minor and is detected early in the LAA, the deployment of the device can seal the leak.
- If the previous measures are not sufficient, surgical intervention may be necessary, although this is rare (0.0–0.24%).
- A case of perforation of the LAA with the device that advanced to the pericardial space has been reported: keeping the sheath, the operators exchanged the device for an ASD closure device, sealing the perforation.

Device Embolization

5.   What is the current incidence of device embolization (DE)?

Current improvements in devices and techniques have made DE a rare complication (0.0–0.5%).

6.   What are the causes of DE, and how can it be prevented?

Inappropriate device size. Undersizing or oversizing can compromise the compression and the device anchor, causing instability or expulsion of the LAA. Planning using CT or 3D TEE can reduce this complication.

Challenging LAA anatomies can increase the risk of embolization: wide ostia, shallow LAA, wide landing zone (LZ), multilobed LAA, etc. Operators must ensure that the device has adequate depth and compression and that the anchoring mechanisms are in contact with the wall (the position must be assessed in several views). Some devices facilitate access to angled or lobed LAAs with difficult coaxiality, using sheaths with different angles or a steerable sheath.

Therapeutic or spontaneous cardioversion has been suggested as a potential mechanism of DE. We consider that this could be a DE trigger in devices with insufficient anchorage.

The "tug test" is recommended. Some devices provide specific stability criteria (PASS criteria for WATCHMAN and CLOSE criteria for the Amulet).

7.   What can be clinical manifestations of DE?

Most DEs are acute, although up to 30% of late cases have been described. Although most are clinically silent, the presentation will depend on the device location, from mild symptoms with palpitations to shock or cardiac arrest. The larger devices will remain in the atrium or ventricle, while the smaller devices tend to migrate toward the aorta. In a systematic review, 14% were in the LA, 43% in the LV, and 43% in the aorta.

8.   How can you perform a device retrieval?

- In cases of hemodynamic instability, the use of catheters to mobilize the device or change the patient's position can be helpful while awaiting device retrieval.
- An activated clotting time (ACT) >250 seconds must be guaranteed.
- A sheath at least 2 Fr larger than the DDS and a snare (e.g. a gooseneck snare with at least a 10 mm loop inside a guide catheter) will be needed.
- Some authors suggest that the Amulet is easier to engage with the end screw of the lobe, while the WATCHMAN 2.5 is best captured by the distal frame struts.

- Retrieval of a trapped device in the ventricle is a risky maneuver that must be performed cautiously to avoid damage to the valves. Some cases will require surgery, especially when the device gets trapped in the mitral valve (Figure 55.1).

Air Embolism (AE)

AE is an avoidable complication generally due to technical failures.

9. What are the manifestations of AE?

AE can manifest as a stroke/TIA that depends on the affected brain territory. However, most patients are under general anesthesia or at least superficial sedation leading to late diagnoses.

Patients with coronary AE can present with ST-segment elevation (more frequently in lower leads due to the position of the right coronary artery), bradycardia, hemodynamic instability, and chest pain in those awake.

10. What are the causes of AE, and how can it be prevented?

Inadequate flushing of sheaths or devices. Preparation should be cautious; continuous flushing is recommended during the advancement of the TSP needle and the device.

Low LA pressure. Avoiding atrial pressure < 10 mmHg by administering intravenous volume can help prevent air from entering the DDS. Changes in intrathoracic pressure

may favor the entry of air, so it is advisable to keep the proximal end of the DDS below the atrium level.

Some authors recommend the use of iodinated contrasts during the advancement of the LAAC device.

11. How do you treat AE?

- Supportive treatment with 100% oxygen. Some cases may require hyperbaric oxygen.
- If air is trapped in the LAA, aspiration with a pigtail catheter can be attempted.
- It may be necessary to keep the patient supine to avoid movement of trapped air.

Periprocedural Ischemic Stroke

12. What is the current incidence of periprocedural ischemic stroke (PIS)?

PIS has decreased, with a current incidence of around 0.1–0.7%. However, LAAC is performed precisely to prevent strokes, so this complication is very unwanted. Fortunately, most can be reversible.

13. What are the causes of PIS, and how can it be prevented?

- *Air embolism.*
- *Previous thrombus.* Ruling out the presence of thrombus before starting the procedure is mandatory. Some

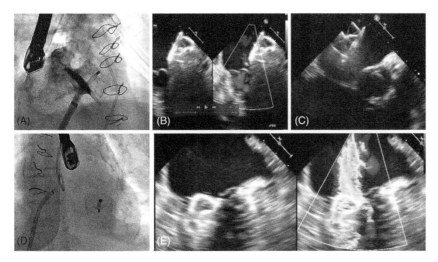

Figure 55.1 Device embolization. (a, b) Final position of the device; not enough compression. (c) The device in the left atrial appendage. (d, e) The device trapped in the mitral valve, causing severe mitral regurgitation.

patients with LAA thrombus can have an OAC contraindication, or the thrombus can be refractory. Some series of LAAC have been reported in patients with thrombus, but this practice should be reserved for special cases. Cerebral embolic protection (CEP) devices can be useful in these cases.

- *New thrombus formation:* Most PISs are due to thrombus formation in relation to catheters. An ACT >250 seconds should be ensured, and close echocardiographic surveillance should be maintained. Some operators administer a low dose of heparin at the beginning of the procedure (before TSP). During the procedure, it is advisable to perform intermittent flushing to avoid blood stasis. If a thrombus is identified during the procedure, some authors suggest aspiration or thrombolysis; we consider that this is a risky practice that should only be performed by experienced operators.

The specific management of strokes exceeds the objective of this chapter.

Complications Related to Vascular Access

14. What are the complications related to access, and how can they be prevented?

Vascular complications are common and similar to those related to other interventional procedures: hematoma, bleeding, pseudoaneurysm, venous thrombosis, arteriovenous fistula, etc. Ultrasound-guided puncture should be considered for all femoral access. The use of vascular closure devices can reduce complications. As an alternative to the use of devices, the closure is usually performed with a "figure-eight suture"; in these cases, we use a three-way "stopcock" that allows us to control the pressure in case of bleeding.

Peri-device Leaks (PDLs)

15. What are the clinical relevance and incidence of PDLs?

A PDL is not in itself a complication. However, it has been proposed that PDLs could be associated with thrombus formation and embolic events, although there is insufficient evidence to demonstrate this association. A study carried out with CT scans has described up to 63% with PDLs, with

a similar rate in the different devices. Only 14% had PDLs in the procedure TEE. By consensus and based on the results of the PROTECT AF (WATCHMAN Left Atrial Appendage System for Embolic PROTECTion in Patients with Atrial Fibrillation) study, a PDL is considered significant above 3–5 mm. Most are posteroinferior.

16. What are the related factors or mechanisms?

Larger LZ, larger LA or larger angle between device lobe and disc, undersizing, off-axis deployment, irregular LAA orifice, incomplete endothelialization, fabric leaks, postimplant migration, etc.

17. What are the treatment options for PDL?

- In patients with significant PDL, continuation of OAC may be considered.
- PDL closure (Figure 55.2) can be considered with different devices (Amplatzer Vascular Plug [AVP], Amplatzer Duct Occluder [ADO], Amplatzer Septal Occluder [ASD], etc.).

Device-Related Thrombus (DRT)

18. What are the incidence and clinical relevance of DRT?

The current incidence of DRT is around 2–4%. Multiple studies associate DRT with embolic events, increasing the risk of stroke three to five times. However, most strokes in patients with LAAC are not associated with DRTs.

19. What factors predispose patients to DRT, and how can it be prevented?

- *Patient factors:* Female sex, CHA2DS2-VASc score, history of stroke/TIA, permanent AF, spontaneous echo contrast, larger LAAs, clopidogrel resistance, smoking, and lower LVEF.
- *Procedure factors:* Both the device being implanted too deep and incomplete LAAC and an uncovered PV ridge have been related to DRT development and should be avoided.

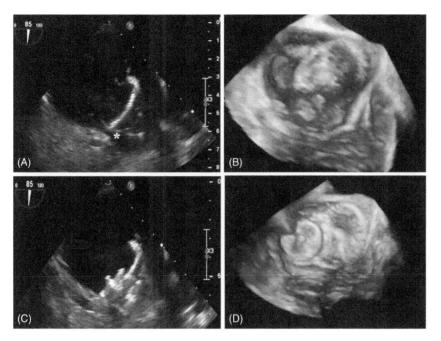

Figure 55.2 (a, b) 3D TEE showing a posteroinferior peri-device leak after left atrial appendage closure. (c, d) An Amplatzer Vascular Plug II device closing the gap.

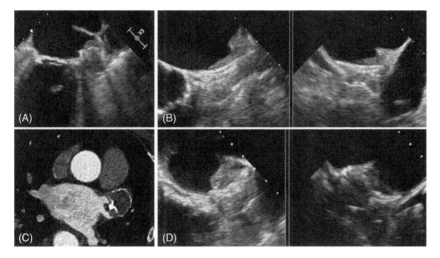

Figure 55.3 Different cases of device-related thrombus.

Antithrombotic treatment after LAAC is controversial and highly variable. A recent propensity-matched comparison suggests that DRT is less frequent in patients with initial OAC compared to antiplatelet therapy; however, thromboembolic events were similar.

20. How do you diagnose DRTs?

It is recommended that a TEE or CT scan be performed in the first 45–90 days and another study at six months. More than 80% of DRTs occur after 45 days; beyond six months, a new thrombus is rare (Figure 55.3). Imaging controls beyond one year in patients without previous alterations is controversial. Most DRTs are located in the anterosuperior region or in relation to leaks or uncovered lobes, and it is important to differentiate the normal endothelialization of the laminar thrombus.

21. How do you treat DRTs?

DRTs should be treated with anticoagulation for a minimum of two to four weeks before attempting to verify dissolution, but there is no consensus on which is the most appropriate regimen, so it is advisable to individualize:

- *Low-molecular-weight heparin (LMWH)* is probably the most effective strategy.
- *Warfarin:* Patients with low bleeding risk and who were already on warfarin can be considered to achieve an INR of 2.5–3.5. Adding a low dose of aspirin can be considered.
- *NOACs:* Evidence is scarce.

Some cases of refractory DRT or recurrent embolisms may require surgery.

22. What other complications have been described?

- *Device erosion with late pericardial effusion:* This is a very rare late complication presenting as PE, cardiac tamponade, or death. Management is that of PE.
- *A recent study reports 1.5% of major complications related to TEE:* Gastrointestinal bleeding, persistent dysphagia/odynophagia, etc.
- *Atrial arrhythmias:* Generally self-limited.
- *Complications related to anesthesia:* Airway trauma or pneumonia.
- *Transient LAA inversion:* Anecdotally.

Bibliography

1 Aminian, A., Lalmand, J., Tzika, A. et al. (2015). Embolization of left atrial appendage closure devices: a systematic review of cases reported with the watchman device and the amplatzer cardiac plug. *Catheter. Cardiovasc. Interv.* 86 (1): 128–135.

2 Berti, S., Santoro, G., Brscic, E. et al. (2017). Left atrial appendage closure using AMPLATZER™ devices: a large, multicenter, Italian registry. *Int. J. Cardiol.* 248: 103–107.

3 Boersma, L., V., Ince, H., Kische, S. et al. (2017). Efficacy and safety of left atrial appendage closure with WATCHMAN in patients with or without contraindication to oral anticoagulation: 1-year follow-up outcome data of the EWOLUTION trial. *Heart Rhythm* 14 (9): 1302–1308.

4 Cruz-González, I., Korsholm, K., Trejo-Velasco, B. et al. (2020). Procedural and short-term results with the new watchman FLX left atrial appendage occlusion device. *JACC Cardiovasc. Interv.* 13 (23): 2732–2741.

5 Eng, M., H., Wang, D.D., Greenbaum, A.B. et al. (2018). Prospective, randomized comparison of 3-dimensional computed tomography guidance versus TEE data for left atrial appendage occlusion (PRO3DLAAO). *Catheter. Cardiovasc. Interv.* 92 (2): 401–407.

6 Enomoto, Y., Gadiyaram, V., Gianni, C. et al. (2017). Use of non-warfarin oral anticoagulants instead of warfarin during left atrial appendage closure with the Watchman device. *Heart Rhythm* 14 (1): 19–24.

7 Freeman, J., V., Varosy, P., Price, M.J. et al. (2020). The NCDR Left aAtrial aAppendage oOcclusion rRegistry. *J. Am. Coll. Cardiol.* 75 (13): 1503–1518.

8 Freitas-Ferraz, A., B., Rodes-Cabau, J., Junqura Vega, L. et al. (2020). Transesophageal echocardiography complications associated with interventional cardiology procedures. *Am. Heart J.* 221: 19–28.

9 Glikson, M., Wolff, R., Hindricks, G. et al. (2019). EHRA/EAPCI expert consensus statement on catheter-based left atrial appendage occlusion – an update. *Europace* euz258.

10 Holmes, D., R., Reddy, V.Y., Turi, Z.G. et al. (2009). Percutaneous closure of the left atrial appendage versus warfarin therapy for prevention of stroke in patients with atrial fibrillation: a randomised non-inferiority trial. *Lancet* 374 (9689): 534–542.

11 Italiano, G., Maltagliati, A., Mantegazza, V. et al. (2020). Multimodality approach for endovascular left atrial appendage closure: head-to-head comparison among 2D and 3D echocardiography, angiography, and computer tomography. *Diagnostics (Basel)* 10 (12): 1103.

12 Lempereur, M., Aminian, A., Freixa, X. et al. (2017). Device-associated thrombus formation after left atrial appendage occlusion: a systematic review of events reported with the watchman, the Amplatzer cardiac plug and the Amulet. *Catheter. Cardiovasc. Interv.* 90 (5): E111–E121.

13 Meier, B., Tarbine, S.G., Costantini, C.R. et al. (2014). Percutaneous management of left atrial appendage perforation during device closure. *Catheter. Cardiovasc. Interv.* 83 (2): 305–307.

14 Meincke, F., Spangenberg, T., Kreidel, F. et al. (2017). Rationale of cerebral protection devices in left atrial appendage occlusion. *Catheter. Cardiovasc. Interv.* 89 (1): 154–158.

15 Mohanty, S., Trivedi, C., Beheiry, S. et al. (2019). Venous access-site closure with vascular closure device vs. manual compression in patients undergoing catheter ablation or left atrial appendage occlusion under uninterrupted anticoagulation: a multicentre experience on efficacy and complications. *Europace* 21 (7): 1048–1054.

16 Osmancik, P., Herman, D., Neuzil, P. et al. (2020). Left atrial appendage closure versus direct oral anticoagulants in high-risk patients with atrial fibrillation. *J. Am. Coll. Cardiol.* 75 (25): 3122–3135.

17 Park, J., W., Bethencourt, A., Sievert, H. et al. (2011). Left atrial appendage closure with Amplatzer cardiac plug in atrial fibrillation: initial European experience. *Catheter. Cardiovasc. Interv.* 77 (5): 700–706.

18 Reddy, V., Y., Gibson, D.N., Kar, S. et al. (2017). Post-approval U.S. experience with left atrial appendage closure for stroke prevention in atrial fibrillation. *J. Am. Coll. Cardiol.* 69 (3): 253–261.

19 Saw, J., Fahmy, P., DeJong, P. et al. (2015). Cardiac CT angiography for device surveillance after endovascular left atrial appendage closure. *Eur. Heart J. Cardiovasc. Imaging* 16 (11): 1198–1206.

20 Sawant, A., C., Seibolt, L., Sridhara, S. et al. (2020). Operator experience and outcomes after transcatheter left atrial appendage occlusion with the watchman device. *Cardiovasc. Revasc. Med.* 21 (4): 467–472.

21 Søndergaard, L., Wong, Y.H., Reddy, V.Y. et al. (2019). Propensity-matched comparison of oral anticoagulation versus antiplatelet therapy after left atrial appendage closure with WATCHMAN. *JACC Cardiovasc. Interv.* 12 (11): 1055–1063.

22 Tarantini, G., D'Amico, G., Latib, A. et al. (2018). Percutaneous left atrial appendage occlusion in patients with atrial fibrillation and left appendage thrombus: feasibility, safety and clinical efficacy. *EuroIntervention* 13 (13): 1595–1602.

23 Thakkar, J., Vasdeki, D., Tzikas, A. et al. (2018). Incidence, prevention, and management of periprocedural complications of left atrial appendage occlusion. *Interv. Cardiol. Clin.* 7 (2): 243–252.

24 Tzikas, A., Gafoor, S., Meerkin, S. et al. (2016). Left atrial appendage occlusion with the AMPLATZER Amulet device: an expert consensus step-by-step approach. *EuroIntervention* 11 (13): 1512–1521.

25 Wilkins, B., Fukutomi, B., De Backer, O. et al. (2020). Left atrial appendage closure: prevention and Management of Periprocedural and Postprocedural Complications. *Card Electrophysiol. Clin.* 12 (1): 67–75.

26 Wunderlich, N., C., Lorch, G., Honold, J. et al. (2020). Why follow-up examinations after left atrial appendage closure are important: detection of complications during follow-up and how to deal with them. *Curr. Cardiol. Rep.* 22 (10): 113.

Part VI

Selected Structural Interventions for Cardiomyopathies

56

The Natural History of Hypertrophic Cardiomyopathy

John S. Douglas, Jr.[1]

[1] *Interventional Cardiology, Emory University School of Medicine, Emory University Hospital, Atlanta, GA, USA*

1. What is hypertrophic cardiomyopathy?

Hypertrophic cardiomyopathy (HCM) is a cardiac disorder characterized by the presence of left ventricular hypertrophy without a secondary cause such as hypertension or valvular heart disease. Left ventricular hypertrophy has been defined as left ventricular end diastolic wall thickness >13 mm based on the CARDIA (Coronary Artery Risk Development in Young Adults) study of young adults or ≥15 mm by the European Society of Cardiology Guidelines. HCM may be inherited or occur as the result of a spontaneous gene mutation. Hypertrophy is often asymmetrical, with the most severe wall thickening occurring in the basal portion of the interventricular septum.

2. What is the prevalence of HCM?

HCM exists in about 1 per 500 individuals in the general population worldwide and about 700 000 people in the United States.

3. Is left ventricular outflow tract obstruction a common occurrence in patients with HCM?

Left ventricular outflow tract (LVOT) obstruction in the resting state is present in about one-third of affected individuals and provocable by Valsalva, exercise, and other maneuvers in an additional one-third of individuals with HCM. The remaining one-third have no LVOT obstruction. The presence of LVOT obstruction is a predictor of adverse outcomes, and treatment strategies are aimed at reducing it.

4. What is the prognosis of an individual with HCM?

HCM has a benign course in a majority of gene-positive individuals, many of whom are unaware of its presence. It is, however, an important cause of sudden cardiac death (SCD), particularly in adolescents and young adults. Many genetically affected individuals who may be unaware of the presence of HCM develop vague symptoms that can negatively impact their quality of life.

5. Are there predictors of sudden cardiac death?

Non-sustained ventricular tachycardia, a family history of sudden cardiac death, unexplained syncope, and severe left ventricular hypertrophy (wall thickness ≥30 mm) are significant risk factors for SCD in patients with HCM. Late gadolinium enhancement assessed by cardiac magnetic resonance imaging, a measure of myocardial fibrosis, is a promising marker for increased risk of SCD.

6. How is a diagnosis of HCM made?

HCM may be suspected due to the presence of a heart murmur, an abnormal electrocardiogram, or a family history of HCM. The use of echocardiography is the most widely available and accurate method of confirming a diagnosis of HCM and is useful in monitoring LVOT obstruction during therapy.

Other imaging techniques such as MRI or cardiac CT may be helpful when the results of echocardiography are equivocal.

7. Is genetic testing helpful?

Genetic testing is a powerful tool in diagnosing and managing HCM patients and their families. A three-generational family history is an important part of the initial evaluation. The HCM-causing gene is most often inherited as an autosomal dominant trait, with offspring having a 50% chance of inheriting the disease-causing genetic variant. In at-risk family members, genetic testing has several benefits, including confirmation of diagnosis, preclinical recognition, and guiding reproductive decisions.

8. Are there multiple HCM-related genes?

Yes. Mutations associated with HCM have been detected in over a dozen genes whose role is encoding sarcomeric proteins. Two genes (MYH7 and MYBPC3) that encode B-myosin heavy chain and myosin-binding protein C are the most common and account for about half of HCM families. In a substantial minority of HCM patients, the responsible gene mutations have not been identified previously.

9. Are all individuals with HCM affected similarly?

No. There is enormous variability in the type and magnitude of heart abnormalities and symptoms experienced. The vast majority of genetically affected individuals are asymptomatic or have mild symptoms. However, to a degree, the specific gene mutation can influence anatomic findings and the degree of LVOT obstruction and symptoms. The commonly encountered variability in anatomy and symptoms, even in individuals with the same gene, is referred to as *variable penetrance*.

10. What kind of symptoms does HCM cause?

Shortness of breath with exertion, chest tightness, and fatigue are common symptoms. Fainting (syncope) or near syncope occur in some patients and is often related to the degree of ventricular outflow tract obstruction present at rest or with exertion.

11. Are there measures that should be undertaken in all individuals with HCM, even those with no symptoms?

The mere presence of HCM dictates a need for three precautionary strategies:

- Competitive athletics such as football, basketball, and track should be avoided.
- Prophylaxis against heart valve infection during dental procedures by antibiotic administration is indicated.
- Dehydration that results in reduced LV volume and increased LVOT obstruction should be avoided.

12. What treatment is available for individuals with symptoms?

Medical therapy, alcohol septal ablation, permanent cardiac pacing, and surgical myectomy each reduce symptoms to a degree and have been utilized in patients with HCM. Medical therapy is the usual initial treatment.

13. What medical therapy is recommended?

HCM has diverse phenotypic expressions and presents primarily in two different forms (obstructive and non-obstructive). In patients with non-obstructive HCM, beta-blockers and non-dihydropyridine calcium channel blockers are guideline recommended. Both slow the heart rate, improve diastolic function, lower LV filling pressure, improve LV filling, and reduce myocardial oxygen demand. Verapamil and diltiazem have been shown to reduce chest pain and improve exercise tolerance. Beta-blockers are used with benefit in non-obstructive HCM, but trial data are lacking. Beta-blockers are generally considered front-line therapy for patients with obstructive HCM and should be titrated to achieve suppression of resting heart rate to 50–60 beats/minute. Diltiazem and verapamil also provide relief of symptoms in obstructive HCM; however, both agents have vasodilating properties that may limit their usefulness.

14. Does medical therapy "cure" the problem of HCM?

No. Medical therapy may, however, reduce symptoms such as exertional shortness of breath and permit patients to be more active, improving quality of life. In some patients, medical therapy remains effective for many years. In others, the severity of the HCM condition may worsen, reducing the effectiveness of medications and increasing symptoms and functional limitations necessitating consideration of septal reduction strategies such as alcohol ablation and myectomy.

15. What is alcohol septal ablation?

Alcohol septal ablation is a cardiac catheterization laboratory procedure aimed at reducing LVOT obstruction in HCM by an alcohol-induced septal myocardial infarction. The septal coronary artery that supplies the basal interventricular septum (the myocardial segment removed by surgical myectomy and the site of systolic anterior motion [SAM]-septal contact) is identified by contrast media injection through an inflated balloon catheter directly into the suspected septal perforating artery. This causes brightening of the myocardium supplied by that septal artery, which can be observed by transthoracic echocardiography. Alcohol injection in the appropriate septal artery results in necrosis of the basal septum, hypokinesis and thinning of the affected wall segment, and reduction in the LVOT pressure gradient.

16. What is septal myectomy?

Septal myectomy is an open-heart procedure during which the surgeon removes a "strip" of heart muscle from the left side of the interventricular septum immediately below the aortic valve. The removal of this muscle tissue relieves the obstruction to outflow from the heart, following which most patients experience substantial relief from symptoms of exertional dyspnea and exercise intolerance. About 5–10% of patients undergoing surgical myectomy require a permanent pacemaker because the electrical wiring of the heart is cut. In a small minority of patients, a second procedure is required due to inadequate initial relief of obstruction or progression of the HCM condition.

17. What is permanent pacing, and how is it helpful to the symptomatic HCM patient?

About 20 years ago, some physicians believed strongly that placement of a permanent cardiac pacemaker offered substantial relief in patients whose symptoms were bothersome in spite of medical therapy. Pacing electrically activates the right side of the septum first in a matter that theoretically should reduce LVOT obstruction. However, two studies were performed during which HCM patients with pacemakers were "blinded" as to whether the pacer was turned on or off, and quality of life was assessed. The outcome of these studies suggested that only a small minority of HCM patients benefited significantly from permanent pacing.

Bibliography

1 Brauwald, E., Lambrew, C.T., Rockoff, S.D. et al. (1964). Idiopathic hypertrophic subaortic stenosis. I. A description of the disease based upon an analysis of 64 patients. *Circulation* 29 (Suppl 4): 3–119.

2 Gersh, B.J., Maron, B.J., Bonow, R.O. et al. (2011). 2011 ACCF/AHA guideline for the diagnosis and treatment of hypertrophic cardiomyopathy: a report of the American College of Cardiology Foundation/American Heart Association Task Force on Practice Guidelines. *J. Am. Coll. Cardiol.* 58: e212–e260.

3 Leonardi, R.A., Kransdorf, E.P., Simel, D.L., and Wang, A. (2010). Meta-analyses of septal reduction therapies for obstructive hypertrophic cardiomyopathy: comparative rates of overall mortality and sudden cardiac death after treatment. *Circ. Cardiovasc. Interv.* 3: 97–104.

4 Maron, M.S., Jr, L., and Maron, B.J. (2010). Management implications of massive left ventricular hypertrophy in hypertrophic cardiomyopathy significantly underestimated by echocardiography but identified by cardiovascular magnetic resonance. AM. *J. Cardiol.* 1051842–1051843.

5 Maron, M.S., Olivotto, I., Zenovich, A.G. et al. (2006). Hypertrophic cardiomyopathy is predominantly a disease of left ventricular outflow tract obstruction. *Circulation* 114: 2232–2239.

57

Alcohol Septal Ablation in Hypertrophic Cardiomyopathy

John S. Douglas, Jr.[1]

[1] Emory University School of Medicine, Emory University Hospital, Atlanta, GA, USA

1. In the group of patients with hypertrophic cardiomyopathy (HCM) who fail medical therapy, what proportion are candidates for alcohol septal ablation?

An overwhelming majority of HCM patients with significant left ventricular outflow tract (LVOT) obstruction who fail medical therapy can safely undergo alcohol septal ablation with an expectation of substantial benefit.

2. Are there patients with drug-refractory obstructive HCM who are not excellent candidates for alcohol ablation?

Yes. Because alcohol ablation may negatively impact the conduction system of the heart, patients who already have some conduction system abnormality are at increased risk of needing permanent pacing. Others at increased risk are very elderly and those with comorbidities.

3. What specific baseline conduction system abnormalities are a problem, and why?

The presence of a left bundle branch block (LBBB) is a significant issue. Alcohol septal ablation causes the development of a right bundle branch block (RBBB) in about 60% of patients. With LBBB at baseline, about 60% of patients will develop complete heart block. There is very little increased procedural risk when this happens but obvious added cost and mild discomfort due to the need for placement of the permanent pacemaker. In addition, there are long-term issues related to battery life and lead failure that are significant, especially in younger patients.

4. Are there other conduction system abnormalities that are caused by alcohol septal ablation?

Yes. About 20% developed left anterior hemiblock, 10% developed LBBB, and transient complete heart block has been seen in 25–55% of patients.

5. What is the time interval for which patients who developed procedural-related conduction system abnormalities must be observed to avoid unnecessary permanent pacemaker insertion?

A European group reported that 55% of patients developed transient atrioventricular (AV) block during alcohol ablation with persisting AV block in 23% at 14 hours, 18% after 3 days, 7% at 1 week, and only 3% at 13 days.

6. Did the European group reporting AV block with alcohol ablation have a recommendation regarding the length of time patients should be observed before inserting a permanent pacemaker?

Yes. They recommended waiting ≥7 days before pacemaker insertion. This rather long waiting period is unacceptable to many US physicians, resulting in a much higher rate of pacemaker implantation in the United States compared to Europe.

7. Are there strategies that may reduce the rate of occurrence of AV block?

Yes. Among nine European centers that minimized the volume of alcohol injected (medium dose 1.5 ml), complete heart block occurred in 18%, but only 9% required a permanent pacemaker. The amount of alcohol injected in a large US experience was 2.9 ml.

8. What complications can be expected in patients undergoing alcohol septal ablation?

Among 874 alcohol ablation procedures performed in nine US centers, dissection of the left anterior descending (LAD) artery occurred in eight patients, cardiac tamponade in four, retroperitoneal bleed in one, and ventricular septal defect in one. Ventricular tachycardia or fibrillation occurred in 14 patients, high-grade AV block in 78, and death in 6.

The 2011 American College of Cardiology/American Heart Association (ACC/AHA) HCM guideline statement is guarded in its recommendations for alcohol ablation, especially in younger patients, in large part due to the paucity of long-term follow-up data at the time that this guideline statement was written (2009–2010). The 2014 European guidelines and 2020 ACC/AHA guidelines give myectomy and alcohol ablation equal status as therapeutic options in drug-refractory patients.

9. Subsequently, have long-term studies been reported?

Yes. Although there are no randomized trials comparing myectomy and ablation (future trials are expected), several studies have reported favorable long-term outcomes after alcohol ablation. Especially important with regard to younger patients, those who underwent alcohol ablation had survival similar to the age-matched general population and age-matched HCM patients without obstruction.

10. What is the first step that the operator takes in performing alcohol ablation?

Following placement of a pacemaker lead, the operator must attempt to identify by coronary arteriography the coronary artery branch most likely to supply the left side of the basal septum (the systolic anterior motion [SAM]-septal contact area) (Figure 57.1b).

11. Does this arterial branch always originate from the LAD?

No. although the arterial supply to the basal septum is commonly the first septal perforating branch of the LAD, this artery may originate from a diagonal branch of the LAD, from the proximal circumflex, left main coronary artery, and rarely even from the right coronary artery.

12. Must the septal artery selected for alcohol ablation be of a certain size?

No. Occasionally the septal perforating artery selected for alcohol ablation is extremely small, barely visible during coronary arteriography. In this case, a very small 1.0–1.5 mm diameter over the wire balloon catheter is inserted. In the presence of an exceptionally large septal artery with early branching, one of the branches of the large septal artery may be selected.

13. How does the operator confirm that the septal artery selected is the correct one?

With a balloon catheter inflated in the proximal part of the selected artery, the operator injects 1–2 ml of contrast media and observes with echocardiography whether the appropriate septal region "brightness" (Figure 57.1c, d).

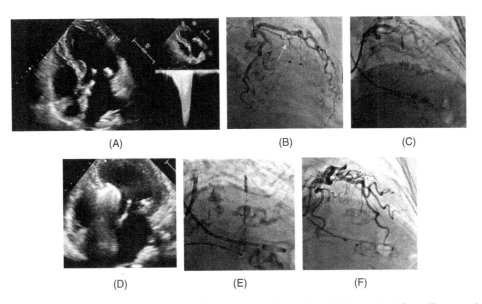

Figure 57.1 (a) Transthoracic echocardiogram image of a patient with hypertrophic cardiomyopathy with a significant gradient across the left ventricular outflow tract (LVOT). (b) First septal perforator arising from the left anterior descending artery. (c) Over-the-wire balloon inflated in the proximal segment of the selected septal perforator for contrast media injection. (d) Brightening of the hypertrophied septal region after contrast media injection through the coronary balloon inflated in the septal artery, matching the selected septal artery with the hypertrophic segment to ablate. (e) Contrast injected through the balloon into the septal artery confirming adequate balloon size and no contrast spillback into the LAD. (f) Angiogram post alcohol septal ablation with absence of the septal perforator.

14. Describe how the proper size of the balloon catheter is determined.

A short balloon (6 mm) is usually preferred. The balloon diameter is determined by the diameter of the septal artery. With the balloon inflated to 4–5 atm of pressure, occlusion of the septal artery occurs. If the balloon is undersized, contrast media injected through the balloon catheter may appear in the LAD simply because the too-small balloon does not occlude the septal artery. An oversized balloon may "melon seed" back into the LAD. With over- or under-sizing, any liquid injected through the balloon catheter may migrate into the LAD (Figure 57.1e).

15. What is the consequence of alcohol being injected into the LAD?

Alcohol entering the LAD causes an infarction in the distribution of this artery, which may be poorly tolerated by the patient. Anterior ST segment elevation, chest pain, hypotension, cardiogenic shock, and death have been observed.

16. Is the usual contrast media suitable for alcohol septal ablation?

Yes. A 50–50 mixture of contrast and saline is agitated with air before injection. This mixture of contrast media, saline, and small air bubbles injected into a coronary artery causes the myocardium to look "bright" on echocardiography.

17. How does the operator determine when the procedure has been successful and should be terminated?

The LVOT pressure gradient is monitored during the procedure, preferably with a catheter placed in the left ventricle and simultaneous measurement of aortic pressure through the guide catheter, which has been placed in the left coronary artery. Some operators prefer to use an LVOT pressure gradient measured by echocardiography. An LVOT pressure gradient of about 50 mmHg is frequently present pre-procedure. An LVOT pressure gradient <20 mmHg is a reasonable target to indicate procedural success.

18. Is reduction of LVOT pressure gradient to <20 mm Hg a reliable indicator of a "successful" alcohol ablation procedure?

Unfortunately, no. Some patients experience a reduction in LVOT pressure gradient after alcohol injection in a septal perforating branch but are later found to have a return of the LVOT pressure gradient. This suggests that transient myocardial dysfunction or "stunning" occurs rather than necrosis in some patients. Whether a second alcohol ablation procedure may produce better results is unclear.

Bibliography

1 Braunwald, E., Lambrew, C.T., Rockoff, S.D. et al. (1964). Idiopathic hypertrophic subaortic stenosis. A description of the disease based upon an analysis of 64 patients. *Circulation* 30: 3.

2 El Sabawi, B., Nishimura, R.A., Barness, G.W. et al. (2020). Temporal occurrence of arrhythmic complications after alcohol septal ablation. *Circ. Cardiovasc. Interv.* 13: e008540. https://doi.org/10.1161/CIRCINTERVENTIONS 119.008540.

3 Elliott, P.M., Anastasakis, A., Borger, M.A. et al. (2014). 2014 European Society of Cardiology guidelines on diagnosis and management of hypertrophic cardiomyopathy. *Eur. Heart J.* 35: 2733.

4 El-Sabawi, B., Nishimura, R.A., Yong-Mri, C. et al. (2020). Transient complete heart block after alcohol septal ablation. *Circulation: CV Interventions* 13: 1–2.

5 Feldman, D.N., Douglas, J.S.J.R., and Naidu, S.S. (2015). Indications for and individualization of septal reduction therapy. In: *Hypertrophic Cardiomyopathy* (ed. S.S. Naidu), 207. London: Spinger-Verlag.

6 Gersh, B., Maron, B.J., Bonow, R.O. et al. (2011). 2011 ACCF/AHA guideline for the diagnosis and treatment of hypertrophic cardiomyopathy: a report of the American College of Cardiology Foundation/American Heart Association Task Force on Practice Guidelines. American College of Cardiology Foundation/American Heart Association Task Force on Practice Guidelines; American Association for Thoracic Surgery; American Society of Echocardiography; American Society of Nuclear Cardiology; Heart Failure Society of American; Heart Rhythm Society; Society for Cardiovascular Angiography and Interventions; Society of Thoracic Surgeons. *J. Am. Coll. Cardiol.* 58: 2703–2738.

7 Leonardi, R.A., Kransdorf, E.P., Simel, D.L. et al. (2010). Meta-analyses of septal reduction therapies for obstructive hypertrophic cardiomyopathy: comparative rates of overall mortality and sudden cardiac death after treatment. *Circ. Cardiovasc. Interv.* 3: 97.

8 Leonardi, R.A., Townsend, J.C., Patel, C.A. et al. (2013). Alcohol septal ablation for obstructive hypertrophic cardiomyopathy: outcomes in young, middle-aged, and elderly patients. *Cather. Cardiovasc. Interv.* 82: 838.

9 Nagueh, S.F., Groves, B.M., Schwartz, L. et al. (2011). Alcohol septal ablation for the treatment of hypertrophic obstructive cardiomyopathy. A multicenter North American registry. *J. Am. Coll. Cardiol.* 58: 2322–2328.

10 Ommen, S.R., Mital, S., and Burke, M.A. (2020). 2020 AHA/ACC guideline for the diagnosis and treatment of patient with hypertrophic cardiomyopathy: a report of the American College of Cardiology/American Heart Association joint committee on clinical practice guidelines. *J. Am. Coll. Cardiol.* 76: 3022–3055.

11 Reihard, W., Ten Cate, F.J., Scholten, M. et al. (2004). Permanent pacing for complete atrioventricular block after nonsurgical (alcohol) septal reduction in patients with obstructive hypertrophic cardiomyopathy. *Am. J. Cardiol.* 93: 1064.

12 Veselka, J., Krejci, J., Tomasov, P. et al. (2014). Survival of patients ≤50 years of age after alcohol septal ablation for hypertrophic obstructive cardiomyopathy. *Can. J. Cardiol.* 30: 634.

58

Transcatheter Edge-to-Edge Repair for Hypertrophic Cardiomyopathy

Camilo A. Gomez[1] and Eduardo J. de Marchena[2]

[1] Department of Cardiology, Jackson Memorial Health System, Miami, FL, USA
[2] Cardiovascular Division, University of Miami Miller School of Medicine, Miami, FL, USA

1. Why is the mitral valve important in hypertrophic cardiomyopathy?

In hypertrophic cardiomyopathy (HCM), left ventricular outflow tract (LVOT) obstruction is the hallmark of the disease. This phenomenon causes the most significant symptoms associated with the disease. The mitral valve has been identified as one of the structures that plays an important role in the pathophysiological process of LVOT obstruction. In particular, the systolic anterior motion (SAM) of the mitral apparatus and its contact with the hypertrophied septum lead to a pressure gradient due to the narrowed LVOT. This phenomenon is dynamic and, in many cases, associated with significant mitral regurgitation (MR).

Increasing interest in this interaction of the mitral valve has led to further research studies. Initially, SAM was believed to be caused only by a Venturi effect from the septal hypertrophy sucking the mitral valve leaflets into the LVOT. Currently, it is understood that left ventricle ejection occurs against an abnormally elongated and positioned anterior mitral valve leaflet. This results in a dragging force to the leaflet into the LVOT, causing obstruction. Additionally, this phenomenon causes a distortion of the mitral valve apparatus, frequently resulting in secondary MR, which may be a major cause of severe symptoms (Figure 58.1).

2. Are mitral valve abnormalities in HCM a primary or secondary phenomenon, or is there primary mitral valve pathology?

Cumulative research and evidence have shown that there are primary mitral valve leaflet abnormalities independent of other disease variables in HCM. An MRI study found that there is an anterior mitral valve leaflet elongation that is independent of the left ventricular wall thickness and age. It likely represents a primary phenotypic expression that is important in the disease process responsible for LVOT obstruction and MR.

3. What are the options for treatment of patients with HCM who fail medical therapy?

Some patients have persistent symptoms from LVOT gradients or MR despite optimal medical therapy; others have an intolerance to the side effect of the medications. These patients can benefit from an invasive intervention such as septal myomectomy or alcohol septal ablation (ASA). However, a residual subset of patients remains persistently symptomatic despite these invasive interventions, mainly due to residual MR from primary mitral valve pathology. The Alfieri technique (edge-to-edge surgical mitral valve

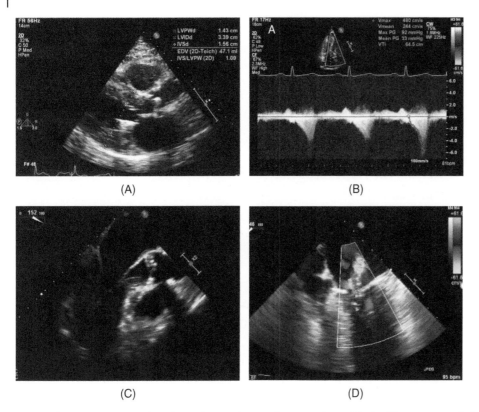

(A) (B)

(C) (D)

Figure 58.1 (a) Transthoracic echocardiogram images from a patient with significant concentric hypertrophy and hypertrophic septum. (b) Significant left ventricular outflow tract gradient of 92 mmHg at rest. (c) Transesophageal echocardiogram (TEE) showing the systolic anterior motion of the mitral valve in contact with the hypertrophic septum. (d) TEE images of the significant mitral regurgitation jet.

repair) has been evaluated for the treatment of HCM in patients undergoing myomectomy and mitral repair to prevent or treat SAM and shown to be effective and durable and to rarely produce significant mitral stenosis. Surgical myomectomy and alcohol septal ablation cannot be used for some patients because of their baseline comorbidities and risk associated with the procedure or non-favorable anatomy. This group of patients has been studied for further interventional therapies.

4. Is percutaneous mitral valve repair with the MitraClip an option in HCM?

There is convincing cumulative evidence for the use of the MitraClip device to mitigate SAM of the anterior mitral leaflet and improve the severity of MR. It is a promising technology for symptomatic HCM patients who are not good candidates for surgical myomectomy or ASA and have intrinsic mitral valve disease amenable to percutaneous repair. Reports have shown that the plication of the anterior and posterior mitral valve leaflets can effectively

relieve SAM and obstruction in the LVOT, improve MR, and lead to a sustained reduction in the LVOT gradient. Observations demonstrated an improvement in symptoms, with improvement in New York Heart Association (NYHA) functional class and exercise tolerance on follow-up.

5. What are the potential benefits of percutaneous mitral valve repair compared to traditional techniques used in HCM?

Currently, the recommendation for patients who are poor surgical candidates for myomectomy is ASA. However, observations and increasing familiarity with the procedure suggest that the MitraClip may be as efficacious as surgical myomectomy or ASA and is a safer option in some cases. It is well described that ASA is associated with the risk of conduction abnormalities and complete heart block in patients with pre-existing left bundle branch block. Hence there is limited evidence available for the use of the MitraClip to treat patients with HCM and LVOT obstruction. It is suggested that it has the potential to accomplish similar results to myomectomy procedures without the risk to the conduction system and myocardial necrosis that has been linked to being a source for potential arrhythmias. Data are still extremely limited in the literature, and there are no comparative studies between the percutaneous minimally invasive techniques.

In patients with favorable anatomy and without significant concomitant mitral valve disease, ASA should be considered first, but the MitraClip is more widely available and is a very attractive technology that can be used in selected patients. This is especially true for those with non-favorable anatomy for ASA, such as a septum thickness of less than 1.6 cm or septal perforators that are not suitable because of their size or lack of supply of the area that needs to be ablated (Table 58.1).

6. What are the technical considerations if the MitraClip is selected as therapy for HCM?

As in every structural procedure, pre-procedural planning is the most important aspect of success. An extensive review of the case by the Heart Team is important; first, assess whether there is room for optimization of the current treatment; and second, evaluate other therapeutic alternatives. If percutaneous mitral valve repair is selected, it is important to always have a pre-procedural transesophageal echocardiogram (TEE) to confirm that the anatomy is favorable for a clip procedure. One of the unique obstacles in these patients that should be considered during the pre-procedural evaluation is the left atrial (LA) size. LA dilation and atrial myopathies are associated with a worse prognosis in HCM, but it is not uncommon that the LA is not dilated to the degree observed in other mitral valve

Table 58.1 Important factors that can be used to decide between percutaneous techniques – alcohol septal ablation or edge-to-edge repair – in patients who are not candidates for surgical myomectomy.

Patient not a candidate for surgical myomectomy	
Alcohol septal ablation candidate	**Edge-to-edge repair candidate**
Significant septal hypertrophy >1.6 cm	Septum less than 1.6 cm
Identifiable septal branch	Severe mitral regurgitation due to primary mitral valve deformity
Septal branch supplies the area that needs to be ablated	Previous myomectomy
Systolic anterior motion-related left ventricular outflow tract obstruction	Severe left ventricular hypertrophy with mid-cavitary gradient as part of a multiple-approach strategy
	Non-favorable septal branches for alcohol septal ablation

disorders, which is important for the navigation of the equipment inside the atrial chamber.

In general, implantation of the clip is performed with the same technique, with the orientation of the clip arms orthogonal to the commissural plane of the valve. Intra-procedural TEE should confirm the improvement in MR and is also important for assessment of the improvement of the SAM in the LVOT view. It is also important to measure the gradients through the LVOT before releasing the clip. Another point for consideration is a detailed assessment of the mitral gradient since the mitral annulus is not as dilated as much as we are used to seeing in other chronic MR cases that we treat with the MitraClip (Figure 58.2).

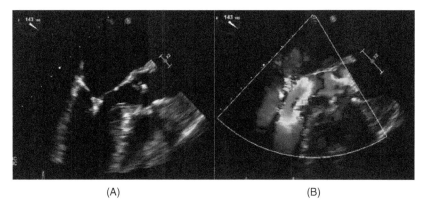

(A)   (B)

Figure 58.2   (a) Transesophageal echocardiography images of post-MitraClip deployment result with improvement in systolic anterior motion. (b) Left ventricular outflow tract gradient and improvement in mitral regurgitation.

7. What are future venues for the percutaneous treatment and repair of the mitral valve with the MitraClip or other technologies in HCM?

As mentioned, the data are limited, but avenues are open for future research on the MitraClip and other percutaneous technologies for the treatment of HCM. More data are needed to determine whether the MitraClip can be used as first- or second-line therapy as an alternative to surgical myomectomy or ASA. We are also unsure whether improvement in the gradient and MR with a clip is long-lasting. Moreover, it would be interesting and important to consider the use of the technology in combination with septal ablation: for example, to try to replicate the positive results shown in surgical studies with concomitant use of surgical myomectomy and mitral valve repair in patients with HCM. Evaluating combined procedures such as surgical myomectomy plus the MitraClip or less invasive ASA plus the MitraClip in the same setting can open future therapeutic venues.

Bibliography

1 Bhudia, S.K., McCarthy, P.M., Smedira, N.G. et al. (2004). Edge-to-edge (Alfieri) mitral repair: results in diverse clinical settings. *Ann. Thorac. Surg.* 77: 1598–1606.

2 Hong, J., Schaff, H., Nishimura, R. et al. (2016). Mitral regurgitation in patients with hypertrophic obstructive cardiomyopathy. *Implicat. Concomitant Valve Proced. JACC* 68 (14): 1497–1504.

3 Long, A. and Mahoney, P. (2020). Use of MitraClip to target obstructive SAM in severe diffuse-type hypertrophic cardiomyopathy: case report and review of literature. *J. Invasive Cardiol.* 32 (9): E228–E232.

4 Maron, M., Olivotto, I., Harringan, C., and Appelbaum, E. (2011). Mitral valve abnormalities identified by cardiovascular magnetic resonance represent a primary phenotypic expression of hypertrophic cardiomyopathy. *Circulation* 124: 40–47.

5 Nishimura, R., Seggewiss, H., and Schaff, H. (2017). Hypertrophic obstructive cardiomyopathy. Surgical myomectomy and septal ablation. *Circ. Res.* 121: 771–783. https://doi.org/10.1161/CIRCRESAHA.116.309348.

6 Sado, D., Flett, A., McGregor, C. et al. (2010). Myomectomy plus Alfieri technique for outflow tract obstruction in hypertrophic cardiomyopathy. *Circulation* 122: 938–939.

7 Schäfer, U., Kreidel, F., and Frerker, C. (2014). MitraClip implantation as a new treatment strategy against systolic anterior motion-induced outflow tract obstruction in hypertrophic obstructive cardiomyopathy. *Heart Lung Circ.* 23: e131–e135.

8 Sorajja, P., Pedersen, W.A., Bae, R. et al. (2016). First experience with percutaneous mitral valve plication as primary therapy for symptomatic obstructive hypertrophic cardiomyopathy. *J. Am. Coll. Cardiol.* 67: 2811–2818. https://doi.org/10.1161/CIRCULATIONAHA.110.969451.

9 Thomas, F., Rader, F., and Siegel, R. (2017). The use of MitraClip for symptomatic patients with hypertrophic bstructive cardiomyopathy. *Cardiology* 137: 58–61. https://doi.org/10.1159/000454800.

59

Interatrial Shunt Creation

Phillip Rubin[1] and Mauricio G. Cohen[1,2]

[1] Cardiovascular Division, Department of Medicine, University of Miami Miller School of Medicine, Miami, FL, USA
[2] Cardiac Catheterization Laboratory, UHealth Tower, University of Miami Hospitals and Clinics, Miami, FL, USA

1. What is the rationale for the creation of interatrial shunts?

Pre-clinical studies in sheep with ischemic cardiomyopathy have demonstrated hemodynamic, echocardiographic, and survival benefits with the creation of small interatrial shunts that selectively unload the left heart. Patients with left-sided valve disease and an atrial septal defect (ASD) have better outcomes than those with valve disease alone, which suggests benefit from left atrial (LA) decompression. Conversely, ASD closure has been observed to precipitate heart failure (HF) symptoms by unmasking elevated LA pressures in previously asymptomatic patients.

2. Which populations may benefit from interatrial shunt devices?

Interatrial shunt creation is an emerging interventional treatment for patients with acute and chronic HF. Interatrial shunting is expected to benefit patients with abnormal LA filling pressures, at rest or upon exertion. HF management guided by pulmonary diastolic pressure (a surrogate for LA pressure) has been shown to reduce HF hospitalizations and improve short- and long-term outcomes. Shunt devices are especially promising in patients with heart failure with preserved ejection fraction (HFpEF) as there is a lack of effective therapies.

3. How is net shunt volume quantified?

A tool for quantifying net shunt is the Qp/Qs ratio, the ratio of total pulmonary blood flow (Qp) to total systemic blood flow (Qs). A ratio of 1 : 1 is normal and indicates that there is no shunting, a ratio of <1 : 1 indicates right-to-left shunting, and a ratio of >1 : 1 indicates the presence of left-to-right shunting.

4. What is the role of shunt creation via atrial septostomy for patients with refractory cardiogenic shock?

Atrial septostomy (AS) is a recently developed option for patients with cardiogenic shock on venoarterial extracorporeal membrane oxygenation (VA-ECMO) who develop refractory pulmonary edema or hypoxemia. LA decompression tends to lead to resolution of pulmonary edema and reduction in ventilator requirements as well as contribute to LV recovery and weaning from ECMO support. Furthermore, AS can prolong patient survival while awaiting LV recovery or heart transplantation.

5. What are the principal steps in performing bedside AS?

The initial step is right-heart catheterization (RHC) with hemodynamic measurements. Using fluoroscopic and echocardiographic guidance, a transseptal puncture is made at the fossa ovalis, followed by advancing a long sheath through the puncture into the LA. A non-compliant balloon is then advanced through a stiff guidewire and dilated at the level of the interatrial septum. Large balloons, usually greater than 10–15 mm and as large as 27 mm (typically an Inoue or peripheral balloon), have been used to create a hemodynamically effective shunt.

6. What are the primary interatrial shunt devices currently under investigation?

There are three primary designs: InterAtrial Shunt Device (IASD), V-Wave device, and the Atrial Flow Regulator (AFR) (Figure 59.1). The IASD is composed of a Nitinol mesh disc with an outer diameter of 19 mm and a fenestration of 8 mm. The V-Wave device is an hourglass-shaped Nitinol frame with a 5 mm inner diameter. The first generation of the V-Wave featured a pericardial valve intended to prevent flow reversal within the shunt to mitigate the risk of paradoxical embolization. However, at six months, approximately 50% of the shunts were stenosed or occluded due to pannus formation, and the valve was removed for the second generation with significant improvement in patency rate. The AFR is composed of two Nitinol discs with a central fenestration 6–10 mm in size, allowing for greater customization of shunt hemodynamics. The AFR has the capacity for bidirectional flow and has also been used for RA decompression in severe pulmonary hypertension.

Shunt creation without device implantation using catheter-directed radioablation or septal tissue removal is currently under investigation.

7. Outline the steps involved in atrial shunt device implantation

The procedure is generally performed under general anesthesia by transfemoral venous approach and with transesophageal echocardiography (TEE) guidance. However, the procedure can also be performed under moderate sedation with intracardiac echocardiography guidance (ICE). After transseptal puncture, a sheath (10–16 Fr, depending on the device) is advanced into the LA, whereupon the device is implanted using a dedicated delivery system by deploying the left side of the device, verifying its position within the

interatrial septum, and finally deploying the right side of the device.

8. Do interatrial shunt devices increase PA pressure and the risk of RV overload?

A concern with interatrial shunts is the potential for increasing pulmonary artery (PA) pressure and overloading the right ventricle (RV). Studies in congenital heart disease have shown that shunts less than 10 mm and/or Qp : Qs ratios <1.5 : 1 are well-tolerated without long-term harmful effects. The devices currently under investigation target shunt diameters and Qp : Qs ratios within these parameters. Initial studies have demonstrated only mild RV dilation at six months that remains stable at one year without evidence of decreased RV function or clinical right-sided HF.

9. What are other long-term concerns with interatrial shunt devices?

There is a small increase in resting central venous pressure (CVP; 1–2 mmHg), which may have long-term effects on hepatic and renal function. There is also concern about rates of device infection and thrombosis development. Furthermore, the presence of a shunt device can complicate or contraindicate other transseptal procedures. The effect of new-onset atrial fibrillation or other changes in LA hemodynamics on shunt function after device implantation has yet to be studied. Finally, the creation of an ASD poses the risk of paradoxical embolization. The trial data to date have not found paradoxical embolization to be a notable risk, but this needs reevaluation as larger trials are performed and longer-term data obtained.

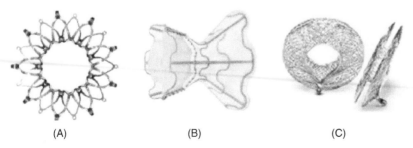

(A)   (B)   (C)

Figure 59.1 Interatrial shunt devices (IASDs). (a) IASD II system (Corvia Medical); (b) V-Wave device; (c) atrial flow regulator (AFR). *Source:* Adapted from Griffin et al. (2020), John Wiley & Sons.

10. What is the recommended antithrombotic therapy after implantation?

The current standard has been aspirin and clopidogrel for six months. In patients already treated with anticoagulation, antiplatelet monotherapy with aspirin has been the standard.

11. What are shunt devices that do not create an ASD?

A device under investigation is the coronary sinus-LA shunt. A channel is created between the coronary sinus and LA with the deployment of the shunt device. This has the advantage of preserving the interatrial septum for other procedures in the future as well as minimizing the risk of embolization.

Bibliography

1 Abraham, W.T., Adamson, P.B., Bourge, R.C. et al. (2011). Wireless pulmonary artery haemodynamic monitoring in chronic heart failure: a randomised controlled trial. *Lancet* 377 (9766): 658–666.

2 Griffin, J.M., Borlaug, B.A., Komtebedde, J. et al. (2020). Impact of interatrial shunts on invasive hemodynamics and exercise tolerance in patients with heart failure. *J. Am. Heart Assoc.* 9 (17): e016760.

3 Guimaraes, L., Del Val, D., Bergeron, S. et al. (2020). Interatrial shunting for treating acute and chronic left heart failure. *Eur. Cardiol.* 27 (15): e18.

Part VII

Selected Adult Congenital Structural Interventions

60

Shunt Hemodynamics and Calculations

Tawseef Dar[1] and Michael D. Dyal[1,2]

[1] *Cardiovascular Division, Department of Medicine, University of Miami Miller School of Medicine, Miami, FL, USA*
[2] *Department of Veterans Affairs, Miami, FL, USA*

1. What is a shunt, and how do we classify shunts?

Abnormal communication between pulmonary (venous) and systemic (arterial) circulation constitutes a *shunt*. Abnormal communication between the right and left heart chambers or great vessels constitutes an *intracardiac shunt*.

Intracardiac shunts are usually the result of an abnormal embryological development but are occasionally acquired as a mechanical complication (e.g. the septal rupture in myocardial infarction, septal perforation post septal myectomy). In the United States, approximately 1.4 million adults are currently living with some form of congenital heart defect. Intracardiac shunts are the most common congenital heart defects encountered in clinical practice.

Based on the direction of the blood flow, intracardiac shunts are usually classified as follows:

- Left-to-right shunt
- Right-to-left shunt
- Bidirectional shunt

Based on the location, intracardiac shunts are classified as follows:

- At the level of the interatrial septum
  a. Atrial septal defects (ASDs)
  b. Partial anomalous pulmonary venous return (pulmonary veins entering the right atrium [RA])

- At the level of the interventricular septum
  a. Ventricular septal defects (VSDs)

- At the level of great arteries
  a. Aortopulmonary window
  b. Patent ductus arteriosus

An abnormal communication between a peripheral artery and vein constitutes an arteriovenous (AV) shunt. These are usually iatrogenic, e.g. AV fistula for dialysis access or AV fistula as a complication of femoral access. In comparison to most large intracardiac shunts or even dialysis shunts (1000 ml/min), AV fistulae are usually low-volume (160–510 ml/min) shunts and therefore rarely symptomatic. AV shunt flows must exceed 30% of the cardiac output to have a hemodynamic impact and produce symptoms.

2. What is a diagnostic shunt study?

A diagnostic shunt study, also called a *saturation run or oximetry run*, is a unique right-heart catheterization procedure in which multiple 1–3 ml labeled blood samples are obtained rapidly and systematically in sequence from the pulmonary artery (PA; left or right), right ventricle (RV; outflow tract level, mid RV, and tricuspid level), RA (low, mid, and high level), superior vena cava (SVC), and inferior vena cava (IVC) on the right side followed by the left ventricle (LV; if feasible) and aorta distal to ductus (or peripheral artery as feasible) to calculate oxygen saturations on each sample. If a right-to-left or bidirectional shunt is suspected, additional samples from the pulmonary veins (or wedge position) and LA are needed to localize the shunt. The goal of the study is to *detect, localize, and quantify* any intracardiac shunts.

Usually, patients referred for a diagnostic shunt study already have a shunt diagnosed or suspected based on their clinical or echocardiographic evaluation prior to the catheterization. The purpose of the diagnostic shunt study in those cases is primarily to quantify the hemodynamic impact of the shunt.

3. During a routine left- or right-heart catheterization, what should prompt an interventional cardiologist to look for an intracardiac shunt?

There are three scenarios where an interventional cardiologist, while doing a routine catheterization procedure, should suspect an intracardiac shunt:

a. **A right-to-left shunt should be suspected** when arterial blood O_2 saturation is <95% despite corrective measures (like propping up with a large wedge/head-up tilt, deep breathing and coughing, and oxygen administration via face mask).

b. **A left-to-right shunt should be suspected** when pulmonary artery blood O_2 saturation is >80%
Note: we recommend routine assessment of systemic and pulmonary arterial saturations in diagnostic cardiac catheterizations.

c. **A shunt should be suspected** if there is a major discrepancy between physical examination findings and catheterization data. For example, a holosystolic murmur on physical exam and a left ventricular cine angiography showing no significant valvular regurgitation should raise suspicion for a possible intracardiac shunt (like VSD, PDA) giving rise to a systolic murmur on examination.

A full diagnostic shunt study is warranted to localize and quantify the shunt.

4. Does it matter if the patient is on oxygen while doing a diagnostic shunt study in the catheterization laboratory?

Yes. Ideally, the patient should be breathing (or ventilated with) room air or a gas mixture with an oxygen concentration of no more than 30% (2 L/minute via nasal canula).

Why does it matter? The dissolved oxygen content becomes significant when a patient is breathing oxygen at >30% concentration. The Fick equation does not factor this excess dissolved oxygen into the calculation because it relies solely on saturation data to calculate oxygen content. The pulmonary blood flow (Q_P) will be overestimated under such circumstances.

Principle

Oxygen consumption $_{ml/min}$ (**VO₂**) = oxygen delivered $_{ml/min}$ (**DO₂**)

Fick equation

Total Oxygen consumption $_{ml/min}$ (**VO₂**) =

[Total incoming blood (arterial) O_2 content $_{ml/min}$] − [Total outgoing blood (venous) O_2 content $_{ml/min}$]

[CO $_{ml/min}$ * arterial blood O_2 content $_{ml/ml}$] − [CO $_{ml/min}$ * mixed venous blood O_2 content $_{ml/ml}$]

CO $_{ml/min}$ * Hb $_{g/ml}$ * O_2 carrying capacity of Hb $_{ml/g}$ * $(SA_{\%satO2} - MV_{\%satO2})$

CO $_{ml/min}$ * Hb $_{g/ml}$ * 1.36$_{ml/g}$ * $(SA_{\%satO2} - MV_{\%satO2})$

$$co(ml/min) = \frac{VO_2(ml/min)}{Hb_{g/ml} * 1.36\,(SA_{\%satO2} - MV_{\%satO2})}$$

$$CO\,(L/min) = \frac{VO_2\,(ml/min)}{Hb_{g/dl} * 1.36 * 10\,(SA_{\%satO2} - MV_{\%satO2})}$$

$$CO\,(L/min) = \frac{VO_{2\,i}\,(ml/min/m^2) * BSA\,(m^2)}{Hb_{g/dl} * 13.6\,(SA_{\%satO2} - MV_{\%satO2})}$$

CO-Cardiac output; VO₂- total oxygen consumption; SA-systemic arterial; MV-mixed venous
$VO_{2\,i}$- Oxygen consumption index (oxygen consumption per unit body surface area); BSA-Body surface area

$$\text{Cardiac Ouput, Systemic (ml/min)}$$

$$\frac{VO_2 (ml/min/m^2) * BSA (m^2)}{\text{Systemic Arterial blood Oxygen content (ml/min)} - \text{Mixed Venous blood Oxygen content (ml/min)}}$$

$$\textbf{Cardiac Ouput, Systemic} (L/min) = \frac{VO_2(ml/min/m^2) * BSA(m^2)}{Hb_{g/dl} * 13.6\,(SA_{\%satO2} - MV_{\%satO2})}$$

$$Q_S\,(L/min) = \frac{125(ml/min/m^2) * BSA(m^2)}{Hb_{g/dl} * 13.6\,(SA_{\%satO2} - MV_{\%satO2})}$$

$$\text{Cardiac Ouput, Pulmonary (ml/min)}$$

$$\frac{VO_2(ml/min/m^2) * BSA(m^2)}{\text{Pulmonary Venous blood Oxygen content (ml/min)} - \text{Pulmonary arterial blood Oxygen content (ml/min)}}$$

$$\textbf{Cardiac Ouput, Pulmonary}\,(L/min) = \frac{VO_2(ml/min/m^2) * BSA(m^2)}{Hb_{g/dl} * 13.6\,(PV_{\%satO2} - PA_{\%satO2})}$$

$$Q_P\,(L/min) = \frac{125(ml/min/m^2) * BSA(m^2)}{Hb_{g/dl} * 13.6\,(PV_{\%satO2} - PA_{\%satO2})}$$

$$\frac{Q_P}{Q_S} = \frac{SA_{\%satO2} - MV_{\%satO2}}{PV_{\%satO2} - PA_{\%satO2}}$$

5. What are the basic principles and equations required for shunt hemodynamics calculation?

In the absence of shunting, the pulmonary blood flow is equal to the systemic blood flow.

A Q_p/Q_s ratio of

- >1 indicates a left-to-right shunt
- <1.5 indicates a small left-to-right shunt
- ≥2.0 indicates a large left-to-right shunt
- 1.5–2.0 indicates a left-to-right shunt of intermediate magnitude

6. How does right-heart catheterization (RHC) data help in the decision-making for ASD closure?

See Table 60.1. Following are some pearls:

- Pulmonary veins are rarely sampled for Q_p calculation in the adult population. Therefore, for Q_P calculation:

- If systemic arterial oxygen saturation is ≥95%, SAO_2 content may be used instead of PVO_2 content.
- If $SAO_{2\,SAT}$ is <95%
  - ○ Scenario 1: There is an intracardiac R-L shunt.
    - ◆ Use the assumed value of 98% $SAO_{2\,sat}$ to calculate PV oxygen content.
  - ○ Scenario 2: The patient limitation in gas exchange due to underlying lung pathology.
    - ◆ Use observed $SAO_{2\,sat}$ to calculate PV oxygen content even if the sampled PVO_2 is higher. This is because the observed $SAO_{2\,sat}$ reflects the summation of all the pulmonary vein saturations.
- For Qs calculation, in the presence of a shunt, the chamber immediately proximal to the shunt should be used for mixed venous blood sampling.
  - For a shunt at the level of the great vessels (e.g. PDA):
    - ○ Use the average saturation of the blood samples obtained from the RV.
  - For a shunt at the level of the ventricles (e.g. VSD):
    - ○ Use the average saturation of the blood samples obtained from the RA.
  - For a shunt at the level of the atria (e.g. ASD):

Table 60.1 Interpretation of right-heart catheterization data in atrial septal defect cases.

ASD				
RHC data			RA or RV enlargement	ASD closure
Q_p/Q_s	PASP	PVR		
>1–1.5	<50% SBP	<1/3 of SVR	−	No
			+	MDT discussion (Yes – if symptomatic, paradoxical embolism, or concurrent cardiac surgery)
>1.5	<50% SBP	<1/3 of SVR	−	MDT discussion (Yes – if symptomatic, paradoxical embolism, or concurrent cardiac surgery)
			+	Yes
>1.5	≥50% to ≤2/3 SBP	<1/3 SVR (or <2.3 WU)	+	Yes
>1.5	≥50% to ≤2/3 SBP	≥1/3 to ≤2/3 SVR (or 2.3–4.6 WU)	+	Case-by-case approach with MDT involving ACHD and PHT specialists
>1.5	≥ 2/3 SBP OR	≥2/3 SVR (or > 4.6 WU)	+	Usually not recommended[a]
<1 (net R-L)	≥2/3 SBP OR	≥2/3 SVR (or > 4.6 WU)	+	Contraindicated[b]

ACHD, adult congenital heart disease; ASD, atrial septal defect; MDT, multidisciplinary team; PASP, pulmonary artery systolic pressure; PHT, pulmonary hypertension; PVR, pulmonary vascular resistance; RA, right atrium; RHC, right-heart catheterization; RV, right ventricle; SBP, systolic blood pressure; SVR, systemic vascular resistance; WU, wood units.

[a] In this group of patients, medical management of severe pulmonary HTN to lower PASP and SVR might render them potential candidates for ASD closure.

[b] In patients with severe PHT and net R-L shunt causing cyanosis (Eisenmenger's syndrome), ASD allows offloading of the RV with preservation of cardiac output at the expense of hypoxemia. ASD closure in such cases can lead to rapid decompensation and is therefore contraindicated.

○ Use Flamm's formula to calculate the average saturation from SVC and IVC samples:

– $Average\,MV_{\%satO2} = \dfrac{\left(3 * SVC_{\%satO2}\right) + \left(1 * IVC_{\%satO2}\right)}{4}$, at rest.

– $Average\,MV_{\%satO2} = \dfrac{\left(1 * SVC_{\%satO2}\right) + \left(2 * IVC_{\%satO2}\right)}{3}$, during exercise.

• In routine RHC with no shunt suspected:
  – Pulmonary artery (PA) saturation represents the true mixed venous (MV) oxygen saturation for the cardiac output (QS) calculation.
  – SVC saturation is the next best surrogate for true MV oxygen saturation.
  – In patients with a transjugular intrahepatic portosystemic shunt (TIPS), PA saturation is usually higher than expected and therefore overestimates the cardia output (CO). It is preferable to use the SVC sample as a surrogate for MV oxygen saturation.

7. What are the criteria for a significant step up to diagnose a left-to-right shunt (assuming Q_S = 3 L/min/m²)?

See Table 60.2. In high-output states with higher Q_S (>3 L/min/m²), inter-chamber variability is blunted, and a minor step up on the right side may indicate a significant left-to-right shunt.

8. What are the criteria for a significant step up to diagnose a right-to-left shunt, and how do you localize it?

• *Diagnosis:* There are no established criteria to diagnose a right-to-left shunt. A right-to-left shunt is present if arterial blood O_2 saturation is <95% despite corrective measures (like propping up with a large wedge/head-up tilt,

Table 60.2 Step-up criteria for left-to-right shunt by oximetry.

| Proximal chamber | Step-up site | | Distal chamber | Level of shunt | Possible diagnosis |
	△ in mean of chamber samples ($O_{2\%sat}$)	△ in highest value of chamber samples ($O_{2\% sat}$)			
SVC	≥7	≥8	PA	Any level	Any of the below Diagnosis
SVC/IVC	≥7	≥11	RA	Atrial	ASD; partial anomalous PV drainage; ruptured sinus of Valsalva; VSD with TR; coronary-to-RA fistula
RA	≥5	≥10	RV	Ventricular	VSD; PDA with PR; primum ASD; coronary to RV fistula
RV	≥5	≥5	PA	Great vessel	PDA; aorta-pulmonic window; aberrant coronary artery origin

ASD, atrial septal defect; IVC, inferior vena cava; PDA, patent ductus arteriosus; PV, pulmonary venous; RA, right atrium; RV, right ventricle; TR, tricuspid regurgitation; VSD, ventricular septal defect.

deep breathing and coughing, and oxygen administration via face mask).

- *Location*: During the oximetry run, blood samples are taken from the PV, LA, LV, and aorta. The site of the first step down (desaturation) is the location of the shunt.
- *Quantification* of right-to-left shunt = Systemic blood flow (Q_s) – Effective blood flow (Q_{eff}).

The challenge is that the PV and LA must be entered.

9. What is a bidirectional shunt, and how do you calculate it?

The simultaneous presence of right-to-left and left-to-right shunts in the same patient constitutes a bidirectional shunt. The direction of the shunt varies with different phases of the cardiac cycle.

$$Effective\ blood\ flow\ (L/min) = \frac{Oxygen\ consumption\ (VO_2)\ ml/min}{PV_{O2\ content}(ml/L) - MV_{O2\ content}(ml/L)}$$

$$Q_{eff}\ (L/min) = \frac{VO_2(ml/min/m^2)\ *\ BSA\ (m^2)}{Hb_{g/dl}\ *\ 13.6\ (PV_{\%satO2} - MV_{\%satO2})}$$

$$Q_{eff}\ (L/min) = \frac{125(ml/min/m^2)\ *\ BSA\ (m^2)}{Hb_{g/dl}\ *\ 13.6\ (PV_{\%satO2} - MV_{\%satO2})}$$

$$\textbf{Left-to-Right shunt} = \textbf{Q}_p - \textbf{Q}_{eff}$$
$$\textbf{Right-to-Left shunt} = \textbf{Q}_s - \textbf{Q}_{eff}$$

MV-Mixed venous; PV-Pulmonary venous; Q_p-Pulmonary blood flow; Q_s- Systemic blood flow

For the purpose of calculations, a hypothetical cardiac output called *effective blood flow* is calculated, which is defined as the flow that would exist in the absence of any shunt.

Please see the online clinical cases accompanying this chapter.

10.   What are the implications of peripheral AV shunts like an AV fistula (AVF) for dialysis access?

High output heart failure: An AV fistula with high shunt volume can lead to right-heart failure symptoms and, if uncorrected, progressive RV dysfunction and pulmonary hypertension.

Patients with a history of dialysis and heart failure with preserved ejection fraction (HFpEF) should be evaluated for a hemodynamically significant AV fistula (high output heart failure) as a potential etiology of their HFpEF.

11.   How can you differentiate between high-output heart failure and other types of heart failure?

- RHC is the gold standard for diagnosing high-output heart failure.
- The cardinal signs are elevated cardiac output or cardiac index (CI; $\geq 4\,L/min/m^2$) and low SVR.
- $CI \geq 3.54\,L/min/m^2$ estimated by transthoracic echocardiography (TTE) identified high-output heart failure patients with 62% sensitivity and 96% specificity.

12.   What is Nicoladoni-Branham sign?

A rapid rise in blood pressure and decrease in heart rate and cardiac output after temporary occlusion of an AVF constitutes a positive Nicoladoni-Branham sign and is indicative of a hemodynamically significant AV fistula.

The mechanism is as follows:

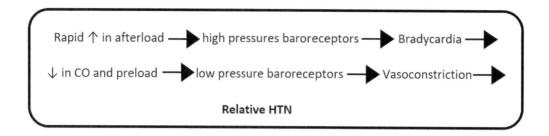

Bibliography

1 Ahmed, S., Lange, R.A., and Hillis, L.D. (2008). Inaccuracies of oximetry in identifying the location of intracardiac left-to-right shunts in adults. *Am. J. Cardiol.* 101 (2): 245–247.

2 Flamm, M.D., Cohn, K.E., and Hancock, E.W. (1969). Measurement of systemic cardiac output at rest and exercise in patients with atrial septal defect. *Am. J. Cardiol.* 23 (2): 258–265.

3 Galie, N., Humbert, M., Vachiery, J. et al. (2016). 2015 ESC/ERS Guidelines for the diagnosis and treatment of pulmonary hypertension: The Joint Task Force for the Diagnosis and Treatment of Pulmonary Hypertension of the European Society of Cardiology (ESC) and the European Respiratory Society (ERS): Endorsed by: Association for European Paediatric and Congenital Cardiology (AEPC), International Society for Heart and Lung Transplantation (ISHLT). *Eur. Heart J.* 37 (1): 67–119.

4 Gilboa, S.M., Devine, O.J., Kucik, J.E. et al. (2016). Congenital Heart Defects in the United States: estimating the Magnitude of the Affected Population in 2010. *Circulation* 134 (2): 101–109.

5 Gutgesell, H.P. and Williams, R.L. (1974). Caval samples as indicators of mixed venous oxygen saturation: implications in atrial septal defect. *Cardiovasc. Dis.* 1 (3): 160–164.

6 Landzberg, M.J. (2001). Closure of atrial septal defects in adult patients: justification of the "tipping point". *J. Interv. Cardiol.* 14 (2): 267–269.

7 Moller, J.H., Patton, C., Varco, R.L. et al. (1991). Late results (30 to 35 years) after operative closure of isolated ventricular septal defect from 1954 to 1960. *Am. J. Cardiol.* 68 (15): 1491–1497.

8 Silversides, C.K., Dore, A., Poirier, N. et al. (2010). Canadian Cardiovascular Society 2009 Consensus

Conference on the management of adults with congenital heart disease: shunt lesions. *Can. J. Cardiol.* 26 (3): e70–e79.

9 Stout, K.K., Daniels, C.J., Aboulhosn, J.A. et al. (2019). 2018 AHA/ACC Guideline for the Management of Adults With Congenital Heart Disease: Executive Summary: A Report of the American College of Cardiology/American Heart Association Task Force on Clinical Practice Guidelines. *J. Am. Coll. Cardiol.* 73 (12): 1494–1563.

10 Whyte, M.K., Hughes, J.M., Peters, A.M. et al. (1998). Analysis of intrapulmonary right to left shunt in the hepatopulmonary syndrome. *J. Hepatol.* 29 (1): 85–93.

11 Wilkinson, J.L. (2001). Haemodynamic calculations in the catheter laboratory. *Heart* 85 (1): 113–120.

61

Persistent Foramen Ovale Closure

Technical Considerations

Pablo Rengifo-Moreno[1,2] and Igor F. Palacios[3,4]

[1] Tallahassee Memorial Hospital, Tallahassee, FL, USA
[2] Florida State University, Tallahassee, FL, USA
[3] Massachusetts General Hospital, Boston, MA, USA
[4] Harvard Medical School, Boston, MA, USA

Devices and Techniques

1. What is the rationale behind the closure of a patent foramen ovale (PFO)?

PFO is common and occurs in 20–34% of the population. In most adults, a PFO appears only as a chance finding during a cardiac investigation or, more likely, remains undetected. Some PFOs may open wide, providing a conduit for thrombus, air, or vasoactive peptides to travel from the venous to arterial circulation, causing a paradoxical embolus. This transfer is associated with several clinical phenomena, including cryptogenic stroke, systemic embolus, migraine with aura, and decompression sickness in divers. Early results from the RESPECT (Randomized Evaluation of Recurrent Stroke Comparing PFO Closure to Established Current Standard of Care Treatment) trial were neutral for PFO closure, but extended follow-up of patients demonstrated a reduction in ischemic stroke compared to medical therapy (hazard ratio [HR] 0.55; 95% confidence interval [CI; 0.31–0.999]; p = 0.046; number needed to treat [NNT] 45). The REDUCE (Gore Septal Occluder Device for PFO Closure in Stroke Patients) clinical study demonstrated that PFO closure significantly improved the clinical ischemic stroke rate (1.4 vs. 5.5%; p = 0.002; NNT = 25) compared with antiplatelet therapy alone. The DEFENSE PFO (Device Closure Versus Medical Therapy for Cryptogenic Stroke Patients with High-Risk PFO) study showed that PFO closure reduced a composite endpoint of stroke, vascular death, and thrombolysis in myocardial infarction (MI) major bleeding at two years compared with medical therapy (0 vs. 12.9%; p = 0.013; NNT = 8). Finally, in the CLOSE (PFO Closure or Anticoagulants Versus Antiplatelet Therapy to Prevent Stroke Recurrence) trial, no patient receiving PFO closure experienced an ischemic stroke compared with 14 in the antiplatelet group (HR 0.03; 95% CI [0–0.26]; p < 0.001; NNT = 17).

2. What devices are available in the United States for the closure of PFOs?

There are two FDA-approved devices for PFO closure: the Amplatzer PFO occluder and the CARDIOFORM occluder device.

The **Amplatzer PFO Occluder** (Abbott) is a self-expanding double-disc device composed of 0.005-in. Nitinol (nickel-titanium) wire with a polyester fabric patch sewn into the two discs (Figure 61.1). The device is compatible with magnetic resonance imaging (MRI) but may create imaging artifacts. The device is available in four sizes (18, 25, 30, and 35 mm), which correspond to the diameters of the right atrial discs. The assorted sizes make the device suitable for challenging anatomies, including PFOs associated with a thickened septum secundum, a long-tunnel, or an atrial septal aneurysm (ASA). Its double-disc design with a smaller left-sided disc decreases the risk of potential complications such as thrombus formation on the prosthetic material and device erosion of the free atrial wall. Both discs are connected by a narrow (3 mm) flexible waist. The waist allows free movement of both discs and

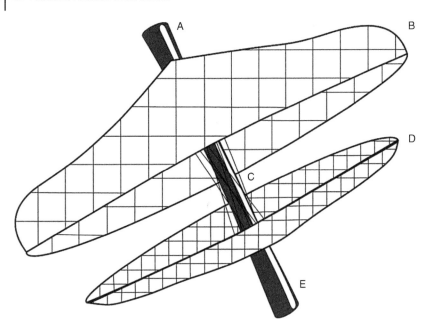

Figure 61.1 Amplatzer PFO Occluder. (a) Right atrial knob/screw; (b) right atrial disc; (c) waist; (d) left atrial disc; (e) left atrial knob.

adaptation to the septum even in a long channel PFO. The flexible waist also allows the discs of the device to be displaced away from the aorta, thereby minimizing the risk of erosion. The device has an end screw in the center of the right disc that attaches to a delivery cable and a pin in the center of the left disc. The device is constrained within an 8 or 9 Fr delivery system. Once delivered, the occluder expands to its double-disc shape. The device is released by unscrewing the delivery system in a counterclockwise fashion. In the event of embolization, a vascular snare may be used to grasp the end screw or pin and retrieve the device using a transcatheter approach.

The **Gore CARDIOFORM Septal Occluder** (GSO) consists of an implantable occluder and a catheter delivery system (Figure 61.2). The occluder comprises five platinum-filled nickel-titanium (Nitinol) wires, which form a frame covered with expanded polytetrafluoroethylene (ePTFE). The ePTFE is treated with a hydrophilic coating to facilitate echocardiographic imaging of the occluder and surrounding tissue during implantation. When fully deployed, the occluder assumes a configuration that prevents the shunting of blood between the right and left atria. The device comes with disc diameters of 15, 20, 25, and 30 mm. The delivery catheter is advanced as a rapid exchange system.

3. What is the appropriate technique for crossing the PFO?

The procedure is usually performed from the right femoral vein. We always recommend access to be performed under ultrasound and fluoroscopy guidance with a micro-puncture needle to avoid vascular complications. The procedure can be performed under fluoroscopy guidance alone; however, the use of transesophageal echocardiography (TEE) or intracardiac echocardiography (ICE) potentially enhances quality and safety. Therefore, if ICE is preferred, a second access in the femoral vein can be obtained inferiorly to the closure site to avoid interactions between the catheters.

The access site can be secure using a 6 Fr sheath followed by the administration of IV heparin with a goal of an activated clotting time (ACT) above 200. A 0.035-in. J-tip wire is advanced, knowing that in about half of the cases, the wire will cross into the left atrium (LA) without any major manipulation. If this is not the case, a Multipurpose catheter at the level of the diaphragm will direct the wire medially. Occasionally, the assistance of TEE or ICE as well as contrast injection can assist the crossing with the wire.

Ideally, the wire can be advanced into the left superior pulmonary vein (LSPV). However, if this is not possible, the Multipurpose catheter can be clock posteriorly to direct the wire away from the left atrial appendage and into the LSPV. The Multipurpose catheter can be advanced into the LSPV for the safe exchange of the J-tip wire for a stiff wire.

4. Are there differences in technique for PFO closure between both approved devices?

The Amplatzer PFO occluder device is mounted loosely onto the pusher wire and retracted submerged in saline into

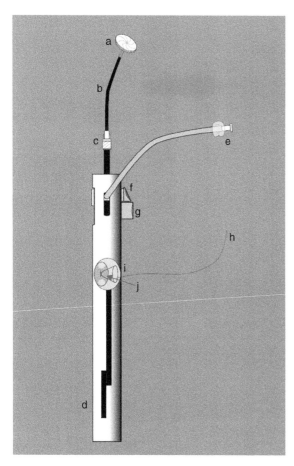

Figure 61.2 CARDIOFORM device and delivery system. (a) CARDIOFORM device; (b) 75 cm delivery catheter; (c) retrieval luer; (d) handle; (e) flush port; (f) occluder lock; (g) packaging insert; (h) retrieval cord; (i) slider; (j) retrieval cord lock.

a short loading sheath to avoid entrapment of air bubbles. A TorqVue sheath (usually 9 Fr) is advanced into the LA over the stiff wire. The sheath dilator is removed as low as possible, allowing bleed-back and removal of potential bubbles, while the short sheath with the device is introduced into the TorqVue sheath. A short loading sheath is connected to the TorqVue sheath, and the device is advanced close to the tip of the sheath. Under fluoroscopy, there should be a separation between the screw on the pusher cable and its female counterpart in the device. The left side of the device is allowed to expand by pulling the sheath while keeping the cable stable. The device and sheath are pulled as a unit until the left disc is stopped by the septum. The sheath is pulled while gently placing forward pressure on the cable. Once the sheath has passed the screw, the entire unit is pushed against the septum, allowing the right disc to rest on the septum. The stability of the device can be checked with a strong wiggle on the cable. Once the stability has been checked, the device is unscrewed (Figure 61.3).

Table 61.1 Special considerations for sizing the Amplatzer PFO device.

PFO morphology	Example anatomical characteristics	Suggested Amplatzer PFO Occluder size (mm)
Simple PFO or PFO with a non-prominent ASA PFO where a secure device position and effective PFO closure can be achieved when using the 25 mm device size	Absence of ASA, long tunnel, and thickened septum secundum Non-prominent ASA (<20 mm total excursion) without a long tunnel (≥10 mm length) and without a thickened septum secundum (≥10 mm thickness)	25
Complex PFO PFO with one or more anatomical characteristics that may complicate the ability to achieve a secure device position and effective PFO closure when using the 25 mm device size	ASA (≥10 mm excursion) with a long tunnel (≥10 mm length) ASA (≥10 mm excursion) with thickened septum secundum (≥10 mm thickness) Prominent ASA with excessive mobility (≥20 mm total excursion) Lipomatous hypertrophy of septum secundum (≥15 mm thickness)	35
PFO with small anatomy Anatomy not suitable for 25 mm device size secondary to interference with adjacent cardiac structures	Septal primum length < 20 mm	18

ASA, atrial septal aneurysm; PFO, patent foramen ovale.
Source: Modified from https://www.accessdata.fda.gov/cdrh_docs/pdf12/P120021c.pdf.

The Gore CARDIOFORM device loading process tends to be simpler as the device is attached to the handle before removal from the packaging, and the device can be advanced as a rapid exchange without a delivery sheath. The device is submerged in a heparinized saline solution. The device should be flushed with heparinized saline until there is no evidence of bubbles. Then the device is loaded into the catheter by pushing the slider down and then to the right until it

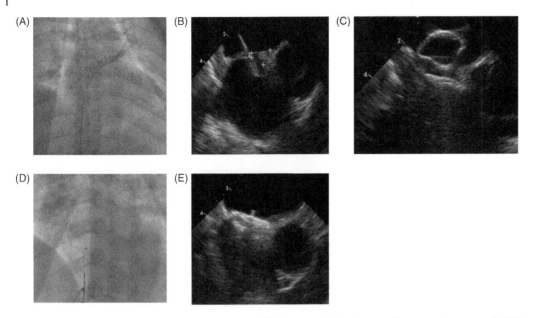

Figure 61.3 (A) Multipurpose catheter crossing the PFO into the left atrium and upper pulmonary vein (B) Intracardiac echocardiogram shows the guidewire crossing the PFO allowing measurements of the interatrial septum (C) Wiggle maneuver under intracardiac echocardiogram guidance (D) Wiggle maneuver under fluoroscopy guidance (E) Amplatzer PFO deployed.

stops. The device should be flushed again to ensure that there is no air in the system. The delivery catheter is loaded on the wire as a rapid exchange system and then introduced through the vascular sheath. This aspect of the design allows avoidance of air embolization. The device can be advanced through a sheath as well; however, the operator should be vigilant about not introducing air at the time of advancement of the device. Once the device reaches the LA, the wire should be removed (if a guidewire was used). Turn the slider to the left to begin deploying the left disc until it stops, then up, and then continue to the left until a flat left disc has formed. At this point, the handle is pulled to contact the septum. Continue pushing the slider to the left until it stops, and then push it down. Once the position is confirmed and satisfactory, lock the device by squeezing and pulling the device occluder lock to the right. If the position of the occluder is appropriate, remove the red retrieval cord. At this point, the device is fully deployed.

5. What is the technique for device retrieval?

If the Amplatzer device is connected to the delivery cable, it can be pulled out of the body without major maneuvers.

The Gore CARDIOFORM requires the retrieval Luer to be unscrewed. Then withdraw the handle to unlock the device, and later bring the device into the catheter.

6. What is the goal of anticoagulation throughout the procedure?

Administer heparin intravenously for a goal-activated clotting time of 200–250 seconds. The patient should receive antiplatelets prior to the procedure.

7. How do you size the device?

Using TEE/ICE measures both the septal length to determine the maximum size of the device that can be used and the defect size using the stop-flow technique. The Amplatzer device is usually sized 2–4 mm more than the stretched length of the defect, while the CARDIOFORM is sized at a ratio of 1.75 : 1.

8. How should multiple shunts associated with a PFO be approached?

If the PFO is associated with one or multiple atrial septal defects (fenestrated septum), a larger device can be used to cover all defects. However, sometimes this is not feasible due to a lack of rims. Then a two-device technique can be used to treat all shunts.

9. Should the device size be modified in the presence of an atrial septal aneurysm?

This is not necessary. The usual sizing is effective if the septum secundum is well captured to establish a stable position, preventing embolization. Given that the presence of an atrial septal aneurysm without PFO is not associated with an increased risk of recurrent embolism, our practice when dealing with a large ASA and a PFO is to close the PFO with a small device and not try to exclude the ASA by using a larger device.

10. Should transseptal puncture be considered when negotiating difficult anatomies?

Only in the case of long tunnels when passing the sheath or wire is unsuccessful or in the case of interfering with the mitral valve in appropriately sized devices.

11. Are there special considerations when closing a PFO associated with a lipomatous atrial septum?

To achieve stability, the arms of the device must be in a divergent conformation rather than a parallel one. The arms will form a "PAC-MAN" sign. This conformation gives stability to the device. This situation may require you to oversize the device or choose an ASD device.

12. Can the PFO closure be performed in the presence of an inferior vena cava (IVC) filter?

The procedure can be performed through an IVC filter. However, the presence of thrombus associated with the filter should be determined prior to attempting the PFO closure. After the long sheath is in place, the PFO closure can be performed in the standard fashion.

13. Can the procedure be performed from other access sites if the femoral access cannot be used?

There are situations in which congenital or acquired obstruction and/or absence of segments of the inferior venous system constitute a challenge for PFO closure.

The right internal jugular vein has been used as an alternative to the femoral approach in patients with congenital absence of portions of the IVC. Palacios et al. reported two cases in which they demonstrated the procedure to be safe and well-tolerated without major technical challenges. The right jugular venous approach provides a simple technical solution in patients requiring PFO closure when femoral venous access is not available. The classic jugular venous approach to PFO closure has always been considered difficult, but the use of the VL catheter enables relatively simple passage across the PFO. The Amplatzer PFO closure device may have characteristics more favorable when the right jugular approach is required.

In other cases, the transhepatic approach can be used to avoid both the femoral and jugular approaches. However, this technique requires coils to achieve hemostasis in the tract made through the liver and is often associated with abdominal discomfort in the subsequent 24 hours due to irritation from peritoneal blood.

Complication Prevention and Management

14. Are there complications related to device preparation?

Air embolism is usually the consequence of air entering the delivery sheath as the dilator is removed from the sheath or as the sheath is prepared. It can also happen when the device is flushed or introduced into the sheath. Therefore, careful attention needs to be paid to the preparation of the equipment. The interventional cardiologist should either supervise the preparation or prepare the device themselves to avoid poor preparation and introduction of air to the delivery sheath. As the device is advanced, careful inspection of the delivery sheath can prevent air from being pushed into the LA. If air is recognized in the delivery sheath, the device can be removed slowly and the delivery sheath allowed to bleed back. If the air bubbles reach the left-side circulation, it could manifest as hypotension, heart block, ventricular tachycardia, inferior ST elevation, and neurological changes. At this point, traditional supportive measures should be taken. The patient should receive 100% oxygen and be placed in the Trendelenburg position, and in some cases the right coronary artery should be aspirated if an airlock is present.

15. How should you manage a device migration?

Migration of the device can occur due to partial deployment of the device inside the PFO tunnel or undersizing the device. This complication can be avoided by careful interrogation of the device's position related to the anatomy of the septum by both fluoroscopy and echocardiography and by performing maneuvers that stress the position of the device. Occasionally, it is necessary to recapture the device to obtain a more favorable position.

Migration of the device can happen immediately after deployment or hours later. The interventional cardiologist performing these procedures needs to be prepared to retrieve an embolized device retrograde or antegrade using a snare. The first step is stabilizing the device; a biotome or snare can be used for this purpose. It is important to know that the biotome will not provide enough tension to pull the device into the sheath, but if used from the right internal jugular vein it can help orient the device so the right atrial knob of the device can be snared. The use of larger sheaths is necessary to accommodate deployed occluders. Usually, a sheath 2 Fr above the delivery sheath size is adequate in the case of the Amplatzer PFO device and a 13 Fr sheath in the case of the CARDIOFORM device. Sometimes, if the device cannot be snared, a stiff coronary wire can be used to cross through the margin of the device and snare the wire; then the wire and device can be retrieved into the sheath.

16. What types of complications can you encounter when treating a PFO in association with multiple atrial septal defects?

This complication is almost exclusive to the closure of large atrial septal defects or when attempting to close multiple defects with a single large device in patients without appropriate rims. If this is to be attempted, meticulous planning and review of the anatomy should precede the closure procedure. In a situation where erosion of the device causes pericardial effusion with tamponade physiology, the patient will require emergency pericardiocentesis and surgical consultation for device removal and repair of the area of erosion.

17. How can device thrombosis be prevented?

Thrombosis of the occluder is an exceedingly rare complication and is usually due to hypercoagulable states. Therefore, a pre-procedural hypercoagulable investigation is extremely important to understand the nature of the paradoxical embolism and anticipate possible thrombotic complications that usually require device removal. Nevertheless, a hypercoagulable state is not a contraindication for PFO closure using appropriate anticoagulation management for up to six months after device closure. Patients with cryptogenic stroke with PFO and hypercoagulable state had an increased risk for recurrent stroke or transient ischemic attack. In an analysis of our cohort of patients, percutaneous PFO closure was a safe and effective therapeutic approach for patients with cryptogenic stroke and an underlying hypercoagulable state.

18. Are there any electrical complications from PFO closure?

The presence of atrial arrhythmias during the first six months of the procedure should be explained to the patient prior to moving on with the procedure, to set expectations. Atrial fibrillation is seen mostly with the CARDIOFORM device, but it tends to be self-limited.

Bibliography

1 Awadalla, H., Boccalandro, F., Majano, R.A. et al. (2004). Percutaneous closure of patent foramen ovale guided by intracardiac echocardiography and performed through the transfemoral approach in the presence of previously placed inferior vena cava filters: a case series. *Catheter. Cardiovasc. Interv.* 63 (2): 242–246. https://doi.org/10.1002/ccd.20174. PMID: 15390345.

2 Ben-Assa, E., Herrero-Garibi, J., Cruz-Gonzalez, I. et al. (2021). Efficacy and safety of percutaneous patent foramen ovale closure in patients with a hypercoagulable disorder. *Catheter. Cardiovasc. Interv.* https://doi.org/10.1002/ccd.29835. Epub ahead of print. PMID: 34132472.

3 Calvert, P.A., Rana, B.S., Kydd, A.C., and Shapiro, L.M. (2011). Patent foramen ovale: anatomy, outcomes, and closure. *Nat. Rev. Cardiol.* 8: 148–160. https://doi.org/10.1038/nrcardio.2010.224.

4 Giblett, J.P., Williams, L.K., Kyranis, S. et al. (2020). Patent Foramen Ovale Closure: State of the Art. *Interv. Cardiol.* 15: e15. Published 2020 Nov 24. https://doi.org/10.15420/icr.2019.27.

5 Hardt, S.E., Eicken, A., Berger, F. et al. (2017). Closure of patent foramen ovale defects using GORE® CARDIOFORM septal occluder: results from a prospective European multicenter study. *Cathet. Cardiovasc. Intervent.* 90: 824–829. https://doi .org/10.1002/ccd.26993.

6 Khosravi, A., Mirdamadi, A., and Movahed, M.R. (2018). Successful retrieval of embolized atrial septal defect occluder and patent foramen ovale closure device using novel coronary wire trap technique. *Catheter. Cardiovasc. Interv.* 92 (1): 189–192. https://doi.org/10.1002/ccd.26955. Epub 2017 Jun 11. PMID: 28603930.

7 Madhkour, R., Wahl, A., Praz, F., and Meier, B. (2019). Amplatzer patent foramen ovale occluder: safety and efficacy. *Expert Rev. Med. Devices* 16 (3): 173–182. https:// doi.org/10.1080/17434440.2019.1581060.

8 McLeod, K.A., Houston, A.B., Richens, T., and Wilson, N. (1999). Transhepatic approach for cardiac catheterisation in children: initial experience. *Heart* 82 (6): 694–696. https://doi.org/10.1136/hrt.82.6.694. PMID: 10573495; PMCID: PMC1729203.

9 Sader, M.A., De Moor, M., Pomerantsev, E., and Palacios, I.F. (2003). Percutaneous transcatheter patent foramen ovale closure using the right internal jugular venous approach. *Catheter. Cardiovasc. Interv.* 60 (4): 536–539. https://doi.org/10.1002/ccd.10702. PMID: 14624437.

10 Zajarias, A., Thanigaraj, S., Lasala, J., and Perez, J. (2006). Predictors and clinical outcomes of residual shunt in patients undergoing percutaneous transcatheter closure of patent foramen ovale. *J. Invasive Cardiol.* 18 (11): 533–537. PMID: 17090816.

62

Atrial Septal Defects Closure

Jose Luis Zunzunegui[1] and Ruth Solana[2]

[1] *Gregorio Marañon Hospital, Madrid, Spain*
[2] *Infanta Leonor Hospital, Madrid, Spain*

1. What are the indications to close an atrial septal defect (ASD)?

Traditionally, the indication for closure is for an ostium secundum type ASD with Qp / Qs > 1.5 obtained by invasive oximetry calculations. Currently, hemodynamic relevance is established by observing dilation of the right cavities on echocardiography, with or without symptoms.

There is abundant literature describing the benefits of closing any ASD with hemodynamic repercussions at any age:

- *Children:* Most units face percutaneous closure from the third year of age (10–15 kg) with or without previous symptoms (lack of growth and frequent respiratory infections).
- *Adults:* The benefits of closure are clear if the indications are well defined. Established atrial arrhythmias rarely return with percutaneous closure of the defect. In contrast, pulmonary hypertension usually returns whenever vascular resistance is <5 Wood units/m^2. Right dysfunction usually improves in the months after closure associated with ventricular remodeling.

2. What are the contraindications to close ASD?

- *Defects > 40 mm or with insufficient margins to anchor the device (<5 mm).* We can tolerate a small retro-aortic rim (2–3 mm), but ASD closure with a total absence of retro-aortic rim in all ultrasound planes ("bald aorta") is not recommended.

- *ASD type ostium primum and venous sinus defect.* They are unapproachable by this technique and must be treated surgically.
- *Existence of a right-left shunt due to established pulmonary hypertension(PHT).* In borderline cases, when pulmonary resistances are close to 5 Wood units/m^2 and the right-left shunt occurs only during an exercise test (↓ transcutaneous SATO$_2$), the patient can be previously treated with pulmonary vasodilators and/or even implanted with a "fenestrated" device. Some companies make this type of endoprosthesis on demand with a fixed fenestration diameter (usually about 5–6 mm).

3. What kind of occluding devices are there?

Self-Centering Devices

These are the most frequently used as they allow most defects to be treated effectively and have a wider range of diameters. Such occluders share the same structure regardless of the company that supplies them. They are self-expanding, Nitinol, retractable, repositionable devices. They have a central occluding waist that expands during implantation and connects the left and right occlusive discs.

The waist length defines the nominal diameter of the device, its range, and the available sizes. The increase in diameter from one occluder to the next higher one depends on the model. The left occluder disc is normally 14 mm larger than the occlusive waist.

The differences between companies lie in the releasing system, the type of prothrombotic fabric they contain inside, and the profile of the discs:

- *Amplatzer (Abbott) atrial septal occluder* (ASO): Nitinol mesh with an occlusive waist ranging from 4 to 40 mm. Thrombogenic Dacron fibers inside. Micro-screw release system.
- *Occlutech Figulla Occluder (Occlutech):* Nitinol mesh with titanium coating (prevents the formation of thrombi on the surface of the discs). The left disc does not present any metallic protrusion, unlike the previous device. Its delivery system consists of a metal ball and a release cable with forceps. This allows the device to pivot on the cable about 180°, adapting to the anatomy of the septum, eliminating the tension and "jump" of the occluder when it is released. It reduces the risk of malposition of the occluder in the septum and its embolization, especially in the smallest patients.
- *CeraFlex Occluder (Lifetech):* Titanium coated Nitinol mesh with a 6–42 mm waist. Its release is carried out with a system of metallic sutures that allow the device to pivot freely on the transporter cable once implanted before releasing it even with a greater angle than the Figulla.

All these devices include their own sheaths with different curvatures and internal diameters to facilitate the implantation of each occluder. They are preloaded "under water" (to avoid air bubbles inside the device) in a short plastic tube, which allows the folded prosthesis to be inserted into the sheath and progressed to the left atrium (LA). All of them are recoverable and repositionable if they have not been released from the delivery cable.

Non-self-Centering Devices

To treat cribriform-like ASDs, companies produce variants of their self-centering devices with a thin, non-occlusive waist that joins the two occluding discs:

- Amplatzer Cribiform Septal Occluder (St Jude)
- Occlutech Cribiform Septal Occluder (Occlutech)
- CeraFlex Cribiform Septal Occluder (Lifetech)

They are designed to cover multiple small defects, typically in the aneurysmal and mobile septum. They cover a large area of the interatrial septum with both discs without restriction by a central core. They are implanted the same way and with the same release system, sheaths, and cables as self-centering devices. The nominal diameter of the device is determined by the length of the occluding discs.

The Gore Septal Occluder is a new device with five Nitinol/platinum wires twisted to form two occluding discs lined with a PTFE membrane. Its structure is softer and allows it to adapt to the heart's inner surface with a very low profile. The device comes preloaded in a 10F sheath with a suture-release system manipulated from the handle. It is only indicated for the closure of ASD < 15 mm (Figures 62.1 and 62.2).

4. What imaging tests should be done before the procedure?

Most units use transthoracic echocardiography (TTE) to establish anatomy and indications initially.

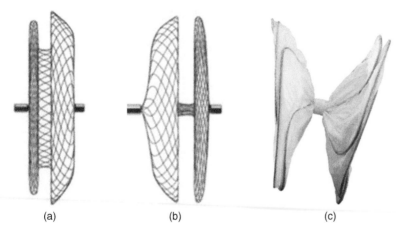

(a)   (b)   (c)

Figure 62.1   (a) Self-centering device (Amplatzer Septal Occluder, Figulla Occluder, Cera Occluder). (b) Non-self-centering device (Amplatzer Cribiform Septal Occluder, Occlutech Cribiform Septal Occluder, CeraFlex Cribiform Septal Occluder). (c) Non-self-centering device, membrane type (Gore Septal Occluder).

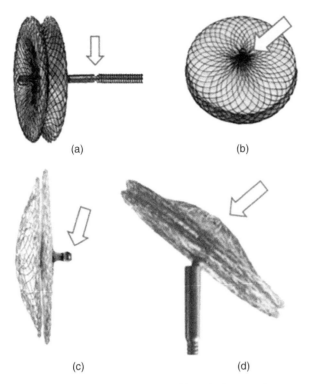

Figure 62.2 Different models of ASD occluders. Amplatzer Septal Occluder: (a) the release system is made up of a micro nut that joins the right disc to the delivery cable (arrow); (b) the left disc presents a slight metallic protrusion that will be insinuated toward the left atrium (arrow). Occlutech Figulla Occluder: (c) the delivery system consists of a ball on the right disc that is attached by forceps on the carrier cable (arrow); (d) the device can pivot on the cable 180° before releasing. The left disc has a lower profile without metallic protrusion (arrow).

In children, with a better ultrasound window, the margins around the defect and its anatomical characteristics can also be studied, as well as the presence of other associated alterations (for example, anomalies in pulmonary venous drainage or alterations of the mitral valve).

In adults, TTE does not have sufficient resolution to accurately determine the dimensions, anatomy, and margins of the ASD. In these cases, it is reasonable to perform transesophageal echocardiography (TEE) to establish the structural characteristics of the defect before performing catheterization. In some cases, magnetic resonance imaging (MRI) can also be useful when determining the volume of the heart chambers and establishing Qp/Qs calculations. It also defines the correct anatomy of the pulmonary venous drains to the LA, although the interatrial septum is better visualized by TEE. Another important point in the precatheterization study in adults is to determine if there is left ventricle (LV) systolic or diastolic dysfunction, which may be masked by the existence of a shunt at the atrial level and could precipitate pulmonary edema immediately after closure. In patients older than 50 years of age, it is

relevant to perform coronary angiography at the initial moment of the procedure to rule out the existence of coronary alterations.

5. What are the steps in a conventional procedure?

1. *Study of the anatomy of the ASD, the interatrial septum, and other cardiac structures*: TEE perfectly defines the position, size, and number of defects, as well as the rest of the cardiac structures (valves and venous drains). However, it is usually necessary to perform it under general anesthesia and intubation. Although TEE is standard practice in children, the use of intracardiac ultrasound (ICE) to guide percutaneous closure is becoming increasingly popular in adults; it allows us to proceed without general anesthesia. In our experience, the use of ICE should be limited to small (<10–15 mm) and central ASDs
2. *Introducer in the femoral vein (5–6F)*: Heparin administration 100 units/kg in children, 4000–5000 units in adults.
3. *Study of pulmonary pressures, resistance, and Qp/Qs*: The determination of these calculations depends on the routine established in each Hemodynamic Unit. In most cases, it is only performed when we have doubts about significant pulmonary hypertension (PHT).
4. *Crossing the ASD with a diagnostic catheter (multipurpose 5F)*: Until the tip is placed inside the left pulmonary veins, the most favorable is the left superior pulmonary vein. Exchange for a long, high-support guidewire (0.035 in.).
5. *Measurement of the defect by image*: For a centered and not very large ASD, most interventionists prefer a simple measurement with TEE, obtaining two perpendicular planes (transversal and longitudinal), measuring the maximum diameter of the flow by color Doppler, and oversizing 2–3 mm the choice of the device with respect to ASD maximum diameter. In children, we use "the rule of 20": we never use devices with a nominal diameter of > 20 mm in patients weighing <20 kg. With ICE, the only plane that can be obtained is transversal, placing the probe at different heights of the RA without the possibility of color Doppler. For this reason, it is believed that ICE should only be used in centered ASDs with good rims, never in cases of complicated defects (for example, with little retro-aortic edge).
6. *In complex cases, balloon measurement can be used*: The "static measurement" technique is generally used, crossing the ASD with a compliant elliptical balloon (Amplatzer Sizing Balloon [St. Jude]) over the guidewire

positioned in a pulmonary vein. A projection should be chosen in which the balloon is completely perpendicular to the interatrial septum, usually in the left anterior oblique with cranial ("four-chamber") projection. The balloon is inflated manually with a 50 cc syringe loaded with contrast diluted with 25% saline. Inflation should be carried out slowly and without applying much pressure, to avoid distension of the defect and, consequently, choosing a device that is too large. Inflation stops as soon as a notch or "waist" appears in the center of the elliptical structure of the balloon.

This will correspond to the diameter of the ASD and can be measured by calibrating the predefined distance between the radiopaque marks that are included in the mast of the balloon. Most operators advise the performance of a simultaneous color Doppler echocardiography during inflation to determine the moment at which the shunt through the ASD is totally blocked ("stop-flow" technique). The nominal diameter of the chosen device should be 2–3 mm more than the waist obtained in the measuring balloon.

7. *Implantation characteristics*: Each device has characteristics, in terms of the deployment of the occluding discs and their placement, that the operator must be aware of. The folded device is advanced through the sheath by pushing it with the delivery cable. The left disc is deployed with ultrasound control, usually in the middle of the left atrial cavity. Subsequently, the sheath and the device are gently pulled until the left occluding disc is close to the septum (but not touching it!) and as parallel to it as possible. You can rotate the sheath slightly clockwise or counterclockwise to modify the orientation of the left disc with respect to the IAS. The right disc is opened by fixing the cable with the right hand and slowly withdrawing the sheath with the left until its complete expansion. Once implanted, its correct position should be checked by ultrasound, and it must be ensured that the margins of the IAS are trapped between both occluding discs. The existence of residual shunts or interference with the surrounding cardiac structures should also be excluded (correct color Doppler flow of the pulmonary veins and absence of AV valve insufficiency).

The stability of the device can be checked by pulling the delivery cable repeatedly and gently. If it is stable, the occlusion discs may separate slightly but return to their initial position upon release of tension (safety maneuvers). The device is then released with different maneuvers depending on the fixation system (micro-screw, forceps, or sutures).

6. What can you do if you cannot get a proper device orientation in relation to the IAS?

Technical modifications. Some maneuvers can be performed if there are difficulties in implantation due to a large defect, difficulties in correctly orienting the discs with respect to the IAS, or deficiency of any of the margins that surround the defect (especially the retroaortic edge):

- Deployment maneuvers:
  - A frequently used technique is to open the left disc insinuated into the left or right superior pulmonary vein. In this way, the occluding disk does not fully expand, acquiring an oval configuration. This allows the waist and the right disc to be deployed in the RA, while the left disc remains anchored within the pulmonary vein, with a perpendicular orientation of the device with respect to the IAS. Then, increasing the traction of the sheath and the releasing cable, with a faster movement, the left disc is released from the pulmonary vein and deployed, allowing correct anchorage most of the time (Figure 62.3).
  - The balloon-assisted technique (BAT). allows you to support the posterior or anterior end of the left occluding disc by using a balloon to maintain the parallel orientation of the disc with respect to the IAS. With an additional femoral venous access, a guidewire (0.018–0.035 in.) is placed in a pulmonary vein through ASD. Subsequently, a balloon catheter (usually a pressure diagnostic catheter) is progressed over the guidewire and inflated with diluted contrast at the level of the interatrial defect. If the device was prolapsing in the RA from its posterior end, the guidewire must be placed into the left upper pulmonary vein; if the prolapse was from the anterior end of the device, the

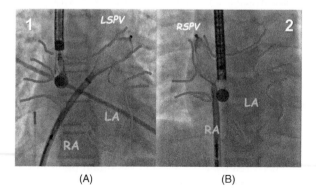

(A) (B)

Figure 62.3 (a) Opening the left disc in the left superior pulmonary vein (LSPV). (b) Opening the left disc in the right superior pulmonary vein (RSPV). LA, left atrium; RA, right atrium.

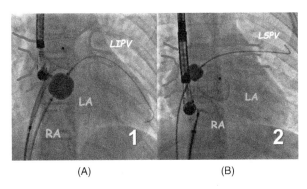

(A)   (B)

Figure 62.4 Balloon Assisted Technique (BAT). (a) Anterior support of the device (small retroaortic rim), guidewire in the left inferior pulmonary vein (LIPV). (b) Posterior support of the device (small posterior-superior rim), guidewire in the left superior pulmonary vein (LSPV).

guidewire should be in the left inferior pulmonary vein. Then the left disc is deployed, and its anterior or posterior end is supported on the inflated balloon, subsequently opening the waist and the right disc in the RA. In this way, the occlusive discs "hug" the balloon, giving it support and avoiding prolapse to the RA. Once the occluder has been stabilized on the IAS, the balloon is deflated and the guidewire is withdrawn slowly before releasing the device, leaving the device, in most cases, correctly positioned (Figure 62.4).

- Releasing cable and sheath modifications:
  – There are modifications available on the market, such as the Hausdorf (Cook) sheath, with a double curvature that alters the approach of the device to the septum.
  – There are other sheaths whose tip is deflectable with a rotation device located on the handle, such as the FuStar (Lifetech) and Agilis (St. Jude), available from 5–14F.
  – The use of sheaths designed for the closure of the ductus arteriosus, which have a 180° curvature, can provide an adequate orientation of the device with respect to the IAS at the time of implantation.
  – The realization of a bevel cut in the tip of the sheath ensures that the left disc can be deployed parallel to the septum (Figure 62.5).
  – You can preform the releasing cable, giving it an angle that allows a parallel orientation of the left disc with respect to the IAS.

7. What should you do when there is more than one defect?

When there are two ASDs, if the distance between the margins of the holes is <7 mm you can try to close it with a single self-centering device, implanted in the larger defect,

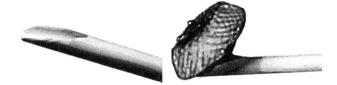

Figure 62.5 Bevel cut of the tip of the sheath to change the orientation of the occluder device when deployed.

slightly oversizing it. The smallest accessory defect can be covered by the occluding disk of the device.

When the distance is >7 mm, the use of two devices is mandatory. In general, the smallest device is implanted first; without releasing it, the largest is implanted through a second venous access. Once its stability has been verified, both occluders are released consecutively, starting with the one with the smallest diameter.

8. What should you do when the device embolizes? When should you try to remove it percutaneously, and when should you send the patient to the operating room?

Device embolization occurs in approximately 1% of cases, depending on the series. Most embolization occurs during the procedure or in the first 24 hours after implantation. Therefore, an ultrasound control is advisable to verify the correct position of the device before discharge.

Tips for an embolized device:

- In our unit, we attempt percutaneous extraction when the embolized device is in the pulmonary trunk or arteries, the aortic arch or descending aorta, or the left or right atrium. We only attempt to remove it when it is in the right ventricle, if it is mobile and free, away from the tricuspid subvalvular apparatus. And in general, we never attempt its extraction when it is in the LV, and we send the patient directly to the operating room.
- Before any extraction attempt, the patient must be fully heparinized, maintaining activated clotting time (ACT) >250 seconds.
- The key to retrieval in the catheterization room is to use as large a sheath as possible to facilitate insertion of the device into the sheath once captured. Reinforced 10–14F sheaths (Cook Flexor Sheath) are used to avoid deformations and folds when trying to pick up the device inside.
- An attempt should be made to capture the device from the nut or ball (in the case of Figulla devices) with a 7–15 mm snare through the sheath. It is almost

impossible to fold and remove the device through the sheath if you capture it by one of the occluding discs.

9. What late complications may occur?

Late cardiac erosion is a worrisome complication; it can occur one to two years after implantation. Many articles have described this complication in relation to the Amplatzer Septal Occluder (Abbott), possibly because it was the first type of device used, although it can also occur with other types of devices. The perforation usually occurs in the roof of the LA or between the aorta and the RA. The clinical debut is characterized by chest pain, dizziness, and the presence of a pericardial effusion that requires urgent surgical intervention to remove the occluder, suture the perforation, and close the ASD. It seems to be related to the use of oversized devices (it is not advisable to use devices larger than 80% of the total length of the IAS) and in the absence of a retro-aortic edge. The total incidence is difficult to estimate since the total number of implants is not recorded, but its incidence is estimated to be <1/1000.

Bibliography

1 Bartel, T. and Müller, S. (2013). Device closure of interatrial communications: peri-interventional echocardiographic assessment. *Eur. Heart J. Cardiovasc. Imaging* 14 (7): 618–624.

2 Faccini, A. and Butera, G.J. (2018). Atrial septal defect (ASD) device trans-catheter closure: limitations. *J. Thorac. Dis.* 10 (Suppl 24): S2923–S2930.

3 Hoashi, T., Yazaki, S., Kagisaki, K. et al. (2014). Management of ostium secundum atrial septal defect in the era of percutaneous trans-catheter device closure: 7-year experience at a single institution. *J. Cardiol.* 65 (5): 418–422. PMID: 25113951.

4 Quereshi, S. and Carminati, M. (2014). *Cardiac Catheterization for Congenital Heart Diseases; from Fetal Life to Adulthood*, 1e. Milan, Heildelberg, New York, Dordrecht, London: Springer.

5 Rigatelli, G. and Zuin, M. (2018). Nghia NT. Interatrial shunts; technical approaches to percutaneous closure. *Expert Rev. Med. Devices* 15, 707–716 (10).

6 Silversides, C.K., Dore, A., Poirier, N. et al. (2010). Canadian cardiovascular society 2009 consensus conference on the management of adults with congenital heart disease: shunt lesions. *Can. J. Cardiol.* 26: E70–E79.

7 Vasquez, A.F. and Lasala, J.M. (2013). Atrial septal defect closure. *Cardiol. Clin.* 31 (3): 385–400.

8 Warnes, C.A., Williams, R.G., Bashore, T.M. et al. (2008). ACC/AHA 2008 guidelines for the management of adults with congenital heart disease: a report of the American College of Cardiology/American Heart Association Task Force on Practice Guidelines (writing committee to develop guidelines on the management of adults with congenital heart disease). Developed in collaboration with the American Society of Echocardiography, Heart Rhythm Society, and International Society for Adult Congenital Heart Disease, Society for Cardiovascular Angiography and Interventions, and Society of Thoracic Surgeons. *J. Am. Coll. Cardiol.* 52: E143–E263.

63

Ventricular Septal Defects Closure

Jose Luis Zunzunegui[1] and Ruth Solana[2]

[1] *Gregorio Marañon Hospital, Madrid, Spain*
[2] *Infanta Leonor Hospital, Madrid, Spain*

Ventricular septal defects (VSDs) are the most common congenital heart disease (20% of cases). Muscular VSDs (MVSDs) account for 20% of interventricular septum defects, being the most common location in the apical portion of the muscular septum, followed by the mid-ventricular and the anterior in the right outflow tract. Many of these muscular defects can be closed percutaneously with self-expanding devices adapted to the ventricular anatomy. On the other hand, perimembranous VSDs (PMVSDs) are the most frequent, and although the proximity of the aortic valve makes them a challenge, the development of new devices has made percutaneous closure possible. In this chapter, we will review the devices used in this therapy, implant techniques, and possible complications, distinguishing the approach for MVSD and PMVSD.

Muscular VSDs

1.   What muscular ventricular septal defects (MVSD) patients should you think about closing percutaneously?

- Diagnosed MVSD by transthoracic echocardiography (TTE) in preliminary evaluation. It is important to determine the size, number, and location. In principle, you can treat MVSDs in the mid-ventricular position and the right ventricle (RV apex). You should not treat anterior defects located in the right ventricular outflow tract (RVOFT). You can treat more than one defect in the septum, combining different occluders.
- A hemodynamically significant left-to-right shunt with clinical symptoms of low cardiac output (no weight gain and respiratory infections in children, and exercise intolerance in adults), dilation of the left chambers by echo, and/or Qp/Qs > 1.5.

2.   What are the contraindications for percutaneous closure of MVSDs?

- Distance < 4 mm between the MVSD and the aortic, mitral, or tricuspid valve.
- Signs of pulmonary hypertension; slight right-to-left shunt, pulmonary resistances > 5 Wood units/m^2.
- Septicemia, or active infectious process.
- Weight < 6 kg. Note that good results have been published even in small children, although this implies greater technical difficulty and incidence of complications. In these cases, the periventricular approach using a hybrid procedure may be an appropriate therapeutic option.

3.   What devices are available?

The Amplatzer Muscular Occluder (AMO; St. Jude) device is specifically designed for the percutaneous treatment of MVSDs and is, without a doubt, the most widely used in clinical practice. It is a self-expanding, self-centering device with an occluding waist that connects the two discs. The waist is 7 mm thick, and the left and right occluder discs are 8 mm longer than the waist. The delivery cable is attached to the device by a micro nut located on the right disc. The nominal diameter of the device corresponds to that of the occlusive waist, and available sizes range from 4 to 18 mm (in 2 mm increments). The sheaths required for implantation range from 6 to 9 Fr and are supplied with the cable and charger.

There is the possibility of implanting other devices to close accessory defects. Narrower-waist self-expanding devices (cribriform occluders) can also be used to cover multiple small defects with larger occlusive discs. There are also smaller self-expanding devices, such as the Amplatzer Ductus Occluder II (ADO II), which can be implanted through 5 f guide catheters, even directly from the left ventricle (LV), without needing to complete the A-V circuit.

4. What are the steps during the procedure?

1. It is preferable to perform the procedure under general anesthesia with intubation and guided by TEE. In the case of single defects with favorable anatomy, it is safe to do so with sedation under TTE-guided fluoroscopy.
2. Canalize the femoral artery and vein. If the location of the MVSD is closer to the apex than the tricuspid valve, it is preferable to canalize the right jugular vein, as it will provide a more favorable orientation. Subsequently, heparin is administered (100 IU/kg, maximum 5000 IU to maintain activated clotting time [ACT] >200 seconds).
3. Obtain hemodynamic data and blood gases to establish pulmonary pressure and vascular resistance, and calculate Qp/Qs. Next, obtain a left ventriculography in a four-chamber projection (35–40° cranial, 35–40° left anterior oblique). Accessory projections are sometimes necessary depending on the anatomy of the septum and VSD.
4. Choose the device size (waist diameter). It should be 1–2 mm oversize with respect to the diameter of the VSD obtained by TEE or ventriculography in end-systole.
5. Canalize the defect with a right coronary catheter (4–5F) from the LV, and place of a soft 0.035-in. exchange guidewire in the pulmonary arteries or the superior cava vein (SCV). Then, with a snare catheter (diameter 10–15 mm for children and 20–25 mm for adults) from venous access (femoral or jugular), catch the exchange guidewire tip. The guidewire is externalized through the venous introducer, completing the arterio-venous loop.
6. On the guidewire and through the vein (jugular or femoral), advance to the ascending aorta, passing the sheath (with a sufficient profile to implant the preselected device) through the MVSD. To facilitate this maneuver, a 4–5F multipurpose catheter is usually inserted from the artery side, which remains in contact with the tip of the sheath dilator ("kissing" technique). Fix the guidewire at the entrance of the sheath and the

entrance of the multipurpose catheter with two clamps so that the guidewire does not move; then, push the sheath through the vein while simultaneously pulling the multipurpose catheter from the artery. This greatly facilitates the placement of the tip of the sheath in the ascending aorta. Once the sheath is in the ascending aorta, the dilator is withdrawn from the venous side, and the guide is maintained (to avoid sheath folds) until the device is ready.

7. The device, screwed to the transport cable through the micro nut located on the right disc, is retracted into a short plastic (loader) tube that adapts to the sheath. This maneuver is performed under saline solution to avoid air bubbles.
8. The guidewire is removed, and the loader is screwed onto the sheath to progress the occluder. It is preferred to deploy the left disc slightly in the ascending aorta before pulling the sheath from the ascending aorta into the LV and removing the LV sheath, thus avoiding the possibility of the sheath with the device "jumping" into the RV during its descent. Once the tip of the sheath is in the middle of the LV cavity, the left disc is fully deployed, and with TEE control, it approaches the interventricular septum by gently pulling simultaneously on the sheath and the transporter cable. It is very important to check that the disc is not trapped in the mitral subvalvular apparatus. If this occurs, the left disc should be retracted back into the sheath and deployed closer to the septum.
9. Once the left disc is in contact with the septum, the waist is deployed by slightly withdrawing the sheath and maintaining tension on the transporter cable. The removal of the sheath continues to deploy the right disc.
10. The correct position of the device is verified by TEE and ventriculography: position of the discs on the right and left side of the septum, detect residual shunts and any interference with cardiac valves.
11. Release the device by turning the carrier cable counterclockwise. Once released, the cable must be introduced quickly into the sheath to avoid the tip of the cable causing any type of injury or perforation. Again, the correct position of the device is checked by TEE and ventriculography (Figure 63.1).
12. There is the possibility of implanting other devices to close accessory defects. Narrower-waist self-expanding devices (cribriform) can also be used to cover multiple small defects with larger occlusive discs.
13. Once the ACT <250 seconds, the femoral or jugular vein sheath is removed. It is almost always possible to discharge the patient in the 24 hours following after performing TTE and ECG.

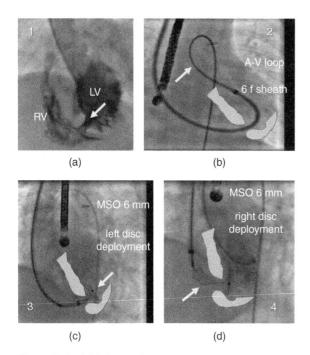

Figure 63.1 (a) Left ventriculography, muscular apical ventricular septal defect (VSD). (arrow). (b) Sheath from the jugular to the ascending aorta through the VSD; placement of a multipurpose catheter in contact with the tip of the introducer (arrow) to facilitate its passage through the septum ("kissing technique"). (c) Deployment of the left disc and approach to the septum (arrow). (d) Deployment of the right disc, which is deformed before release by the tension of the delivery cable (arrow).

5. What are the possible complications of percutaneous closure of MVSDs?

- Embolization is very rare, especially if the procedure is performed by a skilled operator. The device can migrate to the LV, RV, or pulmonary arteries. It can be captured with a snare catheter and retracted into a 2–4F sheath larger than used for implantation. This maneuver is straightforward if the device is in the RV or a pulmonary artery. However, if the occluder is embolized in the LV, the patient should be sent to the operating room for surgical removal: passage with large sheaths through the aortic valve could damage the leaflets or break the chordae tendineae of the mitral subvalvular apparatus.
- Ventricular arrhythmias usually occur during the procedure due to the manipulation of catheters, sheaths, and guides in the ventricular cavity. In most cases, they are benign and transitory. Atrioventricular (AV) block is uncommon.
- Hemolysis is also rare and is related to the existence of residual high-velocity shunts. Some operators immerse the device in a container with a small amount of the

patient's blood for 10–15 minutes before retracting it into the charger. In our opinion, this maneuver promotes intra-device thrombosis once implanted and reduces the incidence of residual shunts.

- To prevent valve insufficiencies (mitral, tricuspid, aortic), it is necessary to check by ultrasound that the device does not interfere with the surrounding structures before releasing it. However, the appearance of mild tricuspid regurgitation is not a contraindication for occluder release since it is usually caused by distortion of the leaflets by the passage of a rigid sheath.
- To prevent stroke, as in all these types of interventions, the correct heparinization of the patient is essential (ACT > 200 seconds).
- Pericardial effusions are usually caused by accidental cardiac perforation when manipulating the catheter, guides, and/or sheaths. You must stop the procedure, monitor for progression with ultrasound, and act accordingly.

Perimembranous VSDs (PMVSDs)

70% of all VSDs are in the membranous septum. Sometimes the upper border does not exist, and the roof of the defect is constituted by the aortic valve leaflets. The technical difficulty for percutaneous closure consists, fundamentally, in that the device must occlude the defect without interfering with the aortic valve.

6. In which patients is percutaneous closure of PMVSDs indicated?

- Ultrasound diagnosis of PMVSD with significant shunt; dilation of the left chambers or clinical symptoms of pulmonary hyperflow.
- The minimum recommended weight is > 10 kg. Smaller patients can be treated if the anatomy of the defect is favorable.
- For most operators, a left chamber dilation on echocardiography is sufficient to establish the indication for closure, although the Qp/Qs is less than 1.5. The argument is that the PMVSD outcome is not free of long-term morbidity (endocarditis, development of aortic insufficiency, and increased incidence of supraventricular arrhythmias from the second/third decade of life), even though it is small. Pulmonary vascular resistance should be < 4–5 Wood units/m².
- The minimum distance to the aortic valve depends on the type of device and the experience of the operator. In most cases, by adapting the implant maneuvers, we can close the PMVSDs even without distance from the aortic valve.

7. What types of devices can be used to close PMVSDs?

The Amplatzer Perimembranous Septal Occluder (APMSO; Abbott) is a self-expanding Nitinol device with asymmetrical discs. The aortic rim of the asymmetric left ventricular disc exceeds the dimensions of connecting waist by only 0.5 mm, to avoid impingement on the aortic valve, whereas the apical end is 5.5 larger than the waist.

This device was first used in clinical practice in 2002. The results described regarding the technical efficacy of the implant, abolition of the shunt, and non-interference with the aortic valve were satisfactory. However, the incidence of AV blocks (sometimes late onset, up to one to two years post-implantation) led to its use being discontinued. A new generation of devices was subsequently created, with a softer structure, but they also did not obtain the desired clinical results.

The off-label use of the Amplatzer Ductus Occluder (ADO I and ADO II) for the closure of PMVSD has been described. The conical structure of the ADO I appears to exert less pressure on the tissue surrounding the septal defect, and it has have a lower incidence of AV block. The self-expanding structure of the ADO II is very soft and low profile (it can be implanted through 5f guide-catheters). Numerous centers have described its use in the closure of PMVSDs with a low incidence of AV block and performing it directly from the left side without the need for an A-V circuit, although it is only used in small PMVSD (Figure 63.2).

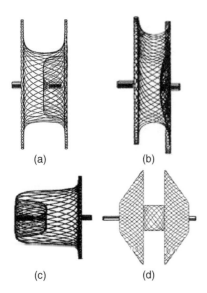

(a)   (b)

(c)   (d)

Figure 63.2 Nitinol self-expanding devices used in the closure of ventricular septal defects: (a) Amplatzer Muscular Septal Occluder (AMSO); (b) Amplatzer Perimembranous Septal Occluder (APMSO); (c) Amplatzer Ductus Occluder I (ADO I); (d) Amplatzer Ductus Occluder II (ADO II).

The Nit-Occlud Coil VSD (PFM) is specially designed for this purpose: its structure is soft, flexible, and adaptable to the anatomy of the defect. The radial force applied to the margins of the PMVSD is minimal, and AV blocks have not been described in the recently published series. In addition, its implantation technique is much less traumatic than the APSO. The device is formed by a series of Nitinol coils that give it a "diabolo" structure when fully expanded: it has a central waist and a larger diameter of coils on the left side than on the right side. The ends of the right and left coils are somewhat more rigid, and they are covered with polyester fibers to increase the thrombogenic capacity of the device.

The device is available in a minimum size of 8×6 mm and a maximum diameter of 16×8 mm. The nomenclature refers to the left coil's diameter followed by the right coil's diameter.

The device comes preloaded on a 6–7 f catheter with a distal radiopaque mark. The transporter cable attached to the coil is the one that allows the coil to be deployed or retracted within the catheter by pushing or pulling it, respectively. This cable has several marks that guide the operator as to what phase of release the device is in. A 6–7F reinforced sheath is required for implantation; the transport catheter is introduced through it.

Although several types of PMVSDs can be closed using the Nit-Occlud VSD, it is specially designed to be implanted in defects with aneurysmal closure tissue, which depends on the subvalvular apparatus of the tricuspid valve. This aneurysmatic tissue is very common, such that the PMVSD has a larger anatomical hole open toward the LV and a smaller hemodynamic hole open toward the RV (which marks the amount of shunt that passes through the LV).

Measurement of the defect is performed by combining TEE and left ventriculography. In this way, the anatomy of the PMVSD is defined with a typically conical morphology due to the aneurysmal closure tissue. The size of the device is calculated knowing that the left coil must be twice the diameter of the hemodynamic hole and at least 1–2 mm larger than the diameter of the anatomical hole. It's about filling a bag, not closing a hole (Figure 63.3).

8. What are the steps of the procedure?

It is advisable to perform the intervention under general anesthesia with intubation and TEE control. The first steps of the procedure are like those described for the closure of MVSDs, until placing the 6–7F sheath in the ascending aorta.

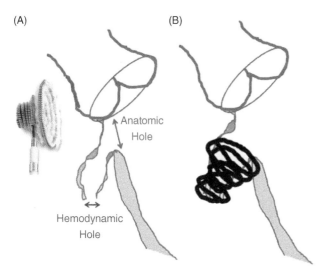

Figure 63.3 (a) Perimembranous VSD with aneurysmal tissue dependent on the tricuspid subvalvular apparatus. (b) Nit-Occlud device implantation within the aneurysm.

- *Nitinol self-expanding devices (APMSO, ADO I, ADO II):* It is important to cross the aortic valve with the left disc partially open. The devices are soft and do not damage the leaflets of the aortic valve, and in this way, it is easier to stabilize it without the sheath jumping to the RV. The rest of the procedure is like that described for MVSDs.
- *Coil-type devices (Nit-Occlud VSD):* For this type of device, there are some technical differences:

1. The transporter catheter with the preloaded coil (attached to the transporter cable) is pushed out of the sheath into the ascending aorta to expose a 1.5–2 cm portion of the catheter.
2. The coil is fully deployed, pushing the transporter cable into the ascending aorta except for the last two coils.

3. The catheter and sheath are then gently pulled until the device "jumps" into the LV in a four-chamber projection (cranial with left anterior oblique).
4. Once the deployed coil is in the left ventricular cavity, under TEE control, the operator pulls on the sheath and catheter until it is accommodated in the aneurysmal tissue. Maintaining tension on the sheath and catheter, the last two turns on the right side are released by withdrawing the catheter and pushing on the carrier wire.
5. The correct position of the coil is verified by TEE and left ventriculography, checking that there is no interference with the aortic and tricuspid valves, as well as for the absence of residual shunt. A mild degree of tricuspid regurgitation is admissible before release, as it is usually caused by the passage of the sheath.

9. What complications may occur in the closure of PMVSDs?

They are like those described for MVSD closure. However, there are two more specific complications:

- Due to the proximity of the AV conduction tissue, AV block can occur at the time of implantation but also months after the procedure. With the reduction in the use of APMSO, the frequency of this complication has decreased dramatically.
- Hemolysis can occur, especially in coil-type devices (Nit-Occlud VSD). For this reason, you must be very demanding in the treatment of residual shunts around the device, with the implantation of a second coil or by removing the implanted coil before releasing it and replacing it with a larger one.

Bibliography

1 Carminati, M., Butera, G., Chessa, M. et al. (2007). Investigators of the European VSD registry transcatheter closure of congenital ventricular septal defects: results of the European registry. *Eur. Heart J.* 28 (19): 2361–2368.

2 Esmaeili, A., Behnke-Hall, K., Schrewe, R., and Schranz, D. (2019). Percutaneous closure of perimembranous ventricular septal defects utilizing almost ideal Amplatzer duct Occluder II: why limitation in sizes? *Congenit. Heart Dis.* 14 (3): 389–395.

3 Haas, N.A., Kock, L., and Bertram, H. (2017). Interventional VSD-closure with the Nit-Occlud () Le VSD-Coil in 110 patients: Early and midterm results of

the EUREVECO-Registry. *Pediatr. Cardiol.* 38 (2): 215–227.

4 Nguyen, H.L., Phan, Q.T., Dinh, L.H. et al. (2018). Nit-Occlud Lê VSD coil versus Duct Occluders for percutaneous perimembranous ventricular septal defect closure. *Congenit. Heart Dis.* 13 (4): 584–593.

5 Nguyen, H.L., Phan, Q.T., Doan, D.D. et al. (2018). Percutaneous closure of perimembranous ventricular septal defect using patent ductus arteriosus occluders. *PLoS One* 13 (11): e0206535.

6 Quereshi, S. and Carminati, M. (2014). *Cardiac Catheterization for Congenital Heart Diseases; from Fetal*

Life to Adulthood, 1e. Milan, Heildelberg, New York, Dordrecht, London: Springer.

7 Quereshi, S. and Carminati, M. (2014). *Cardiac Catheterization for Congenital Heart Diseases; from Fetal Life to Adulthood*, 1e. Milan, Heildelberg, New York, Dordrecht, London: Springer.

8 Rigatelli, G., Zuin, M., and Nghia, N.T. (2018). Interatrial shunts; technical approaches to percutaneous closure. *Expert. Rev. Med. Devices* 707–716.

9 Silversides, C.K., Dore, A., Poirier, N. et al. (2010). Canadian cardiovascular society 2009 consensus conference on the management of adults with congenital heart disease: shunt lesions. *Can. J. Cardiol.* 26: E70–E79.

10 Solana-Gracia, R., Mendoza Soto, A., Carrasco Moreno, J.I. et al. (2021). **Spanish** registry of percutaneous **VSD** closure with NitOcclud Le **VSD** coil device: lessons learned after more than a hundred implants. *Rev. Esp. Cardiol. (Engl. Ed.)* 74 (7): 591–601.

11 Walavalkar, V., Maiya, S., Pujar, S. et al. (2020). Percutaneous device closure of congenital isolated ventricular septal defects; a single-center retrospective database study amongst 412 cases. *Pediatr. Cardiol.* 41 (3): 591–598.

12 Warnes, C.A., Williams, R.G., Bashore, T.M. et al. (2008). ACC/ AHA 2008 guidelines for the management of adults with congenital heart disease: a report of the American College of Cardiology/American Heart Association task force on practice guidelines (writing committee to develop guidelines on the management of adults with congenital heart disease). Developed in collaboration with the American Society of Echocardiography, Heart Rhythm Society, and International Society for Adult Congenital Heart Disease, Society for Cardiovascular Angiography and Interventions, and Society of Thoracic Surgeons. *J. Am. Coll. Cardiol.* 52: E143–E263.

64

Percutaneous Treatment of Aortic Coarctation

Yuen Yee Lo Yau Leung, Fahad Alfares, and Satinder K. Sandhu

[1] *Division of Pediatric Cardiology, Department of Pediatrics, University of Miami Miller School of Medicine, Miami, FL, USA*

1. What is coarctation of the aorta?

Coarctation of the aorta occurs in 5.1–8.1% of patients with congenital heart disease. It is a heterogeneous defect of the aortic arch that can present as a simple stricture at the juxtaductal region or as a complex defect with varying degrees of hypoplasia of the transverse arch and isthmus and rarely may present as an isolated abdominal coarctation. Decompression via collateral vessels from the proximal to the segment distal to the stenosis is common in severe stenosis.

Pathologically, the stricture occurs because of thickening and infolding of the media with superimposed neointimal tissue. Medial wall degeneration in pre- and post-stenotic specimens is consistent with general arteriopathy. Arteriopathy may be secondary to systemic hypertension and flow abnormalities across the coarctation, resulting in aortic arch dissection and aneurysm formation.

2. What other conditions is coarctation of the aorta associated with?

In the majority of individuals, coarctation of the aorta occurs as a sporadic mutation; however, arterial flow abnormalities in the fetus have also been attributed to its causation. Mutations in the *NOTCH1* gene have been identified in patients with coarctation. Chromosomal anomalies like Turner's, Noonan's, PHACE, DiGeorge, and velocardiofacial syndrome have a high incidence of coarctation. A bicuspid aortic valve is present in 30–40% of patients, and it can occur in association with multiple left-sided lesions, including Shone's complex and other complex congenital heart lesions. The Baltimore Washington Infant study linked the maternal intake of sympathomimetic medications to coarctation of the aorta.

Intracranial aneurysms (berry aneurysms) have been reported in 10% of patients with coarctation of the aorta, and screening should be recommended in adults. It is unclear whether the intracranial aneurysms are a primary associated defect or occur in response to long-standing systemic hypertension.

3. What is the clinical presentation?

Patients can present as critically ill neonates requiring emergent surgery, or they may present in childhood or as adults as an incidental finding during a routine exam. Patients presenting as adults can present with a history of systemic hypertension, claudication of the lower extremities, or abdominal angina. Physical examination would reveal weak to absent femoral pulses and radial artery to femoral artery delay. A suprasternal notch thrill may be appreciated. A systolic murmur that may spill into diastole is best heard along the dorsal spine at the interscapular region. A continuous murmur may be auscultated over the thorax in patients with collateral decompression of the segment proximal to the stenosis. Other heart sounds and murmurs may be heard related to the associated heart defects, with the most common being the constant systolic ejection click of the bicuspid aortic valve.

4. What diagnostic imaging is recommended?

Successful transcatheter intervention relies on a complete anatomical assessment of the aortic arch prior to the procedure. Echocardiogram is invaluable in the diagnosis of coarctation of the aorta. Further anatomy of the aortic arch is better defined with advanced cardiac imaging utilizing a cardiac magnetic resonance imaging (C-MRI) or CT angiogram. Imaging evaluation should focus on the site of the coarctation, the length of the stenotic segment, the diameter of the stenosis, the isthmus, and the transverse arch. The presence or absence of an aneurysm and the proximity of the lesion to the brachiocephalic vessels should be evaluated.

- *Electrocardiogram:* The typical finding is left ventricular hypertrophy secondary to systemic hypertension (Figure 64.1).
- *Chest X-ray:* The "three sign" occurs because of indrawing of the aortic wall at the site of obstruction and post-stenotic dilation distal to the obstruction. The blood flow in moderate to severe coarctation is diverted across the stenotic segment via collaterals and dilated and pulsatile intercostal vessels of the fourth to eighth ribs bilaterally, resulting in "rib notching" of the inferior edge of the ribs.
- *Transthoracic echocardiography (TTE):* A suprasternal notch view can define the aortic arch anatomy. Doppler interrogation of the arch in the suprasternal notch view can assess the degree of obstruction. The lack of pulsatility on Doppler interrogation of the aorta in the subcostal view should suggest the diagnosis (Figure 64.2).
- *C-MRI:* C-MRI defines the anatomic and hemodynamic characteristics of coarctation, including the site and length

of the obstruction and its proximity to the brachiocephalic vessels, and the presence or absence of collateral vessels. 3D reconstruction of the image is invaluable in procedure planning (Figure 64.3). This modality has the advantage of not using ionizing radiation or a contrast agent.

- *Computed tomography angiography (CTA):* CTA can be done in the presence of metal implants and offers high spatial resolution and shorter acquisition time but does not provide hemodynamic data. As such, CTA is invaluable for follow-up of patients with stent placement across the site of obstruction (Figure 64.4). Similar to C-MRI, 3D reconstruction of images is invaluable in pre-procedural planning.

5. What are the types of transcatheter interventions in a patient with coarctation?

- *Balloon angioplasty:* Balloon dilation of the aortic arch results in varying degrees of disruption of the tunica intima and the media layer of the artery, allowing for relief of stenosis. Balloon angioplasty is indicated for discrete re-coarctation. In patients with native coarctation, there is a high rate of restenosis with balloon angioplasty, but it can be considered in patients older than six months

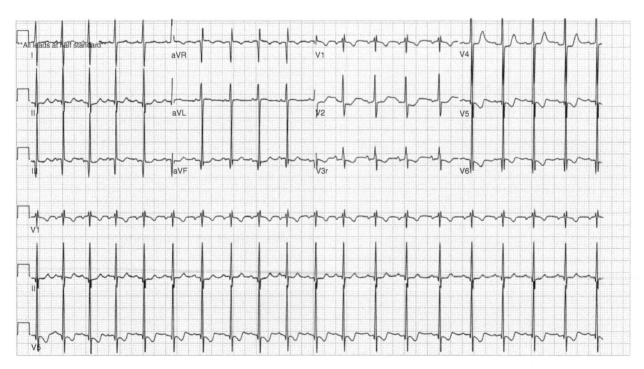

Figure 64.1 ECG demonstrating left ventricular hypertrophy in a patient with coarctation of the aorta.

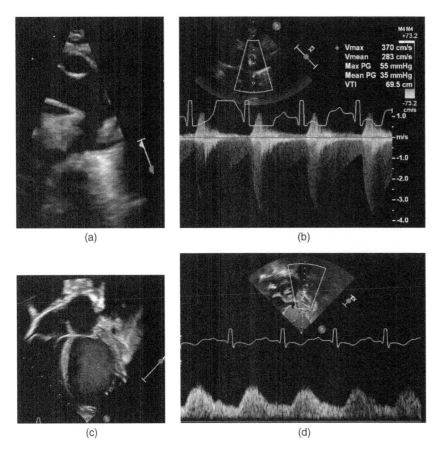

Figure 64.2 Echocardiogram images demonstrating severe discrete coarctation of the aorta with severely depressed left ventricular function. (a) Severe discrete coarctation of the aorta. (b) Sawtooth Doppler pattern noted with peak gradient 55 mmHg and mean gradient 35 mmHg. (c) Severely dilated left ventricle. (d) Dampened systolic upstroke with antegrade flow noted on descending aorta Doppler.

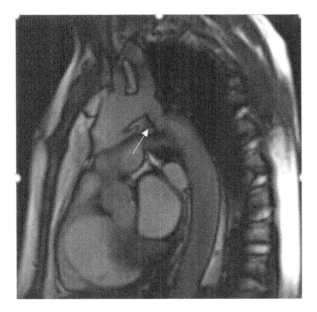

Figure 64.3 C-MRI.

of age with native coarctation and depressed ventricular function.

- *Bare-metal stent placement:* The bare-metal stent, when placed across the stenotic vessel, dilates the stenotic vessel and provides an endoprosthesis to prevent recoil of the arterial wall. The bare-metal stent is a therapeutic alternative in patients with native or recurrent coarctation in whom balloon angioplasty has failed and also in high-risk surgical patients with complex arch anatomy.

- *Covered endovascular stent placement:* The PTFE fabric covering the stent is impermeable and provides additional structural support, thereby creating a protective barrier at the site of stent placement. A covered stent can be considered in complex arch anatomy like a near interruption or tortuous aortic arch. Patients with aortic wall injury would also benefit from the placement of a covered stent (Figure 64.5).

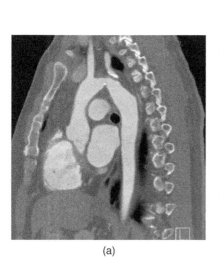
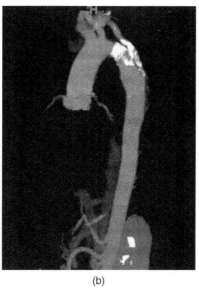
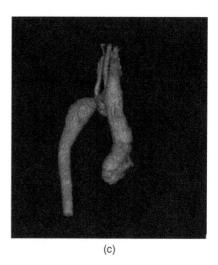

(a) (b) (c)

Figure 64.4 Computed tomography angiography images of (a) coarctation of the aorta; (b) bare-metal stent at the coarctation site; (c) 3D reconstruction.

Acute outcomes reported by the Congenital Cardiovascular Interventional Study Consortium on the treatment of native coarctation showed higher dissection tear and aneurysm formation with balloon angioplasty alone versus stent implantation (9.8% to 0%, respectively). Balloon rupture was higher in stent implantation than balloon angioplasty (0.5% and 0%). Stent migration was reported at 1.4% in the study population. The advantages and limitations of the therapeutic interventions are outlined in Table 64.1.

6. How is balloon angioplasty performed?

The procedure is done under general anesthesia using biplane fluoroscopy. An activated clotting time of > 250 seconds is maintained once access has been obtained. Venous access is obtained from the femoral vein for right heart catheterization and the possibility of right ventricular pacing during stent placement. The femoral artery is accessed for the procedure; however, if crossing the stenosis

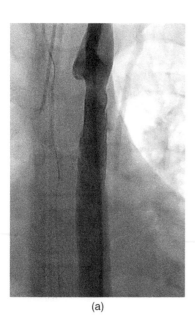
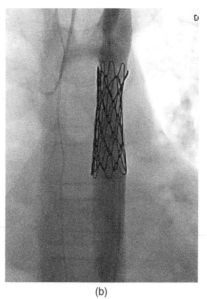

(a) (b)

Figure 64.5 (a) Patient with an aneurysm following bare-metal stent placement. (b) A covered stent is placed, excluding the aneurysm.

Table 64.1 Comparison of transcatheter interventions.

	Balloon angioplasty	**Endovascular stent**	**Covered stents**
Year of introduction	1982	1991	1999
Benefits	• Shorter hospitalization time • Short-term success in 80–90%	• Sustained relief of obstruction • Lower acute complications (aneurysm) • Short-term success of 96% • Does not require overdilation of the aortic wall	• Decreased shear stress. Reduces the risk of acute vascular trauma as well as longer-term aneurysm formation. • It is the salvage therapy for previous aortic wall injury, stent fracture, complex anatomy, and calcified aortic wall.
Disadvantages	• Greater propensity to arterial wall injury • Higher restenosis rate • Less likely to achieve treatment success	• Patient must be big enough to receive an adult-size stent • Requires multiple interventions as the patient grows • Risk of stent malposition	• Require larger sheath sizes, which limits their use in small children • Cases reported of aneurysm • Possible occlusion of spinal arteries (around T9–T12 vertebrae)

retrograde is challenging, the carotid artery or radial artery access can be obtained to cross the lesion. Once the stenosis is crossed antegrade, the wire is snared and externalized from the femoral artery, thereby obtaining retrograde access for the intervention. A complete right and left heart hemodynamic assessment is performed, which should include cardiac output, the gradient across the coarctation site, the left ventricular end-diastolic pressure, the gradient across the mitral valve, and the left ventricular outflow tract. Biplane imaging of the aortic arch anatomy should be performed in the right anterior oblique (RAO) angulation and lateral projection (Figure 64.6a,d). Measurements should include the minimal diameter and length of the coarctation segment, diameter of the transverse arch proximal to the site of coarctation, and descending aorta diameter at the diaphragm. Evaluation of the brachiocephalic vessels and their relationship with the stenotic segment, presence or absence of aneurysm, and presence of any collateral vessels should also be included in the angiographic evaluation.

For angioplasty, the balloon diameter should be two to three times the diameter of the stenosis but should not exceed the diameter of the aorta at the diaphragm or that of the adjacent transverse arch. A super-stiff wire is positioned in the right subclavian artery or the ascending aorta to ensure the stability of the balloon catheter during inflation. Rapid right ventricular pacing of the right ventricle to maintain the aortic pressure between 40 and 50 mm Hg can help with balloon stability in select cases. The balloon is inflated, and attention is paid to the presence or absence of a "waist" at full inflation (Figure 64.6b,e). Repeat hemodynamics is performed to assess cardiac output and the gradient across the coarctation site. An angiogram of the aorta is performed to assess relief of stenosis and the absence of dissection or aneurysm (Figure 64.6c,f). A stepwise approach starting with a low-pressure balloon can minimize the risk of vessel aortic wall injury.

7. Should a low-pressure balloon or high-pressure balloon be used?

Low-pressure balloons are more compliant and have a low burst pressure. They are usually indicated for balloon angioplasty in young children to avoid potential injury to the vessel wall. If there is a complete loss of waist at low pressure with angiographic evidence of stenosis, then a high-pressure balloon can be considered in select patients.

8. How is stent implantation performed?

The selection of the stent is based on the final inflated diameter of the stent and the length of the stenotic segment (Figure 64.7a,d). The stent selected should be re-expandable to a minimum diameter of 20 mm, and the balloon should not exceed the diameter of the aorta at the

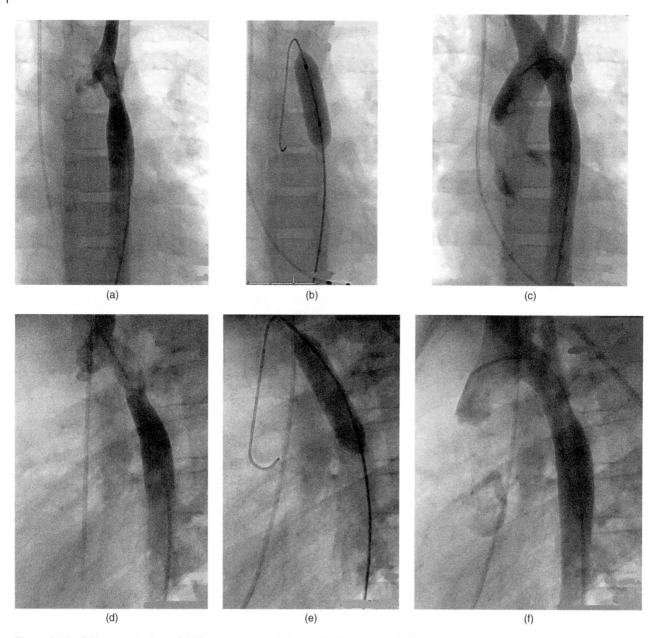

Figure 64.6 Balloon angioplasty: (a) AP projection pre-balloon; (b) AP projection balloon dilation; (c) AP projection post-balloon; (d) lateral projection pre-balloon; (e) lateral projection balloon dilation; (f) lateral projection post-balloon dilation.

diaphragm and the diameter of the segment proximal to the coarctation segment. For stent delivery, a high-pressure balloon or a BIB balloon (NuMed) can be used. The BIB balloon has an outer balloon diameter ranging from 12 to 30 mm and is delivered through an 8–16 Fr sheath. The inner balloon is 1 mm shorter than the outer balloon, and the diameter of the inner balloon is half the diameter of the outer balloon. Inflating the inner balloon first allows for repositioning the stent if needed and minimizes injury to the aortic wall. A super-stiff wire is positioned in the ascending aorta or the right subclavian artery to ensure the

stability of the balloon/stent. A long sheath is positioned across the coarctation, and the mounted stent is advanced over the wire and positioned across the coarctation site. Hand injections through the sheath are performed to position the stent prior to complete unsheathing of the stent (Figure 64.7b,e). The inner balloon is inflated, and the stent position is assessed followed by the outer balloon inflation with rapid right ventricular pacing. Following stent placement, repeat hemodynamics and aortic angiograms should be performed, and further dilatation of the stent can be performed if needed. Flaring of the distal stent struts can

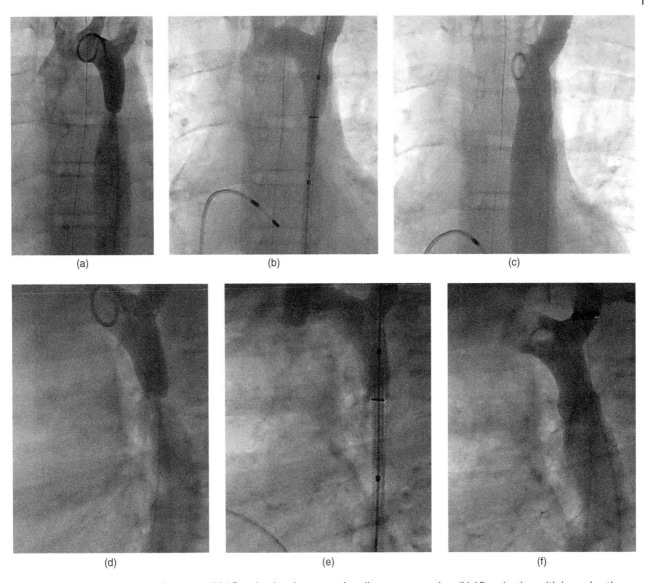

Figure 64.7 Bare-metal stent placement: (a) AP projection demonstrating discrete coarctation; (b) AP projection with long sheath across the coarctation and positioning of stent. Pacing catheter in RV; (c) AP projection post-stent placement; (d) lateral projection demonstrating discrete coarctation with post-stenotic dilation; (e) lateral projection with long sheath across the coarctation and positioning of stent; (f) lateral projection with the stent across the coarctation.

be performed so that the stent is opposed to the vessel wall at its post-stenotic site, followed by angiographic and hemodynamic assessment (Figure 64.7c,f). Patients with severe coarctation can have a staged approach where further dilatation of the stent following the initial intervention.

9. Should a bare-metal or covered stent be used?

There are insufficient data to prefer a bare-metal or covered stent. Some studies have reported that covered stents have a lower risk of aneurysm formation; others have found that long-term outcomes with non-covered stents provide better results. Self-expanding stents have demonstrated good results in a select patient population with suitable anatomy.

A randomized trial of 120 patients following placement of bare-metal or covered stents in severe native coarctation reported no difference in the rate of re-coarctation or pseudoaneurysm formation. The COAST II (Coarctation of Aorta Stent Trial) trial was a multicenter, single-arm study of 158 patients who underwent covered Cheatham Platinum (CP) stent (Numed) placement for the treatment/prevention of aortic wall injury in patients with acute or chronic aortic wall injury, coarctation measuring $\leq 3\,\text{mm}$

in diameter, genetic syndromes at a high risk of aortic wall injury, or patients ≥60 years of age. Following CP stent implantation, the success rate was 92%, with a reduction in gradient from 27 to 4 mmHg. There was no aortic wall injury, repeat intervention, or death. The authors concluded that the covered stent protects from aortic wall injury related to stretch-induced wall trauma and aortic rupture.

10. What are the most common complications?

Procedure-related complications are related to vascular access, aortic wall injury with aortic dissection (0.9%), and aortic rupture (0.4%). The stent may overlap and obstruct the brachiocephalic vessels, and stroke has been reported. Stent embolization has been reported in 2.4%. Death is uncommon.

Transcatheter intervention for coarctation of the aorta can be associated with re-coarctation, aneurysm, pseudoaneurysm, dissection, stent fracture, and death. Aneurysm formation is most often seen after balloon angioplasty of a native lesion rather than in a patient with recurrent stenosis. It usually occurs within the first year following the procedure and has an incidence of 5–9%. The mechanism of aneurysm formation is unclear and multifactorial but may be related to cystic medial necrosis or the use of a larger balloon size, causing tears of the intima-media. Balloon angioplasty alone is associated with a higher rate of intimal tears and aneurysm formation compared with stent placement. Aneurysm formation has been reported following bare metal and covered stent placement. Following covered stent placement, the pseudoaneurysm occurs at the proximal ends of the stent and can be treated with a second covered magnetic resonance imaging (MRI) or CT. Angiography is recommended at intervals following transcatheter intervention.

The COAST study evaluated the safety and efficacy of CP stents placed across the coarctation site. Assessment of efficacy was measured by a reduction in upper to lower extremity systolic blood pressure measurements and the hospital length of stay. There was an immediate reduction in gradient following the procedure, which persisted at an average follow-up of two years. The rate of hypertension and medication use decreased from intervention to 12 months with no significant change at two years. Safety outcome variables assessed were the occurrence of any serious or somewhat serious adverse events attributed to the stent or implantation and the occurrence of paradoxical hypertension. There were no procedural deaths, serious adverse events, or surgical interventions. There were six

aortic aneurysms at follow-up: five underwent covered stent placement, and one resolved without intervention. Stent fractures were noted in 2 patients at one year, 11 patients at two years, and 12 patients after two years, with evidence of fracture progression. No fracture has resulted in the loss of stent integrity, stent embolization, aortic wall injury, or restenosis. There was an association between a larger stent diameter and stent fracture. There were 19 stent re-dilations, mostly related to somatic growth. Stent fracture usually occurred along with the sigma hinge point of the two pieces. This has been an incidental finding, and thus far there have been no reports of fragment embolization.

Aortic dissection is the most catastrophic complication, with an incidence of 1.6% and mortality of around 30%. It is usually in the setting of uncontrolled hypertension.

11. What is the follow-up for patients who undergo percutaneous intervention?

Following transcatheter intervention, a chest X-ray, ECG, and transthoracic echocardiogram are done within 24 hours. Documentation of four extremity blood pressure immediately post-procedure and before discharge is routinely performed.

For follow-up, patients are divided into four groups based on their physiologic state. Patients in New York Heart Association (NYHA) state I with no hemodynamic or anatomic sequelae, no arrhythmias, and normal hepatic, renal, and pulmonary function should have follow-up every two years with an ECG and echocardiogram. An exercise stress test is recommended every three years, and a CTA/C-MRI can be done every three to five years. Patients in NYHA state II with mild hemodynamic or anatomic sequelae (mild enlargement of the aorta, ventricle or ventricular dysfunction, mild valvular disease, trivial or small shunt) and arrhythmias that do not require treatment should have follow-up every two years with ECG and echocardiogram and exercise stress test done every two years and a CTA/C-MRI done every three to five years. Patients in NYHA state III with significant (moderate or greater) valvular disease; moderate or greater ventricular dysfunction (systemic, pulmonic, or both), moderate anatomical sequelae (moderate aortic enlargement, venous or arterial stenosis, hemodynamically significant shunt), and pulmonary hypertension, moderate cyanosis, and end-organ dysfunction should be followed up every 6–12 months with an ECG and echocardiogram, an exercise stress test every two years, and a CTA/C-MRI every one to two years. Patients in NYHA state IV with severe aortic enlargement, arrhythmias refractory to treatment, severe hypoxemia, severe pulmonary hypertension, Eisenmenger syndrome, and refractory end-organ dysfunction should be followed up every three to six months with an ECG, echocardiogram and exercise stress test recommended every year, and a CTA/C-MRI every one to two years.

Lifelong surveillance is mandatory due to the risk of re-coarctation and aneurysm formation. Other comorbidities are hypertension, coronary atherosclerosis, aortic dissection, stroke, and congestive heart failure. Hypertension (baseline or exercise-induced) is endemic in this population secondary to underlying arteriopathies, decreased aortic wall compliance, and renal abnormalities. Exercise is encouraged for those who are normotensive, without an aneurysm, and with no other associated heart defect. Endocarditis prophylaxis is recommended for six months following the transcatheter intervention.

12. What are the short- and long-term results?

A successful outcome is a decrease in peak-to-peak gradient following intervention to ≤ 20 mmHg across the coarctation. Patients with coarctation who survive beyond infancy without treatment have poor outcomes, with 75% mortality rate by 43 years of age secondary to heart failure, aortic dissection or rupture, endocarditis, or intracranial bleeding.

Balloon angioplasty. For balloon angioplasty, the short-term effective relief of gradient occurs in 75–79% of patients with a low mortality rate of 0.7–2.5%. For discrete lesions following balloon angioplasty at long-term follow-up of 20 years, the freedom from intervention was 87%.

Stent implantation. In 2007, the Congenital Cardiovascular Consortium (CCISC) reported the results of 565 stent implantations at the coarctation site between 1989 and 2005. The gradient decreased to ≤ 20 mmHg in 98% of the patients, with a decrease in gradient from 31.6 ± 16 (mean $\pm$ SD) to 2.7 ± 4.2 mmHg and an increase in the diameter of the stenotic vessel from 7.4 ± 3 to 14.3 ± 3.2 mm. Forbes et al. reported persistence of relief of gradient at a median follow-up of 12 months. Following stent placement, 92.2% of the patient had a successful short-term outcome. The rate of re-intervention is about 22%, mostly related to somatic growth.

Conclusion

Transcatheter treatment for coarctation of the aorta is a safe and effective treatment. Close follow-up with advanced imaging is recommended at frequent intervals after successful treatment to monitor for aortic wall injury. Systemic hypertension may persist in patients after successful relief of gradient.

Bibliography

1 Alkashkar, W., Albugami, S., and Hijazi, Z. (2019). Management of coarctation of the aorta in adult patients: State of the Art. *Korean Circ. J.* 49 (4): 298–313.

2 Bruckheimer, E., Birk, E., Santiago, R. et al. (2010). Coarctation of the aorta treated with the Advanta V12 large diameter stent: acute results. *Catheter. Cardiovasc. Interv.* 75 (3): 402–406.

3 Campbell, M. (1970). Natural history of coarctation of aorta. *Br. Heart J.* 32: 633–640.

4 Fawzy, M.E., Fathala, A., Osman, A. et al. (2008). Twenty-two years of follow-up results of balloon angioplasty for discrete native coarctation of the aorta in adolescents and adults. *Am. Heart J.* 156: 910–917.

5 Firoozi, A., Mohebbi, B., Noohi, F. et al. (2018). Self-expanding versus balloon-expandable stents in patients with isthmic coarctation of the aorta. *Am. J. Cardiol.* 122 (6): 1062–1067.

6 Forbes, T.J., Garekar, S., Amin, Z. et al. (2007). Procedural results of acute complications in stenting native and recurrent coarctation of the aorta in patients over 4 years of age: a multi-institutional study. *Catheter. Cardiovasc. Interv.* 70: 276–285.

7 Forbes, T.J. and Gowda, S.T. (2014). Intravascular stent therapy for coarctation of the aorta. *Methodist Debakey Cardiovasc. J.* 10 (2): 82–87.

8 Forbes, T.J., Kim, D.W., Du, W. et al. (2011). Comparison of surgical, stent, and balloon angioplasty treatment of native coarctation of the aorta. An observational study by the CCISC. *J. Am. Coll. Cardiol.* 58 (25): 2664–2674.

9 Forbes, T.J., Moore, P., Pedra, C.A. et al. (2007). Intermediate follow-up following intravascular stenting for treatment of coarctation of aorta. *Catheter. Cardiovasc. Interv.* 70: 569–577.

10 Haji Zeinali, A.M., Sadeghian, M., Qureshi, S.A., and Ghazi, P. (2017). Midterm to long-term safety and efficacy of self-expandable nitinol stent implantation for coarctation of aorta in adults. *Catheter. Cardiovasc. Interv.* 90 (3): 425–431.

11 Hartman, E.M., Groenendijk, J.M., Heuvelman, H.M. et al. (2015). The effectiveness of stenting of coarctation of the aorta: a systematic review. *EuroIntervention* 11: 660–669.

12 Kische, S., D'Ancona, G., Stoeckicht, Y. et al. (2015). Percutaneous treatment of adult isthmic aortic coarctation. *Circ. Cardiovasc. Interv.* 8: e001799.

13 Lin, A.E., Basson, C.T., Goldmuntz, E. et al. (2008). Adults with genetic syndromes and cardiovascular abnormalities. Clinical history and management. *Genet. Med.* 10: 469–494.

14 Luijendijk, P., Bouma, B.J., Groenink, M. et al. (2012). Surgical versus percutaneous treatment of aortic coarctation. New standards in an era of transcatheter repair. *Expert Rev. Cardiovasc. Therapy* 10 (12): 1517–1531.

15 McCrindle, B.W., Jones, T.K., Morrow, W.R. et al. (1996). Acute results of balloon angioplasty of native coarctation versus recurrent aortic obstruction are equivalent. Valvulplasty and angioplasty for congenital anomalies (VACA) registry investigators. *J. Am. Coll. Cardiol.* 28: 1810–1817.

16 Meadows, J., Minahan, M., McElhinney, D.B. et al.: COAST Investigators(2015). Intermediate outcomes in the prospective, multicenter coarctation of the aorta stent trial (COAST). *Circulation* 131: 1656–1664.

17 Preventza, O., Livesay, J.J., Cooley, D.A. et al. (2013). Coarctation associated aneurysms: a localized disease or diffuse arteriopathy. *Ann. Thorac. Surg.* 95: 1961–1970.

18 Qureshi, S.A. (2009). Use of covered stents to treat coarctation of the aorta. *Korean Circ. J.* 39 (7): 261–263.

19 Sasikumar, D., Sasidharan, B., Rashid, A. et al. (2020). Early and late outcome of covered and non-covered stents in the treatment of coarctation of aorta – a single centre experience. *Indian Heart J.* 72 (4): 278–282.

20 Sohrabi, B., Jamshidi, P., Yaghoubi, A. et al. (2014). Comparison between covered and bare Cheatham-Platinium stent for endovascular treatment of patients with native post-ductal aortic coarctation. *JACC* 7 (4).

21 Sohrabi, B., Jamshidi, P., Yaghoubi, A. et al. (2014). Comparison between covered and bare Cheatham-Platinum stents for endovascular treatment of patients with native post-ductal aortic coarctation: immediate and intermediate-term results. *JACC Cardiovasc. Interv.* 7: 416–423.

22 Stout, K.K., Daniels, C.J., Aboulhosn, J.A. et al. (2018, 2019). AHA/ACC Guideline for the Management of Adults With Congenital Heart Disease. *Circulation* 139: e698–e800.

23 Taggart, N.W., Minahan, M., Cabalka, A.K. et al. (2016). Immediate outcomes of covered stent placement for treatment or prevention of aortic wall injury associated with coarctation of the aorta (COASTII). *JACC Cardiovasc. Interv.* 9: 484–493.

24 Torok, R.D., Campbell, M.J., Fleming, G.A., and Hill, K.D. (2015). Coarctation of the Aorta: Management from infancy to adulthood. *World J. Cardiol.* 7 (11): 765–775.

25 Tzifa, A., Ewert, P., Brzezinska-Rajszys, G. et al. (2006). Covered cheatham-platinum stents for aortic coarctation: early and intermediate-term results. 47 (7): 1457–1463.

26 Wilson, P.D., Loffredo, C.A., Correra-Villasenor, A., and Ferenez, C. (1998). Attributable fraction for cardiac malformations. *Am. J. Epidemiol.* 148: 414–423.

65

Percutaneous Pulmonary Valve Replacement (PPVR)

Jose Luis Zunzunegui and Alejandro Rodríguez Ogando

[1] *Gregorio Marañon Hospital, Madrid, Spain*

1. In what anatomical settings can we perform percutaneous pulmonic valve replacement (PPVR)?

Prosthetic conduits. Surgical correction of certain congenital heart diseases (almost all in the setting of Tetralogy of Fallot (TOF)) involves the reconstruction of the right ventricular outflow tract with the interposition of homograft, manufactured valved conduits (made with Dacron or Goretex), and bovine jugular grafts (Contegra, Medtronic[R]), between the right ventricle (RV) and the trunk of the pulmonary artery. Even though these reconstructive surgeries for the right ventricle outflow tract (RVOT) can be performed with low mortality, the useful life of implanted valvulated conduits is normally short (<10 years) because of the degeneration and/or calcification of the materials used to make them, especially if they are implanted in very young patients. Added to this, in the pediatric field, is the impossibility of the prosthetic material itself to follow the growth of the patient and the possible progressive extrinsic compression of the conduit by other anatomical structures during development (sternum, posterior ascending aorta, etc.), which also limits its durability.

Congenital heart defects that typically require implantation of a valved conduit between the RV and the pulmonary arteries for surgical correction include:

- TOF with an absence of pulmonary valve
- Double outlet RV
- Pulmonary atresia
- Truncus arteriosus
- Transpositions of great arteries with ventricular septal defect and pulmonary stenosis (PS) or atresia, with Rastelli-type surgical correction
- Ross surgery

Aortic or pulmonary homografts can be dilated a few millimeters (with balloons and/or stents) with respect to their nominal size. Those manufactured with Dacron or Goretex are practically indistensible. The bovine jugular Contegra is the most distensible of all, being able to dilate ducts from 12–14 to 20–22 mm without difficulty.

Native RVOT. The term "native RVOT" is used when there is no conduit or biological prosthesis between the RV and the pulmonary branches. This is the case when the surgeon has repaired the infundibular stenosis with the placement of an enlargement patch (normally autologous pericardium), this enlarges the muscular infundibulum and the pulmonary ring (transannular patch). Patients with native RVOT represent more than 80% of the possible candidates for PPVR. Congenital heart defects that are usually repaired with a transannular patch are:

- TOF with adequate pulmonary branches.
- Congenital pulmonary valvular stenosis; normally, very dysplastic valves that have not responded to percutaneous valvuloplasty (for example, PS associated with Noonan syndrome)

The term "native outflow tract" is also used in patients who did not undergo surgery, in patient whom a percutaneous valvuloplasty was performed during childhood and currently have residual insufficiency or stenosis.

This native outflow tract is highly compliant, changing dimensions during the cardiac cycle. Thus, it is difficult to determine the maximum diameters of the area to be valved. Computed tomography (CT) and magnetic resonance imaging (MRI) often do not accurately determine these maximum dimensions, and there is risk of stent and/or valve embolization.

Biological pulmonary valves. Biological valves have been widely used by surgeons in the repair of enlarged

Mastering Structural Heart Disease, First Edition. Edited by Eduardo J. de Marchena and Camilo A. Gomez.
© 2023 John Wiley & Sons Ltd. Published 2023 by John Wiley & Sons Ltd.
Companion website: www.wiley.com/go/deMarchena/Mastering-Structural-Heart-Disease

RVOTs with a transannular patch. It is the ideal anatomical substrate for the percutaneous implantation of a pulmonary prosthesis; it is one of the easiest scenarios to start with the PPVR protocol in any center.

2. When is PPVR indicated?

The definition of objective parameters to undertake valve replacement in the setting of chronic pulmonary insufficiency/stenosis has been complex. At the present time, we can say the following regarding PPVR:

- PPVR is the first treatment option (before surgery) if the anatomy is adequate.
- Any symptomatic patient with residual pulmonary insufficiency/stenosis has an indication for pulmonary valve replacement (surgical or percutaneous).
- The tendency to indicate PPVR is increasingly earlier; in this way, we increase the chances of recovery of RV function.
- In asymptomatic patients with residual RVOT dysfunction, there has been great controversy regarding the time to indicate PPVR. (Figures 65.1 and 65.2) describe the decision-making diagram that we apply in our environment.

3. What diagnostic tests should be performed before doing the PPRV?

The goals of cardiac magnetic resonance imaging (cMRI) examination in patients with repaired heart disease and residual RVOT dysfunction include:

- Establishing the RVOT dimensions during the cardiac cycle to determine the "landing zone"
- Quantitative measurement of volumes and systolic function of both ventricles
- Obtaining anatomical images of the RVOT, pulmonary branches, aorta, and possible aortopulmonary collaterals
- Quantitative assessment of pulmonary or tricuspid regurgitation or any other valvular abnormality and calculation of the pulmonary/systemic flow ratio
- Evaluating myocardial viability

In recent years, CT has been incorporated for the evaluation of the RVOT, with very good results, especially in the analysis of the RVOT dimensions, the anatomical study of the pulmonary branches, and especially the relationship of the coronary arteries with the area of the possible implant.

4. What kind of valves are available?

Currently, two types of prostheses are mainly used for pulmonary position, both balloon-expandable: the Melody valve (Medtronic) and the SAPIEN 3 prosthesis (Edwards Lifesciences), both of which have CE marks to be implanted in pulmonary position (Figure 65.3).

The Melody valve consists of an 18 mm bovine jugular valve segment that is sutured onto a Cheatham Platinum (CP) stent (NuMED) made of platinum and iridium. The initial length of the valve is 28 mm (34–36 mm crimped), but it is shortened in accordance with the final implanted

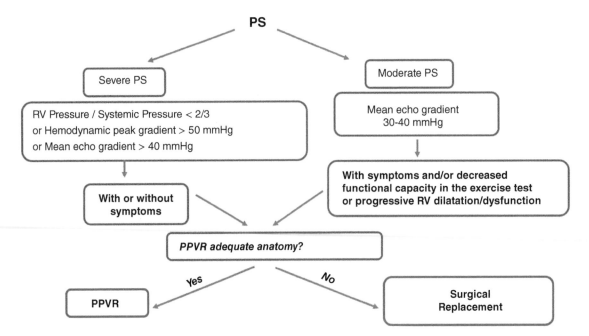

Figure 65.1 Decision-making diagram for RVOT with pulmonary stenosis. *Source:* Adapted from Alkasshkari and Albusubei (2018).

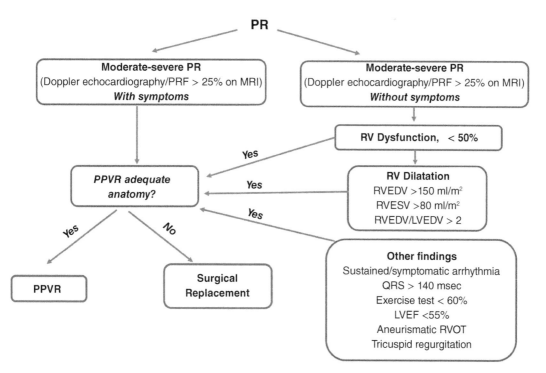

Figure 65.2 Decision-making diagram for RVOT with pulmonary regurgitation. LVEF; left ventricle ejection fraction. LVEDV; left ventricle end diastolic volume. Left ventricle PRF; pulmonary regurgitation fraction. RVEDV; right ventricle end diastolic volume. RVESV; right ventricle end systolic volume. *Source:* Adapted from Alkasshkari and Albusubei (2018).

diameter. The valve can be expanded from 16 to 22 mm in diameter and, in some instances, up to 24 mm. The valve is delivered via a 22 F Ensemble transcatheter delivery system (Medtronic). This consists of a balloon-in-balloon (BiB) system (available in 18, 20, 22 mm), which enables

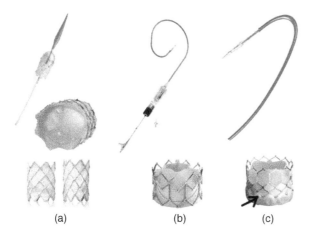

Figure 65.3 Types of balloon-expandable percutaneous pulmonary valves. (a) Medtronic Melody valve and Ensemble delivery system. (b) Edwards SAPIEN XT valve and the NovaFlex delivery system. (c) SAPIEN S3 valve and Commander delivery system. The SAPIEN S3 (last generation) valve has a pericardium skirt (arrow), which prevents periprosthetic leaks. *Source:* J. Gales et al (2018), Elsevier.

the valve to be repositioned, if needed, after the inner balloon has been inflated.

The SAPIEN 3 valve implant kit includes the Commander delivery system (which is deflectable and includes the balloon where the valve is crimped), a crimper, and a hydrophilic introducer with a different profile depending on the size of the valve that we are going to implant. As fundamental differences, it should be noted that it reaches up to 29 mm (20, 23, 26, and 29 mm) and is a bovine pericardium bioprosthesis mounted on a cobalt-chromium stent with great radial strength, so breakages of its struts are exceptional. The largest external diameter that the 29 SAPIEN valve can achieve is 31 mm (if we add 4–8 cc of saline to the nominal inflation volume).

It is a valve with poorer navigability, which is used in older patients, its implantation being more complicated in patients weighing <30 kg. In addition, jugular access is not recommended by manufacturers, although it can be done if necessary.

5. How is the procedure performed?

With an angiography catheter (pigtail 5–6 F), injections are made in the pulmonary artery (PA) with cranial and lateral angulation, and measurements are made, comparing them with those of previous imaging studies (cMRI, CT).

It is important to rule out the risk of coronary compression (especially of the left coronary artery) with the inflation of a non-compliant balloon in the RVOT (native outflow tract or conduits) (Figure 65.4). To do this, and taking advantage of the arterial access, we perform selective coronary angiography while inflating a non-compliant balloon with a diameter similar to the final diameter, which we intend to achieve with the Melody or SAPIEN 3 valve. The risk of coronary compression is much higher in adult patients with highly calcified stenotic ducts, especially in Ross surgery, where the surgeon has to surgically translocate the coronary arteries, and their origin may be displaced toward the most anterior portion of the aortic wall.

Finally, the high support guidewire is placed, It is used to advance the valve crimped on the delivery system. The guidewire must be "impacted" in the distal lung bed. Probably the best option for this procedure is the Lunderquist (Cook), which has a very "floppy" or flexible distal segment and is undoubtedly the first choice for the procedure.

In recent years, prior stent implantation *(pre-stenting)* in the RVOT has been routinely recommended:

- *In the native outflow tract,* to create a rigid and stable landing zone that improves valve anchorage and reduces the risk of embolization
- *In valved prosthetic conduits;* to avoid the risk of strut valve rupture during follow-up (especially in the Melody valve), especially in highly calcified, very anterior (directly retrosternal), or very tortuous ducts

The most-used stents are the NuMED CP in dysfunctional conduit (covered or not covered) or the AndraStent XL and XXL (Andramed) in native RVOT (Figure 65.5).

With the landing zone of the future pulmonary valve ready, the valve and delivery system are prepared. Finally, the delivery system (Ensemble for the Melody valve, Commander for the SAPIEN 3 valve) is introduced with its crimped valve in the access vein, and it is advanced to the implantation area, where it will be expanded by inflating balloons.

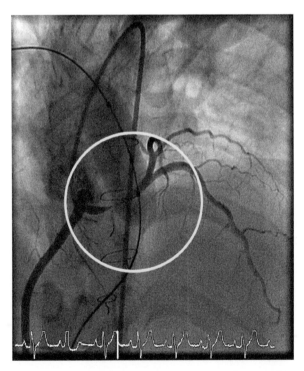

Figure 65.4 Coronary compression test in a patient with Ross surgery. Valved homograft between the right ventricle and the pulmonary branches. Inflation of a 20-mm Mullins balloon with simultaneous left coronary angiography. Left trunk compression. *Source:* Courtesy of Dr. Gerad Marti.

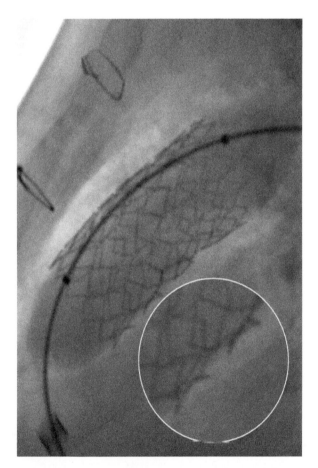

Figure 65.5 Pre-stenting in the native right ventricle outflow tract with a 57 mm AndraStent XXL. The metal struts open outward, improving anchorage to the smooth walls of the native RVOT. *Source:* Zunzunegui et al. Gregorio Marañón Children´s Hospital, Madrid.

6. What technical differences do you have to consider depending on the type of dysfunctional RVOT?

PPVR in Dysfunctional Prosthetic Conduits

For conduit predilation and pre-stenting, it is recommended to select a balloon size that does not exceed 110% of the nominal size of the conduit so as not to unnecessarily increase the risk of rupture. In pre-stenting, we recommend always using a covered stent (Covered CP Stent, NuMED). This way, in addition to reducing the risk of bleeding due to rupture of the conduit, perivalvular leaks and small accumulations of blood between the valve and the internal surface of the conduit are avoided, which could be an adequate substrate for bacterial growth and endocarditis.

PPVR in Dysfunctional Native RVOT

The native outflow tract (transannular patch enlargement or dysplastic pulmonary valves) is a very distensible structure, and sometimes the end-systolic diameter cannot be accurately determined by CT and/or MRI. To choose the sizes of balloons, stents, and valves, a sizing balloon is always used before implantation. It consists of inflating a compliant balloon in the native RVOT (usually with a large diameter > 24 mm) while contrast is injected through the lateral port of a long introducer with its tip placed in the RV. At that time, we check whether the passage of contrast to the pulmonary branches is blocked and whether there is any "waist" in the balloon (which will correspond to the narrowest area of the native outflow tract). The diameter of the balloon and the diameter of the balloon indentation serve as a reference to choose which balloons and/or stents we use for pre-stenting (Figure 65.6). In clinical practice, if the RVOT is not completely occluded with a 30 mm balloon, it is recommended that the patient undergo surgical valve replacement.

To perform the pre-stenting, we use the AndraStent or the Optimus stent (AndraTec). It is common practice to perform the valve implantation two to three months after pre-stenting, waiting for stent endothelialization.

Finally, depending on the pre-stenting diameter, one prosthesis diameter and model are chosen.

PPVR in Dysfunctional Biological Valves

A dysfunctional biological valve is the ideal anatomical substrate for the percutaneous implantation of a pulmonary

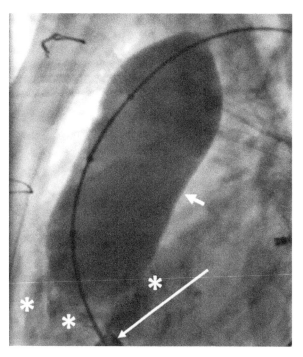

Figure 65.6 30 mm sizing balloon in a native outflow tract. Balloon inflation, simultaneous angiography through the lateral port of the 14 f Mullins sheath, sheath tip located in the right ventricle (long arrow). Slight indentation (waist) in the balloon (short arrow) Contrast (*) is retained in the right ventricle without opacifying the pulmonary arteries. *Source:* Zunzunegui et al. Gregorio Marañón Children's Hospital, Madrid.

prosthesis. In general, it is not necessary to perform prestenting or the coronary compression test. The diameter of the valve is chosen depending on the nominal internal diameter of each prosthesis (the implanted model must be known). If the pulmonary valve is small and restrictive, its diameter can be increased by fracturing the metal ring (cracking technique) with an ultra-high-pressure balloon (Atlas Gold, Bard) 1–2 m larger than the internal diameter nominal value of the biological bioprosthesis, with an inflation pressure > 10 atm.

7. What do you do if you cannot advance the prosthesis to the implant area?

On some occasions, despite having the high support guidewire well positioned, there are serious difficulties in bringing the delivery system with the crimped valve up to the landing zone. Some suggestions are as follows:

- *Modify the position of the guidewire* from one pulmonary branch to the other (Figure 65.7).

- *Change the type of guidewire.* The most frequently used guides are Back-Up Meier (Boston Scientific), Lunderquist

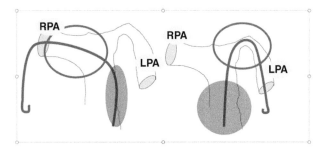

Figure 65.7 The guidewire in the right pulmonary artery can be placed more distally and provides more support. The guidewire in the left pulmonary artery provides a more centered position and less friction with the anterior wall of the right ventricle outflow tract. *Source:* Zunzunegui et al. Gregorio Marañón Children's Hospital, Madrid.

(Cook Medical), and Amplatz Super Stiff (Boston Scientific). All of them are 0.035 in., and they are listed from most to least stiff, although our first choice is always the Lunderquist.

- *Change the femoral access for the jugular access.* The right jugular pathway undoubtedly offers a more favorable orientation to reach the RVOT. It must be remembered that the jugular route is not recognized for the SAPIEN 3 valve, although it can be performed in case of extreme need.
- *The SAPIEN 3 valve has a deflectable delivery system.* It can be of some use in RVOT to direct the valve posteriorly and avoid contact of the system with the anterior walls of the RVOT.

8. What complications are associated with the procedure?

The most important are as follows:

- *Conduit rupture:* Risk factors for conduit rupture with or without serious bleeding are the need for prior balloon dilation in severe stenosis and very calcified ducts, especially with distal calcified stenosis.
- *Coronary compression:* 5–6% of all potential PPRV candidates have coronary anatomy susceptible to compression during implantation. Surgeries that have required a coronary translocation (Ross surgery) and highly calcified conduits in adult patients are two of the risk factors for this severe complication.
- *Others:* Damage in pulmonary branches (including perforation of lobar arteries) or the tricuspid valve.

The global peri-procedural complication rate is around 6%, but only 2.7% are major complications.

9. What is the result of PPVR during follow-up?

At the present time, we can say that the durability of the percutaneous valves is at least similar to that of surgical prostheses; 86% of patients undergoing PPVR do not need any type of reintervention, with a mean follow-up of 24 months.

The incidence of endocarditis can range between 1% and 4% and seems to be associated more with the Melody valve than with the SAPIEN valve. Interruption of antiplatelet therapy and post-procedural residual gradients > 25 mmHg have been identified as risk factors.

10. What technical innovations in PPVR are available in clinical practice?

Direct implantation of the SAPIEN 3 valve without pre-stenting. Performing pre-stenting in native RVOT can be technically challenging, and many times it is necessary to defer valve implantation to a second procedure. Some centers are directly implanting the SAPIEN 3 valve without pre-stenting in patients with native outflow tract. In our experience, this technique should be used in native RVOT < 28 mm, with simultaneous overpacing.

Self-expanding valves. All self-expanding valves are implanted directly in the native outflow tract without the need for pre-stenting. There are several models: The Venus P-valve (Venus Medtech), the Harmony valve (Medtronic; the only one with FDA approval), and the Pulsta valve (Taewong). All of them have an hourglass shape, with larger diameters at their proximal and distal ends, to confer greater stability. The valve is made of porcine pericardium and is housed in the central portion of the self-expanding Nitinol structure. Diameters range from 18 to 34 mm, and native outflow tracts of up to 32 mm can theoretically be treated, although in clinical practice, the limit is usually 30 mm. Due to their low radial force, all of these valves are only indicated in native outflow tracts with severe pulmonary regurgitation without stenosis (Figure 65.8).

PPVR in pyramidal outflow tract or clover lesions. The combination of bilateral stenosis of the branches and distal stenosis of the duct or the enlargement patch is called *pyramidal RVOT*, although we prefer to call it *clover lesion* (Figure 65.9). This RVOT morphology is common and very challenging. We treat these injuries using the "jailing technique" (Figure 65.10).

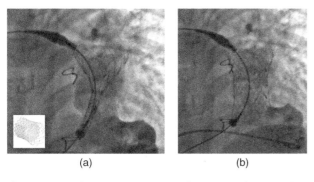

Figure 65.8 32 mm autoexpandable Pulsta valve implantation in the native right ventricle outflow tract, and severe pulmonary regurgitation.(a) Deployment of the distal portion in the pulmonary bifurcation. (b) Full valve deployment. *Source:* Zunzunegui et al. Gregorio Marañón Children's Hospital, Madrid.

Use of the DrySeal sheath for SAPIEN 3 valve implantation. The DrySeal sheath (Gore) is a reinforced, flexible, hydrophilic introducer originally designed for the implantation of stents in the treatment of abdominal aneurysms. It is available from 14–26 F, in lengths of 33.45 and 65 cm. The hemostatic valve can be inflated and deflated with a 2 cc syringe filled with saline. The 29 mm SAPIEN 3 can be implanted through the 26 F sheath and the 23 and 26 mm SAPIEN through a 24 F DrySeal. This improves the navigability of the delivery system, decreases the risk of tricuspid damage, and decreases the chances that the prestent be mobilized, even when performed in the same procedure. At the present time, its use has become a standard in most implantation centers and has greatly simplified the implant technique (Figure 65.11).

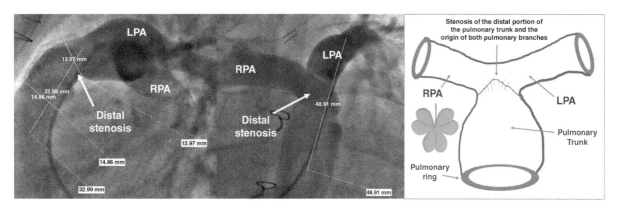

Figure 65.9 Clover lesion, also called pyramidal right ventricle outflow tract or bifurcated stenosis. The distal stenosis of the conduit or the enlargement patch is combined with stenosis of the origin of both pulmonary arteries. *Source:* Zunzunegui et al. Gregorio Marañón Children's Hospital, Madrid.

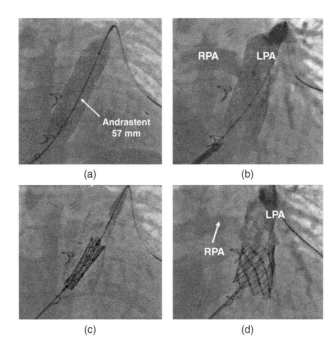

Figure 65.10 Jailing technique in the same patient as in Figure 65.9. (a) AndraStent implanted on a 20×60 mm balloon, insinuated in the left pulmonary artery. (b) AndraStent overdilated with a 22 × 40 mm balloon; flow in the right pulmonary artery preserved. (c) Melody valve crimped on Ensemble 22. (d) Final result without pulmonary insufficiency and good flow in the right pulmonary artery. *Source:* Zunzunegui et al. Gregorio Marañón Children's Hospital, Madrid.

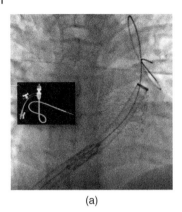
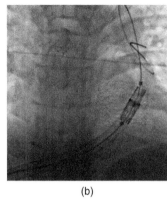
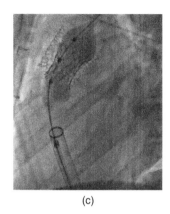

(a)   (b)   (c)

Figure 65.11 Implantation of a 29 mm SAPIEN 3 valve in the native right ventricle outflow tract that was previously pre-stented (two months before), using a DrySeal sheath. (a) DrySeal crossing the stent. (b) Positioning of the crimped SAPIEN 3 valve within the stent, removing the sheath. (c) SAPIEN 3 valve expansion. *Source:* Zunzunegui et al. Gregorio Marañón Children´s Hospital, Madrid.

Bibliography

1 Alkashkari, W., Albugami, S., Abbadi, M. et al. (2020). Transcatheter pulmonary valve replacement in pediatric patients. *Expert Rev. Med. Devices* 17 (6): 541–554.

2 Alkasshkari, W. and Albusubei, H.Z. (2018). Transcatheter pulmonary valve replacement; current state of art. *Curr. Cardiol. Rep.* 20: 27.

3 Baumgartner, H., De Backer, J., Babu-Narayan, S.V. et al. (2020). 2020 ESC guidelines for the management of adult congenital heart disease. *Eur. Heart J.* 42 (6): 563–645.

4 Boudjemline, Y., Malekzadeh-Milani, S., Patel, M. et al. (2016). Predictors and outcomes of right ventricular outflow tract conduit rupture during percutaneous pulmonary valve implantation: a multicentre study. *EuroIntervention* 11 (9): 1053–1062.

5 Cheatham, J.P., Hellenbrand, W.E., Zahn, E.M. et al. (2015). Clinical and hemodynamic outcomes up to 7 years after transcatheter pulmonary valve replacement in the US Melody valve investigational device exemption trial. *Circulation* 131: 1960–1970.

6 Curran, L., Agrawal, H., Kallianos, K. et al. (2020). Computed tomography guided sizing for transcatheter pulmonary valve replacement. *J. Cardiol. Heart Vasc.* 29: 100523.

7 DB, M.E. et al. (2021). Multicenter study of endocarditis after transcatheter pulmonary valve replacement. *J. Am. Coll. Cardiol.* 78 (6): 575–589.

8 Giugno, L., Faccini, A., and Carminati, M. (2020). Percutaneous pulmonary valve implantation. *Korean Cir. J.* 50 (4): 302–316.

9 Kenny, D., Morgan, G.J., Murphy, M. et al. (2019). Use of 65 cm calibrer DrySeal sheaths to facilitate delivery of Edwards SAPIEN valve to dysfunctional right ventricular outflow tracts. *Catheter. Cardiovasc. Interv.* 94 (3): 1–5.

10 Morgan, G.J., Sadeghi, S., Salem, M.M. et al. (2019). SAPIEN valve for percutaneous transcatheter pulmonary valve replacement without "pre-stenting": a multi-institutional experience. *Catheter. Cardiovasc. Interv.* 93: 324–329.

11 Morray, B.H., McElhinney, D.B., Cheatham, J.P. et al. (2013). Risk of coronary compression among patients referred for transcatheter pulmonary valve implantation; a multicenter experience. *Circ. Cardiovasc. Interv.* 6: 535–542.

12 Sinha, S., Aboulhosn, J., and Levi, D. (2019). Transcatheter pulmonary valve replacement in congenital heart diseases. *Intervent. Cardiol. Clin.* 8: 59–71.

13 Tanase, D., Grohmann, J., Schubert, S. et al. (2014). Cracking the ring of edwards perimount bioprosthesis with ultrahigh pressure balloons prior to transcatheter valve in valve implantation. *Int. J. Cardiol.* 176: 1048–1049.

14 Zahn, E.M. (2019). Self-expanding pulmonary valves for large diameter right ventricular outflow tracts. *Intervent. Cardiol. Clin.* 8: 73–80.

Part VIII

Miscellaneous

66

Hemodynamic Pearls in Adult Structural Heart Disease

Juan G. Lopez[1] and Michael D. Dyal[1,2]

[1] Cardiovascular Division, Department of Medicine, University of Miami Miller School of Medicine, Miami, FL, USA
[2] Department of Veterans Affairs, Miami, FL, USA

Hemodynamic Assessment of the Aortic Valve

1. When is an invasive hemodynamic assessment required?

An invasive hemodynamic assessment should not be considered for all patients with aortic valve disease. If noninvasive velocities, area, and clinical evaluation (symptoms plus physical examination) are consistent with severe aortic stenosis (AS), an invasive assessment is not necessary and can increase risks such as stroke and left ventricular perforation.

When there are discrepancies, however, accurate invasive hemodynamics are required.

2. How do you calculate the aortic valve area using invasive hemodynamics?

To calculate valve area, three tools are needed:

a. Transvalvular pressure gradient
b. An accurate cardiac output
c. Gorlin or Hakki formulas

The Gorlin formula, first described in 1951, states

$$\text{Aortic valve area} = F / \left(Cc \cdot Cv\right)\sqrt{2gh}$$

where F is the flow or cardiac output. Cc and Cv are the coefficients of orifice contraction and velocity loss and are estimated to be 1, making the more useful equation

$$\text{Aortic valve area} = CO / \sqrt{2gh}$$

where CO is cardiac output, g is acceleration from gravity, and h is the mean transvalvular pressure gradient.

3. Does the Hakki formula accurately estimate the valve area when compared to the more complex Gorlin formula?

The aortic valve area is calculated automatically using the Gorlin formula by most modern hemodynamic monitoring systems. However, there are common human input errors and inaccurate automated inputs that should be checked by the interventional cardiologist. The Hakki formula is a well-validated, accurate, simple assessment that should be done by hand in every case to confirm the automated results:

$$\text{Aortic valve area} = CO / \sqrt{Pressure\ gradient}$$

4. How do you accurately measure cardiac output?

Accurate assessment of cardiac output (CO) is critical to understanding cardiovascular physiology, particularly in valvular heart disease. The two main ways to measure CO invasively are the Fick and thermodilution techniques. Fick is the gold standard

$$CO(L/\text{min}) = \frac{VO_2(ml/\text{min})}{Hb_{g/dl} * 1.36(SA_{\%satO2} - MV_{\%satO2})} * \frac{1}{10}$$

Mastering Structural Heart Disease, First Edition. Edited by Eduardo J. de Marchena and Camilo A. Gomez.
© 2023 John Wiley & Sons Ltd. Published 2023 by John Wiley & Sons Ltd.
Companion website: www.wiley.com/go/deMarchena/Mastering-Structural-Heart-Disease

where CO is cardiac output, VO_2 is total oxygen consumption, and Hb is hemoglobin.

Measurement of total oxygen consumption can be done, but in most labs, it is cumbersome, and therefore this value is estimated by multiplying the body surface area by the oxygen consumption index ($VO_{2i} = 125 \, ml/min/m^2$). Therefore, Fick is most often calculated using the following formula

$$CO \, (L/min) = \frac{VO_{2i} \, (ml/min/m^2) * BSA \, (m^2)}{Hb_{g/dl} * 13.6 \, (SA_{\%satO2} - MV_{\%satO2})}$$

where CO is cardiac output, VO_{2i} is the oxygen consumption index (oxygen consumption per unit body surface area), BSA is the body surface area, and Hb is hemoglobin.

There are clear inherent errors when estimating total oxygen consumption, particularly in patients with advanced structural heart disease. Therefore, most laboratories have moved toward using the thermodilution technique. Just as with Fick, it is important to be aware of the limitations of the thermodilution technique, such as low CO states, severe tricuspid insufficiency, irregular rhythms, and intracardiac shunts.

5. How do you appropriately measure the transvalvular gradient?

The most accurate method for assessing the aortic transvalvular pressure gradient involves measuring simultaneous left ventricular and aortic pressures and superimposing their waveforms. This is performed using two side-hole catheters with one in the ascending aorta and the other in the left ventricle (LV). Another commonly used tool is a catheter with two lumens, either a dual-lumen pigtail or multipurpose. It is critical to constantly flush the smaller second lumen to avoid damping, which results in an overestimation of the pressure gradient.

Once the waveforms are superimposed, the area between the two waveforms is automatically calculated by the hemodynamic monitoring system and provides the mean pressure gradient. While we can use the peak-to-peak gradient, as is often used for the quick manual calculation in the Hakki equation, it is important to note that this is a non-physiological marker because the two peaks occur at different time points (Figure 66.1).

6. How do you assess the transvalvular aortic valve gradient in atrial fibrillation?

Atrial fibrillation in the setting of severe AS remains an independent risk factor for poor outcomes. This is further compounded by the difficulty of assessing the aortic valve gradient while the patient is in atrial fibrillation due to the beat-to-beat variation in stroke volume. Current guidelines recommend obtaining five continuous-wave peak and mean gradients. However, whether to use the average gradient versus the largest gradient remains a mystery.

7. Can a single-catheter pullback from the LV into the aorta be used to assess the transvalvular gradient?

The pullback is a simplified and less accurate alternative for evaluating the transvalvular pressure gradient. Furthermore, it is quite inaccurate in patients with any rhythm irregularities including atrial fibrillation and atrial or ventricular ectopy (ventricular ectopy is commonly encountered when pulling a catheter from the LV).

8. Can the left ventricular and femoral pressures be used to evaluate the gradient?

We strongly discourage using this method as it both over- and underestimates the transvalvular gradient. Underestimation occurs due to peripheral amplification of the aortic pressure waveform, and overestimation occurs if

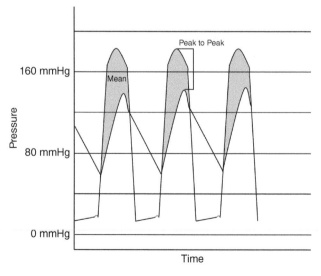

Figure 66.1 Hemodynamic measurement using simultaneous left ventricle and aortic measurements in aortic stenosis showing differences in mean gradient calculation versus peak-to-peak gradient. This demonstrates how peak to peak occurs at different times in severe aortic stenosis.

there is large-vessel stenosis or the Carabello sign. The Carabello sign occurs when the catheter (usually $\geq 7\,F$) contributes to the fixed obstruction of AS (usually with valve areas $\leq 0.7\,cm^2$).

9. How can you use the pressure waveforms to better understand the degree of aortic valve stenosis?

Pressure waveform analysis remains a critical piece to the invasive assessment of AS, with increasing evidence that the time to peak aortic pressure is an independent marker of severity. The delayed (tardus) and reduced (parvus) peak aortic pressure also suggests a fixed stenosis over the dynamic stenosis caused by the obstructive subtype of hypertrophic cardiomyopathy.

10. What other features suggest that the pressure gradient is due to a static or dynamic obstruction?

The waveform in AS shows a late (tardus) peaking upstroke of the central aortic pressures that occur at valve opening, while dynamic obstructions the hemodynamic tracing is of a "spike and dome" appearance. Furthermore, in the presence of premature ventricular

contractions, static obstructions keep the same transvalvular gradient, while dynamic obstructions have exacerbation of the gradient (Figure 66.2). This is known as Brockenbrough-Braunwald-Morrow sign and is discussed in more detail later in this chapter.

11. What is low-flow, low-gradient AS?

The evaluation of the valve area via the Gorlin or Hakki equations is derived from direct measurement of the transvalvular gradient. It is possible to have severe AS with pressure gradients less than 40 mmHg, and this is often the direct result of decreased transvalvular flow. Two entities contribute to low-flow, low-gradient AS:

- Stroke volume can be decreased in the setting of reduced left ventricular contractility, most commonly due to severe systolic dysfunction and decreased left ventricular ejection fraction (LVEF). By definition, low flow is a calculated stroke volume index of $< 35\,ml/m^2$.
- Stroke volume is "paradoxically" low ($SV_i < 35\,ml/m^2$) when the LVEF is normal or increased. This condition is known as *paradoxical low-flow, low-gradient AS* and occurs most commonly in severe diastolic dysfunction due to either infiltrative diseases or small left ventricular cavities in the setting of marked left ventricular hypertrophy.

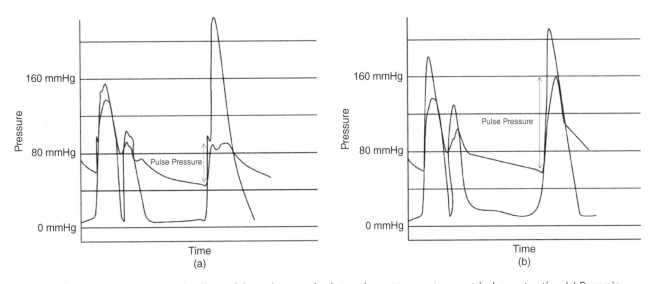

Figure 66.2 Different hemodynamic effects of dynamic vs. static obstruction post-premature ventricular contraction. (a) Dynamic obstruction with the characteristic spike and dome appearance, with augmentation of the gradient and reduction in pulse pressure. (b) Static obstruction in aortic stenosis with increased pulse pressure and a relatively unchanged gradient.

12. How do you differentiate true low-flow AS from pseudo-AS or a severe cardiomyopathy without contractile reserve?

Due to the difference in mortality benefit and long-term survival, differentiating between these three groups is important. In these cases, using a dobutamine challenge during transthoracic echo or invasive hemodynamics to increase stroke volume can aid in a proper diagnosis and treatment. This carries a Class 2a recommendation from the 2020 American College of Cardiology/American Heart Association (ACC/AHA) guidelines. Flow reserve or contractile reserve is defined as the ability to increase stroke volume by at least 20% at peak dobutamine dosing, a maximum of 20 µg/kg/min. This creates the following three categories (Figure 66.3):

- *True low-flow AS* is defined as an increasing mean pressure gradient ≥ 40 mmHg with or without adequate flow reserve.
- *Pseudo-severe low-flow AS* is defined as those patients who have adequate flow reserve but whose gradients remain < 40 mmHg.
- *Indeterminate low-flow AS* is used to describe patients without flow reserve for whom mean gradients remain < 40 mmHg. These patients are unable to augment their CO with dobutamine, and the severity of AS needs to be differentiated by other means, including calcium score or planimetry by computed tomography (CT). Outcomes and long-term survival have been difficult to assess and have had mixed results. We recommend utilizing your local Heart Team or referring to large structural heart centers to make difficult decisions in these complex cases.

13. How does hypertension affect the invasive hemodynamic assessment of AS?

Discordantly low transvalvular gradients can be caused by valvulo-arterial interactions. Decreased arterial compliance and increased systemic vascular resistance impact transvalvular flow and can result in an underestimation of transvalvular pressure gradients and therefore stenosis severity. Patients undergoing cardiac catheterization for evaluation of aortic valve disease are often hypertensive for a myriad of reasons with increased systemic vascular resistance and have, given the nature of this patient population, decreased arterial compliance.

When invasive transvalvular gradients are surprisingly lower than anticipated by clinical (symptoms and physical examination) and noninvasive imaging evaluations, we recommend cautious and quick afterload reduction with an arterial vasodilator. Modifying vascular resistance will in essence reveal a more representative and accurate transvalvular gradient and therefore stenosis severity. An alpha-agonist must be ready to give due to the fixed nature of AS and unpredictable decrease in CO with possible hemodynamic compromise caused by the acute afterload reduction and blood pressure drop. We recommend, if possible, avoiding less predictable afterload reducers such as hydralazine or longer-acting such as nicardipine. Nitroprusside is the preferred agent, given at a starting dose of 0.5 µg/min/kg and increased by 0.5–1 µg/min/kg every five minutes until one of the predefined endpoints is achieved:

a. Maximum dose of 10 µg/min/kg
b. Aortic mean gradient > 40 mmHg
c. MAP < 60 mmHg
d. Development of intolerable symptoms or side effects

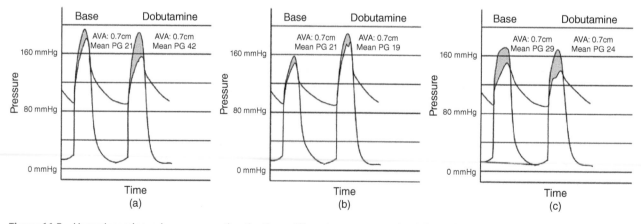

Figure 66.3 Hemodynamic tracings representing the three different responses to the dobutamine challenge. (a) True low-flow severe aortic stenosis with worsening of pressure gradient post dobutamine challenge. (b) Pseudo-low-flow aortic stenosis with the gradient staying about the same, with adequate flow reserve. (c) A patient without flow reserve, with mean pressure gradient remaining unchanged.

14. What are the expected hemodynamic changes that occur post-transcatheter aortic valve replacement?

Immediately after transcatheter aortic valve replacement (TAVR) and termination of rapid pacing, you should anticipate near-complete resolution of the transvalvular gradient and restoration of normal aortic pressure waveform morphology. Specifically, the aortic upstroke parallels that of the LV; the pulse pressure should increase, reflecting an increase in stroke volume; and you might even see the dicrotic notch reappear (Figure 66.4).

15. What hemodynamic findings are concerning post-TAVR?

Hemodynamic abnormalities after deploying a transcatheter heart valve (THV) that require immediate assessment include:

- A persistently elevated transvalvular gradient with a delay in the aortic upstroke. This could be due to under-expansion of the THV, and we recommend assessment in multiple orthogonal views. If the THV is under-expanded, subsequent inflations with a non-compliant balloon are likely needed.
- A persistently elevated transvalvular gradient with dynamic features and a normal aortic upstroke. This could represent what has been referred to as a "suicide ventricle" resulting from persistently increased contractility and a functional left ventricular outflow tract obstruction. The treatment of this condition involves IV fluids to increase preload, α-agonist to increase afterload (to simulate what the ventricle was accustomed to prior to the relief of AS with the THV), and β-blockade to

increase diastolic filling time and decrease contractility. This is usually self-limited and resolves in a matter of minutes to hours. Emergent alcohol septal ablation is a last resort but has been employed if this condition persists.

- Newly or worsened left ventricular end diastolic pressure (LVEDP) in conjunction with a wide pulse pressure and low aortic diastolic pressure. This is possibly due to severe aortic insufficiency from a central or perivalvular leak. It could also be due to disruption of the aortic valve annulus.
- Hypotension. Post–rapid ventricular pacing blood pressure is usually low with a rapid recovery without the need for vasopressors or inotropes, even in patients with decreased systolic function. If hypotension persists or requires significant vasopressor support, this requires immediate attention. Assessment of annular or ventricular perforation, aortic dissection, coronary obstruction, iliofemoral bleeding, or any other possible complications during THV deployment should be investigated and managed emergently and using all available tools.

Hemodynamics of the Mitral Valve

16. What are the main hemodynamic principles of the left atrium (LA)?

The LA pressure-volume curve is determined by the incoming pulmonary venous flow entering the LA from the lungs, the transmitral valve outflow, and the back pressure from the LV. The lower the compliance of the ventricle, the stiffer the chamber becomes. This causes small changes in flow to result in large changes in pressure.

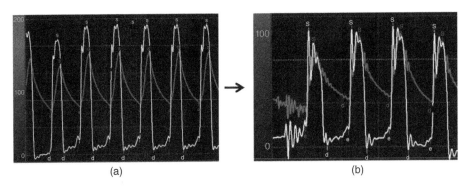

(a)   →   (b)

Figure 66.4   Hemodynamic tracing of severe aortic stenosis (a) with complete resolution of gradient and (b) restoration of the dicrotic notch post-transcatheter aortic valve replacement.

17. How do you adequately evaluate the pressure across the mitral valve (MV)?

The most accurate approach for evaluating mitral stenosis (MS) involves an atrial transseptal puncture and left atrial pressure measurement with simultaneous measurement from a catheter placed in the LV.

18. Can you use the pulmonary capillary wedge pressure (PCWP) to measure the left atrial pressure and transmitral gradient?

PCWP has been shown to correlate well with left atrial pressure when wedge pressures are low; however, the diastolic mitral gradient using PCWP is likely to overestimate the degree of stenosis when phase lag is not appropriately corrected. Vinayakumar et al. demonstrated that when phase is appropriately corrected, PCWP and left atrial pressure as well as diastolic gradient have great correlation. However, Nishimura et al. found that even with phase correction, there can remain a 30–50% overestimation of gradient severity. Furthermore, in the setting of severe pulmonary hypertension, the ability to wedge catheters becomes difficult, leading to hybrid PCWP and PA pressures.

Therefore, if the mitral transvalvular pressure gradient and the degree of MS remain unclear after transesophageal and transthoracic echocardiography, we recommend proceeding with a diagnostic transseptal LA catheterization and simultaneous LA-LV pressure measurement.

19. How do you correct the phase lag between the LV pressure tracing and PCWP tracing?

The left atrial pressure waveform is divided into three phases, including atrial systole (*a*), ventricular contraction (*c*), and atrial filling (*v*) wave. LVEDP is calculated at the end of the *a* wave as LVEDP includes atrial contraction as well as passive filling (Figure 66.5).

Mitral Stenosis

20. When should you do invasive hemodynamic measurements for MS?

Grading of MS is dependent on symptomatology, valve anatomy, and hemodynamic measurements. Severe MS is defined as a MV area ≤ 1.5 cm² with a transmitral mean gradient > 5 mmHg per ACC/AHA 2020 valvular heart disease guidelines. Echocardiographic evaluation has continued to improve, now having an accurate diagnosis and gradient evaluation prior to valvuloplasty. However, in cases where discordance is present between symptoms, transmitral gradient, or pulmonary pressure, invasive hemodynamics are critical for the accurate evaluation of MS. Furthermore, invasive exercise hemodynamics can prove useful in evaluating mean mitral gradient and changes in pulmonary artery pressures.

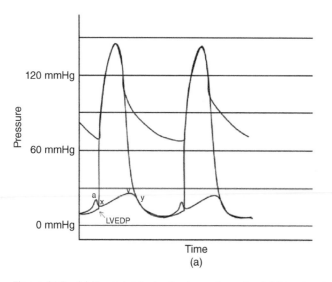

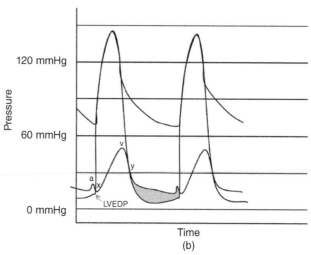

Figure 66.5 (a) Normal mitral valve hemodynamics. (b) A tracing demonstrating an elevated "*v*" wave in a setting of severe mitral regurgitation and a diastolic transmitral pressure gradient (blue shading) consistent with mitral stenosis.

21. What invasive hemodynamic findings are suggestive of severe MS?

- Calculated valve area $\leq 1.5\,cm^2$ based on the Gorlin formula
- Transmitral gradient $> 5\,mmHg$
- Shallow slope y descent secondary to delayed left atrial emptying
- Low CO/cardiac index
- Elevated LA pressure or PCWP relative to LVEDP
- Pulmonary hypertension and elevated pulmonary vascular resistance

22. How are the hemodynamics affected in patients with atrial fibrillation?

Atrial fibrillation poses two main problems during MS. The irregularly irregular rhythm leads to inconsistent diastolic filling times, which lead to decreased flow and increased LA pressure, as mentioned earlier. Furthermore, the loss of effective atrial contraction further decreases flow and increases LA pressure. The combination of these two mechanisms results in an increase in the transmitral gradient (increased LA pressure and decreased LV end diastolic pressure) and further decreases CO, which makes assessment of the transmitral gradient difficult and brings into question the accuracy of the valve area.

23. What is considered a successful percutaneous mitral balloon valvuloplasty (PMBV) via hemodynamic measurements?

PMBV is considered successful if the gradient decreases by 50% or more with a valve area of at least $1.5\,cm^2$. Ideally, the calculated valve area is $1.8\,cm^2$ or more. However, while striving for gradients of success, each PMBV should have echo evaluation for worsening mitral regurgitation (MR). Should the gradient decrease by 50% or MR worsen by one grade, further inflations should not be performed.

24. How can you detect worsening MR during the procedure if you cannot get an adequate echocardiographic assessment?

Immediate concern should arise if LA pressure increases post-PMBV instead of the expected decrease. Furthermore, the development of a large prominent *v* wave with steep *y* descent is consistent with severe MR. Early hemodynamic recognition of severe MR can lead to timely surgical assessment prior to hemodynamic instability.

Mitral Regurgitation

The hemodynamics of MR are complex and susceptible to moment-to-moment variations in cardiovascular physiologic changes, including heart rate, preload, afterload, contractility, and even lusitropy. Understanding an individual patient's MV anatomy and physiology often requires multiple modalities and an in-depth knowledge of how and when each assessment was made relative to the patient's condition at that specific time point. Careful attention to medical therapy and adherence to that medical regimen is critical in decision-making and the outcomes of structural interventions on the MV.

25. How can you differentiate between acute and chronic MR?

Acute, severe MR is associated with large *v* waves, severely elevated LVEDP, and low peak LV systolic pressure with low forward CO. Clinical manifestations of acute MR include acute pulmonary edema with respiratory distress and hemodynamic instability. In contrast, the peak *v* wave and LVEDP are relatively low in chronic MR. However, if the patient presents with decompensated chronic MR, the *v* waves and LVEDP will clearly increase from baseline.

26. What else can cause an elevated *v* wave on PCWP or LA pressure tracings?

a) Ventricular septal defect
b) MS as discussed
c) Heart failure
d) Tachycardia leading to inadequate atrial emptying
e) Decrease LA compliance (constriction, infiltrative disease, tumors)

27. How does atrial fibrillation affect the hemodynamics of MR?

Loss of effective atrial contraction leads to inadequate emptying of the LA and an increase in LA pressure.

28. How does the MitraClip affect LA pressure, and should continuous pressure measurement be used?

Given that most patients undergoing the MitraClip procedure will have low CO, elevated LA pressure, and large *v* waves, successful MitraClip placement results in decreased *v* wave and LA pressures and increased CO. Pulmonary hypertension may not necessarily improve acutely, given secondary remodeling of the vasculature from prolonged elevated pressures.

Initial MitraClip steerable sheath systems were not equipped with real-time continuous pressure measurement; as a result, many initial measurements were done using a "buddy catheter" system. The MitraClip NT MDS system provides real-time left atrial measurement by allowing for a 5 Fr catheter to be placed in the LA. Kuwata et al. demonstrated in 50 consecutive patients that real-time continuous measurement provided prognostic data that is not otherwise available when using echocardiography alone. In particular, elevations in left atrial mean pressure (LAmP) result in worse short-term clinical outcomes independent of echocardiographic findings.

Hypertrophic Cardiomyopathy and Septal Ablation

29. What is the adequate way to measure gradient in patients with left ventricular outflow tract (LVOT) obstruction?

Invasive measurements of LVOT obstruction require a great amount of care and diligence to adequately evaluate the severity of obstruction due to frequent entrapment of catheters and pressure dampening. The best method to obtain adequate gradients involves transseptal catheterization with direct antegrade measurement of the LV so catheter entrapment is avoided. However, given the relative increase in complexity with transseptal puncture, a retrograde approach for measurements can be performed. Catheters with side holes are typically avoided as they make accurate localization of the LVOT obstruction challenging. Catheters with a distal side-hole or end-hole configuration allow precise location of the gradient. Care should be taken to ensure that catheters are well flushed and not entrapped in order to avoid diagnostic errors.

30. The gradient of LVOT obstruction remains <50 mmHg at rest. What should you do next?

Hypertrophic cardiomyopathy is a dynamic obstruction; thus, provocation maneuvers can be used to unmask the gradient. The use of exercise (increase in contractility) or the Valsalva maneuver (decrease in preload volume) are simple ways to exacerbate the obstruction and reveal gradient severity. You can also manipulate the catheter in the LV to provoke a premature ventricular beat. The post-extrasystolic beat should have a marked increase in LV-Ao gradient, a decrease in aortic pressure, and narrowing of the pulse pressure – this is known as the Brockenbrough-Braunwald-Morrow sign (Figure 66.2). Should the gradient remain low yet be discordant with the clinical presentation and physical examination, an isoproterenol infusion can be used to further induce LVOT obstruction.

31. How does atrial fibrillation affect the gradient in hypertrophic cardiomyopathy?

Loss of effective atrial contraction results in impaired filling of the LV and can reduce preload, exacerbating dynamic obstruction. Furthermore, longer RR intervals in atrial fibrillation can precipitate dynamic obstruction due to a combination of the Frank-Starling mechanism and increased calcium availability, leading to increased contractility and a greater degree of obstruction. The beat-to-beat variability changes LV filling, contractility, and stroke volume, making adequate gradient evaluation quite challenging.

32. How do you determine success after alcohol septal ablation?

Procedural success is defined as >50% reduction in resting and provoked gradients.

33. There was intra-procedural relief of obstruction after septal ablation, but the echocardiogram two days post-procedure showed an increase in the LVOT gradient. Does this mean the procedure was a failure?

Alcohol septal ablations often result in immediate resolution of the LVOT dynamic gradient. This is due to the myocardial stunning that occurs after the injection of alcohol and the acute injury that ensues. The pathological sequence of events includes, at ~24–72 hours, myocardial edema. The swelling of the LVOT can result in transient obstruction to flow and increased gradients observed on echocardiograms performed during this time period. The edema and resulting obstruction are transient. Over time, the myocardium thins due to secondary remodeling, and gradients improve or resolve permanently within 3–12 months.

Bibliography

1 Assey, M.E., Zile, M.R., Usher, B.W. et al. (1993). Effect of catheter positioning on the variability of measured gradient in aortic stenosis. *Catheter. Cardiovasc. Diagn.* 30 (4): 287–292.

2 Hildick-Smith, D.J., Walsh, J.T., and Shapiro, L.M. (2000). Pulmonary capillary wedge pressure in mitral stenosis accurately reflects mean left atrial pressure but overestimates transmitral gradient. *Am. J. Cardiol.* 85 (4): 512–515, A11. https://doi.org/10.1016/s0002-9149(99)00785-7. PMID: 10728964.

3 Kern, M.J., Goldstein, J.G., and Lim, M.J. (ed.) (2017). *Hemodynamic Rounds: Interpretation of Cardiac Pathophysiology from Pressure Waveform Analysis*, 4e. New York, NY: Wiley-Liss.

4 Kuwata, S., Taramasso, M., Czopak, A. et al. (2019). Continuous direct left atrial pressure: intraprocedural measurement predicts clinical response following MitraClip therapy. *JACC Cardiovasc. Interv.* 12 (2): 127–136. https://doi.org/10.1016/j.jcin.2018.07.051. PMID: 30594511.

5 Lloyd, J.W., Nishimura, R.A., Borlaug, B.A., and Eleid, M.F. (2017). Hemodynamic response to nitroprusside in patients with low-gradient severe aortic stenosis and preserved ejection fraction. *J. Am. Coll. Cardiol.* 70 (11): 1339–1348. https://doi.org/10.1016/j.jacc.2017.07.736. PMID: 28882231.

6 Monin, J.L., Quere, J.P., Monchi, M. et al. (2003). Low-gradient aortic stenosis: operative risk stratification and predictors for long-term outcome: a multicenter study using dobutamine stress hemodynamics. *Circulation* 108: 319–324.

7 Nishimura, R.A., Rihal, C.S., Tajik, A.J., and Holmes, D.R. (1994). Accurate measurement of the transmitral gradient in patients with mitral stenosis: a simultaneous catheterization and doppler echocardiographic study. *J. Am. Coll. Cardiol.* 24: 152–158.

8 Otto, C.M., Nishimura, R.A., Bonow, R.O. et al. (2020). ACC/AHA Guideline for the Management of Patients With Valvular Heart Disease: A Report of the American College of Cardiology/American Heart Association Joint Committee on Clinical Practice Guidelines.

9 Sato, K., Kumar, A., Jobanputra, Y. et al. (2019). Association of time between left ventricular and aortic systolic pressure peaks with severity of aortic stenosis and calcification of aortic valve. *JAMA Cardiol.* 4 (6): 549–555. https://doi.org/10.1001/jamacardio.2019.1180.

10 Sato, K., Sankaramangalam, K., Kandregula, K. et al. (2019). Contemporary outcomes in low-gradient aortic stenosis patients who underwent dobutamine stress echocardiography. *J. Am. Heart Assoc.* 8: e011168.

11 Veselka, J., Duchonová, R., Procházková, S. et al. (2004). The biphasic course of changes of left ventricular outflow gradient after alcohol septal ablation for hypertrophic obstructive cardiomyopathy. *Kardiol. Pol.* 60 (2): 133–136; discussion 137. PMID: 15116158.

12 Vinayakumar, D., Bijilesh, U., Sajeev, C.G. et al. (2016). Correlation of pulmonary capillary wedge pressure with left atrial pressure in patients with mitral stenosis undergoing balloon valvotomy. *Indian Heart J.* 68: 2, 143–6. https://doi.org/10.1016/j.ihj.2015.07.050 PMID: 27133321; PMCID: PMC4867958.

13 Wigle, E.D., Sasson, Z., Henderson, M.A. et al. (1985). Hypertrophic cardiomyopathy: the importance of the site and the extent of hypertrophy: a review. *Prog. Cardiovasc. Dis.* 28: 1–83.

14 Yoerger, D.M., Picard, M.H., Palacios, I.F. et al. (2006). Time course of pressure gradient response after first alcohol septal ablation for obstructive hypertrophic cardiomyopathy. *Am. J. Cardiol.* 97 (10): 1511–1514.

67

Percutaneous Closure of Coronary Artery Fistulas

Diego Celli[1], Fahad Alfares[2], Satinder K. Sandhu[2], and Cesar E. Mendoza[3]

[1] Department of Medicine, University of Miami Miller School of Medicine, Miami, FL, USA
[2] Division of Pediatric Cardiology, Department of Pediatrics, University of Miami Miller School of Medicine, Miami, FL, USA
[3] Department of Cardiology, Jackson Memorial Health System, Miami, FL, USA

1. What is the incidence of coronary artery fistulas?

The true incidence of coronary fistulas in the general population is unknown as most of these abnormalities are small and clinically irrelevant. However, the published angiographic data reveals an incidence of 0.08–0.22%.

2. Describe how coronary artery fistulas are currently classified

Coronary artery fistulas (CAFs) can be divided into congenital and acquired depending on their origin. The acquired fistulas have been described after chest trauma, cardiac surgery, endomyocardial biopsy, Takayasu arteritis, and some complicated electrophysiologic and coronary percutaneous procedures. There is no consensus on specific size ranges to classify CAFs; some classification proposals have been published. Said et al. defined small-sized fistulas as communications with a vessel diameter of less than 2 mm, medium-sized fistulas with a vessel diameter between 2 and 8 mm, and large-sized fistulas with a vessel diameter over 8 mm. Alternatively, Latson et al. classified CAFs as small-sized (less than twice the normal proximal diameter of the coronary artery), medium-sized (larger than twice but less than three times the proximal diameter of the coronary artery), and large-sized (larger than three times the proximal normal coronary artery diameter).

When transcatheter intervention is considered, the angiographic classification by Sakakibara et al. is helpful. They classify the fistulas as

- *Type A (proximal type):* The coronary fistula arises from the proximal segment of the coronary artery. The proximal coronary artery is dilated, but the distal coronary artery is relatively normal in diameter.
- *Type B (distal type):* The coronary artery is dilated along its length and terminated as a fistula on the right side of the heart. Proximal to the Type B fistula, there are regular branches of the coronary artery.

3. What is the coronary steal phenomenon?

The *coronary steal phenomenon* is defined as a reduction of myocardial perfusion due to alteration of blood flow to the myocardium resulting in myocardial ischemia. In CAFs, this phenomenon can occur when the blood diverts from the proximal coronary artery through the fistula (lower resistance) and reduces blood flow to the distal high resistance coronary branches. Rarely, myocardial infarction due to steal syndrome has been reported.

4. What diagnostic modalities are used in establishing the diagnosis of CAF?

2D transthoracic echocardiography (TTE) and color Doppler echocardiography are valuable tools for diagnosing CAF in children and adults. However, in adults, transesophageal echocardiography (TEE) is more sensitive in delineating the anatomy of CAF with more precision. Less invasive methods, such as 64-slice multidetector computed tomography (CT; Figure 67.1a,b), can characterize the anatomy, the course of the fistula, and the surrounding structure with high accuracy. Coronary magnetic resonance angiography with 3D rendering is also a beneficial noninvasive tool that can meticulously identify CAF and aid in surgical or transcatheter repair. Coronary angiography is the gold standard in diagnosing due to its ability to identify the coronary artery, the communicating chambers, and the locations of the communications involved in the fistula.

5. Describe the clinical presentation of hemodynamically significant CAFs

Most patients with CAFs are asymptomatic with a normal cardiac exam. Some patients with CAFs present with a murmur described as a continuous murmur. Patients with large hemodynamically significant fistulas can present with symptoms of left to right shunt and congestive heart failure, myocardial ischemia, and have a higher risk of coronary atherosclerotic disease and bacterial endocarditis. Left CAF that terminates into the right side of the heart is associated with an increased risk of developing pulmonary hypertension.

6. What are the indications and contraindications for device closure of a CAF?

The 2008 American College of Cardiology/American Heart Association (AHA/ACC) guidelines for managing adults with congenital heart disease recommend the repair of large fistulas in all patients and small fistula in patients with symptoms. The updated 2018 AHA/ACC guidelines recommend an individual approach. Options to repair CAFs are surgical and transcatheter. The transcatheter approach appears to be effective, with a high success rate in more than 80% of cases. The success of transcatheter closure depends largely on the anatomy of the fistula; number of fistulas; size, origin, and termination of the fistula; and landing zone for deploying the device without affecting the distal coronary perfusion. To achieve a satisfactory and successful transcatheter closure, the fistula must be single and narrow without large branches. Transcatheter closure is contraindicated in very small infants or children, in large and wide fistulas, in distal fistulas or fistulas with multiple communications, or if the patient needs a surgical repair for an additional cardiac pathology.

7. Describe the devices currently available for occlusion of CAF

No head-to-head trials have sought to compare efficacy and outcomes between closure devices; selection is performed based on the size and complexity of the fistula, the desired vascular approach, and the center's preference and availability; these include coils, detachable balloons, vascular plugs, ductal occluders, embolization particles, and covered stents (Table 67.1).

8. Describe the technical principles for device occlusion of CAFs: surgical vs. percutaneous approach

The optimal treatment for CAFs remains unclear, as the literature has only provided case reports and series. Given that for any given patient, multiple factors could impact the multidisciplinary Heart Team's management option, an individualized approach is pivotal to maximizing successful outcomes; however, the preferred approach will heavily rely on each institution's expertise in the elimination of fistulas.

Surgical management is generally reserved for patients with reasonable predicted surgical mortality and high-risk anatomical characteristics, including symptomatic patients with large fistulas, multiple communications and drainage sites, high tortuosity, presence of aneurysms within the fistula, and large vascular branches that can be accidentally embolized; moreover, a surgical closure is the preferred approach in patients who are undergoing operative repair of other cardiovascular problems. The general objective is

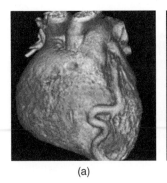 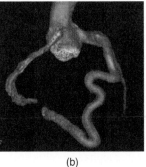

(a) (b)

Figure 67.1 Computed tomography with 3D reconstruction shows a large coronary artery fistula: (a) dilated coronary artery fistula; (b) left coronary artery to right ventricle fistula.

Table 67.1   Devices for transcatheter closure of coronary artery fistulas.

	Coils	Detachable balloon	Covered stent	Chemical agent	Amplatzer duct occluder	Amplatzer vascular plug
Fistula size	Small to medium	Medium to large	Small to medium	Small to medium	Medium to large	Medium to large
Transcatheter approach	Anterograde or retrograde	Retrograde	Retrograde	Retrograde	Anterograde	Anterograde or retrograde
Clinical experience	High	Low	Moderate	Low	High	High

Source: Modified from Oto et al. 2011.

to obliterate the fistulous tract while preserving the blood flow to the myocardium, generally obtained through simple ligation.

Percutaneous transcatheter closure has emerged as a feasible and noninvasive alternative that does not require median sternotomy or cardiopulmonary bypass. Given its excellent outcomes, this is the default route for patients with amenable anatomy for closure. Special attention must be given to pre-procedural planning on the landing site; if the device is placed too proximal to the branching vessel, there is an increased risk for sub-optimal occlusion of the shunt with higher rates of distal embolization with distal deployments. The branches supplying the myocardium and coming off proximal to the fistula must be identified prior to device placement.

9. Describe the technical principles for device occlusion of CAFs: retrograde arterial vs. antegrade venous approach

As mentioned previously, transcatheter closure is a suitable and valuable alternative for conventional surgery in most cases of CAF. Despite the limitations of small procedural volume, a systematic approach to its treatment has shown excellent results. The retrograde arterial approach has been mainly used in small to medium CAFs without extreme tortuosity; access is achieved through the femoral or radial artery with catheter advancement into the desired position for delivery. Moreover, the anterograde venous approach has been used in patients with complex and tortuous fistulas in whom the venous end of the fistula could be cannulated through its drainage point. In CAFs that requires a large sheath size for device delivery, the wire advanced through the fistula can be snared and a large sheath placed antegrade over the snared wire.

A coronary artery angiogram is done (Figure 67.2a,b) to outline the fistula and the coronary artery anatomy. Particular attention is paid to the vessels supplying the myocardium, which may arise from the fistulous vessel (Figure 67.1c,d). Selective cannulation of the fistula is done and angiography performed to identify the vessel size, its entry point into the heart, and any vessels arising from the fistula.

The vessel is then crossed with a wire (IIe), and a stable catheter or sheath is advanced for device delivery. If possible, an angiographic catheter with the balloon inflated is placed as close to the drainage point, and a hand injection is done to identify myocardial vessels arising from the fistula. If a balloon catheter cannot be advanced, the fistula is closed as close to the drainage point (Figure 67.2f,g), and a repeat angiogram is done to identify viable vessels. The vessel is then closed just distal to the viable vessel, and a repeat angiogram is done to define the anatomy (Figure 67.2h,i). It is important to not have any "dead space" proximal to the occlusion device because this would be a nidus for thrombus formation and propagation, resulting in occlusion of the viable branches.

10. What are the results of device closure of CAFs?

Given the rarity and heterogeneity of CAFs, experience with transcatheter closure remains limited. Nevertheless, multiple case reports and series, including multicenter studies, have suggested its association with a high rate of procedural success and relatively low morbidity in selected patients.

11. What other coronary problems involving a steal flow phenomenon can be treated using these occlusion devices?

Although still controversial, these devices have been used in the treatment of coronary steal syndrome due to unligated side branches of the left internal mammary artery in

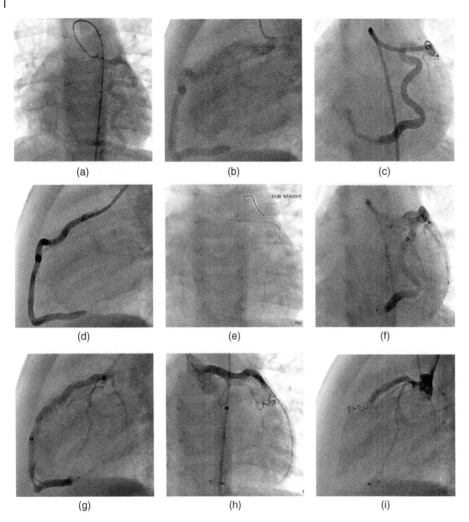

Figure 67.2 Four-year-old with a large distal left coronary artery to the right ventricle: (a) left coronary artery angiogram (anteroposterior projection); (b) left coronary artery angiogram (lateral projection); (c) selective angiogram in the coronary artery fistula (anteroposterior projection); (d) selective angiogram in coronary fistula (lateral projection) showing myocardial branches arising from the fistula; (e) retrograde placement of a wire across the fistula into the right atrium; (f, g) 4 mm Amplatzer Vascular Plug II positioned and released at the insertion of the fistula into the right ventricle; occlusion of the vessel now outlines the coronary artery vessels not seen prior to occlusion. (h, i) 0.035-3-4 MReye delivered, and a second 0.035-3-4 MReye placed because of a persistent shunt.

patients with myocardial ischemia post-coronary artery bypass graft. The use of these devices has been documented in isolated case reports for patients with progressive worsening angina that is clearly related to competitive run-off into the side branches and has objective evidence of ischemia.

Bibliography

1 Abdo, N., Curran, P.J., Kumar, V., and Tobis, J.M. (2005). Coronary steal syndrome with coil embolization of a large LIMA side branch: radionuclide evidence for reversible ischemia. *Catheter. Cardiovasc. Interv.* 66 (3): 360–363. https://doi.org/10.1002/ccd.20501.

2 Ahmed, M.F., Mubin, A., Syed, R. et al. (2020). Multivessel coronary artery fistula presenting as coronary steal syndrome leading to cardiac arrest. *Cureus* 12 (5): e8358. https://doi.org/10.7759/cureus.8358.

3 Angelini, P., Velasco, J.A., and Flamm, S. (2002). Coronary anomalies: incidence, pathophysiology, and clinical relevance. *Circulation* 105 (20): 2449–2454. https://doi.org/10.1161/01.cir.0000016175.49835.57.

4 Armsby, L.R., Keane, J.F., Sherwood, M.C. et al. (2002). Management of coronary artery fistulae. Patient selection and results of transcatheter closure. *J. Am. Coll. Cardiol.* 39 (6): 1026–1032. https://doi.org/10.1016/s0735-1097(02)01742-4.

5 Baltaxe, H.A. and Wixson, D. (1977). The incidence of congenital anomalies of the coronary arteries in the adult population. *Radiology* 122 (1): 47–52. https://doi.org/10.1148/122.1.47.

6 Duerinckx, A.J., Shaaban, A., Lewis, A. et al. (2000). 3D MR imaging of coronary arteriovenous fistulas. *Eur. Radiol.* 10 (9): 1459–1463. https://doi.org/10.1007/s003309900273.

7 El-Sabawi, B., Al-Hijji, M.A., Eleid, M.F. et al. (2020). Transcatheter closure of coronary artery fistula: A 21-year experience. *Catheter. Cardiovasc. Interv.* 96 (2): 311–319. https://doi.org/10.1002/ccd.28721.

8 Endo, M., Tomizawa, Y., Nishida, H. et al. (2003). Angiographic findings and surgical treatments of coronary artery involvement in Takayasu arteritis. *J. Thorac. Cardiovasc. Surg.* 125 (3): 570–577. https://doi.org/10.1067/mtc.2003.39.

9 Fukuda, K., Handa, S., Ogawa, S. et al. (1988). Noninvasive evaluation of right coronary artery-right atrial fistula using two-dimensional echocardiography, pulsed Doppler echocardiography and color flow mapping. *Cardiology* 75 (5): 375–380. https://doi.org/10.1159/000174402.

10 Gillebert, C., Van Hoof, R., Van de Werf, F. et al. (1986). Coronary artery fistulas in an adult population. *Eur. Heart J.* 7 (5): 437–443. https://doi.org/10.1093/oxfordjournals.eurheartj.a062086.

11 Härle, T., Kronberg, K., and Elsässer, A. (2012). Coronary artery fistula with myocardial infarction due to steal syndrome. *Clin. Res. Cardiol.* 101 (4): 313–315. https://doi.org/10.1007/s00392-011-0405-1.

12 Hu, X., Wu, L., Liu, F. et al. (2013). Coronary artery fistulas in children. Evaluation with 64-slice multidetector CT. *Herz* 38 (7): 729–735. https://doi.org/10.1007/s00059-013-3786-2.

13 Huang, Z., Liu, Z., and Ye, S. (2020). The role of the fractional flow reserve in the coronary steal phenomenon evaluation caused by the coronary-pulmonary fistulas: case report and review of the literature. *J. Cardiothorac. Surg.* 15: https://doi.org/10.1186/s13019-020-1073-x.

14 Ilkay, E., Celebi, O.O., Kacmaz, F., and Ozeke, O. (2015). Percutaneous closure of coronary artery fistula: long-term follow-up results. *Postep. Kardiol. Inter.* 11 (4): 318–322. https://doi.org/10.5114/pwki.2015.55603.

15 Jama, A., Barsoum, M., Bjarnason, H. et al. (2011). Percutaneous closure of congenital coronary artery fistulae: results and angiographic follow-up. *JACC Cardiovasc. Interv.* 4 (7): 814–821. https://doi.org/10.1016/j.jcin.2011.03.014.

16 Kádár, K., Vázsonyi, J., Kiss, A., and Bendig, L. (1991). Coronary artery anomalies studied by Doppler echocardiography in infancy and childhood – possibilities and limitations. *Orv. Hetil.* 132 (29): 1581–1586.

17 Kahraman, S., Agac, M.T., Demirci, G. et al. (2018). Successful percutaneous treatment of coronary steal syndrome with the amplatzer vascular plug 4 and coil embolization. *Intractable Rare Dis. Res.* 7 (4): 287–290. https://doi.org/10.5582/irdr.2018.01083.

18 Khurana, R., Mittal, T., Qasim, A. et al. (2009). Coronary steal with unstable angina secondary to a coronary artery fistula. *EuroIntervention* 4 (4): 542–548. https://doi.org/10.4244/i4a91.

19 Latson, L.A. (2007). Coronary artery fistulas: how to manage them. *Catheter. Cardiovasc. Interv.* 70 (1): 110–116. https://doi.org/10.1002/ccd.21125.

20 Liu, X., Zhang, L., Qi, Z. et al. (2019). The characteristics of coronary-pulmonary artery fistulas and the effectivity of trans-catheter closure: a single center experience. *J. Thorac. Dis.* 11 (7): 2808–2815. https://doi.org/10.21037/jtd.2019.06.60.

21 Loukas, M., Germain, A.S., Gabriel, A. et al. (2015). Coronary artery fistula: a review. *Cardiovasc Pathol* 24 (3): 141–148. https://doi.org/10.1016/j.carpath.2014.01.010.

22 Mangukia, C.V. (2012). Coronary artery fistula. *Ann. Thorac. Surg.* 93 (6): 2084–2092. https://doi.org/10.1016/j.athoracsur.2012.01.114.

23 Natarajan, A., Khokhar, A.A., Kirk, P. et al. (2013). Coronary-pulmonary artery fistula: value of 64-MDCT imaging. *QJM* 106 (1): 91–92. https://doi.org/10.1093/qjmed/hcr254.

24 Noble, S., Frangos, C., and Roméo, P. (2009). Coronary artery-middle cardiac vein fistula after endomyocardial biopsy in a heart transplant patient. *Can. J. Cardiol.* 25 (9): e334. https://doi.org/10.1016/s0828-282x(09)70150-3.

25 Pattee, P.L. and Chambers, R.J. (1992). Acquired postoperative coronary arteriovenous fistula. *Catheter. Cardiovasc. Diagn.* 26 (2): 140–142. https://doi.org/10.1002/ccd.1810260213.

26 Qureshi, S.A. and Tynan, M. (2001). Catheter closure of coronary artery fistulas. *J. Interv. Cardiol.* 14 (3): 299–307. https://doi.org/10.1111/j.1540-8183.2001.tb00336.x.

27 Rangel, A., Badui, E., Verduzco, C. et al. (1990). Traumatic coronary arteriovenous fistula communicating the left main coronary artery to pulmonary artery, associated with pulmonary valvular insufficiency and endocarditis: case report. *Angiology* 41 (2): 156–160. https://doi.org/10.1177/000331979004100211.

28 Said, S.A. (2016). Congenital coronary artery fistulas complicated with pulmonary hypertension: analysis of 211 cases. *World J. Cardiol.* 8 (10): 596–605. https://doi.org/10.4330/wjc.v8.i10.596.

29 Said, S.A.M. and van der Werf, T. (2006). Dutch survey of coronary artery fistulas in adults: congenital solitary fistulas. *Int. J. Cardiol.* 106 (3): 323–332. https://doi.org/10.1016/j.ijcard.2005.01.047.

30 Sakakibara, S., Yokoyama, M., Takao, A. et al. (1966). Coronary arteriovenous fistula. Nine operated cases. *Am. Heart J.* 72 (3): 307–314. https://doi.org/10.1016/s0002-8703(66)80004-2.

31 Sanghvi, A.B., Diaz Fernandez, J.F., and Gomez Menchero, A.E. (2011). Transradial occlusion of a large intercostal branch of a left internal mammary artery graft with the novel amplatzer vascular plug 4 using a 4 French diagnostic catheter: treatment of coronary steal phenomenon. *J. Invasive Cardiol.* 23 (5): E113–E116.

32 Serçelik, A., Mavi, A., Ayalp, R. et al. (2003). Congenital coronary artery fistulas in Turkish patients undergoing diagnostic cardiac angiography. *Int. J. Clin. Pract.* 57 (4): 280–283.

33 Stout, K.K., Daniels, C.J., Aboulhosn, J.A. et al. (2019). 2018 AHA/ACC Guideline for the Management of Adults With Congenital Heart Disease: Executive Summary: A Report of the American College of Cardiology/American Heart Association Task Force on Clinical Practice

Guidelines. *Circulation* 139 (14): e637–e697. https://doi.org/10.1161/CIR.0000000000000602.

34 Vitarelli, A., De Curtis, G., Conde, Y. et al. (2002). Assessment of congenital coronary artery fistulas by transesophageal color Doppler echocardiography. *Am. J. Med.* 113 (2): 127–133. https://doi.org/10.1016/s0002-9343(02)01157-9.

35 Warnes, C.A., Williams, R.G., Bashore, T.M. et al. (2008). ACC/AHA 2008 guidelines for the management of adults with congenital heart disease: a report of the American College of Cardiology/American Heart Association Task Force on Practice Guidelines (Writing Committee to Develop Guidelines on the Management of Adults With Congenital Heart Disease). Developed in Collaboration With the American Society of Echocardiography, Heart Rhythm Society, International Society for Adult Congenital Heart Disease, Society for Cardiovascular Angiography and Interventions, and Society of Thoracic Surgeons. *J. Am. Coll. Cardiol.* 52 (23): e143–e263. https://doi.org/10.1016/j.jacc.2008.10.001.

36 Xiao, Y., Gowda, S.T., Chen, Z. et al. (2015). Transcatheter closure of coronary artery fistulae: considerations and approaches based on fistula origin. *J. Interv. Cardiol.* 28 (4): 380–389. https://doi.org/10.1111/joic.12212.

37 Yamanaka, O. and Hobbs, R.E. (1990). Coronary artery anomalies in 126,595 patients undergoing coronary arteriography. *Catheter. Cardiovasc. Diagn.* 21 (1): 28–40. https://doi.org/10.1002/ccd.1810210110.

68

Renal Denervation Therapy

Available Evidence, Catheters, and Techniques

Sergio A. Perez[1,2], and Eduardo J. de Marchena[3]

[1] Cardiovascular Service, Baptist Health Medical Center, Cardiovascular Service, Montgomery, AL, USA
[2] Jackson Health System, Miami, FL, USA
[3] Division of Cardiovascular Medicine, University of Miami Miller School of Medicine, University of Miami Hospital, Miami, FL, USA

1.   What is renal denervation?

Renal denervation (RDN) is a catheter-based therapy for arterial hypertension that aims to interrupt the activity of sympathetic nerves located in the adventitia and perivascular fat tissue of the renal artery. Denervation can be performed by applying radiofrequency energy, ultrasound energy, cryoablation, or injected alcohol. Historically, catheter-based RDN is based on experience from several decades ago of surgical lumbodorsal splanchnicectomy to treat severe hypertension.

2.   What did first-generation trials on RDN show?

Figure 68.1 summarizes the timeline of trials in device therapies for arterial hypertension. In 2009, the Symplicity HTN-1 (Renal Denervation in Patients with Refractory Hypertension) trial provided data for the feasibility of RDN using radiofrequency energy. Soon after that, the non-blinded Symplicity HTN-2 trial randomized patients to RDN plus medical therapy or medical therapy alone. Both trials were done with the use of the mono electrode Symplicity radiofrequency catheter system (Medtronic). The Symplicity catheter system is a 6 French radiofrequency catheter that delivers energy (8 W) to the endoluminal surface of the renal artery. Both studies showed an unexpectedly significant drop in office systolic blood pressure (BP) with no significant adverse events. In Symplicity HTN-2, the mean office BP at six months dropped by 32/12 mmHg in the RND group (p < 0.001) but increased by 1/0 mmHg in the control group (p > 0.70). However, multiple limitations of both studies were noticed, including lack of blinding, selection and observer bias, and the placebo effect.

To overcome some of those limitations, the Symplicity HTN-3 trial incorporated a sham treatment group. For Symplicity HTN-3, the Symplicity Flex catheter (Medtronic) iteration eliminated the fixed arch of its predecessor and enabled the physician to alter the angle of attack of the lead. This trial showed no significant difference in BP reduction between the RDN and sham procedure groups (−2.39 mmHg, 95% confidence interval [CI] −6.89 to 2.12 mmHg, $P = 0.26$ for superiority, with a margin of 5.00 mmHg) despite a significant decrease from baseline at six months both groups. Issues related to patient selection, medication adherence, and suboptimal procedural performance may have explained these results. At the time, the findings of this study halted the clinical development of RDN. However, other studies showed the opposite results. For example, the DENER-HTN (Renal Denervation in Hypertension) trial included 106 patients and showed that RDN reduced BP more than standardized antihypertension therapy alone.

3.   What did second-generation trials on RDN show?

Following the renewed interest sparked by the results of DENER-HTN, international expert groups provided

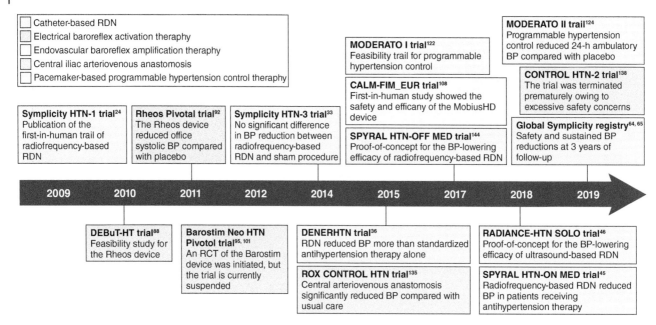

Figure 68.1 Milestones in device-based treatment of arterial hypertension. During the past decade, several device-based treatments for hypertension were introduced. The timeline depicts the landmark trials for different device-based therapies for hypertension. BP, blood pressure; RCT, randomized controlled trial; RDN, renal denervation. *Source:* Lauder et al 2020 / with permission of Springer Nature.

recommendations on optimal trial design and methodology. As a result, three adequately designed trials (SPYRAL HTN-OFF MED [Global Clinical Study of Renal Denervation with the Symplicity Spyral Multi-electrode Renal Denervation System in Patients with Uncontrolled Hypertension in the Absence of Antihypertensive Medications], SPYRAL HTN-ON MED [Global Clinical Study of Renal Denervation with the Symplicity Spyral Multi-electrode Renal Denervation System in Patients with Uncontrolled Hypertension on Standard Medical Therapy], and RADIANCE-HTN [A Study of the ReCor Medical Paradise System in Clinical Hypertension]) demonstrated a convincing significant reduction of in-office BP in comparison with respective sham procedure groups. SPYRAL HTN-OFF MED and SPYRAL HTN-ON MED were two proof-of-concept trials using the new-generation Symplicity Spyral (Medtronic) radio frequency (RF) ablation catheter system in the absence or presence of antihypertensive medications. The new Spyral is a multi-electrode 4 French catheter that creates four simultaneous lesions in a helical pattern, allowing a more circumferential ablation and theoretically more complete denervation. The catheter is 6 French guide compatible and delivered over a 0.014-in. wire in a rapid-exchange fashion. The RADIANCE-HTN trial investigated endovascular ultrasound-based RDN with the Paradise catheter system (ReCor Medical).

4. What are other RDN ablation systems?

Figure 68.2 depicts different catheters and technologies used for RDN. The latest iteration of the Symplicity catheter system is the Spyral catheter system. As mentioned previously, the Spyral is a multipolar catheter 6 French guide catheter compatible, delivered over a 0.014-in. wire that delivers RF energy from four electrodes simultaneously, generating 360° of ablation. The catheter can be used to treat arteries between 3 and 8 mm in diameter. Other RF-based devices under development are the EnligHTN RDN system (St. Jude Medical), which has a basketlike catheter design to optimize endoluminal contact, and the Vessix V2 catheter (Boston Scientific).

The Paradise (ReCor) RDN system is a 6 French catheter that delivers ultrasound energy circumferentially to ablate the sympathetic nerves. The catheter consists of a piezoelectric transducer located at the distal end and a distal balloon pressurized using sterile circulating water. The transducer emits acoustic energy, which is delivered through the cooling balloon into the renal artery. Other ultrasound-based systems under investigation include the TIVUS system (Cardiosonic) and Kona Medical Surround Sound system that externally delivers ultrasound energy.

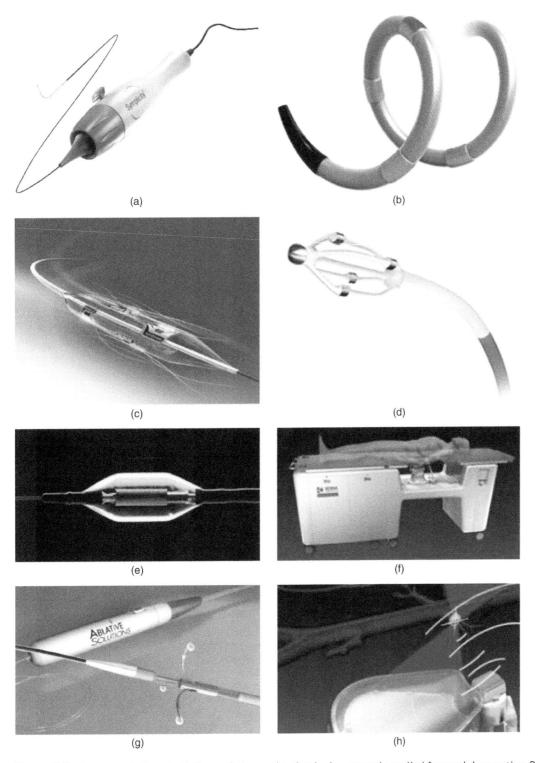

Figure 68.2 A representation of ablation catheters and technologies currently applied for renal denervation. RF energy: (a) Symplicity Flex; (b) Symplicity Spyral; (c) Vessix; (d) EnligHTN. Ultrasound: (e) intravascular by ReCor Medical's Paradise catheter; (f, h) extravascular by Kona. (g) Perivascular chemical ablation by Ablative Solutions' Peregrine catheter. *Source:* Reproduced from *Textbook of Interventional Cardiology*, Eighth Edition, Topol, Eric J., MD / Elsevier.

The Peregrine system infusion catheter (Ablative Solutions) is an investigational device to inject ethanol into the periarterial space through the arterial wall via three needles that extend from an intra-arterial catheter.

RDN Procedure: Technique and Steps

5. Describe the use of antiplatelet thereapy and anticoagulation

Although there is no universally accepted standard protocol, most physicians recommend the use of antiplatelet therapy before the procedure (e.g. aspirin 81–325 mg or clopidogrel 300–600 mg) and for a few weeks after the procedure (e.g. aspirin 81–100 mg or clopidogrel 75 mg) until healing of endothelial injury occurs. In addition, intravenous anticoagulation with Heparin or direct thrombin inhibitors should be performed during the procedure.

6. What is the preferred vascular access?

Most procedures are performed from a femoral approach. If alternative access is needed (e.g. brachial access), the length of the catheter (90 cm for the Symplicity and 100 cm for the Spyral) needs to be considered. The Symplicity Flex is compatible with a 6 French introducer, whereas the Symplicity Spyral is compatible with a 4 French. If there is significant iliac tortuosity, a long sheath is recommended to facilitate manipulation of the catheter.

7. How do you engage the renal artery?

Initial non-selective angiography can be performed with a pigtail or Omni flush catheter in the abdominal aorta. Slight left anterior oblique (LAO) angulation is recommended to better visualize the slightly more anterior take-off of the right renal artery than the left. Alternatively, selective angiography can be done using a 6 French guide catheter that is also used to advance the denervation catheter. If the takeoff of the artery is inferiorly oriented, an internal mammary (IM) catheter may be suitable. Conversely, for a superiorly oriented takeoff, a multipurpose catheter may be helpful. For horizontal courses, a JR-4 or renal double curve (RDC) catheter is recommended. The size, course, tortuosity, and branching of the renal arteries should be carefully examined. Ideally, the guide catheter should be carefully advanced 3–4 cm into the renal artery. If the advancement of the catheter is difficult, it can be delivered over a Glidewire or a smaller catheter in a telescoping fashion.

8. Should you use vasodilators before RDN?

Although not standard practice, many physicians routinely administer a vasodilator to prevent vasospasm before denervation. Options include 100–400 mcg of intra-arterial nitroglycerine, 100 mcg of verapamil, or 100–200 mcg of nicardipine.

9. What additional medication may be needed?

Severe visceral pain can be experienced after the application of energy for denervation. For this reason, most operators recommend routine administration of IV analgesics (e.g. Fentanyl) and sedatives (e.g. midazolam) before energy application. As in any other case using benzodiazepines and opiates, reversing agents should be available. Additionally, atropine should be available in the event of a vagal reaction.

10. How do you deliver the RDN catheter?

Following engagement with the guide catheter, the denervation catheter is delivered into the renal using a rapid exchange system over a 0.014-in. wire. The Spyral catheter is used to treat arteries with a diameter between 3 and 8 mm. When the guidewire is removed, the Spyral catheter shape naturally conforms to the renal artery.

11. How do you deliver the RDN therapy?

Once the catheter is in the desired location, a foot pedal is pushed to deliver RF energy. The generator allows the physician to monitor the impedance and temperature of each electrode. After a single 60-second ablation, the catheter can be removed, and the same process is repeated in the contralateral artery.

12. What are some of the potential complications of RF RDN?

Overall, the rate of serious complications is low. Potential complications include vasospasm, severe visceral pain, renal artery dissection or stenosis, and vascular access complications. Bailout equipment, including stents, covered stents, and 0.014-in. and 0.018-in. wires should be available.

Bibliography

1 Azizi, M., Sapoval, M., Gosse, P. et al. (2015). Optimum and stepped care standardised antihypertensive treatment with or without renal denervation for resistant hypertension (DENERHTN): a multicentre, open-label, randomised controlled trial. *Lancet* 385: 1957–1965.

2 Azizi, M., Schmieder, R.E., Mahfoud, F. et al. (2018). Endovascular ultrasound renal denervation to treat hypertension (RADIANCE-HTN SOLO): a multicentre, international, single-blind, randomised, sham-controlled trial. *Lancet* 391: 2335–2345.

3 Bhatt, D.L., Kandzari, D.E., O'Neill, W.W. et al. (2014). A controlled trial of renal denervation for resistant hypertension. *N. Engl. J. Med.* 370: 1393–1401.

4 Epstein, M. and de Marchena, E. (2015). Is the failure of Symplicity HTN-3 trial to meet its efficacy endpoint the "end of the road" for renal denervation? *J. Am. Soc. Hypertens.* 9: 140–149.

5 Kandzari, D.E., Bohm, M., Mahfoud, F. et al. (2018). Effect of renal denervation on blood pressure in the presence of antihypertensive drugs: 6-month efficacy and safety results from the SPYRAL HTN-ON MED proof-of-concept randomised trial. *Lancet* 391: 2346–2355.

6 Kiuchi, M.G., Esler, M.D., Fink, G.D. et al. (2019). Renal denervation update from the international sympathetic nervous system summit: JACC state-of-the-art review. *J. Am. Coll. Cardiol.* 73: 3006–3017.

7 Krum, H., Schlaich, M., Whitbourn, R. et al. (2009). Catheter-based renal sympathetic denervation for resistant hypertension: a multicentre safety and proof-of-principle cohort study. *Lancet* 373: 1275–1281.

8 Lauder, L., Azizi, M., Kirtane, A.J. et al. (2020). Device-based therapies for arterial hypertension. *Nat. Rev. Cardiol.* 17: 614–628.

9 Smithwick, R.H. and Thompson, J.E. (1953). Splanchnicectomy for essential hypertension; results in 1,266 cases. *J. Am. Med. Assoc.* 152: 1501–1504.

10 Symplicity HTNI, Esler, M.D., Krum, H. et al. (2010). Renal sympathetic denervation in patients with treatment-resistant hypertension (the Symplicity HTN-2 trial): a randomised controlled trial. *Lancet* 376: 1903–1909.

11 Townsend, R.R., Mahfoud, F., Kandzari, D.E. et al. (2017). Catheter-based renal denervation in patients with uncontrolled hypertension in the absence of antihypertensive medications (SPYRAL HTN-OFF MED): a randomised, sham-controlled, proof-of-concept trial. *Lancet* 390: 2160–2170.

69

Acute Pulmonary Embolism Interventions: Data and Indications

Michael McDaniel, and Wissam A. Jaber

[1] *Interventional Cardiology,, Emory University School of Medicine, Grady Memorial Hospital, Atlanta, GA, USA*
[2] *Interventional Cardiology, Emory University Hospital, Atlanta, GA, USA*

1. How do you risk-stratify patients with acute pulmonary embolism?

Risk-stratification is the most important step in the management of patients with acute pulmonary embolism (PE) and requires assessing the ability of the right ventricle (RV) to overcome the acute afterload caused by acute obstruction to the pulmonary vasculature. While there is no single best way to perform risk stratification, usually a variety of clinical, imaging, and/or laboratory data are used. Based on the patient's risk, the treatment can range from anticoagulation alone to catheter-directed thrombolysis, systemic thrombolysis, catheter or surgical embolectomy, and/or mechanical circulatory support.

Patients presenting with acute PE and cardiogenic shock and/or cardiac arrest are defined as high-risk or massive PE. Shock is typically defined as systolic blood pressure <90 mmHg for more than 15 minutes and/or requiring inotropic support. Patients with massive PE have up to 50% early mortality but fortunately represent only about 5% of all acute PE.

Patients with evidence of RV dysfunction but normal blood pressure are classified as intermediate-risk or submassive PE. About 40% of patients with acute PE are classified as submassive, and these patients are at higher risk for adverse advents and mortality than patients with normal RV function. RV dysfunction can be identified on computed tomography angiogram (CTA) as an increased ratio of the RV to the left ventricle (LV). On echocardiography, RV dysfunction is defined by RV dilation and/or RV hypokinesis or the presence of McConnell's sign (RV free wall dysfunction with sparing of the apex).

The European Society of Cardiology (ESC) guidelines further subdivides intermediate-risk PE based on the cardiac biomarkers. The combination of RV dysfunction and abnormal biomarkers is classified as high-risk submassive PE, while patients with RV dysfunction and normal biomarkers are classified as low-risk submassive PE. Patients with both RV dysfunction and abnormal biomarkers have much higher in-hospital mortality compared to either of these findings in isolation. The most common biomarkers for risk stratification in acute PE are cardiac troponin, brain natriuretic peptide (BNP), and lactic acid. In a meta-analysis of 1132 patients with acute PE, patients with elevated BNP had a 10% (95% confidence interval [CI] 8.0–13%) risk of early death. In a separate meta-analysis of 1985 patients with acute PE and normal blood pressure, there was significantly higher mortality with an elevated troponin (odds ratio [OR] 5.9; 95% CI 2.68–12.95). Adding lactate levels to these biomarkers may identify an even higher risk for early decompensation. In 496 normotensive patients with acute PE, the combination of elevated lactic acid, RV dysfunction, and elevated troponin was associated with an 18% incidence of in-hospital mortality or hemodynamic collapse.

The majority (55%) of acute PEs are classified as low-risk or minor PE. Patients with low-risk PE have normal blood pressure, normal RV size and function, and normal biomarkers. These patients have low mortality and morbidity and can be managed with anticoagulation alone.

2. Is anticoagulation alone enough for patients with high-risk submassive PE?

The 2019 ESC and 2016 CHEST PE guidelines recommend anticoagulation alone with rescue systemic thrombolysis for most patients with submassive PE. Although anticoagulation alone is sufficient for many patients with submassive PE, several studies question this conservative approach, given a higher incidence of hemodynamic decompensation, mortality, and poor functional status in patients who receive only anticoagulation. In the PEITHO (PE International Thrombolysis) trial, 1006 patients with high-risk submassive PE were randomized to anticoagulation alone or systemic thrombolysis. Patients randomized to anticoagulation alone had a higher incidence of death and hemodynamic collapse within seven days of randomization (5.6 vs. 2.6%, p = 0.002) compared to patients randomized to systemic thrombolysis. More importantly, in a meta-analysis of 1775 patients from eight randomized trials of submassive PE, patients receiving anticoagulation alone had a high risk for mortality (2.92% vs. 1.39%, NNH = 65, p = 0.03) compared to patients who received systemic thrombolysis. While the absolute mortality benefit with systemic thrombolysis in the analysis was modest, these randomized trials enrolled selected patients, and real-world registries suggest that mortality with high-risk submassive PE is two to three times greater than in randomized trials. Finally, small trials suggest that more aggressive removal of thrombus in acute PE could help return patients to their baseline quality of life faster than with anticoagulation alone. In the 83-patient TOPCOAT (Tenecteplase or Placebo: Cardiopulmonary Outcomes at Three months) trial, patients randomized to anticoagulation alone had a higher rate of the composite of death, shock, recurrent PE, or poor functional status at three months (37% vs. 15%, p = 0.017) compared to patients randomized to systemic thrombolysis. This was primarily driven by worse New York Heart Association (NYHA) functional class and six-minute walk times in patients who received anticoagulation alone.

Together, these studies challenge the current treatment guidelines, as anticoagulation alone may have worse outcomes in patients with high-risk submassive PE. Patients treated only with anticoagulation have a higher risk for clinical decompensation, mortality, and worse functional status in early follow-up. However, these data do not mean that systemic thrombolysis is the optimal treatment for these patients. Systemic thrombolysis is unfortunately limited by a high incidence of major bleeding complications. In the same meta-analysis, major bleeding was significantly more common with systemic thrombolysis compared to anticoagulation alone (OR 3.19; 95% CI, 2.07–4.92), with a number needed to harm (NNH) of only 18 patients. More concerning, thrombolysis was associated with greater intracranial hemorrhage (ICH) risk (OR 4.63; 95% CI, 1.78–12.04, NNH = 78 patients).

3. What is the role of catheter-directed thrombolysis in submassive PE?

Given the poor efficacy of anticoagulation alone and high bleeding complications with systemic thrombolysis, catheter-directed thrombolysis (CDL) has been proposed to provide a better balance of safety and efficacy than anticoagulation or systemic thrombolysis. With CDL, the total thrombolytic dose is usually 10–20% of the systemic dose and given locally into the pulmonary thrombus at about 10% of the rate of systemic thrombolysis. This results in much lower doses of thrombolytics at any given time for the patient.

Several studies suggest that CDL may be more effective than anticoagulation and safer than systemic thrombolysis. In the 59-patient ULTIMA (Ultrasound Accelerated Thrombolysis of PE) trial, patients with submassive PE randomized to ultrasound-facilitated CDL (CDL-US) unloaded the RV more rapidly than anticoagulation alone without increasing bleeding complications. In the SEATTLE II (Submassive and Massive Pulmonary Embolism Treatment with Ultrasound Accelerated Thrombolysis Therapy) trial, 150 patients with submassive and massive PE treated with CDL-US had significant early reductions in pulmonary pressures, RV size, and obstruction index with low complication rates. In a meta-analysis of 860 patients from 16 observational studies undergoing CDL for acute PE, there were consistent early improvements in RV/LV ratio and pulmonary artery pressures with CDL. On average, the RV/LV ratio improved by 0.34, and right ventricular systolic pressure (RVSP) improved by 16 mmHg within 24–48 hours. These improvements are similar to that achieved with systemic thrombolysis (Table 69.1). Importantly, in this analysis, there were very low rates of ICH (0.35%), mortality (0.74%), and major vascular complications (4.65%).

While the data for CDL is intriguing, these studies are mostly retrospective observational non-randomized studies. Larger randomized trials are warranted to investigate the impact of CDL on clinical outcomes. Hopefully, the HI-PEITHO (Ultrasound-facilitated, Catheter-directed, Thrombolysis in Intermediate-high Risk Pulmonary Embolism) trial will provide some answers as it will be randomizing patients with high-risk submassive PE to anticoagulation alone or CDL-US

4. Does CDL-US improve outcomes compared to standard CDL?

CDL-US has theoretical advantages over CDL without ultrasound. *in vitro* studies suggest that ultrasound may

Table 69.1 Comparison of studies on RV/LV ratio and major bleeding.

Study	N	Treatment	tPA	Reduction in RV/LV ratio (24–48 hours)	Major bleeding
FLARE	104	FlowTriever embolectomy	0 mg	0.39 (25%)	0.9%
EXTRACT-PE	119	Indigo embolectomy	0 mg	0.43 (27%)	1.7%
SEATTLE II	150	CDL-US	24 mg	0.42 (24%)	11.4%
ULTIMA	30	CDL-US	10–20 mg	0.29 (22%)	0.0%
SUNSET	81	CDL-US and CDL	18–19 mg	0.45 (28%)	2.5%
Becattini et al.	23	Systemic thrombolysis	30–50 mg (Tenecteplase)	0.31 (24%)	8.7%
Fasullo et al.	37	Systemic thrombolysis	100 mg (Alteplase)	0.38 (27%)	5.4%
Mi et al.	79	Systemic thrombolysis	50 mg (Alteplase)	0.11 (8%)	6.3%
ULTIMA	29	Anticoagulation	0 mg	0.03 (2.5%)	0.0%
Becattini et al.	28	Anticoagulation	0 mg	0.1 (8%)	3.6%
Fasullo et al.	35	Anticoagulation	0 mg	0.2 (14%)	2.9%
Mi et al.	57	Anticoagulation	0 mg	0.04 (2.9%)	1.8%

CDL, catheter-directed thrombolysis; CDL-US, ultrasound-assisted catheter-directed thrombolysis.

improve fibrin disaggregation and enhance thrombolytic penetration and thus enhance thrombolysis efficacy. Moreover, much of the data supporting CDL in acute PE utilizes CDL-US using the EkoSonic Endovascular System (EKOS, Boston Scientific). This system is the only catheter with FDA clearance for CDL in acute PE.

Several studies question the need for ultrasound facilitation in CDL. The SUNSET-sPE (Standard vs. Ultrasound-assisted Catheter Thrombolysis for Submassive Pulmonary Embolism) trial randomized 81 patients to catheter-directed thrombolysis with CDL-US or to standard CDL without ultrasound. In this trial, the majority of the patients presented with high-risk submassive acute PE, and about two-thirds also had acute deep venous thrombosis. The average total TPA infusion in SUNSET-PE was just under 20 mg in both arms. In this trial, changes in thrombus burden from baseline to 48-hour follow-up were similar with CDL and CDL-US. Changes in RV/LV ratio were actually better without ultrasound, but this may be related to differences in baseline RV/LV ratios. Importantly, there

were no differences in bleeding complications or mortality, suggesting that ultrasound facilitation may not provide an additional advantage in CDL. These findings are similar to those from a larger retrospective registry analysis of 2060 patients treated with CDL from the 2016 National Readmissions Database. In this analysis, 417 (20.2%) received CDL-US and 1643 (79.8%) received standard CDL. After adjustment in baseline demographics, the in-hospital mortality (OR, 1.19; 95% CI, 0.63–2.26; $P = 0.59$) and 30-day readmission rates (OR, 0.75; 95% CI, 0.47–1.22; $P = 0.25$) were similar with CDL-US and standard CDL. Moreover, the rates of bleeding events, intracranial hemorrhage, vasopressor use, and mechanical ventilation were similar between these two strategies. Other small single-arm registries have noted similar improvements in right ventricular systolic pressure (RVSP) from baseline to follow-up between CDL-US and standard CDL.

In total, the current data questions the benefit of ultrasound facilitation in CDL. As ultrasound-facilitated catheter systems are significantly more expensive than non-ultrasound catheters, these findings suggest there could be significant cost savings with the omission of the ultrasound in CDL.

5. What is the role of mechanical thrombectomy in patients with submassive PE?

Currently, there are two catheters with FDA approval for mechanical thrombectomy in patients with acute PE: the FlowTriever system (Inari Medical) and the Indigo aspiration system (Penumbra).

The FlowTriever catheter system consists of 16–24 Fr aspiration guide catheters. In the multicenter single-arm FLARE (FlowTriever Pulmonary Embolectomy Clinical) trial, 106 patients with submassive PE underwent embolectomy using the FT device. The primary endpoint was the change in RV/LV ratio at 48 hours, which improved by 0.39 from baseline. Importantly, the adverse event rate was only 3.8%, and there were no cases of ICH, access-site major bleeding, or device-related deaths. The mean intensive care unit (ICU) stay was about one day, and 42% of patients had no time in the ICU. To put the results of the FLARE trial in context, the change in RV/LV ratio with FT is similar to those noted in other trials investigating CDL and systemic thrombolysis and better than that of anticoagulation alone (Table 69.1). Importantly, the low rate of adverse events with FT is similar to that of anticoagulation (Table 69.1). Although limited by its single-arm nature and lack of long-term outcome data, the FLARE trial demonstrates that mechanical thrombectomy using the FlowTriever is feasible and safe.

Similar findings have been noted with FlowTriever embolectomy in the FLASH (FlowTriever All-Comer Registry for Patient Safety and Hemodynamics) Registry. While this prospective registry is ongoing, an interim analysis was presented at the American Heart Association 2020 scientific sessions. In this interim analysis of 230 intermediate-risk patients with acute PE, there was a very low access site complication rate of only 0.5%. Interestingly, the total FlowTriever device time was only 46 minutes, and the estimated blood loss with the procedure was only 250 ml. The average length of stay was 3 days, and the 30-day mortality was only 0.5%. Finally, FlowTriever embolectomy was associated with an average 7.2 mmHg immediate reduction in mean pulmonary artery pressure, and the RV/LV ratio improved by an average of 0.42.

The indigo aspiration embolectomy system is an 8 Fr aspiration catheter connected to a vacuum pump. The indigo system was investigated in the EXTRACT-PE (Evaluating the Safety and Efficacy of the Indigo Aspiration System in Acute Pulmonary Embolism) trial. This was a prospective, multicenter, single-arm trial that enrolled 119 patients with submassive PE at 22 sites. In this trial, there was a significant 27.3% reduction in the RV/LV ratio (absolute change of 0.43) at 48 hours. This change in RV/VL ratio is similar to that of FT, CDL, and systemic thrombolysis (Table 69.1). Importantly, there was only a 1.7% incidence of major adverse events within 48 hours, and the median procedure time was only 37 minutes, with an average stay of one day in the ICU. Since the publication of this trial, Penumbra has released a larger Lightning 12 Fr version of this catheter system. How this larger catheter with improved aspiration compares clinically to the 8 Fr version or the FT catheter is unknown. Randomized trials are warranted comparing the embolectomy catheters as well as comparing catheter embolectomy to CDL and anticoagulation alone in intermediate-to-high risk acute PE.

6. What is the role of catheter-directed therapy in massive PE?

While systemic thrombolysis is the standard of care for many patients with high-risk PE, many patients with massive PE fail to receive this life-saving therapy due to absolute or relative contraindications. For patients with contraindications to and/or failure of thrombolysis, CDL, surgical or catheter embolectomy and/or hemodynamic support should be considered.

Patients with massive PE have very high in-hospital mortality, around 50%. In an analysis of 58 784 patients with massive PE presenting from 1999 to 2017, mortality improved over time. However, this improvement resulted from changes in the treatment of shock and cardiac arrest and not necessarily from advances in the treatment of acute PE. Sadly, patients treated with systemic thrombolytics still had around a 40% mortality rate despite thrombolysis, and only 16% of patients with massive PE received systemic thrombolytics. These findings suggest that patients with massive PE still have very high mortality despite treatment and that little progress has been made over the last two decades in the treatment of these highest-risk patients.

Systemic thrombolysis is a class I recommendation in the 2019 ESC PE Guidelines and a 2B recommendation in the 2016 CHEST PE Guidelines. However, these recommendations are largely based on observational studies with very little randomized data. No large randomized trials are investigating systemic thrombolysis in patients with massive PE, and only 254 patients from five randomized trials have had massive PE. While patients randomized to systemic thrombolysis in these five trials had lower rates of the combination of recurrent PE and death (OR 0.45, 95% CI 0.22–0.92), there was also a 22% risk for major bleeding complications.

Given the high incidence of contraindications to thrombolysis, the poor outcomes despite thrombolysis, and the lack of progress in the treatment of massive PE, there is renewed interest in the use of endovascular treatments for massive PE. Much like the evolution of acute myocardial infarction and acute stroke, there is hope of moving from a systemic thrombolytic era to an endovascular era. In support of this idea is a small analysis of 34 patients undergoing FlowTriever embolectomy with massive PE, intubated, or normotensive with cardiac indexes less than 1.8 l/min/m². In this analysis, there were consistent and rapid on-table improvements in the mean pulmonary artery pressures, cardiac index, blood pressure, and heart rate. Given the low bleeding risk with embolectomy and these significant immediate improvements in hemodynamics, there is interest that such an approach would be more effective and safer than systemic thrombolysis. Currently, the FLAME (FLowTriever for Acute Massive Pulmonary Embolism) trial is enrolling patients with massive PE and investigating the outcomes of FlowTriever embolectomy in these patients compared to the current standard of care.

Mechanical circulatory support should also be considered for patients with massive PE with failure or contraindications to other advanced therapies. While there are no randomized trials examining the role of mechanical circulatory support in PE, several uncontrolled case series have demonstrated favorable outcomes with the use of veno-arterial extracorporeal membrane oxygenation (ECMO) in massive PE. Although survival rates vary greatly in the literature, 15–17 Fr arterial cannulas and 25–29 Fr venous cannulas can be rapidly placed in experienced centers, which rapidly unload the RV with an oxygenator that is independent of pulmonary flow.

7. What is the role of PE response teams in the interventional management of patients with acute PE?

Given the various treatment options for acute PE and the paucity of randomized trials to guide clinicians and patients, multidisciplinary PE response teams (PERTs) have been developed at many hospitals to help guide treatment for these complex patients. These teams are modeled on the Heart Team approach and aim to provide multidisciplinary input to avoid the biases of any individual physician or specialty. While every PERT is different, there is usually a single activation to an on-call physician who gathers information and then facilitates discussion with the team to generate shared decision-making recommendations. There are no randomized data for such an approach, but the 2019 ESC guidelines recommend the use of a PERT as a 2A recommendation. Clinicians and hospital systems interested in learning more about PE response teams can visit the PERT Consortium website at www.pertconsortium.com.

Bibliography

1 Ain, D.L., Albaghdadi, M., Giri, J. et al. (2018). Extracorporeal membrane oxygenation and outcomes in massive pulmonary embolism: two eras at an urban tertiary care hospital. *Vasc. Med.* 23: 60–64.

2 Becattini, C., Agnelli, G., Salvi, A. et al. (2010). Bolus tenecteplase for right ventricle dysfunction in hemodynamically stable patients with pulmonary embolism. *Thromb. Res.* 125: e82–e86.

3 Becattini, C., Vedovati, M.C., and Agnelli, G. (2007). Prognostic value of troponins in acute pulmonary embolism: a meta-analysis. *Circulation* 116: 427–433.

4 Beyer, S.E., Shanafelt, C., Pinto, D.S. et al. (2020). Utilization and outcomes of thrombolytic therapy for acute pulmonary embolism: a Nationwide cohort study. *Chest* 157: 645–653.

5 Bloomer, T.L., El-Hayek, G.E., McDaniel, M.C. et al. (2017). Safety of catheter-directed thrombolysis for massive and submassive pulmonary embolism: Results of a multicenter registry and meta-analysis. *Catheterization and Cardiovascular Interventions* 89 (4): 754–760.

6 Braaten, J.V., Goss, R.A., and Francis, C.W. (1997). Ultrasound reversibly disaggregates fibrin fibers. *Thromb. Haemost.* 78: 1063–1068.

7 Casazza, F., Bongarzoni, A., Capozi, A., and Agostoni, O. (2005). Regional right ventricular dysfunction in acute pulmonary embolism and right ventricular infarction. *Eur. J. Echocardiogr.* 6: 11–14.

8 Chatterjee, S., Chakraborty, A., Weinberg, I. et al. (2014). Thrombolysis for pulmonary embolism and risk of all-cause mortality, major bleeding, and intracranial hemorrhage: a meta-analysis. *Jama* 311: 2414–2421.

9 Fasullo, S., Scalzo, S., Maringhini, G. et al. (2011). Six-month echocardiographic study in patients with submassive pulmonary embolism and right ventricle

dysfunction: comparison of thrombolysis with heparin. *Am. J. Med. Sci.* 341: 33–39.

10 George, B., Parazino, M., Omar, H.R. et al. (2018). A retrospective comparison of survivors and non-survivors of massive pulmonary embolism receiving veno-arterial extracorporeal membrane oxygenation support. *Resuscitation* 122: 1–5.

11 Jaff, M.R., McMurtry, M.S., Archer, S.L. et al. (2011). Management of massive and submassive pulmonary embolism, iliofemoral deep vein thrombosis, and chronic thromboembolic pulmonary hypertension: a scientific statement from the American Heart Association. *Circulation* 123: 1788–1830.

12 Kearon, C., Akl, E.A., Ornelas, J. et al. (2016). Antithrombotic therapy for VTE disease: CHEST guideline and expert panel report. *Chest* 149: 315–352.

13 Kline, J.A., Nordenholz, K.E., Courtney, D.M. et al. (2014). Treatment of submassive pulmonary embolism with tenecteplase or placebo: cardiopulmonary outcomes at 3 months: multicenter double-blind, placebo-controlled randomized trial. *J. Thrombosis. Haemost. : JTH* 12: 459–468.

14 Klok, F.A., Mos, I.C., and Huisman, M.V. (2008). Brain-type natriuretic peptide levels in the prediction of adverse outcome in patients with pulmonary embolism: a systematic review and meta-analysis. *Am. J. Respirat. Critic. Care Med.* 178: 425–430.

15 Konstantinides, S.V. and Meyer, G. (2019). The 2019 ESC guidelines on the diagnosis and Management of Acute Pulmonary Embolism. *Euro. Heart J.* 40: 3453–3455.

16 Kucher, N., Boekstegers, P., Muller, O.J. et al. (2014). Randomized, controlled trial of ultrasound-assisted catheter-directed thrombolysis for acute intermediate-risk pulmonary embolism. *Circulation* 129: 479–486.

17 Kuo, W.T., Banerjee, A., Kim, P.S. et al. (2015). Pulmonary embolism response to fragmentation, embolectomy, and catheter thrombolysis (PERFECT): initial results from a prospective Multicenter registry. *Chest* .

18 McConnell, M.V., Solomon, S.D., Rayan, M.E. et al. (1996). Regional right ventricular dysfunction detected by echocardiography in acute pulmonary embolism. *Am. J. Cardiol.* 78: 469–473.

19 Meyer, G., Vicaut, E., Danays, T. et al. (2014). Fibrinolysis for patients with intermediate-risk pulmonary embolism. *N. Engl. J. Med.* 370: 1402–1411.

20 Mi, Y.H., Liang, Y., Lu, Y.H. et al. (2013). Recombinant tissue plasminogen activator plus heparin compared with heparin alone for patients with acute submassive pulmonary embolism: one-year outcome. *J. Geriatr. Cardiol.* 10: 323–329.

21 Piazza, G., Hohlfelder, B., Jaff, M.R. et al. (2015). A prospective, single-arm, Multicenter trial of ultrasound-facilitated, catheter-directed, low-dose fibrinolysis for acute massive and submassive pulmonary embolism: the SEATTLE II study. *JACC Cardiovasc. Interv.* 8: 1382–1392.

22 Sista, A.K., Horowitz, J.M., Tapson, V.F. et al. (2021). Indigo aspiration system for treatment of pulmonary embolism: results of the EXTRACT-PE trial. *JACC Cardiovasc. Interv.* 14: 319–329.

23 Stein, P.D. and Matta, F. (2012). Thrombolytic therapy in unstable patients with acute pulmonary embolism: saves lives but underused. *Am. J. Med.* 125: 465–470.

24 Stein, P.D., Matta, F., Hughes, P.G., and Hughes, M.J. (2021). Nineteen-year trends in mortality of patients hospitalized in the United States with high-risk pulmonary embolism. *Am. J. Med.* .

25 Stein, P.D., Matta, F., Janjua, M. et al. (2010). Outcome in stable patients with acute pulmonary embolism who had right ventricular enlargement and/or elevated levels of troponin I. *Am. J. Cardiol.* 106: 558–563.

26 Toma, C. (2020). ABSTRACT: interim acute and 30-day results of the Flash registry. *Circulation* 142: A16623.

27 Toma, C., Khandhar, S., Zalewski, A.M. et al. (2020). Percutaneous thrombectomy in patients with massive and very high-risk submassive acute pulmonary embolism. *Catheter Cardiovasc Interv : Offic. J. Soc. Cardiac. Angiog. Intervent.* 96: 1465–1470.

28 Tu, T., Toma, C., Tapson, V.F. et al. (2019). A prospective, single-arm, multicenter trial of catheter-directed mechanical thrombectomy for intermediate-risk acute pulmonary embolism: the FLARE study. *JACC Cardiovasc. Interv.* 12: 859–869.

29 Vanni, S., Jimenez, D., Nazerian, P. et al. (2015). Short-term clinical outcome of normotensive patients with acute PE and high plasma lactate. *Thorax* 70: 333–338.

30 Wan, S., Quinlan, D.J., Agnelli, G., and Eikelboom, J.W. (2004). Thrombolysis compared with heparin for the initial treatment of pulmonary embolism: a meta-analysis of the randomized controlled trials. *Circulation* 110: 744–749.

70

Acute Pulmonary Embolism Intervention: Devices and Techniques

Wissam A. Jaber[1] and Catalin Toma[2]

[1] Interventional Cardiology, Emory University School of Medicine, Grady Memorial Hospital, Atlanta, GA, USA
[2] Interventional Cardiology, University of Pittsburg Medical Center, Pittsburgh, PA, USA

1. What devices are currently available to treat acute pulmonary embolism?

There are currently three devices on the market that are FDA approved for the treatment of acute pulmonary embolism (PE). These are the EkoSonic ultrasound-assisted thrombolysis catheter (EKOS; Boston Scientific, Figure 70.1a), the FlowTriever system (Inari Medical, Figure 70.1b), and the Indigo catheter (Penumbra, Figure 70.1c.) Although not specifically indicated for the treatment of acute PE, simple multi-side-hole infusion catheters without ultrasound core have been extensively used for that indication.

Conceptually, these devices can be categorized as either means to deliver thrombolytics locally or devices used for thrombus retrieval/aspiration. The EKOS catheter belongs to the first category and consists of a 5.4 Fr infusion catheter with distal side holes spread over a specific treatment zone. Once delivered over a 0.035-in. guide wire, the central lumen is then occupied by an ultrasonic core with transducers spanning the treatment zone and emitting acoustic pulses. The ultrasound pulses are meant to loosen the fibrin sheets, allowing for better exposure to the infused thrombolytic agent (typically TPA) and thus a faster thrombolysis. The treatment zone ranges from 6 to 50 cm in length, but the most commonly used lengths for PE treatment are 6 and 12 cm. A similar TPA infusion can be delivered through commercially available, cheaper catheters without the use of ultrasound. Examples include the Uni-Fuse (AngioDynamics) 4Fr or 5Fr and Cragg-McNamara (Medtronic) 5Fr catheters. Both catheters are 0.035 in. guidewire-compatible, and both have multiple treatment zone lengths, with the 10 cm being the most useful length for treating PE.

The new Bashir thrombolytic infusion catheter (Thrombolex, Figure 70.1d) is available on the market for the treatment of deep venous thrombosis and is currently under investigation in a prospective trial for the treatment of acute PE. It consists of a 7Fr shaft, with the tip being equipped with a basket of multiple mini-infusion catheters with side holes designed to infuse lytics over a larger three-dimensional area.

The second category of devices is represented by aspiration thrombectomy tools that do not utilize thrombolytics, such as the FlowTriever and Indigo systems. The main component of the FlowTriever system is a 95 cm guide catheter (available in 20 and 24 Fr) equipped with a large-bore syringe used to create a vacuum through manual pull, exerting aspiration pressure on the thrombus. An optional self-deployed Nitinol disk can be used to help macerate or drag a more distal thrombus for better aspiration. The 16 Fr and 20 Fr curved-tip catheters can also be intussuscepted inside a bigger-bore catheter to reach distal thrombi in smaller vessels if needed.

The Indigo system is a smaller catheter, originally available in 8Fr and recently in 12Fr. As opposed to the FlowTriever, where the aspiration is manual, the aspiration in the Indigo system is continuous through a connected pump, with aspirated blood collected in a canister. The catheter is equipped with a separator to facilitate clearing the thrombus from the tip of the catheter. To minimize blood loss related to continuous aspiration, an intelligent aspiration tubing has been added to the system, equipped with a sensor that monitors blood flow and automatically controls a valve.

Finally, the AngioVac (AngioDynamics) catheter is a large aspiration catheter that uses a continuous pump with filtered blood returned through a closed venovenous circuit.

Mastering Structural Heart Disease, First Edition. Edited by Eduardo J. de Marchena and Camilo A. Gomez.
© 2023 John Wiley & Sons Ltd. Published 2023 by John Wiley & Sons Ltd.
Companion website: www.wiley.com/go/deMarchena/Mastering-Structural-Heart-Disease

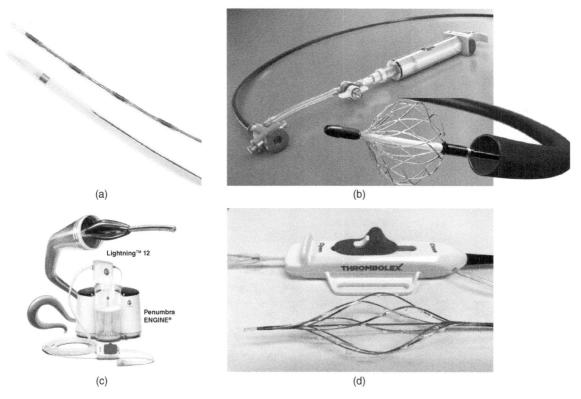

(a)

(b)

Lightning™ 12

Penumbra
ENGINE®

THROMBOLEX

(c)

(d)

Figure 70.1 Different catheters available for the treatment of acute pulmonary embolism: (a) EKOS; (b) FlowTriever; (c) Penumbra Indigo; (d) Bashir catheter.

Although it has been tried in the pulmonary artery (PA), the catheter's stiffness and bulkiness limit its use for intracardiac or intravenous thrombi. A proposed smaller AngioVac catheter is not yet on the market as of the writing of this chapter.

2. How do you choose between the different treatment options?

There are currently limited data or guidelines to help answer this question. Treatment choice depends on local expertise, preferences, and catheter availability. Some operators prefer catheter-directed thrombolysis for its ease of use. When the thrombolysis is chosen, simple infusion catheters are an acceptable alternative to the ultrasound-assisted catheter EKOS. On the other hand, catheter thrombolysis requires a stay in the intensive care unit and has an associated increased risk of bleeding. PE is commonly seen in post-surgical, trauma, or stroke patients who are at high risk for bleeding. Thus, for these types of patients, or for patients where more rapid hemodynamic improvement is desired, catheter embolectomy may be preferable over thrombolysis. Performing catheter embolectomy would not preclude catheter thrombolysis if the former did not lead to satisfactory thrombus removal.

3. Is acute PE treatment similar to chronic PE treatment?

Acute PE treatment bears no similarities to chronic PE treatment. The former deals with acute, non-wall-adherent thrombi that can be fragmented, thrombolyzed, or surgically or percutaneously aspirated. Chronic PE is a condition where thrombi have organized and been replaced by fibrous tissue, adherent to the wall and forming bands and variable obstructions to the arterial lumen, with associated chronic pulmonary hypertension. The treatment of the latter condition is surgical endarterectomy or balloon angioplasty for nonsurgical cases, preferably performed in highly specialized centers with a comprehensive experience in chronic thromboembolic disease management.

By definition, chronic PE is a PE present for more than three months. On the other hand, acute PE that has a reasonable chance to respond to treatment, whether medical or mechanical, is typically one that is of less than two weeks duration. For example, a patient with progressive dyspnea and cough of several weeks duration is unlikely to benefit from interventional management (systemic thrombolysis, catheter thrombolytic, or catheter aspiration) unless there has been a clear sudden, recent deterioration in symptoms suggestive of an acute component.

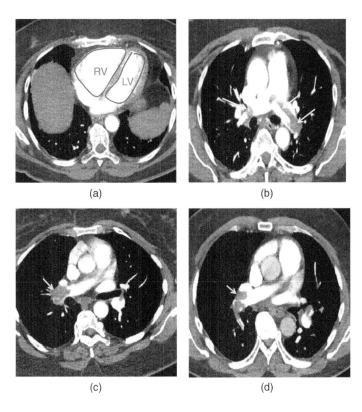

4. How safe is the interventional treatment of acute PE?

The most common complications of catheter intervention relate to access site injury and bleeding, with an incidence of around 1.5–10%. Pulmonary vascular injury is uncommon and is typically related to wire perforation. Treatment of a pulmonary segment with a large downstream infarct may lead to hemorrhage in the infarcted territory. With catheter thrombolysis, although the TPA dose is low, intracranial bleeding has been reported at a rate of around 0.3–0.6%, the risk increasing with increasing age. With catheter embolectomy, the volume of blood aspirated should be tracked to avoid excessive loss, but the latter is rare with careful techniques, as described later in the chapter.

5. What patient and what artery do you treat?

As described in the previous chapter, patients with massive PE (especially when contraindicated for thrombolytic use) and patients with submassive PE and increased risk features (e.g. large right ventricle, elevated cardiac biomarkers, elevated lactate level, tachycardia, severe hypoxemia,

increased work of breathing, low cardiopulmonary reserve) are reasonable candidates for intervention.

Besides the clinical features, review of the computed tomography (CT) angiogram is crucial in deciding on treatment options. The clinical picture must be associated with a corresponding large thrombus burden to warrant intervention. The main PA, main PA branches, and proximal lobar arteries are locations amenable to intervention (Figure 70.2). Thrombi in distal locations (segmental and subsegmental branches) are typically not associated with hemodynamic compromise and rarely require an interventional treatment.

6. What is the most efficient technique for catheter placement for directed thrombolysis?

Access can be obtained in the jugular, femoral, or brachial veins using ultrasound for guidance to avoid vascular complications. For bilateral PA treatments, the same vein can be accessed twice with two 5 or 6 Fr sheaths. Next, a 6 Fr balloon-tipped catheter or a pigtail catheter is used to perform a right heart catheterization and access the PA. In general, we recommend obtaining basic hemodynamic data at baseline, such as PA pressures and mixed central venous oxygen saturation to calculate cardiac output.

From a femoral approach, catheters usually enter the left PA when advanced. To access the right PA, a directional catheter like a pigtail is used. A soft J-tipped guide wire usually follows the interlobar and basilar branches, where most of the thrombi are typically located. If the thrombus to be treated is located in the main PA branches, angiography frequently is not necessary as the infusion catheter advanced over the wire will typically traverse the thrombus. For more distal thrombi, manual injection of contrast in selective branches may be necessary to direct the wire and catheter into the occluded branches. The use of angled or straight hydrophilic wires (for example, Glidewire; Terumo) generally is not recommended as they may cause distal perforations.

Once an appropriate distal branch is selected, an exchange-length soft-tipped wire is used to advance the infusion catheter. An infusion length of 10 or 12 cm is appropriate for most cases. The catheter can then be connected to the TPA pump. The lumen of the catheter can also be used to monitor PA pressure and inject contrast if needed.

7. How long do you infuse TPA?

There is significant uncertainty regarding the answer to such a question. In the ULTIMA (ULTrasound Accelerated ThrombolysIs of PulMonAry Embolism) trial, TPA infusion was run for 15 hours and in the SEATTLE II (Submassive and Massive Pulmonary Embolism Treatment with Ultrasound Accelerated Thrombolysis Therapy) study for 12–24 hours, with an infusion rate of 0.5 mg per hour per catheter for bilateral treatments and 1 mg per hour when a single PA is treated. The OPTALYSE PE (Optimum Duration of Acoustic Pulse Thrombolysis Procedure in Acute Pulmonary Embolism) randomized trial evaluated infusion lengths ranging from two to six hours with similar clinical outcome regardless of the infusion length, although the thrombus burden on CT scan was higher in the shortest infusion group compared to the other groups. Most operators treat for at least 6 hours, and rarely for more than 18 hours, for a total TPA dose of less than 20 mg.

It is also important to continue anticoagulation for the duration of TPA infusion. Most operators use a fixed dose of 500 U/hr or a low-dose nomogram without boluses.

8. What are the safe techniques to perform large-bore aspiration?

The most common access point is the femoral vein, and using ultrasound to guide access is crucial to avoid vascular complications and rule out femoral or iliac thrombi at the access site. Once access is obtained, a large sheath is placed over a stiff wire: 10 Fr sheath for the 8 Fr Indigo system, 12–14 Fr sheath for the 12 Fr Indigo system, and 22–26 Fr sheath for the FlowTriever catheter. Almost all femoral veins can accommodate a 26 Fr sheath, allowing for the easy advancement of the 24 Fr FlowTriever catheter. Anticoagulation is administered with a target activated clotting time of around 250 seconds. A balloon-tipped catheter is then advanced through the tricuspid valve and up to the PA. Crossing with straight catheters or guidewires should be avoided as they may cross behind a papillary muscle, leading to potential injury to the tricuspid valve upon advancement of the large catheter. Once in the PA, a baseline PA pressure and PA saturation are obtained, and the PA branch to be treated is selected. A selective pulmonary angiogram may be necessary to identify the areas to be treated. In case of a large thrombus burden with significant RV dysfunction or low cardiac output, a manual injection of less than 10 ml of contrast is usually sufficient for visualization. Although the initial injection can be performed in the anteroposterior projection for the right PA and in a shallow left anterior oblique for the left PA, different right or left oblique projections may be necessary to identify distal bifurcations. The next step is to navigate safely to a distal occluded branch, so a stiff wire is delivered. This step can be achieved using diagnostic catheters like a multipurpose or a Judkins right curve. Gentle test injections of contrast distally can identify branches of acceptable sizes to place the stiff wire. To advance the 24 Fr FlowTriever, the authors use the Amplatz Super Stiff wire with a 1 cm soft distal tip (Boston Scientific). Softer wires like the Rosen wire (Cook Medical) are usually supportive enough for smaller catheters. Exchange should not happen over straight or angled wires with hydrophilic coated tips (Glidewire) to avoid distal perforations.

The 24 Fr FlowTriever catheter can be advanced safely to the branch PA in almost all acute PE cases. A critical step is the actual engagement of the thrombus by the catheter tip. We typically advance the catheter with the dilator to the distal interlobar branch, where aspiration can be initiated after removal of the dilator. The catheter can also be withdrawn to engage thrombi upstream. If the suction syringe does not fill with blood or thrombi, and in the presence of continuous vacuum, the catheter should be withdrawn and flushed outside the body.

The 12 Fr Indigo catheter (Penumbra) is advanced in a similar manner but is used without a guidewire once in the PA. The slight angle at the tip allows changing the direction of the tip for more reach. Continuous suction is applied using a pump, and a separator is used to keep the tip free of occlusive thrombi. The operator should be careful not to advance the catheter blindly, especially when using the

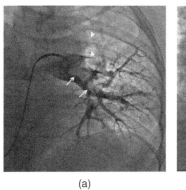

(a)

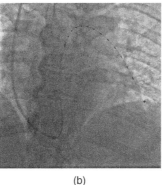

(b)

Figure 70.3 (a) Selective left pulmonary artery (PA) angiogram showing central filling defects (arrows) and reduced flow in multiple segments, particularly in the upper lobe (arrowheads). (b) EKOS catheter placed in the left PA with treatment zone seen as the dashed radiopaque line representing the ultrasound emitters.

separator, as the latter can be introduced in small arteries increasing the perforation risk.

Once finished, the venotomy site can usually be closed using a figure-eight or mattress suture with immediate hemostasis (Figures 70.3 and 70.4).

9. What are the endpoints for percutaneous thrombectomy?

It is rare to be able to remove all pulmonary emboli. When multiple passes have been performed and a reasonable amount of thrombus removed, the PA pressure and PA saturation should be repeated. Normalization or a significant improvement in either or both, together with improvement in other clinical signs like oxygen saturation and cardiac output, are reasonable indicators of the end of the

procedure. At times, angiographic normalization of flow in most segments can be seen and signal the end of the intervention. On the other hand, if multiple attempts achieve no thrombus removal and no hemodynamic improvement, leaving catheters for TPA infusion for a few hours may be helpful in achieving better results. This is rarely necessary and should prompt the physician to reconsider the possibility of subacute or chronic thrombi.

10. How do you manage hemodynamically unstable patients?

Massive as well as high-risk submassive PE patients can be hemodynamically unstable and continue to deteriorate during the intervention. In these patients, mechanical thrombectomy is favored, given the more rapid impact on

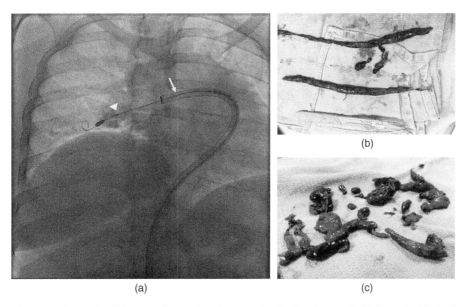

(a)

(b)

(c)

Figure 70.4 (a) FlowTriever catheter placed over a wire in the right main PA (arrow) with deployed distal disks (arrowheads.) (b)≈Examples of retrieved emboli.

hemodynamics. Pharmacological or mechanical circulatory support needs should be evaluated before the procedure.

In addition to the natural progression of right ventricular dysfunction, other procedure-related elements can lead to decompensation. The operator must be able to recognize and treat hemodynamic deterioration that can occur during these procedures. PE patients are very preload dependent, so excessive aspirations can lead to worsening hemodynamics. Volume resuscitation or autotransfusion of filtered blood can prevent this. The same preload dependence is why elective intubation for the procedure must be avoided at all costs and the procedure should be performed with minimal sedation with avoidance of cardiodepressive drugs (such as propofol).

Prolonged manipulation of a large-bore catheter over a stiff wire traversing the right heart can alter right ventricular performance and should be avoided. Finally, thrombus shifting from one side to the contralateral side can lead to prompt hemodynamic collapse and should be treated with immediate aspiration on the opposite side.

It is important that these high-risk patients are treated in a setting with immediate access to an extracorporeal membrane oxygenator (ECMO). A conversation with the ECMO team may be necessary before taking the patient to the angiography suite, and occasionally obtaining fluoroscopy and ultrasound-guided arterial placeholder access for potential ECMO should be contemplated. PE patients respond favorably to ECMO support as the right ventricular function often recovers over the course of two to three days. However, the cannulation should be achieved in a controlled fashion with distal perfusion in place to avoid vascular complications.

11.   How do you manage thrombus in transit?

Free-floating thrombus in the right-heart chambers can be seen in 4% of patients presenting with acute PE and is associated with a worse prognosis when compared with patients without such findings. Targeted therapy beyond anticoagulation is warranted, especially when there is a concomitant right ventricular dysfunction, given the associated risk of sudden deterioration. Options include systemic thrombolysis, surgical embolectomy, and large-bore catheter aspiration. We favor the catheter therapy option, including AngioVac or FlowTriever thrombectomy with echocardiographic guidance – transesophageal, transthoracic, or intracardiac. The thrombus should be approached with great care to avoid embolization, minimizing the manipulation of wires and catheters in the right heart and around the thrombus. For AngioVac thrombectomy, a stiff wire is usually brought to the vena cava just outside the right atrium; once the wire is retrieved and the circuit initiated, the catheter is advanced slowly under continuous suction until it engages the thrombus. For FlowTriever thrombectomy, the 20 Fr curved catheter placed inside the 24 Fr catheter is helpful in directing the aspiration to the desired location. Manual aspiration is started as soon as the catheter tip appears close to the thrombus on echocardiography. PE thrombectomy, if indicated, can be performed during the same setting.

Before advancing the catheter into the inferior vena cava, a venogram is indicated to rule out concomitant central venous thrombus and avoid pushing such a thrombus toward the heart.

For the thrombus in transit through a patent foramen ovale, surgical treatment is the preferred treatment option to avoid systemic embolization. Catheter aspiration can break the thrombus and leave fragments on the left atrial side.

12.   How do you manage anticoagulation around treatment?

For catheter lysis, low-dose subtherapeutic anticoagulation is usually continued during the TPA infusion. Once the infusion is finished, standard anticoagulation is resumed. For long infusions – for example, lasting more than 10 hours – monitoring fibrinogen levels may be necessary to avoid bleeding. The infusion is usually stopped if the fibrinogen level is lower than 50–100 mg/dl, and anticoagulation is not restarted until the fibrinogen and the activated partial thromboplastin time are back to safe levels.

For thrombectomy without thrombolysis, anticoagulation is usually continued without interruption. If there are no bleeding complications and the patient is stable, oral anticoagulation can usually be started the next day. An echocardiogram prior to discharge is important in determining the degree of residual right ventricular dysfunction and pulmonary hypertension.

13.   What outpatient follow-up is needed?

Clinical follow-up post-acute PE interventions is very important and often missed. The main objectives are to ensure compliance with anticoagulation therapy for at least three months for a provoked PE and long-term for unprovoked events. The second is to monitor these patients for the development of long-term sequelae of PE. Most patients post PE on anticoagulation undergo an efficient thrombus resorption process; however, in smaller proportions, some degree of residual thrombus persists long-term and can be associated with symptoms and objective perfusion-ventilation mismatch. When the obstruction is extensive, chronic thromboembolic pulmonary hypertension ensues. A follow-up echocardiogram at three to six months post procedure, particularly in patients with residual right ventricular dysfunction/pulmonary hypertension on discharge and in patients with persistent symptoms, is a useful screening tool. If abnormal, or if symptoms persist despite a normal echocardiogram, a ventilation-perfusion scan is indicated to rule out residual perfusion defects.

Bibliography

1 Bloomer, T.L., El-Hayek, G.E., MC, M.D. et al. (2017). *Safety of catheter-directed thrombolysis for massive and submassive pulmonary embolism: results of a multicenter registry and meta-analysis. Catheter. Cardiovasc. Interv.* 89 (4): 754–760.

2 Chartier, L., Delomez, J.B., Asseman, P. et al. (1999). *Free-floating thrombi in the right heart: diagnosis, management, and prognostic indexes in 38 consecutive patients. Circulation* 99 (21): 2779–2783.

3 Kucher, N., Boekstegers, P., Muller, O.J. et al. (2014). *Randomized, controlled trial of ultrasound-assisted catheter-directed thrombolysis for acute intermediate-risk pulmonary embolism. Circulation* 129 (4): 479–486.

4 Piazza, G., Hohlfelder, B., Raff, M.R. et al. (2015). *A prospective, single-arm, multicenter trial of ultrasound-facilitated, catheter-directed, low-dose fibrinolysis for acute massive and submassive pulmonary embolism: the SEATTLE II study. JACC Cardiovasc. Interv.* 8 (10): 1382–1392.

5 Sista, A.K., Horowitz, J.M., Tapson, V.F. et al. (2021). *Indigo aspiration system for treatment of pulmonary embolism: results of the EXTRACT-PE trial. JACC Cardiovasc. Interv.* 14 (3): 319–329.

6 Tapson, V.F., Sterling, N., Elder, M. et al. (2018). *A randomized trial of the optimum duration of acoustic pulse thrombolysis procedure in acute intermediate-risk pulmonary embolism: the OPTALYSE PE trial. JACC Cardiovasc. Interv.* 11 (14): 1401–1410.

7 Torbicki, A., Galie, N., Covezzoli, A. et al. (2003). *Right heart thrombi in pulmonary embolism: results from the international cooperative pulmonary embolism registry. J. Am. Coll. Cardiol.* 41 (12): 2245–2251.

8 Tu, T., Toma, C., Tapson, V.F. et al. (2019). *A prospective, single-arm, multicenter trial of catheter-directed mechanical thrombectomy for intermediate-risk acute pulmonary embolism: the FLARE study. JACC Cardiovasc. Interv.* 12 (9): 859–869.

71

Transseptal Puncture Technique in the ERA of Structural Heart Disease

Joao Braghiroli and Alexandre C. Ferreira

[1] *Jackson Health System, Miami, FL, USA*
[2] *Department of Cardiology, Jackson Memorial Health System, Miami, FL, USA*

Introduction

Obtaining catheter-driven access to the left atrium across the interatrial septum was first described by Constantine Cope in 1959. Shortly after, the development of dedicated equipment and the step-by-step procedure was described by Ross, Braunwald, and Brockenbrough, using principles of the Seldinger technique and fluoroscopic guidance.

Although less precise, the capability to estimate the left atrial pressure with non-invasive imaging and the utilization of a balloon tip pulmonary wedge pressure catheter led to a significant decline in the need for transseptal puncture for diagnostic purposes. In contrast, percutaneously crossing the interatrial septum for therapeutic interventions, approached by both electrophysiology and interventional cardiology, became by far the most common reasons for transseptal puncture.

The transseptal puncture maneuvers have undergone only minor modifications, but imaging, particularly the utilization of echocardiographic guidance, with either transesophageal or intracardiac echo, has increased the safety of the procedure and allowed a precise site-specific puncture that markedly increases the success of some of the contemporary structural heart procedures.

The role of 3D echocardiography, computed tomography (CE), and fusion of different imaging modalities, particularly fluoroscopy and transesophageal echocardiography (TEE), has been increasing exponentially.

1. What constitutes the fossa ovalis and the interatrial septum?

The interatrial septum accounts for the area interposed by the right and left atria. Only approximately 20% of that area can be safely crossed without accessing the extracardiac space, which is referred to as the *true interatrial septum*.

The fossa ovalis, composed of thin fibrous tissue, is located in the lower and posterior part of the true interatrial septum and typically has an oval shape. The anatomy of the fossa ovalis can become significantly distorted depending on changes in the size and pressure of both atria.

In the era of structural heart interventions requiring precise and site-specific punctures, the fossa ovalis has been schematically subdivided into four quadrants (superior/inferior–anterior/posterior) for proper anatomical reference (Figure 71.1).

2. What are the current indications for accessing the left atrium

Although it remains the gold standard for left atrium pressure measurement, a transseptal puncture is rarely required for diagnostics purposes. Those are scenarios with equivocal hemodynamics obtained with a balloon tip catheter and to assess the transaortic gradient in patients with mechanical aortic prostheses.

Currently, percutaneous access to the left atrium has become far more relevant for electrophysiology catheter-based ablation, structural heart interventions, and hemodynamic circulatory support.

Following is a list of the current indications:

- Direct atrial pressure measurement
- Pulmonary vein isolation
- Left atrial appendage (LAA) closure
- Mitral valve paravalvular leak repair
- Edge-to-edge transcatheter mitral valve repair
- Transcatheter mitral valve-in-valve

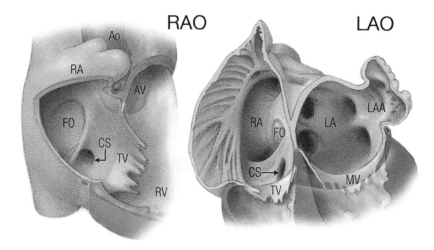

Figure 71.1 Anatomy of the interatrial septum in RAO and LAO projections. RAO, right anterior oblique; LAO, left anterior oblique; Ao, aorta; AR, aortic root; AV, aortic valve; CS, coronary sinus; LAA, left atrial appendage; LAO, left anterior oblique; PA, pulmonary artery; RAO, right anterior oblique; TV, tricuspid valve. *Source:* Alkhouli et al., 2016 / With permission of Elsevier.

- Transcatheter mitral valve implantation
- Percutaneous balloon mitral valvuloplasty
- Antegrade treatment of left ventricular and aortic valve disease
- Percutaneous closure of patent foramen ovale with a long tunnel
- Percutaneous left ventricular assist devices
- Balloon atrial septostomy

3.   Why is it relevant to access specific locations of the interatrial septum?

If the patient has suitable anatomy, accessing the left atria at a site-specific location allows safer manipulation of the equipment, particularly when large-bore catheters typically used for structural heart interventions are involved.

The success of complex structural procedures such as edge-to-edge mitral valve repair, percutaneous closure of paravalvular leaks (particularly when the leak is located at a septal/posterior location), and LAA closure may be significantly impacted by proper axial alignment of the catheters with the anatomical area of interest.

The ability to safely steer the equipment to achieve the desired co-axial alignment can be significantly affected by the site of transseptal puncture.

4.   What are the typical site-specific locations for the most common procedures requiring transseptal puncture?

Most patients who require interventions associated with transseptal puncture may suffer comorbidities that affect the left atrium loading condition and, potentially, distort the cardiac anatomy. Pre-planning procedures, particularly with the assistance of structural imaging expertise, incorporating multi-imaging modalities, allows precision and adaptation for each patient's anatomical variances.

Site-specific puncture locations are as follows (Figure 71.2):

- LAA closure
  - Posterior/inferior
- Mitral valve paravalvular leak repair
  - Lateral: posterior/mid
  - Septal: posterior/superior
- Edge-to-edge transcatheter mitral valve repair
  - MitraClip: posterior/superior. With the newer devices, a mid/posterior puncture is occasionally required.
- Transcatheter mitral valve-in-valve
  - Mid/posterior
- Transcatheter mitral valve implantation
  - Mid/posterior
- Percutaneous balloon mitral valvuloplasty
  - Mid/posterior

5.   How is a site-specific transseptal puncture performed?

1. Fluoroscopic and echocardiographic guidance is strongly suggested.
2. Ultrasound-guided venous access is recommended. Although not essential, a right-side puncture is usually preferred due to the more linear trajectory. Typically, an 8 Fr sheath is introduced. Administer 1000–2000 U of heparin to avoid device thrombosis.
3. Advance a 0.032-in. J-tip guidewire under fluoroscopic guidance to the superior vena cava.

Figure 71.2 Site-specific locations for transseptal puncture for various intracardiac interventions. *Source:* Alkhouli et al. 2016 / with permission of Elsevier.

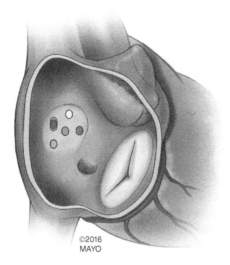

Red: MitraClip, paravalvular leak closure (a higher crossing site is recommended for medial leaks, and a lower crossing site is recommended for lateral leaks).

Yellow: transseptal patent foramen ovale closure.

Blue: percutaneous left ventricular assist device placement, hemodynamic studies.

Green: left atrial appendage closure.

Orange: pulmonary vein interventions.

©2016 MAYO

4. Exchange the venous sheath for the transseptal sheath and dilator, which is subsequently advanced over the guidewire to the superior vena cava (SVC).
5. Remove the 0.032-in. J-tip guidewire, keeping the tip of the sheath facing left on the AP projection.
6. Advance the transseptal needle under fluoroscopy, and allow free rotation of the needle. At this step, do not advance the needle distal to the sheath to avoid inadvertent perforation.
7. Park the needle 4 cm proximal to the tip of the sheath. (If using a Brockenbrough, BRK, or BRK1 needle, use the stylet when advancing the needle to avoid scraping the lumen of the sheath, and remove it when it is adjacent to the tip of the sheath.)
8. Rotate the entire system (needle and sheath) as a unit until the needle arrow reaches 4 to 6 o'clock. At times, more clockwise rotation is required, especially in very dilated atria. Clockwise rotation directs the system more posteriorly.
9. Under echocardiographic guidance (midesophageal 90° to 110° bicaval view on TEE), slowly retrieve the system caudally with the needle arrow pointing to 4 to 6 o'clock. Be careful to prevent inadvertent advancement of the needle distal to the sheath. Observe on fluoroscopy and echocardiography the location of the system moving from the SVC to the right atrium and then the tenting of the septum once the tip of the sheath falls in the fossa ovalis. Further retrieval of the system will lead to a more inferior location at the fossa.
10. Under echocardiographic guidance (midesophageal 20° to 40° short aortic axis [SAX] view), check the site of tenting at the fossa with regard to an anterior–posterior axis.
11. Under echocardiographic guidance (midesophageal 0° four-chamber view), measure the height of the puncture – the distance from the fossa tenting and mitral annulus.

12. Adjust the site of the puncture location by providing gentle traction of the system combined with a clockwise rotation for a posterior location or counterclockwise rotation for an anterior location.
    If tenting of the fossa is already too inferior and the procedure requires a more superior puncture, restart with the placement of the 0.032″ wire at the SVC.
13. Once the site-specific tenting location is achieved with bicaval, SAX, and four-chamber views, it can also be confirmed with a TEE 3D reconstruction of the fossa from the left atria.
14. Under fluoroscopic guidance, slowly advance the needle to the distal tip while maintaining the sheath in place. In situations where there is a small left atrium chamber, fibrotic or lipomatous interatrial septum, presence of a surgical patch, or requirement for a precise puncture, the utilization of a diathermy surgical system or radiofrequency transseptal system (NRG RF transseptal kit, Baylis Medical Company) may enhance safety.
15. Crossing the septum is followed by the release of tenting and direct visualization echocardiography. Before the advancement of the sheath, confirmation of successful puncture into the left atrium can be achieved by monitoring the pressure, administration of iodinated contrast under fluoroscopy or microbubbles, or echocardiographic contrast.
16. Administer 100 U/kg of heparin, targeting an activated clotting time of 250–300 seconds.
17. Under TEE guidance, advance the entire system 1–2 cm into the left atrium.
18. Stabilize the needle together with the dilator, and gently slide the sheath over the dilator.
19. Slowly retrieve the needle and dilator.
20. Advance the guidewire into the left atria.

6. What transseptal needles are commercially available?

- The Brockenbrough needle is made of stainless steel and has a stylet inside the lumen to prevent injuries to the sheath. It is slightly modified from the original device with a tapered 21-gauge needle tip and a proximal end flange with an arrow that points to the needle tip.
- The adult BRK needle (Abbott Vascular) is a variation of the Brockenbrough and has a 19° angle between the distal curved region and the needle shaft. The adult BRK-1 needle has an increased curvature: a 53° angle between the distal curved region and the needle shaft. These needles are available in different adult and pediatric lengths (Figure 71.3).
- The NRG transseptal needle (Baylis Medical Company) uses radiofrequency energy (delivering 5–10W energy for two to five seconds) for transseptal puncture. It can increase the success rate compared to mechanical alternatives in challenging cases such as fibrotic septums. It can be used inside a TorFlex transseptal guiding sheath or a SureFlex steerable guiding sheath.
- A VersaCross RF wire (Baylis Medical Company) can be used, without exchanges, as a guidewire, a transseptal puncture device, or an exchange rail for delivering therapy sheaths (Figure 71.4).
- The TSP Crosser (Transseptal Solutions) is made of a stabilizing loop wire that locates and defines the fossa ovalis boundaries and a steerable system that allows pre-puncture steering and adaptation to the patient anatomy (Figure 71.5).
- The SafeSept needle-free transseptal guidewire (Pressure Products Medical Supplies) is a 180cm, 0.0315-in. diameter Nitinol guidewire with a sharp tip. When unsupported by a dilator and sheath, the tip of the SafeSept needle assumes a J shape, making it incapable of further tissue penetration (Figure 71.6).
- The SafeCross transseptal radiofrequency (RF) puncture and steerable balloon introducer system is a three-in-one system that includes a steerable introducer sheath with an ultra-visible positioning balloon and RF puncture dilator. The contrast-filled balloon is visible under echocardiography and X-ray to facilitate precise puncture site selection, while the bi-directional steerable introducer sheath allows for safe maneuvering and perpendicular placement on the septum (Figure 71.7).

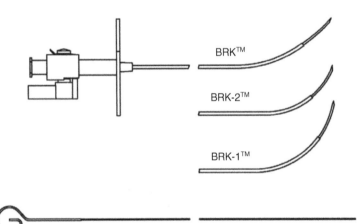

Figure 71.3 BRK needle with different curves. *Source:* Grayline Medical, Abbott Swartz Braided Transseptal Introducers - Swartz Braided Transseptal Introducers, BRK, 18G, 71 cm - 407200. Last accessed August 02, 2022.

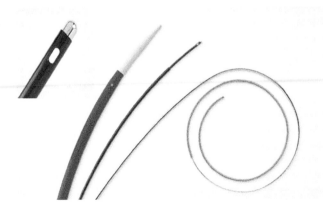

Figure 71.4 NRG transseptal needle and VersaCross RF wire. *Source:* Baylis Medical Company, Inc., https://www.baylismedical.com/products/nrg-transseptal-platform/nrg-rf-transseptal-kit/, last accessed July 28, 2022.

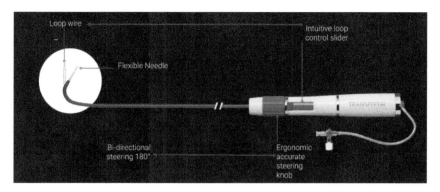

Figure 71.5 The TSP Crosser (Transseptal Solutions) is made of a stabilizing loop wire that locates and defines the fossa ovalis boundaries and a steerable system that allows pre-puncture steering and adaptation to the patient anatomy. *Source:* Transseptal Solutions, https://www.transseptalsolutions.com/, last accessed July 29, 2022.

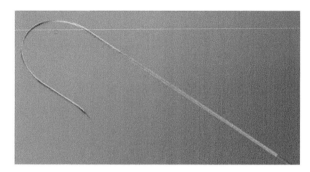

Figure 71.6 SafeSept needle-free transseptal guidewire (Pressure Products Medical Supplies). *Source:* Pressure Products Medical Supplies, Inc., https://www.pressure-products.com/wip/safesept.html, last accessed July 29, 2022.

7. What recent advances in imaging can assist with transseptal puncture?

Cross-sectional imaging modalities such as electrocardiogram-gated CT with 3D and 4D reconstructions allow detailed visualization of the heart structures and aid in the understanding of anatomical considerations, including the ideal location for transseptal puncture. Some centers use software that fuses fluoroscopic and 3D TEE images to guide structural procedures. TEE images are combined in real time with images from fluoroscopy to produce a single image. Fiduciary markers for the transseptal puncture can be added.

8. What are the most common complications associated with transseptal puncture?

The most frequent complications are cardiac tamponade, embolic events, and iatrogenic atrial septal defects.

Cardiac tamponade may result from these scenarios:

- Inadvertent manipulation of gear, particularly with premature protrusion of the needle over the sheath, leading to perforation of the right atrial free wall.
- Transseptal puncture through the intrapericardial space (stitch phenomena).
- Puncture of the left atrium free wall, typically when there is either a small left atrium chamber or abnormalities affecting the interatrial septum.

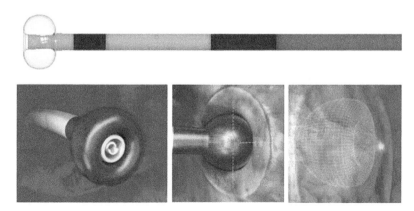

Figure 71.7 SafeCross transseptal radiofrequency puncture and steerable balloon. *Source:* East End Medical I LLC., https://safecrossdevice.com/, last accessed July 29, 2022.

- Hyperplastic septal tissue that can be stretched close to the left atrium wall or extreme fibrotic septum leading to high resistance to advancement of the equipment can lead to traumatic injury.

Embolic events may occur in the setting of inappropriate anticoagulation, heparin resistance, failure to appreciate intracardiac thrombus, poor de-airing of the system, or inappropriate injection of air.

Persistent iatrogenic atrial septal defects (iASDs) after structural transseptal interventions are not uncommon, especially when larger transseptal sheaths are used. Historically, the majority of residual iASDs following transcatheter transseptal interventions have been thought to close spontaneously and therefore have not been routinely closed. However, there is growing evidence that iASDs resulting from the placement of larger-diameter devices may persist beyond six months.

9. What is the stitch puncture complication?

The *stitch effect* is a rare complication where the needle pierces the intrapericardial space from the right atrial side and re-enters the left atria. This usually happens in extreme superior or posterior aspects of interatrial septum puncture. This complication may not be recognized until the sheath is withdrawn and a cardiac tamponade ensues after removal.

10. Is it always required to close the interatrial communication after every transseptal procedure?

No. The majority of procedures that involve a transseptal puncture, with the development of an iatrogenic atrial septal defect, do not require percutaneous closure. The clinical significance of the iatrogenic atrial septal defect will determine the need for closure. Patients with severe pulmonary hypertension, leading to a right-to-left shunt associated with hypoxemia, large residual defects (more than 8 mm) with high Qp: Qs, and increased risk for paradoxical embolism (history of DVT, prior cryptogenic stroke, presence of pacemaker lead) are the most frequent scenarios where percutaneous closure are indicated.

11. Is it feasible to cross the interatrial septum in the presence of a percutaneous septal occluder (PFO/ASD)?

Yes. The transseptal puncture can be performed around the device (if small). Most of the atrial occlusion devices are located in the anterior superior location; therefore, the puncture can be performed inferior or posterior to the device. In scenarios where devices cover the entire surface of the true interatrial septum, crossing can be carefully done through the occluder Dacron patches. This is not recommended if the occluder is a Gore CARDIOFORM Septal Occluder.

Bibliography

1 Cope, C. (1959). Technique for the transseptal catheterization of the left atrium: a preliminary report. *J. Thorac. Surg.* 37: 482486.

2 Ross, J. Jr., Braunwald, E., and Morrow, A.G. (1959). Transseptal left atrial puncture: a new technique for the measurement of left atrial pressure in man. *Am. J. Cardiol.* 3: 653–655.

3 Brockenbrough, E.C., Braunwald, E., and Ross, J. Jr. (1962). Transseptal left heart catheterization: a review of 450 studies and description of an improved technic. *Circulation* 25: 15–21.

4 Brockenbrough, E.C. and Braunwald, E. (1960). A new technic for left ventricular angiocardiography and transseptal left heart catheterization. *Am. J. Cardiol.* 6: 1062–1064.

5 Klimek-Piotrowska, W., Hołda, M.K., Koziej, M. et al. (2016). Anatomy of the true interatrial septum for transseptal access to the left atrium. *Ann. Anat.* 205: 60–64.

6 Mohamad Alkhouli, M.D., Mohammad Sarraf, M.D., David, R. Holmes, MD (2016). Circulation: Cardiovascular Interventions. 9(4).

7 Chen, K., Sang, C., Dong, J., and Ma, C. (2012). Transseptal puncture through Amplatzer septal occluder device for catheter ablation of atrial fibrillation: use of balloon dilatation technique. *J. Cardiovasc. Electrophysiol.* 23 (10): 1139–1141.

8 Honarbakhsh, S., O'Brien, B., and Schilling, R.J. (2017). A simplified trans-septal puncture technique using a needle free approach for cryoablation of atrial fibrillation. *J. Atr. Fibrillation.* 10: 1628.

9 Sherman, W., Lee, P., Hartley, A., and Love, B. (2005). Transatrial septal catheterization using a new radio-frequency probe. *Catheter. Cardiovasc. Interv.* 66: 14–17.

10 Smelley, M.P., Shah, D.P., Weisberg, I. et al. (2010). Initial experience using a radiofrequency powered transseptal needle. *J. Cardiovasc. Electrophysiol.* 21: 423–427.

11 Alkhouli, M., Rihal, C.S., Holmes, D.R. Jr. (2016). Transseptal Techniques for Emerging Structural Heart Interventions. *JACC Cardiovasc. Interv.* 9(24): 2465–2480. doi: 10.1016/j.jcin.2016.10.035. PMID: 28007198.

72

ECMO for Structural Interventions

Ali Ghodsizad[1], Matthias Loebe[1] and Tomas Salerno[2]

[1] Miami Transplant Institute, University of Miami Miller School of Medicine, Miami, FL, USA
[2] Cardiothoracic Surgery, University of Miami Miller School of Medicine, Miami, FL, USA

Following partner trials and recent trends, transaortic valve implantation/transaortic valve replacement (TAVI/TAVR) has become standard of care in different age groups. The significant frailty of structural heart disease patients has been an ongoing challenge and will remain so. Hemodynamic variability during the TAVR procedure may be challenging, interfering with end-organ perfusion. At any time during the procedure, challenging hemodynamics may cause low cardiac output and shock physiology. Critical steps are described in Table 72.1.

Peripheral or central venoarterial extracorporeal membrane oxygenation (VA-ECMO) should be considered as a rescue pump in such cases. One of the important aspects that the structural Heart Team has to consider is the maintenance of end-organ perfusion by timely communication, avoiding or limiting low coronary perfusion episodes.

Table 72.1 Critical steps during transcatheter aortic valve replacement (TAVR). Any time during TAVR, arrhythmia and cardiac arrest can happen. Understanding comorbidities and the frailty of TAVR and minimizing low cardiac output episodes remains a major goal.

- Pacemaker insertion
- Crossing the aortic valve (straight wire or pigtail catheter)
- Wire exchange using a pigtail catheter
- Crossing the aortic valve with the loaded device
- Deployment phase – using a balloon-expandable valve system
- Deployment phase – using a self-expandable valve system until the valve achieves annular contact and allows flow through the valve
- Pre- and postimplantation balloon-aortic valvuloplasty

1. What is the ideal access strategy to initiate VA-ECMO in TAVR patients?

TAVR patients have an established vascular access site during the entire procedure. When hypotensive episodes cannot be managed using IV medication, proactive management and decision-making are required. Once the patient requires advanced cardiovascular life support (ACLS) following asystole or pulseless electrical activity (PEA) arrest, VA-ECMO insertion becomes a far more demanding step. The main goal is to ensure femoral arterial and venous accesses as long as a pulse pressure can be recognized on the monitor.

2. What is the anticoagulation goal following VA-ECMO insertion and initiation?

In TAVR patients, the activated clotting time (ACT) is routinely used for anticoagulation management. ACT in TAVI patients is usually maintained at over 300. These patients already have therapeutic partial thromboplastin time (PTT) levels >70 seconds. Depending on how late myocardial and end-organ perfusion is restored, shock patients have a known risk of going into extensive disseminated intravascular coagulation (DIC). The structural team is advised to be more careful while applying additional IV heparin infusion, as extensive groin or neck bleeding may require mass transfusion. Transfusion-related acute lung injury (TRALI) and respiratory failure in patients with flash pulmonary edema usually worsen the expected outcome. Novel oxygenator

Mastering Structural Heart Disease, First Edition. Edited by Eduardo J. de Marchena and Camilo A. Gomez.
© 2023 John Wiley & Sons Ltd. Published 2023 by John Wiley & Sons Ltd.
Companion website: www.wiley.com/go/deMarchena/Mastering-Structural-Heart-Disease

technology allows for long-term ECMO support with low and intermittent IV heparin. A lower heparin dosage will also decrease the risk of developing heparin-induced thrombocytopenia (HIT), understanding that novel ECMO devices include heparin-coated cannulae and ECMO circuits.

3. What VA-ECMO flow goal should be maintained in adult patients?

In general, 55–60 cc/kg/min flows result in 3–5 l of flow/min in adult patients. Routine lactate levels should be monitored to confirm sufficient end-organ perfusion. The goal is to maintain lactate levels <10 mg/dl. Higher lactate levels have been associated with worse outcomes in our experience. Depending on hemodynamic instability, flow fluctuations can be challenging, and the perfusionist or bedside team has to be ready to administer an IV fluid bolus and/or IV inotropic and vasopressor support.

4. Following VA-ECMO insertion, is flow >5.5 liters/min indicated in adult patients?

Up to 5 l/min flows in VA-ECMO usually allow for sufficient end-organ perfusion, well reflected in fluctuations in lactate dynamics. Higher flows, maintained by VA-ECMO, can cause too much afterload and cause left ventricle (LV) overdistension. Understanding that peripheral arterial cannula insertion may interfere with peripheral limb perfusion, a limb reperfusion cannula should be inserted into the superficial femoral artery (SFA) distal to the arterial cannulation site. The cannulation site should be the common femoral artery (CFA), confirmed by using ultrasound and fluoroscopy.

5. Following balloon aortic valvuloplasty (BAV), the patient goes into extensive cardiogenic shock and requires CPR. How high should VA-ECMO flows be maintained?

Following BAV, there is usually significant aortic insufficiency (AI), and VA-ECMO flows should not exceed 2–3 l/min, as that can worsen AI in patients on peripheral VA-ECMO. It is critical to maintain sufficient coronary perfusion and end-organ perfusion until the valve can be successfully deployed. Considering the large number of cases that require pre-implantation balloon-aortic valvuloplasty,

a critical moment can be immediately post balloon-aortic valvuloplasty.

6. Will emergency sternotomy and open cardiac massage improve survival in case of cardiac arrest?

Open cardiac massage has not been shown to improve outcomes in patients undergoing ACLS. Considering that a fair number of TAVR patients have had prior sternotomy, emergency sternotomy is associated with hemorrhage and interruptions during CPR and may not be beneficial. While groin cannulation is performed, a second team can maintain ongoing CP, which is a very important aspect while performing ACLS.

In patients with no previous sternotomy and no groin access, experienced surgical teams may be able to establish central cannulation quickly and effectively. Central VA cannulation is associated with less peripheral vascular and thromboembolic complications and can provide better myocardial unloading. Usually a 32F dual-stage cannula or 2×28F straight venous cannula and a 17F arterial cannula can easily be used for central cannulation. An earlier application of peripheral VA-ECMO in a "crash and burn" case may prevent mechanical CPR, avoiding damage to the valve frame.

7. What is the preferred cannula size used for peripheral ECMO cannulation in CPR patients (ECPR)?

A 15–17F flat wound arterial cannula and 19–23F venous cannula are preferred choices for peripheral cannulation during CPR. The ideal cannula sizes to maintain perfusion in a 70 kg ideal patient are a 21F venous cannula and a 19F arterial cannula. Depending on the anatomy and urgency, inserting larger cannula sizes during CPR may cause peripheral limb ischemia, thromboembolic events, and extensive vessel injuries, thereby delaying maintenance of restoration of end-organ perfusion. A 15–17F arterial/21–23F venous cannula usually enables 2–3 l/min of VA-ECMO flow with acceptable line pressure.

8. What can be done in emergency situations during TAVR when no arterial access is easily available?

If no arterial femoral access can be secured using ultrasound, ongoing attempts should be continued while

ACLS is being performed. Ultrasound and transesophageal echocardiography (TEE) can be extremely helpful, as TAVR patients with excessive comorbidity may have excessive hypoxia before or shortly after requiring CPR, and observed arterial vessels may contain very dark hypoxic blood. Femoral vein access can usually be established even in the most challenging cases. When the patient is in cardiac arrest, even with two different access sites on each groin, or one groin and right internal jugular vein, it is advisable to establish ECMO flow even without identifying femoral vessels as vein and/or artery. Once ECMO flow has been established, unless two cannulas are positioned in the same arterial vessel, a reasonable color exchange can be observed. Providing venovenous extracorporeal membrane oxygenation (VV-ECMO) support to the patient with intended VA-ECMO support can be helpful. CPR helps maintain perfusion, while VV-ECMO support enables the delivery of oxygenated blood into the right atrium. Once better oxygenation is achieved, an arterial cannula can be added.

9. What is the inotropic management following VA-ECMO insertion?

The goal is to avoid an "inotropic holiday" during VA-ECMO support, effective myocardial unloading, and prevention of myocardial over-distension in patients with advanced cardiogenic shock. Endocardial ischemia must be avoided, and end-organ perfusion must be maintained. The goal is to always have the heart ejecting. Especially after BAV and before deploying the valve in the right position, there will be extensive AI, which causes increasing left ventricular end diastolic pressure (LVEDP). Flows sufficient to maintain mean arterial pressures (MAPs) >55 mmHg as long as no higher MAPs are needed to avoid cardiac arrhythmia (Figures 72.1 and 72.2).

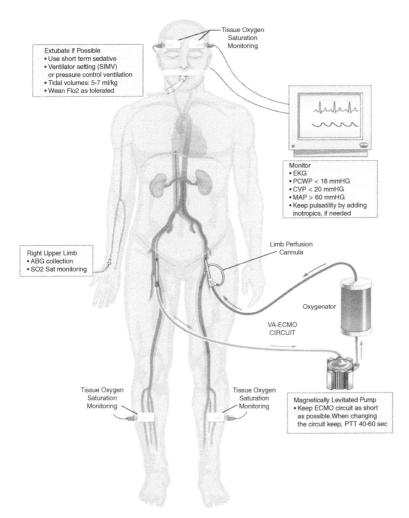

Figure 72.1 Venoarterial extracorporeal membrane oxygenation (VA-ECMO) in place as well as ECMO management details. Recent advances in ECMO circuits and smart oxygenator technology enable safe use of low anticoagulation. The goal remains to reduce the circuit length and minimize systemic inflammatory response syndrome (SIRS).

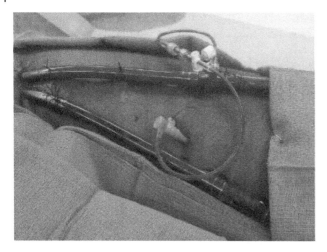

Figure 72.2 Venoarterial extracorporeal membrane oxygenation (VA-)ECMO cannula inserted using a 21F venous cannula and a 19F arterial cannula, as well as a 5F wire enforced antegrade limb perfusion cannula. The color exchange always confirms oxygenated blood going into the arterial system. *Sources:* Ekos Software Inc., INARI Medical, Penumbra, Inc., Thrombolex.

10. A TAVR patient with patent foramen ovale (PFO) presents with low cardiac output and hypoxia. What should be done?

Establishing VA-ECMO support in patients with PFO has been shown to prevent hypoxia. A 50 cm venous cannula is usually inserted into the femoral vein, and the tip is positioned at the level of the right atrium or inferior cavo-atrial junction. In hemodynamically challenging patients, shunting can be observed secondary to pulmonary hypertension, causing the flow of deoxygenated blood into the aorta. VA-ECMO can prevent such intermittent shunting of deoxygenated blood, helping unload the LV by venting through the PFO.

Bibliography

1 Alzaga-Fernandez, A.G. and Varon, J. (2005). Open-chest cardiopulmonary resuscitation: past, present and future. *Resuscitation* 64 (2): 149–156.

2 Ghodsizad, A., Koerner, M.M., Brehm, C.E., and El-Banayosy, A. (2014). The role of extracorporeal membrane oxygenation circulatory support in the 'crash and burn' patient: from implantation to weaning. *Curr. Opin. Cardiol.* 29 (3): 275–280.

3 Prasad, A., Ghodsizad, A., Brehm, C. et al. (2018). Refractory pulmonary edema and upper body hypoxemia during Veno-arterial extracorporeal membrane oxygenation-a case for atrial septostomy. *Artif. Organs* 42 (6): 664–669.

73

Best Practices for Mechanical Circulatory Support with Impella for Acute Myocardial Infarction Cardiogenic Shock and Selected Structural Interventions

William W. O'Neill[1] and Solomon A. Seifu[2]

[1] Division of Cardiology, Center for Structural Heart Disease, Henry Ford Hospital, Detroit, MI, USA
[2] Department of Medicine, Division of Cardiovascular Medicine, University of Miami Miller School of Medicine, Miami, FL, USA

1. What is the historical background of acute myocardial infarction shock intervention?

In the early 1980s, mechanical reperfusion therapy for acute myocardial infarction (STEMI) was developed to manage this morbid condition. Early feasibility trials conducted by Hartzler et al. in Kansas City, as well as O'Neill at the University of Michigan in Ann Arbor, demonstrated the feasibility of emergency percutaneous transluminal coronary angioplasty (PTCA) therapy for acute myocardial infarction (MI). In the mid-1980s, because of these interventions, approaches were taken to use PTCA for the treatment of acute MI causing cardiogenic shock. Early studies in the mid-1980s demonstrated that survival was substantially improved in patients with cardiogenic shock who were treated with early revascularization. Survival rates increased from 20% in a historical control to 50% in a study conducted by Lee et al.

Over a decade, there was interest in the performance of PTCA for acute myocardial infarction cardiogenic shock (AMICS); however, no randomized studies were completed until Hochman et al. conducted the Shock (Early Revascularization in Acute Myocardial Infarction Complicated by Cardiogenic Shock) trial. In this trial, early revascularization was shown to substantially improve survival for patients with AMICS. Initially, the study demonstrated no substantial improvement in survival at 30 days, but one-year survival was substantially improved. To date, this is the only randomized controlled study of AMICS with early revascularizations, and it has led to a 1B American College of Cardiology/American Heart Association (ACC/AHA) guidelines recommendation.

Since the publication of the Hochman study, no further randomized trials have demonstrated an improvement in survival. The field has basically stalled. In 2018, Scholtz et al. published a large European registry of patients treated with mechanical reperfusion for AMICS (Figure 73.1). Survival was substantially improved in 10 000 patients who were treated without shock. A mortality rate of under 5% occurred. However, when patients with cardiogenic shock were analyzed, those who had cardiogenic shock and no out-of-hospital cardiac arrest had 80% mortality. So, this demonstrates that in the last 30 years, there has been no improvement in the survival of AMICS patients. Reperfusion therapy has improved survival, but only to 50%. No further improvement has occurred because no other therapy besides primary angioplasty has been employed. The mainstay of therapy for patients with AMICS is the use of vasopressor therapy. When patients

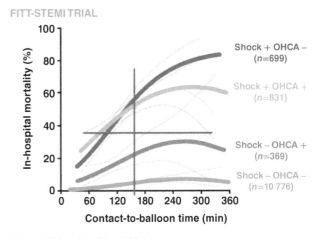

Figure 73.1   Fitt-Stemi Trial

report to an emergency room or become hypotensive in the intensive care unit (ICU), the first therapies offered are vasopressors and inotropes. Samuelson et al. demonstrated in 1999 that increasing doses of vasopressors increased mortality in patients with AMICS. We have confirmatory data that we will discuss further.

In addition to vasopressors and inotropes, clinicians have used intra-aortic balloon counterpulsation to treat cardiogenic since the 1970s. Numerous randomized trials have failed to prove the efficacy of this adjunctive therapy in decreasing infarct size or improving ejection fraction. The IABP-SHOCK (Intraaortic Balloon Pump in Cardiogenic Shock II) trial by Thiele et al. demonstrated that balloon pumps did not substantially improve survival in patients with AMICS. The mortality rate was the same at one year when patients were treated with balloon-pump support or control.

In summary, vasopressor therapy increases mortality, the balloon pump does not improve survival, and no other active therapies have been tested, so survival for these patients has not changed dramatically since 1987 (Figure 73.2).

More powerful circulatory support agents, specifically the Impella catheter (Abiomed), allowed for rapid transfemoral access and transvalvular left ventricular support for patients with AMICS. This device was approved in the United States in 2007 for general circulatory support, and subsequently, in April 2016, the FDA approved the use of Impella catheters for AMICS. There is now a great deal of interest in and enthusiasm for using these support devices for AMICS. An overview of the history demonstrates that between 1988 and 2016, very little improvement in survival occurred. More recently, the Detroit Cardiogenic Shock Initiative and the National Cardiogenic Shock Initiative have shown substantial improvement in survival in patients with AMICS who are treated with Impella mechanical circulatory support (Figure 73.3). These studies must be confirmed by randomized trials, but before randomized trials can be conducted, optimal use of mechanical circulatory support is required; to optimize the benefits, best practices needed to be determined. This is the topic of this chapter.

2. What hemodynamic variables help diagnose and optimize the treatment of cardiogenic shock?

First, the basic hemodynamic concept of cardiac power output (CPO) needs to be understood. This is the mean arterial pressure times the cardiac output divided by 451, and a normal value should be greater than 0.6 W. CPO represents watts of power. One watt of power is normal; less than 0.5 is associated with a significant increase in mortality. Fincke et al. demonstrated that a clear linear relationship with lower survival occurs in patients with lower CPO (Figure 73.4). Balloon pumps have not substantially improved survival because when hemodynamic data are calculated, CPO is not substantially improved with an intra-aortic balloon pump. Although diastolic pressure is augmented, forward CPO is not improved by more than 0.5 watts, which appears insufficient to improve survival.

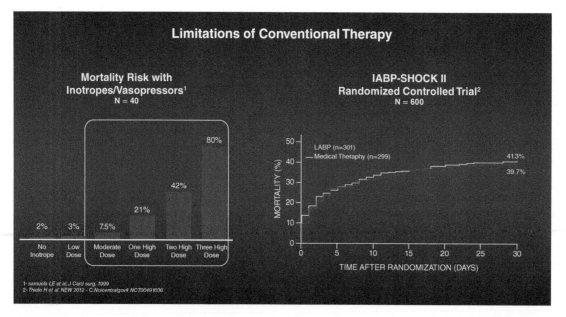

Figure 73.2 Limitations of conventional therapy. Graph in the left shows that vasopressor therapy increases mortality, it has a linear relationship with the dose requirements and the number of pressors used. Graph in the right from the IABP-SHOCK II, shows that balloon pump does not improve survival compared to medical therapy.

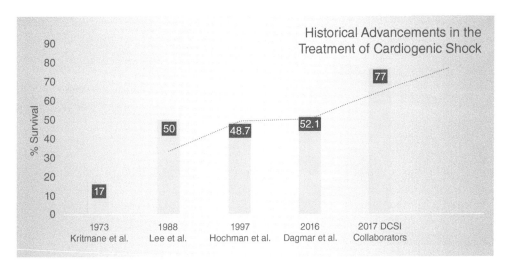

Figure 73.3   Historical advancements in the treatment of cardiogenic Shock. The Detroit Cardiogenic Shock Initiative (DCSI) has shown substantial improvement in survival in patients with AMICS who are treated with Impella mechanical circulatory support.

To optimize therapy in patients treated with mechanical circulatory support, an understanding of the hemodynamic power calculations of both the right heart and left heart is required. Again, the most commonly used term for left ventricular power is CPO. In addition, a pulmonary artery (PA) pulsatility index is calculated for right ventricular power. This is the systolic PA pressure minus the diastolic PA pressure, divided by the mean right atrial pressure, and a normal value should be greater than 2. When these numbers are abnormal, problem-solving must occur to maximize the benefit of the mechanical circulatory support devices.

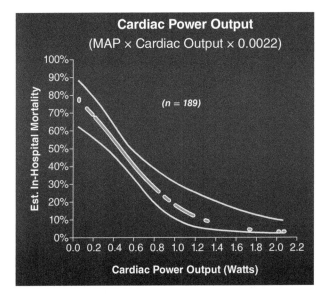

Figure 73.4   Cardiac power is the strongest hemodynamic correlate of mortality in cardiogenic shock. Fincke et al. demonstrated that a clear linear relationship with lower survival occurs in patients with lower CPO. Unadjusted estimated in-hospital mortality by cardiac power output (n = 189) with pointwise 95% confidence bands.

3.   What types of Impella devices are available for mechanical circulatory support?

A family of Impella catheters are available for circulatory support for both the left and right sides (Figure 73.5). The Impella 2.5 is a 9 Fr shaft that goes through a 13 Fr sheath and provides up to 2.5 l of flow per minute. The Impella CP also has a 9 Fr shaft through a 14 Fr sheath and provides 4.3 l of flow. Larger devices such as the 5.0 and the LD device are available for surgical cutdown and implantation; and the new 5.5 catheter, which is available for surgical implant, will provide 5.5 l of flow. In addition, the Impella RV uses a venous access with a 22 Fr sheath inserted in a femoral vein. That allows catheterization of the PA and right ventricular support by allowing flow to go from the right atrium across the pulmonic valve and providing flow for right ventricular failure. Thus, both right ventricular failure and left ventricular failure can now be supported with the Impella transvalvular pumps. The outcomes of 15 529 patients treated with AMICS in the US between 2007 and 2016 have been reported.

4.   What are the hemodynamic benefits of Impella devices?

The design of the Impella device allows superb hemodynamic improvement in patients with cardiogenic shock. It is a transvalvular pump in the left ventricle (LV), pulling blood from the LV through the aortic valve; thus, flow occurs in the normal direction of the cardiac circulation.

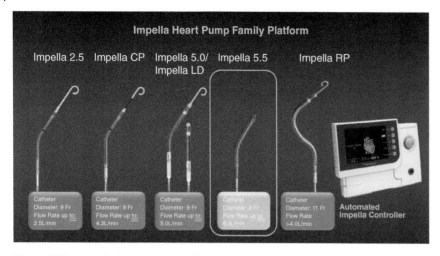

Figure 73.5 Impella heart pump family platform. Impella 2.5, Impella CP, Impella 5.0/Impella LD, Impella 5.5, Impella RP.

Hemodynamics have demonstrated that left ventricular and diastolic pressure and volumes are decreased. This decrease in end diastolic pressure and volume causes a marked decrease in wall tension, substantially decreasing myocardial oxygen demand. In addition, decreasing the left ventricular end diastolic pressure (LVEDP) while increasing aortic pressure increases the transmyocardial gradient to flow and improves oxygen supply to the ischemic myocardium (Figure 73.6). Finally, increasing forward cardiac output provides blood flow to the systemic circulation. The improved peripheral perfusion ameliorates the secondary complications that can occur from peripheral shock. The design is ideal for improving hemodynamics and metabolics in patients with AMICS.

Hemodynamic studies have demonstrated that the cardiac index increased by 1.9 liter per minute. Compared to an index less than 0.5 with a balloon pump, patients who are treated with an Impella have an increase in mean arterial pressure from 60 to 90 mmHg. They have a decrease in systemic vascular resistance from 2.2 to 1.5 and an improvement in wedge pressure from 28 to 21 mmHg; thus patients can have a forward increase in cardiac flow, an increase in arterial pressure with a decrease in systemic vascular resistance, and a decrease in wedge pressure ideal hemodynamics for patients who are in AMICS (Figure 73.7).

5. What are the invasive hemodynamic variables to identify right ventricular cardiogenic shock?

Right-sided involvement in acute MI shock occurs in up to 50% of shock patients. Classically, right ventricular failure and right ventricular shock occur when proximal occlusion of the right coronary artery proximal to the acute marginal

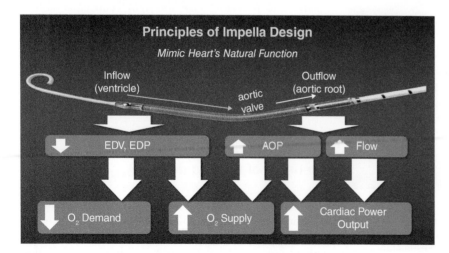

Figure 73.6 Principles of Impella Design

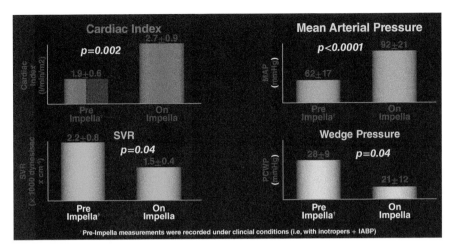

Figure 73.7   Impella improves immediately the hemodynamics in AMI shock. Decrease the cardiac index, there is a decrease in the systemic vascular resistance (SVR), an increase in the mean arterial pressure, and decrease in the wedge pressure.

branches occurs. Right ventricular infarction can be identified by the VR4 lead on the electrocardiogram.

When patients with acute inferior wall infarctions come into the hospital and are markedly hypotensive, or when their blood pressure (BP) drops dramatically with the use of intravenous nitroglycerin, then a high level of suspicion should occur for a right ventricular infarction. This can be rapidly confirmed by hemodynamics: a PA catheter is inserted, and right atrial, right ventricular, and PA pressures are calculated. Right ventricular failure can be defined as central venous pressure (CVP) >16, right atrial to pulmonary capillary pressure ratio of <0.8, or pulmonary artery pulsatility index (PAPI) ratio <1.

6.   How is cardiogenic shock with right ventricular infarction and failure clinically managed?

Right ventricular failure leads to right-sided congestion and lack of forward blood flow. The severe lack of blood flow to the left side causes severe hypotension. It is critical to identify these patients early on because the use of a left-sided support device with an Impella catheter may be suboptimal in acute right heart failure since there is inadequate filling of the LV. Patients present in relative hypovolemic shock. Bowers et al. demonstrated that acute inferior wall shock responds very rapidly to primary angioplasty. In 1998, he demonstrated that when patients are treated with acute primary angioplasty with successful reperfusion, the echocardiographic wall motions substantially improve quite rapidly: right ventricular function starts to improve within an hour of reperfusion and normalizes over a period of one to three days. Conversely, in patients who do not have successful reperfusion or have delayed reperfusion of

the right ventricle (RV), the RV remains remarkably impaired over the first week and then, over the first month, finally improves. So, patients admitted with acute right ventricular shock need support very early on: if successful reperfusion happens early, the RV will rapidly recover.

7.   Is mechanical circulatory support an option for cardiogenic shock related to right ventricular failure?

If profound RV shock occurs, Impella RP mechanical support often provides outstanding hemodynamic benefits. BP is dramatically increased, urine output increased, and vasopressor dosage decreased in recovered RV shock patients with acute MI shock who were treated with Impella RP, and survival was 50%.

It is important to emphasize that RV shock can also occur in the presence of left coronary occlusion. The intraventricular septum provides a large portion of the mechanical power of the RV. If the septum is akinetic or dyskinetic due to a left anterior descending (LAD) infarction, RV shock may develop. Recognizing RV shock is essential to normalizing hemodynamics. If RV shock is not recognized, persistent hypotension is treated with increasing doses of vasopressors, which raise the BP by activating alpha receptors. Importantly, not only are systemic alpha receptors activated – so are pulmonary alpha receptors. A failing RV faces a dramatic increase in pulmonary vascular resistance and ultimately fails entirely. Often, clinicians respond to this crisis by adding venoarterial extrcorporeal membrane oxygenation (VA-ECMO). This therapy can improve hemodynamics by bypassing the RV. Unfortunately, it does so at the expense of requiring two more large-bore access sites and the hematologic perturbations of the oxygenator. Early recognition of RV shock can circumvent all these abnormal hemodynamics, and RV Impella support can rapidly reverse unstable left-sided hemodynamics.

It is critical that the right ventricular catheter be placed in an appropriate position. The catheter is advanced over a guidewire into the PA. As it is advanced into the PA, it is gently torqued in a clockwise direction, and the catheter advances across the pulmonary valve. Once the catheter is in place, the device can be activated, and up to 4 liters of flow can occur with this device; this will dramatically decrease the patient's hemodynamics issues. Again, it is essential that RV shock is identified and treated as quickly as possible to optimize the benefit for the left ventricular device. Recently, Basir et al. have demonstrated that a specific pattern of diastolic suction occurs in the left-sided device when RV shock develops. In patients with substantial diastolic suction, mortality is more than doubled compared to patients who do not have diastolic suction. Thus it is critical to identify and problem-solve patients with RV shock so they can be optimally supported.

8. What is the role of right-heart catheterization in the management of cardiogenic shock?

To further understand and tailor therapy, it is essential that a right-heart catheterization be performed in patients who present in cardiogenic shock and are treated with the left-sided Impella. After the Impella has been placed in the LV,

a right-heart catheterization should occur, and the correct findings will help dictate further action that might be required (Figure 73.8). Once the right-heart cath is performed, cardiac pressures and cardiac output are calculated. CPO and PAPI should be calculated, and a CPO >0.6 and PAPI >1 demonstrate adequate right- and left-sided hemodynamics. These patients can then be watched in the ICU, and over a period of time, the support devices can be down-titrated and then removed. Usually this happens within the first 48 hours.

However, problem-solving is essential when the CPO is less than 0.6. Again, when a patient has a CPO <0.6, survival is markedly depressed, and immediate therapy is required. First you must determine whether the decrease in the forward flow of the LV is related to primary left ventricular dysfunction or right ventricular dysfunction. Specifically, patients with PAPI <1 should be treated aggressively, and strong consideration should be given to using the Impella RP device. This will allow for a decrease in vasopressors used in these patients. If the patient has right heart hemodynamics that are not severely depressed, then strong consideration should be given to upgraded left-sided support. The left side can be supported by an increase in the catheter from a 3.5 to a 5 liters device or by the use of ECMO in hospitals that cannot use a 5 liters device. In any event, hemodynamics must be optimized early in the course of patient therapy to improve survival. Ideally, the patient should leave the cath lab with a mean arterial pressure greater than 60 mmHg, CPO >0.6, and PAPI >1.

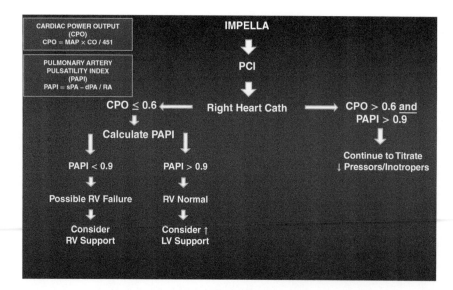

Figure 73.8 After the Impella has been placed in the LV, a right-heart catheterization should be performed. Carrdiac pressures and cardiac output are calculated. CPO and PAPI should be calculated, and a CPO >0.6 and PAPI >1 demonstrate adequate right- and left-sided hemodynamics. Abnormal values will help dictate further action that might required further mechanical support.

9. What is the optimal approach for a cardiogenic shock patient in the emergency room?

To optimize survival, a rapid, well-planned strategy is required for the treatment of patients with AMICS. The flow starts in the emergency department or the ICU when AMICS is first identified. These patients have a dramatic time-dependent gradient to survival. Ideally, these patients must be supported within 90 minutes of the onset of cardiogenic shock. Patients with chest pain, ST elevation, or ST depression and severe hypotension should be identified. Patients with BP less than 90 for over 30 minutes or needing vasopressors to maintain a BP of 90 should be considered in AMICS and rapidly transported to the heart catheterization laboratory.

10. What is the optimal approach for a cardiogenic shock patient in the cardiac catheterization laboratory?

Once the patient is prepped and draped, a sonosite-guided catheterization of the common femoral artery and femoral vein should occur. A pigtail catheter is advanced into the LV. If the left ventricular diastolic pressure exceeds 15 mmHg, LV support should be initiated. If the LVEDP is low, other causes of shock must be considered: in particular, RV shock must be ruled out. The Impella CP catheter is placed over the 14 Fr sheath, which should already be in place. Before the insertion of the sheath, femoral angiography is performed to ensure that the femoral vessels are large enough to accommodate the 14 Fr sheath. Once the Impella is properly placed and therapy is initiated, left-heart catheterization with identification of the culprit vessel occurs. Patients should have therapy of the culprit vessel; in addition, if other vessels have flow less than thrombolysis in myocardial infarction (TIMI) grade 3, they should be treated.

Recently, Lemor et al. demonstrated in the National Cardiogenic Shock Initiative that culprit vessel angioplasty can be safely performed and showed a trend of increased survival. This is counter to the randomized CULPRIT-SHOCK (Culprit Lesion Only PCI Versus Multivessel PCI in Cardiogenic Shock) trial, in which unsupported angioplasty in the setting of cardiogenic shock with multivessel therapy was associated with an increase in 30-day mortality. It is believed that patients supported with Impella have better hemodynamic support and less contrast nephropathy as a mechanism by which survival is enhanced compared to unsupported or balloon pump-supported percutaneous coronary intervention (PCI).

Once the PCI has been completed, the right-heart catheterization occurs. Hemodynamic evaluation is required for the assessment of both right- and left-heart function. If patients have adequate left-heart and right-heart function, they should be transferred to the coronary care unit. Prior to transfer, it is essential that the blood flow to the instrumented femoral artery be assessed. Patients cannot leave the cath lab with limb ischemia, which is associated with a marked increase in mortality. To assure adequate limb perfusion, a small contrast angiogram can be obtained through the repositioning sheath. After the flow is demonstrated, patients can be transferred; however, if there is any question, an antegrade femoral access for perfusion for the superficial femoral artery should occur. The instrumented leg should have an orthopedic splint placed so that the leg is immobilized so that the patient cannot move the position of the Impella catheter.

11. What is the optimal approach for a cardiogenic shock patient in the ICU?

In the ICU, the patient should have serial CPO determinations as well as serial lactate determinations at 6 and 12 hours. This allows analysis of the hemodynamic trajectory and status of the patient. Ideally, lactates that were elevated initially should continue to trend down and normalize within the first 24 hours; in addition, the CPO should increase to over 1. In this scenario, consideration of removing the Impella at 48 hours should be entertained.

12. What is the survival of cardiogenic shock?

When the Impella IQ registry was analyzed, 15 259 patients had been treated in the United States with AMICS between 2007 and 2016. When outcomes were analyzed, it was apparent that there was a large variation in outcomes of shock among the various centers (Figure 73.9). While the average survival was around 50%, many centers had significantly lower survival rates: one-third of the centers had survival of 23%, and one-third had survival of over 78%. There was a wide variation in outcomes because of the lack of consistency in the treatment of patients. When these data were analyzed, some factors were associated with a significant improvement in survival. The use of the PA catheter, the use of the Impella prior to PCI, and the use of the CP devices as opposed to the 2.5 devices were associated with better survival. These three best practices, in

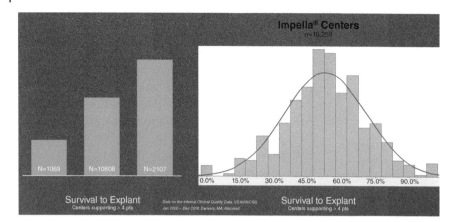

Figure 73.9 Impella IQ registry outcomes analysis. There was a large variation in outcomes of shock among the various centers.

addition to the rapid use of the Impella, were the basis for developing the Detroit Cardiogenic Shock Initiative/National Cardiogenic Shock Initiative.

In April 2016, upon approval of the Impella by the FDA for the treatment of cardiogenic shock, a group of investigators in Detroit began treating patients systematically. The five centers in Detroit initially started treatment of patients and demonstrated 78% survival. Improvement appeared to occur because of this systematic use of early catheterization, early Impella placement, systematic use of right-heart catheterization, and rapid down-titration of vasopressors.

This led to the development of the National Cardiogenic Shock Initiative (NCSI): 406 patients were enrolled in 80 participating hospitals, of which 32 of the hospitals were academic centers and 48 were community hospitals. The protocol is summarized in Figure 73.10. Patients are rapidly brought to the cath lab, hemodynamics are identified, the Impella is placed, and then angioplasty is performed. When the results were presented in 2021, the use of the Impella occurred prior to PCI in 72% of the cases. The door-to-support was 109 minutes, 90% of patients had established a TIMI 3 flow, and survival to discharge was 70%. One of the early observations was a dramatic impact of the Impella on patient survival after cardiac arrest. A total of 26 patients who were treated had active CPR at the time of insertion of the Impella, and of these 26 patients, 18 survived (69%).

In addition, Goldsweig et al. demonstrated that in patients with out-of-hospital cardiac arrest, survival of 85% occurred, and in patients with in-hospital cardiac arrest, a 72% survival occurred. These patients are in Class E cardiogenic shock, and the survival was outstanding. In addition, Hanson has demonstrated in the NCSI that survival is substantially enhanced when Society for Cardiovascular Angiography and Intervention (SCAI) classification is adjudicated. No patients were treated in either Class A or Class B (preshock); however, in patients with classic Class C shock, 76% survival occurred even in patients with significant deterioration. In Class D, shock survival was 76%; finally, for patients in extremis, such as those treated with active CPR, survival was 58%. When these data were analyzed and compared to two other databases (the Mayo Clinic database and the Schrage Acute MI database), it can be demonstrated that survival with the Impella is substantially improved in patients with severe levels of shock (Figure 73.11). A dramatic increase in survival in patients with Class E shock occurs. Thus, patients with the most important benefit for acute MI shock are those in the direst distress. This should be used in risk stratification for patients and deciding when mechanical circulatory support is considered.

While patients are actively supported initially, it is important to follow them over time. Substantial changes can occur within the first 12–24 hours. At 12 hours, it is important to reassess the patient in terms of whether lactate washout is occurring and whether CPO can be maintained. When patients have a lactate level less than 4 and a CPO greater than 0.6, they have 90% survival, whereas patients with CPO less than 0.6 and lactate that remains elevated have 29% survival. In patients who have impaired hemodynamics at 12–24 hours, escalation of care should be

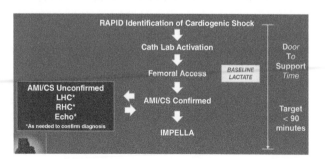

Figure 73.10 National Cardiogenic Shock Initiative (NCSI). *Source:* NCSI Investigators - September 2019.

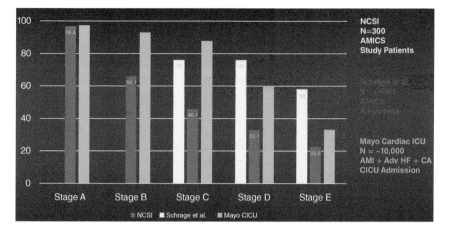

Figure 73.11 Survival based on the SCAI Shock in AMI-CS. The data comparison shows that when the NCSI data analyzed and compared to two other databases (the Mayo Clinic database and the Schrage Acute MI database), demonstrated that survival with the Impella is substantially improved in patients with severe levels of shock.

considered. Specifically, the escalation should be driven by the determination of the presence of right-heart dysfunction, left-heart dysfunction, or both. If the patient appears to have severe right-heart dysfunction, early placement of the Impella RP should occur; in patients with left-heart failure, upgrade from a CP device to a 5.0 device or even to a 5.5 surgical implant should be considered. If patients have combined shock and evidence of hypoxemia, ECMO can be added as a combination called ECpella. Ideally, these therapies should be initiated very early; once the patient improves, they can be down-titrated. If the patient remains in persistent shock for more than 12 hours, long-term survival is unlikely.

13. What is the impact on survival of vasopressors for cardiogenic shock?

Basir et al. recently reviewed the NCSI data on survival based on vasopressor use. Classically, it has been difficult to determine whether patients have a poor outcome because of high doses of vasopressors alone or because they require high doses of vasopressors due to severe hemodynamic compromise. Basir has calculated survival based on baseline CPO and found that when patients have a high CPO greater than 0.8, survival is diminished with increasing doses of vasopressors. In patients with a low CPO, vasopressor use dramatically increases mortality. Thus, it is likely that high doses of vasopressors independently increase mortality. Understandably, vasopressors cause an increase in heart rate, wall tension, and contractility, all of which dramatically escalate myocardial oxygen demand at a time when the myocardial oxygen supply is quite limited. For these reasons, vasopressors likely increase infarction size and worsen survival. Therefore, down-escalation of vasopressors as soon as possible should be associated with improved outcomes.

The NCSI has reported that patients treated in the medical arm of the SHOCK trial in 1998 had 44% 30-day survival; patients who were revascularized had survival of 53%. In the CULPRIT-SHOCK trial, survival was 57%. In the IABP-SHOCK (Intraaortic Balloon Pump in Cardiogenic Shock II) trial, survival was 60%. For all patients in the NCSI, survival is 68%; in Class C and Class D, survival is 77%. Thus, over time, survival is substantially improved compared to historical control and PCI supported with an intra-aortic balloon pump.

All of these data will require further confirmation. Currently, a large randomized trial is being planned: RECOVER IV. In this trial, patients will be randomized to the Impella-driven protocol discussed as a best practice in the NCSI trial. Patients will be rapidly identified and taken to the cath lab and have the Impella placed, after which stenting of the culprit vessels (or further vessels at the operator's discretion) will occur. Patients will then be transferred to the coronary care unit, where rapid de-escalation of support should occur; in patients requiring escalation of care, the Impella RP device will be used in patients with severe right-sided dysfunction, and LV support will increase to a 5.0 device. The control arm will be treated using the standard of care: currently, in the United States, the standard of care requires the use of PCI alone, potentially augmented by an intra-aortic balloon pump. If patients deteriorate and have further shock, then the control arm can be escalated to care with ECMO therapy. The primary endpoint will be six-month survival. It is hoped that this trial will prove that Impella support improves survival in shock; in addition, the The DanGer Shock trial will be completed within a year and a half. Thus two major studies aim to prove that Impella therapy improves survival. Until the publication of these trials, the best practices for using Impella appear to be associated with substantial improvement in survival compared to historical control.

14. Describe the National Cardiogenic Shock Initiative.

In April 2016, the FDA approved the use of Impella catheter for the treatment of acute MI shock. Investigators in the Detroit area gathered from St. Joseph's Hospital in Pontiac, MI, St. John's Hospital in Detroit, MI, the Detroit Medical Center in Detroit, MI, Providence Hospital in Southfield, MI, and Henry Ford Hospital in Detroit, MI. We initiated a region-wide initiative where patients were systematically treated using the best practices that have been previously determined. The three pillars of the practice were (i) early identification of patients with acute MI and use of the Impella as soon as possible to support those patients, (ii) using the Impella prior to angioplasty (pre-PCI angioplasty), and (iiii) rapid de-escalation of inotropic therapy once patients were supported.

Initially, a preliminary report from the group demonstrated an 80% survival rate for the first small subgroup of treated patients. The first major report was completed by Basir et al and included 41 patients with an average age of 65; 71% of patients were male. 27% of patients suffered from cardiac arrest, and 17% patients were under active CPR when the Impella catheter was being implanted. Before PCI, the CPO was 0.57W; after the Impella was implanted and PCI was performed, it was 0.95 (p < 0.01). Survival to explant was 85%, and survival to discharge was 76%.

Based on this initial report from the Detroit Cardiogenic Shock Initiative, the National Cardiogenic Shock Initiative was initiated: 83 hospitals throughout the United States and Canada agreed to use the same common protocol and the same common database in a single-arm prospective registry. Patients were recruited if they met guidelines of having cardiogenic shock, systolic BP less than 90, or use of vasopressors to sustain a BP of 90. Patients were also suffering from acute MI, and no other causes of shock were present. If patients met these criteria, they were treated systematically with rapid initiation of Impella support, use of the Impella prior to angioplasty, and de-escalation of therapy after they were adequately supported.

Between July 2016 and February 2019, 25 sites participated in the NCSI. A total of 171 patients were enrolled; they had an average age of 63, 77% were male, and 68% were admitted with acute MI shock. At the time of therapy, 83% of patients were on vasopressors for inotropes, 20% had a witnessed out-of-hospital cardiac arrest, and 29% had an in-hospital cardiac arrest. Catheterization was performed in 92% of patients, and 78% presented with ST segmented elevation of MI. Survival to discharge was 72%. The study was completed in December 2020. 300 patients had one-year follow-up data, and 406 patients were recruited. Survival continued to be over 70%; in particular, patients who had SCAI Class C and Class D had 75% survival. Thus, the NCSI investigators have demonstrated systematically that when patients are identified rapidly and a systematic protocol is used for early Impella support, survival of over 70% can be obtained.

During the NCSI registry, a total of 118 patients suffered cardiac arrest; this data was reported by Goldsweig et al. Investigators found that in patients who had out-of-hospital cardiac arrest, 85% survival was achieved, and in patients with an in-hospital cardiac arrest, 72% survival was achieved. Patients with out-of-hospital cardiac arrest have an excellent prognosis if they can be identified and treated rapidly. It is important to emphasize that patients who had prolonged resuscitation and had signs of anoxic brain injury at the time of evaluation were not included in the protocol.

15. What is the role of multivessel PCI in cardiogenic shock?

During the investigation, operators were requested to use their judgment concerning the treatment of non-culprit lesions. Initially, the treatment of the culprit vessel with stenting and establishment of TIMI 3 flow was required; if operators found that other vessels had interluminal thrombus that also appeared to be a culprit, those vessels definitely needed to be treated, especially if they had TIMI flow less than 3. Patients with other blood vessels identified could be treated, but it was imperative that less contrast be used and that the patient not have recanalization of chronic total occlusion. Lemor has demonstrated that among 300 patients with acute infarction in the NCSI, 198 patients had multivessel coronary disease and 102 patients had single-vessel disease. Patients with single-vessel disease had 74% survival. Patients with multivessel disease had lower survival; in patients where multivessel angioplasty was performed, 69.8% survival occurred, whereas patients with only culprit vessels and single-vessel disease had 65% survival. Importantly, there was no excess risk of contrast nephropathy in these patients. Thus the NCSI concludes that multivessel procedures can be safely performed and may allow for a trend toward improved survival. In the first 12 hours post-procedure, there seems to be a transient decrease in power output for these patients, and it is likely that distal embolization in non-infarct culprit artery occurs, but patients are adequately supported with mechanical support, so at 24 hours, they improve. These results will have to be corroborated by other investigators.

16. What is the SCAI classification of cardiogenic shock?

During the NCSI, the SCAI shock classification was published. This has been a major advance in risk stratification for patients with cardiogenic shock. There are five stages: A, B, C, D, and E. Classes A and B are considered pre-shock, meaning patients do not meet the hemodynamic criteria for shock. Class C is classic shock: BP below 90 or the use of vasopressors to keep BP above 90. Class D is for patients requiring multiple pressors, and Class E patients are in extremis.

This risk classification was employed by Hanson et al. for the 300 patients included in the NCSI: 61% of patients presented in Class C, 8% in Class D, and 31% in Class E. No patients in Class A or B were treated. Survival to discharge was 76% for Class C, 76% for Class D, and 58% for Class E. Thus it was apparent that survival was excellent for those patients who would have classically fit the protocol for a randomized trial. Class E patients in extremis had almost 60% survival. These data suggest that patients in extremis have an extraordinary benefit to survival (Figure 73.11).

Basir has reported that vasopressors used in patients significantly and independently increase mortality. In the report from the NCSI, the 400 patients who were treated were randomized, and an outcome was determined based on the CPO as well as the number of vasopressors. The overall survival for patients with CPO <0.6 was 77%, 45%, and 35% (p<0.02) when zero, one, or two inotropes were used. Similarly, survival was significantly lower in patients with CPO >0.6: 81% for no vasopressors, 72% for one, and 56% for two or more (p<0.01). Multiple linear regression analysis demonstrated that increasing requirements for vasopressors were independently associated with an increase in mortality (p<0.02); thus the rapid de-escalation of vasopressors was crucial for the long-term survival of patients.

Finally, Lemor et al. have published the impact of age on survival of patients treated in the NCSI. The first 300 patients who were treated were analyzed. Patients younger than 50 years old had over 97% survival. Patients between 50 and 59 years old had 74% survival, 60–69 had 68% survival, 70–79 had 61% survival, and older than 80 had 57% survival. Thus, the operators demonstrated that survival is dramatically impacted by age, but overall survival still appears to be excellent even in patients older than age 80. When SCAI classification was employed to analyze patients by age who were younger or older than 75, patients older than age 75 in Class E had 38% survival and in Class D had 50% survival. Thus, in elderly patients who are markedly compromised in Class E shock, strong risk/benefit consideration should be given to whether the patients should be aggressively treated. Conversely, it is imperative for patients under the age of 50 to be treated with maximal hemodynamic support.

17. What is the role of the Impella during aortic balloon valvuloplasty?

The Impella device can be used for hemodynamic support during balloon aortic valvuloplasty in patients with high-risk features. In particular, patients with severe multivessel coronary artery disease or severe left main disease will better tolerate the rapid ventricular pacing needed during valvuloplasty as a continuous blood flow through the Impella is guaranteed throughout the valvuloplasty procedure. There are theoretical concerns that the presence of the Impella device across the severely stenotic aortic valve might cause a reduction in the effective orifice area, but multiple reports have demonstrated that Impella implantation is safe and feasible in patients with severe aortic stenosis and may improve the tolerability of the procedure. The balloon valvuloplasty can be performed with the Impella device in situ across the aortic valve with no loss of function of the device. Once the aortic valve is crossed, the 0.018 Impella wire and a 5 Fr pigtail catheter are placed in the LV (Figure 73.12a). Then, over the 0.018 wire, the Impella device is advanced and placed across the aortic valve in a proper position and turned on to the appropriate level of support (Figure 73.12b). Once the Impella device is fully functional, the 0.035 wire is advanced to the LV through the 5 Fr pigtail. The pigtail catheter is removed, and the appropriately sized valvuloplasty balloon is advanced. The balloon is then inflated, and valvuloplasty is performed under rapid pacing while the Impella is fully functional (Figure 73.12c).

18. What is the utility of the Impella in transcatheter aortic valve replacement (TAVR)?

Sudden onset of severe hypotension in patients undergoing transcatheter aortic valve replacement (TAVR) can occur due to coronary artery obstruction, valve misplacement/migration, ventricular perforation, cardiac tamponade, severe paravalvular regurgitation, stunned myocardium, ventricular arrhythmia, and annulus rupture. In most such circumstances, a mechanical hemodynamic assist device can be used to stabilize the patient while the primary problem is addressed. The use of the Impella device for such indications with successful outcomes has been reported in the past. Impella device can also be used in patients with cardiogenic shock and severe aortic stenosis prior to TAVR.

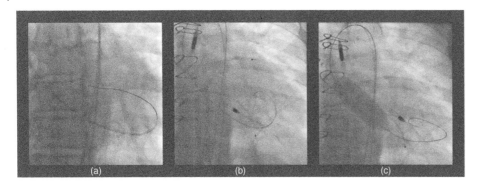

Figure 73.12 Hemodynamic support during balloon aortic valvuloplasty. A. Impella wire in the LV for the Impella device advancement. B. Impella device in the LV, in addition to a 0.035 stiff wire for the balloon advancement. C. Balloon inflation for aortic valvuloplasty with impella device.

19. What is the utility of the Impella in transcatheter edge-to-edge mitral valve repair (TEER)?

Acute mitral regurgitation caused by papillary muscle rupture or dysfunction during acute MI causes severe hemodynamic imbalance. Such patients have hypoxic respiratory failure and cardiogenic shock, making them unstable for acute surgical intervention. In such circumstances, left ventricular support with the Impella device can be used for initial stabilization. TEER can then be performed on critically sick patients once they are stabilized from the initial phase of shock. Case reports have shown that combined left Impella and TEER procedures can be an option for such patients.

Bibliography

1 Anderson, M., Morris, D.L., Tang, D. et al. (2018). Outcomes of patients with right ventricular failure requiring short-term hemodynamic support with the Impella RP device. *J. Heart Lung Transplant.* 37 (12): 1448–1458. https://doi.org/10.1016/j.healun.2018.08.001. Epub 2018 Aug 8. PMID: 30241890.

2 Basir, M., Taylor, A., Lemor, A. et al. (2020). TCT CONNECT-29 vasopressors have independent adverse impact on survival in patients with acute myocardial infarction cardiogenic shock. *J. Am. Coll. Cardiol.* 76: B13. https://doi.org/10.1016/j.jacc.2020.09.060.

3 Basir, M.B., Kapur, N.K., Patel, K. et al. (2019). Improved outcomes associated with the use of shock protocols: updates from the National Cardiogenic Shock Initiative. *Catheter. Cardiovasc. Interv.* 93 (7): 1173–1183. https://doi.org/10.1002/ccd.28307.

4 Basir, M.B., Schreiber, T., Dixon, S. et al. (2018). Feasibility of early mechanical circulatory support in acute myocardial infarction complicated by cardiogenic shock: the Detroit cardiogenic shock initiative. *Catheter. Cardiovasc. Interv.* 91 (3): 454–461. https://doi.org/10.1002/ccd.27427. Epub 2017 Dec 20. PMID: 29266676.

5 Basir, M., Gorgis, S., Lemor, A. et al. (2020). TCT CONNECT-176 diastolic suction alarms are an early marker for right ventricular failure in the setting of left ventricular mechanical circulatory support. *J. Am. Coll.* Cardiol. 76: B76. https://doi.org/10.1016/j.jacc.2020.09.189.

6 Bowers, T.R., O'Neill, W.W., Grines, C. et al. (1998). Effect of reperfusion on biventricular function and survival after right ventricular infarction. *N. Engl. J. Med.* 338 (14): 933–940. https://doi.org/10.1056/NEJM199804023381401. PMID: 9521980.

7 Fincke, R., Hochman, J.S., Lowe, A.M. et al. (2004). Cardiac power is the strongest hemodynamic correlate of mortality in cardiogenic shock: a report from the SHOCK trial registry. *J. Am. Coll. Cardiol.* 44 (2): 340–348. https://doi.org/10.1016/j.jacc.2004.03.060. PMID: 15261929.

8 Goldsweig, A.M., Tak, H.J., Alraies, M.C. et al. (2021). Mechanical circulatory support following out-of-hospital cardiac arrest: insights from the National Cardiogenic Shock Initiative. *Cardiovasc. Revasc. Med.* 32: 58–62. https://doi.org/10.1016/j.carrev.2020.12.021. Epub 2020 Dec 23. PMID: 33358390.

9 Hanson, I.D., Tagami, T., Mando, R. et al. (2020). SCAI shock classification in acute myocardial infarction: insights from the National Cardiogenic Shock Initiative. *Catheter. Cardiovasc. Interv.* 96: 1137–1142. https://doi.org/10.1002/ccd.29139.

10 Hartzler, G.O., Rutherford, B.D., and McConahay, D.R. (1984). Percutaneous transluminal coronary angioplasty: application for acute myocardial infarction.

Am. J. Cardiol. 53 (12): 117C–121C. https://doi .org/10.1016/0002-9149(84)90763-x. PMID: 6233873.

11 Hochman, J.S., Sleeper, L.A., Webb, J.G. et al. (1999). Early revascularization in acute myocardial infarction complicated by cardiogenic shock. SHOCK Investigators. Should we emergently revascularize occluded coronaries for cardiogenic shock. *N. Engl. J. Med.* 341 (9): 625–634. https://doi.org/10.1056/NEJM199908263410901. PMID: 10460813.

12 Kuchibhotla, S., Esposito, M.L., Breton, C. et al. (2017). Acute biventricular mechanical circulatory support for cardiogenic shock. *J. Am. Heart Assoc.* 6 (10): e006670. https://doi.org/10.1161/JAHA.117.006670. PMID: 29054842; PMCID: PMC5721869.

13 Lee, L., Bates, E.R., Pitt, B. et al. (1988). Percutaneous transluminal coronary angioplasty improves survival in acute myocardial infarction complicated by cardiogenic shock. *Circulation* 78 (6): 1345–1351. https://doi .org/10.1161/01.cir.78.6.1345. PMID: 2973377.

14 Lemor, A., Basir, M.B., Gorgis, S. et al. (2021). Impact of age in acute myocardial infarction cardiogenic shock: insights from the national cardiogenic shock initiative. *Crit. Pathw. Cardiol.* 20 (3): 163–167. https://doi .org/10.1097/HPC.0000000000000255. PMID: 33606413.

15 Lemor, A., Basir, M.B., Patel, K. et al. (2020). Multivessel versus culprit-vessel percutaneous coronary intervention in cardiogenic shock. *JACC Cardiovasc. Interv.* 13 (10): 1171–1178. https://doi.org/10.1016/j.jcin.2020.03.012. Epub 2020 Apr 29. PMID: 32360256.

16 O'Neill, W., Basir, M., Dixon, S. et al. (2017). Feasibility of early mechanical support during mechanical reperfusion of acute myocardial infarct cardiogenic shock. *JACC Cardiovasc. Interv.* 10 (6): 624–625. https://doi .org/10.1016/j.jcin.2017.01.014. PMID: 28335901.

17 O'Neill, W., Timmis, G.C., Bourdillon, P.D. et al. (1986). A prospective randomized clinical trial of intracoronary streptokinase versus coronary angioplasty for acute myocardial infarction. *N. Engl. J. Med.* 314 (13): 812–818. https://doi.org/10.1056/NEJM198603273141303. PMID: 2936956.

18 O'Neill, W.W., Grines, C., Schreiber, T. et al. (2018). Analysis of outcomes for 15,259 US patients with acute myocardial infarction cardiogenic shock (AMICS) supported with the Impella device. *Am. Heart J.* 202: 33–38. https://doi.org/10.1016/j.ahj.2018.03.024. Epub 2018 Apr 7. PMID: 29803984.

19 O'Neill, W.W., Weintraub, R., Grines, C.L. et al. (1992). A prospective, placebo-controlled, randomized trial of intravenous streptokinase and angioplasty versus lone angioplasty therapy of acute myocardial infarction. *Circulation* 86 (6): 1710–1717. https://doi.org/10.1161/01 .cir.86.6.1710. PMID: 1451242.

20 Patel, M.R., Smalling, R.W., Thiele, H. et al. (2011). Intra-aortic balloon counterpulsation and infarct size in patients with acute anterior myocardial infarction without shock: the CRISP AMI randomized trial. *J. Am. Med. Assoc.* 306 (12): 1329–1337. https://doi.org/10.1001/ jama.2011.1280. Epub 2011 Aug 29. PMID: 21878431.

21 Prondzinsky, R., Unverzagt, S., Russ, M. et al. (2012). Hemodynamic effects of intra-aortic balloon counterpulsation in patients with acute myocardial infarction complicated by cardiogenic shock: the prospective, randomized IABP shock trial. *Shock* 37 (4): 378–384. https://doi.org/10.1097/SHK.0b013e31824a67af. PMID: 22266974.

22 Samuels, L.E. and Darzé, E.S. (2003). Management of acute cardiogenic shock. *Cardiol. Clin.* 21 (1): 43–49. https://doi.org/10.1016/s0733-8651(03)00003-1. PMID: 12790043.

23 Scholz, K.H., Maier, S.K.G., Maier, L.S. et al. (2018). Impact of treatment delay on mortality in ST-segment elevation myocardial infarction (STEMI) patients presenting with and without haemodynamic instability: results from the German prospective, multicentre FITT-STEMI trial. *Eur. Heart J.* 39 (13): 1065–1074. https://doi. org/10.1093/eurheartj/ehy004. PMID: 29452351; PMCID: PMC6018916.

24 Stone, G.W., Marsalese, D., Brodie, B.R. et al. (1997). A prospective, randomized evaluation of prophylactic intraaortic balloon counterpulsation in high risk patients with acute myocardial infarction treated with primary angioplasty. Second primary angioplasty in myocardial infarction (PAMI-II) trial investigators. *J. Am. Coll. Cardiol.* 29 (7): 1459–1467. https://doi.org/10.1016/ s0735-1097(97)00088-0. PMID: 9180105.

25 Thiele, H., Akin, I., Sandri, M. et al. (2017). PCI strategies in patients with acute myocardial infarction and cardiogenic shock. *N. Engl. J. Med.* 377 (25): 2419–2432. https://doi.org/10.1056/NEJMoa1710261. Epub 2017 Oct 30. PMID: 29083953.

26 Thiele, H., Zeymer, U., Neumann, F.J. et al. (2012). Intraaortic balloon support for myocardial infarction with cardiogenic shock. *N. Engl. J. Med.* 367 (14): 1287–1296. https://doi.org/10.1056/NEJMoa1208410. Epub 2012 Aug 26. PMID: 22920912.

27 Unverzagt, S., Buerke, M., de Waha, A. et al. (2015). Intra-aortic balloon pump counterpulsation (IABP) for myocardial infarction complicated by cardiogenic shock. *Cochrane Database Syst. Rev.* 2015 (3): CD007398. https:// doi.org/10.1002/14651858.CD007398.pub3. PMID: 25812932; PMCID: PMC8454261.

28 Webb, J.G., Lowe, A.M., Sanborn, T.A. et al. (2003). Percutaneous coronary intervention for cardiogenic shock in the SHOCK trial. *J. Am. Coll. Cardiol.* 42 (8):

1380–1386. https://doi.org/10.1016/s0735-1097(03)01050-7. PMID: 14563578.

29 Londoño, J.C., Martinez, C.A., Singh, V., and O'Neill, W. W. (2011). Hemodynamic support with Impella 2.5 during balloon aortic valvuloplasty in a high-risk patient. *J. Interv. Cardiol.* 24 (2): 193–197.

30 Singh, V., Yarkoni, A., and O'Neill, W.W. (2015). Emergent use of Impella CP™ during transcatheter aortic valve replacement: transaortic access. *Catheter. Cardiovasc. Interv.* 86 (1): 160–163. https://doi.org/10.1002/ccd.25784.

74

Transcatheter Interventions for Aortic Valve Insufficiency in Patients with Left Ventricular Assist Devices

Gabriel A. Hernandez, JoAnn Lindenfeld and Sandip Zalawadiya

Cardiovascular Division, Department of Medicine, University of Mississippi Medical Center, Jackson, MI, USA

1. Describe LVADs and the current devices encountered in clinical practice

Left ventricular assist devices (LVADs) represent perhaps the greatest paradigm shift in the history of advanced heart failure (HF) therapies. Compared with the first-generation pulsatile LVADs, current devices have continuous flow (CF) and the benefits of being smaller in size with minimal or no bearings for improved durability. With the growing number of patients living with LVADs for a prolonged time, especially those implanted as destination therapy (DT), the burden of LVAD-associated adverse events, including the risk of aortic insufficiency (AI), increases.

The HeartMate II LVAD (HMII; Thoratec, now Abbott), a second-generation axial flow device, was the first CF device to receive approval for bridge to transplant (BTT) and DT. This device is no longer routinely used; however, it has been the most widely implanted LVAD. A third-generation system, the HVAD (HeartWare, now Medtronic), gained popularity due to its smaller size and intra-pericardial position; as of June 2021, this pump has been withdrawn from the market. Currently, the fourth-generation HeartMate 3 (HM3; Abbott), a fully magnetically levitated centrifugal-flow pump with intrinsic artificial pulsatility (interval change in speeds), is the only commercially available pump approved for use in advanced HF patients. Normal pump parameters are shown in Table 74.1.

2. What is the underlying mechanism for AI in patients with LVAD, and how often is it seen?

CF-LVAD often impairs the normal functioning of the aortic valve (AV), limiting its aperture and closure for each

Table 74.1 Left ventricular assist device characteristics.

	HeartMate II	HVAD	HeartMate 3
Pump type	Axial	Centrifugal	Centrifugal, full MagLev
Typical speed range, rpm	8000–10000	2400–3200	5000–6000
Flow, l/min	4–7	4–6	4–6
Lowest speed, rpm	6000	1800	4000
Speed adjustment increment, rpm	200	20	100
Power, W	5–8	3–7	4.5–6.5
Artificial speed change	N/A	Lavare cycle	Intermittent pulsatility

cardiac cycle, resulting in a non-physiological perfusion profile that manifests as minimal to no peripheral pulse. This phenomenon leads to asymmetric leaflet fusion and myxoid degeneration. Due to the constant ventricle unloading, which creates pressure changes across the valve, a pancyclic regurgitant flow, also known as a *blind circulatory loop*, is generated. Although small amounts of AI are generally well tolerated, more severe forms can lead to increased left-sided filling pressures and a reduction in forward cardiac output, which often results in end-organ malperfusion. With longer durations of LVAD support, there is a higher risk of developing and/or worsening AI.

During the first year of CF-LVAD support, the development of more than mild AI has been reported in up to 25–50% of patients, and the cumulative incidence of at least moderate AI is approximately 30% by the second year of support.

Mastering Structural Heart Disease, First Edition. Edited by Eduardo J. de Marchena and Camilo A. Gomez.
© 2023 John Wiley & Sons Ltd. Published 2023 by John Wiley & Sons Ltd.
Companion website: www.wiley.com/go/deMarchena/Mastering-Structural-Heart-Disease

3. Is post-LVAD AI preventable?

Prevention of AI starts at the time of LVAD implant with the surgical correction of more than mild AI. This can be achieved with a partial closure of the valve with a central stitch (Park's stitch or modified Park's stitch), complete closure with a circular patch (which should generally be avoided), or an AV bioprosthesis. Postoperatively, physicians should try to adjust the LVAD speed to maintain sufficient organ perfusion while keeping intermittent AV opening.

4. What interventions are available for LVAD-related AI?

Non-invasive or invasive hemodynamic ramp studies can be useful for optimizing speeds (AV opening and septal position) and evaluating the function of the right ventricle (RV). As a general rule, an increase in LVAD speed will ameliorate symptoms of low output but worsen pre-existing AI over time, ultimately leading to congestion and RV failure. Decreased speed may improve the AI severity but may lead to organ hypoperfusion. Diuresis and vasodilators can also be used judiciously to manage volume and afterload, respectively.

Figure 74.1 outlines the variety of management options for LVAD patients with AI. In general, direct heart transplantation (HT) is recommended for patients who are listed or are eligible to be listed; current United Network for Organ Sharing (UNOS) guidelines allow for a status upgrade (to status 3) for these patients. Any surgical or percutaneous intervention should be ideally done before there is evidence of RV failure.

Surgical interventions (the same as those described at implant time) are challenging due to the need for redo sternotomy, especially in this group of patients with significant comorbidities, which may render them at high peri-operative risk.

5. Which percutaneous interventions are available?

In the last decade, percutaneous interventions such as AV exclusion using an occluder device and transcatheter valve replacement (TAVR) have been used in an attempt to treat LVAD-associated AI. In a systematic review of 29 LVAD patients undergoing percutaneous intervention for AI (67% HMII, 25% HVAD, and non-specified system in the remaining patients) with a median duration of support of 423 days, the majority (72.4%) underwent valve exclusion with an occluder device (Amplatzer Cribriform Septal Occluder),

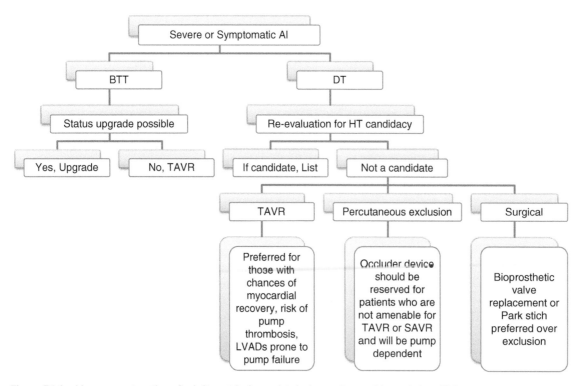

Figure 74.1 Management options for left ventricular assist device patients with aortic insufficiency.

whereas 9 patients (27.6%) received TAVR (50% Edwards Lifesciences SAPIEN, 37.5% Medtronic CoreValve, and 12.5% Medtronic Melody valve). Although AI improved in all patients, significant peri-procedural mortality (31%) and morbidity were observed during the index hospitalization; two patients developed hemolysis, and two device migrations into the ventricle occurred with the occluder device. Among patients who underwent TAVR, one patient developed significant perivalvular leakage, and two had device migration (one patient required surgical explanation and AV suture, and the other required percutaneous valve-in-valve placement); interestingly, all three complications occurred with the self-expanding valve.

It is important to mention that AV exclusion with an occluder makes the patient completely dependent upon the LVAD flow, and if the pump is compromised (for example, thrombus, electromechanical fault or controller exchange, etc.), the patient will not have forward perfusion. For that reason, the complete exclusion of the AV valve is not recommended for patients being bridged to transplant or with potential myocardial recovery.

6. What technical considerations are important and differ from non-LVAD TAVR?

There are no standardized technical considerations for TAVR in LVAD patients. We suggest that valve sizing should be done according to the expertise of each center and/or interventionalist (computed tomography scan and/or transesophageal echocardiography).

One key concept to remember is that aortic stenosis is far better tolerated in LVAD patients than in AI; a restricted valve tends not to be a problem (i.e. need for valve-in-valve). The biggest limitation for TAVR is adequate valve sizing to allow anchoring in patients without significant leaflets or annular calcification.

Even though self-expandable valves may offer an advantage at the time of deployment compared to balloon-expandable valves, given less risk of suction and the possibility of valve recapture, no data are available to support this practice. On the contrary, prior reports showed that self-expandable valves were more prone to migration.

In our unpublished experience with six consecutive patients (four HVAD, two HMII) who underwent self-expandable valves (29–34 mm CoreValve Evolut R), there were no significant procedural complications. The first case required recapturing of the CoreValve due to deeper migration when the patient was paced at 180 bpm; subsequent cases were done with no pacing or pacing at 120 bpm (Figure 74.2).

Some considerations to have in mind during the procedure:

- Flow through all CF-LVADs is directly proportional to pump speed and inversely related to the pressure gradient across the inlet (LV) and outlet (aorta). At a given pump speed, pump flow increases as the pressure gradient across the inflow and outflow cannula decreases (i.e. systole). When rapid pacing is performed, the native cardiac output and aortic-to-ventricular pressure gradient decrease (due to shortening of diastolic time), leading to enhanced LVAD flows, which can ultimately cause more suction. In our experience, pacing at 120 bpm seems sufficient to achieve adequate self-expandable valve positioning.
- We suggest lowering the LVAD speed to the minimum allowed parameter (see Table 74.1) for the shortest period (while maintaining appropriate anticoagulation) to minimize device suction. If an HVAD is used, we also recommend turning off the Lavare cycle (artificial speed changes for circuit washing) during the procedure to avoid sudden changes in flows.

Recently, Yehya et al. reported their experience with self-expandable valves (CoreValve or Evolut R) in nine HMII patients with more than moderate AI. They reported that no speed adjustments were made at the time of deployment (speed was adjusted only in the first two cases) and rapid pacing was performed (180 bpm), and they recommended letting the valve sit for 10 minutes at 75% deployment before full release. They successfully

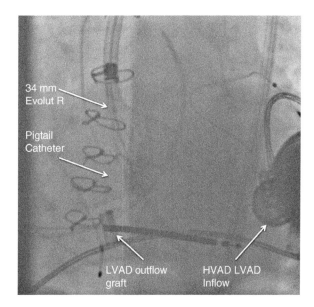

Figure 74.2 Transcatheter intervention for severe aortic insufficiency using a 34 mm CoreValve Evolut R on a patient supported with an HVAD left ventricular assist device.

eliminated AI in all patients. In two patients, the 31 mm CoreValve migrated toward the ventricle and required emergent snaring and a valve-in-valve. It is important to mention that the HMII pump, being an axial pump, has a different HQ curve (flow/pressure gradient behavior) than centrifugal pumps.

Bibliography

1 Cowger, J., Rao, V., Massey, T. et al. (2015). Comprehensive review and suggested strategies for the detection and management of aortic insufficiency in patients with a continuous-flow left ventricular assist device. *J. Heart Lung Transplant.* 34 (2): 149–157. https://doi.org/10.1016/j.healun.2014.09.045.

2 Cowger, J.A., Aaronson, K.D., Romano, M.A. et al. (2014). Consequences of aortic insufficiency during long-term axial continuous-flow left ventricular assist device support. *J. Heart Lung Transplant.* 33 (12): 1233–1240. https://doi.org/10.1016/j.healun.2014.06.008.

3 Feldman, D., Pamboukian, S.V., Teuteberg, J.J. et al. (2013). The 2013 International Society for Heart and Lung Transplantation guidelines for mechanical circulatory support: executive summary. *J. Heart Lung Transplant.* 32 (2): 157–187. https://doi.org/10.1016/j.healun.2012.09.013.

4 Fried, J.A., Nazif, T.M., and Colombo, P.C. (2019). A new frontier for TAVR: aortic insufficiency in CF-LVAD patients. *J. Heart Lung Transplant.* 38 (9): 927–929. https://doi.org/10.1016/j.healun.2019.06.024.

5 Goodwin, M.L., Bobba, C.M., Mokadam, N.A. et al. (2020). Continuous-flow left ventricular assist devices and the aortic valve: interactions, issues, and surgical therapy. *Curr. Heart Fail. Rep.* 17 (4): 97–105. https://doi.org/10.1007/s11897-020-00464-0.

6 Holtz, J. and Teuteberg, J. (2014). Management of aortic insufficiency in the continuous flow left ventricular assist device population. *Curr. Heart Fail. Rep.* 11 (1): 103–110. https://doi.org/10.1007/s11897-013-0172-6.

7 Jorde, U.P., Uriel, N., Nahumi, N. et al. (2014). Prevalence, significance, and management of aortic insufficiency in continuous flow left ventricular assist device recipients. *Circ. Heart Fail.* 7 (2): 310–319. https://doi.org/10.1161/CIRCHEARTFAILURE.113.000878.

8 Mehra, M.R., Uriel, N., Naka, Y. et al. (2019). A fully magnetically levitated left ventricular assist device — final report. *N. Engl. J. Med.* 380 (17): 1618–1627. https://doi.org/10.1056/nejmoa1900486.

9 Molina, E.J., Shah, P., Kiernan, M.S. et al. (2021). The Society of Thoracic Surgeons Intermacs 2020 annual report. *Ann. Thorac. Surg.* 111 (3): 778–792. https://doi.org/10.1016/j.athoracsur.2020.12.038.

10 Pal, J.D., McCabe, J.M., Dardas, T. et al. (2016). Transcatheter aortic valve repair for management of aortic insufficiency in patients supported with left ventricular assist devices. *J. Card. Surg.* 31 (10): 654–657. https://doi.org/10.1111/jocs.12814.

11 Patel, A.C., Dodson, R.B., Cornwell, W.K. et al. (2017). Dynamic changes in aortic vascular stiffness in patients bridged to transplant with continuous-flow left ventricular assist devices. *JACC Heart Fail.* 5 (6): 449–459. https://doi.org/10.1016/j.jchf.2016.12.009.

12 Phan, K., Haswell, J.M., Xu, J. et al. (2017). Percutaneous transcatheter interventions for aortic insufficiency in continuous-flow left ventricular assist device patients: a systematic review and meta-analysis. *ASAIO J.* 63 (2): 117–122. https://doi.org/10.1097/MAT.0000000000000447.

13 Sacks, C.A., Jarcho, J.A., and Curfman, G.D. (2014). Paradigm shifts in heart-failure therapy — a timeline. *N. Engl. J. Med.* 371 (11): 989–991. https://doi.org/10.1056/nejmp1410241.

14 Sayer, G., Sarswat, N., Kim, G.H. et al. (2017). The hemodynamic effects of aortic insufficiency in patients supported with continuous-flow left ventricular assist devices. *J. Card. Fail.* 23 (7): 545–551. https://doi.org/10.1016/j.cardfail.2017.04.012.

15 Yehya, A., Rajagopal, V., Meduri, C. et al. (2019). Short-term results with transcatheter aortic valve replacement for treatment of left ventricular assist device patients with symptomatic aortic insufficiency. *J. Heart Lung Transplant.* 38 (9): 920–926. https://doi.org/10.1016/j.healun.2019.03.001.

Index

Page locators in **bold** indicate tables. Page locators in *italics* indicate figures. This index uses letter-by-letter alphabetization.

a

AA *see* aortic angle
abdominal aortic aneurysm
  optimal selection of TAVR
    devices, 57
  transfemoral access, 173, *175*
AccuCinch system, 323, *323*
ACD *see* arteriotomy closure devices
ACP *see* Amplatzer Cardiac Plug
activated clotting time (ACT),
    64, 567–568
ACTIVATION trial, 110–111
ACURATE *neo* valve
  challenging anatomy scenarios
    in TAVR, 78
  native aortic valve
    regurgitation, 90–91
  optimal selection of TAVR
    devices, 51
  present generation of THVs, 34, *34*
  transfemoral access, 170
acute kidney injury (AKI), 111
acute limb ischemia, 187–188
acute mitral regurgitation (MR),
    227, 531
acute myocardial infarction cardiogenic
    shock (AMICS), 571–584
  balloon aortic valvuloplasty, 581, *582*
  hemodynamics, 572–573, *573*
  historical development,
    571–572, *571–572*
  Impella mechanical circulatory
    support, 572, 573–582, *573–574*
  multivessel PCI, 580
  National Cardiogenic Shock
    Initiative, 578–581
  optimal approaches, 577

percutaneous transluminal coronary
    angioplasty, 571
right-heart catheterization, 576, *576*
right ventricular infarction/
    failure, 575–576
Society for Cardiovascular
    Angiography and Intervention,
    578, 581
survival rates, 577–579, *578–579*
transcatheter aortic valve
    replacement, 581
transcatheter edge-to-edge mitral
    valve repair, 582
vasopressor therapy, 571–572, *572*,
    579, 581
acute procedural success (APS), 251
acute pulmonary embolism
  acute PE vs. chronic PE
    treatment, 554–555
  anticoagulation for high-risk
    submassive PE, 547–548
  anticoagulation therapy, 556, 558
  available devices, 553–554, *554*
  catheter-directed thrombolysis in
    massive PE, 550–551
  catheter-directed thrombolysis in
    submassive PE, 548, **549**
  catheter placement technique,
    555–556
  data and indications, 547–552
  devices and techniques, 553–559
  endpoints for percutaneous
    thrombectomy, 556–557
  follow-up, 558
  hemodynamically unstable patients,
    557–558
  infusion length, 556

large-bore aspiration, 556, *557*
mechanical thrombectomy in
    submassive PE, 550
outcomes with CDL-US vs. standard
    CDL, 548–550
patient selection, 555, *555*
risk-stratification, 547
role of PE response teams, 551
safety of interventional
    treatment, 555
thrombus in transit, 558
adjunctive repair, 340
adjunct pharmacology, 100
AFMR *see* atrial functional mitral
    regurgitation
air embolism
  complications from MitraClip
    procedure, 282–284
  left atrial appendage occlusion, 451
  patent foramen ovale closure, 488
AKI *see* acute kidney injury
alcohol septal ablation (ASA)
  artery selection, 464–465
  atrioventricular block, 464
  catheter and contrast media
    specifications, 465
  complications and long-term
    outcomes, 464
  conduction system abnormalities, 463
  determinants of success, 465–466
  hemodynamics in adult structural
    heart disease, 532–533
  hypertrophic cardiomyopathy, 461,
    463–466, 467–470, **469**
  patient selection, 463
  post-procedural monitoring, 463–464
  stepwise procedure, 464

ALLEGRA valve, 34

AMICS *see* acute myocardial infarction cardiogenic shock

Amplatzer Atrial Septal Occluder, 494, *494–495*

Amplatzer Cardiac Plug (ACP), 433–434

Amplatzer Cribiform Septal Occluder, 494, *494*

Amplatzer Ductus Occluder I/II, 500, 502, *502*

Amplatzer Muscular Occluder, 499, *502*

Amplatzer Perimembranous Septal Occluder, 502, *502*

Amplatzer PFO Occluder, 485–489, *486*, **487**

Amulet device, 433–437, *436*, *438*, 445–446

anchor wire technique, 413

angina, 3–4, 6, 538

angiography
    acute myocardial infarction cardiogenic shock, 581, *582*
    acute pulmonary embolism, *557*
    alternative access, 178–179, *180*
    aortic paravalvular leak closure, *398*, *400*
    caval valve implantation, 391–392, *392*
    coronary artery disease, 109
    coronary artery fistulas, 536, 537, *538*
    left atrial appendage occlusion, *446*
    percutaneous pulmonary valve replacement, 517–518, *518–519*, *521–522*
    structural mitral valve interventions, 243, *243*
    TAVR-related stroke, *159*
    transcatheter aortic valve replacement, 33
    ventricular septal defect closure, 500, *501*
    see also fluoroscopy; *individual modalities*

AngioVac system, 553–554

annular calcification, 75, 270

annular evaluation/sizing
    bicuspid aortic valve, 85
    challenging anatomy scenarios in TAVR, 77

computed tomography for TAVR planning, 40–41, *41*, 48

mechanical complications of TAVR, 131, 137

optimal selection of TAVR devices, 53

annular reduction/reshaping, 354, 357

annular rupture, 41, 131–133, *132*

antegrade venous access, 537, *538*

anterograde transseptal approach, 408, *409*

anti-calcification technology, 32

anticoagulation therapy
    acute pulmonary embolism, 547–548, 556, 558
    ECMO for structural interventions, 567–568
    left atrial appendage occlusion, 417–420, 435, 450, 453–454
    mechanical complications of TAVR, 133
    mitral regurgitation, 198
    mitral stenosis, 195
    patent foramen ovale closure, 488
    pathology of valve degeneration and thrombosis, 141
    TAVR-related stroke, 158
    transcatheter mitral valve replacement, 306–307
    valve thrombosis and early thickening, 151–153

antiplatelet therapy
    left atrial appendage occlusion, 435
    TAVR-related stroke, 158
    transcatheter mitral valve replacement, 306–307
    valve thrombosis and early thickening, 151–152

antithrombotic therapy
    interatrial shunt devices, 473
    left atrial appendage occlusion, 435–436, 453

aortic aneurysm
    challenging anatomy scenarios in TAVR, 79
    percutaneous treatment of aortic coarctation, 512
    transfemoral access, 173, *173*

aortic angle (AA), 53, 56, 76, 84–85, *84*

aortic coarctation
    associated conditions, 505

balloon angioplasty procedure, 508–509, *510*

clinical presentation, 505

complications, 512

diagnostic imaging, 505–506, *506–508*

follow-up, 512–513

percutaneous treatment, 505–514

short- and long-term results, 513

stent placement, 509–512, *511*

transcatheter intervention types, 506–508, *508*, **509**

aortic dissection, 512

aortic paravalvular leak closure, 397–401
    available devices, 399
    complications, 400, *400*
    crossing the PVL defect, 397, *398*
    delivering occluder device, 397–399, *398*
    indications and contraindications, 397
    negotiating uncrossable defects, 99
    post-transcatheter aortic valve replacement, 399–400
    pre-procedural planning, 397, *398*

aortic regurgitation (AR), 6–9
    chronic aortic regurgitation, 7
    diagnosis, 7–8
    ECMO for structural interventions, 568
    etiology, 6–7, 11, **12**
    hemodynamics, 7, *8*
    indications and treatment, 8
    left ventricular assist device-related AI, 585–588
    percutaneous mitral valve intervention, 246
    prognosis, 8
    severe acute aortic regurgitation, 8–9
    severe aortic regurgitation, 7, **7**
    symptoms and physical signs, 7
    transcatheter aortic valve implantation, 27
    see also native aortic valve regurgitation

aortic root rupture
    challenging anatomy scenarios in TAVR, 76–77
    mechanical complications of TAVR, 131, 133
    valve-in-valve TAVR, 81

aortic stenosis (AS), 3–6
  bicuspid aortic valve, 83–87
  diagnosis, 5, *5–6*
  etiology, 3
  hemodynamics, 3–5
  hemodynamics in adult structural
      heart disease, 525–529, *526–529*
  indications and treatment, 6
  low-flow aortic stenosis, 5–6
  normal aortic valve anatomy, 11
  prognosis, 6
  severity grading, 3, **4**
  symptoms and physical signs,
      3–5, *4*
  transcatheter aortic valve
      implantation, 19–29
  transfemoral access, 169–170, *170*
  see also calcific aortic stenosis; severe
      aortic stenosis
aortic valve area (AVA)
  aortic stenosis, 3, **4**, 5
  balloon aortic valvuloplasty, 69
aortic valve calcium score, 39–40
APOLLO trial, 248
APS *see* acute procedural success
AR *see* aortic regurgitation
arterial dissection, 187
arterial hypertension, 541–545
arterial perforation, 187
arteriotomy closure devices (ACD),
      185, *186*
arteriovenous (AV) fistula, 477, 482
ARTO system, 322
AS *see* aortic stenosis; atrial
      septostomy
ASA *see* alcohol septal ablation; atrial
      septal aneurysm
ascending aorta, 41–42, *42–43*
ascending aortic aneurysm, 79
ASD *see* atrial septal defect
aspirin
  interatrial shunt devices, 473
  left atrial appendage occlusion, 436
  valve thrombosis and early
      thickening, 151
atrial arrhythmias, 490
atrial decalcification, 229
atrial fibrillation (AF)
  hemodynamics in adult structural
      heart disease, 526, 531–532
  left atrial appendage occlusion,
      417, 449

mitral stenosis, 195
  surgical techniques for mitral valve
      repair, 233
  TAVR-related stroke, 157–158
  valve thrombosis and early
      thickening, 152
atrial functional mitral regurgitation
      (AFMR), 207–208, *208*
atrial septal aneurysm (ASA),
      485–486, 488
atrial septal defect (ASD)
  available devices for closure,
      493–494, *494–495*
  closure, 493–498
  complications from MitraClip
      procedure, 288–289
  device embolization, 497–498
  edge-to-edge mitral valve
      repair, 259
  indications and contraindications for
      closure, 493
  interatrial shunt devices, 471–473
  late complications post-closure, 498
  left atrial appendage occlusion, 445
  multiple defects, 497
  orientation in relation to IAS,
      496–497, *496–497*
  patent foramen ovale
      closure, 488–490
  pre-closure imaging, 494–495
  shunt hemodynamics and
      calculations, 477, 479–480, **480**
  surgical trials in mitral valvular
      disease, 230
  technique for ASD closure,
      495–496
  transseptal puncture, 566
  transseptal transcatheter mitral
      valve-in-valve replacement, 314
atrial septostomy (AS)
  interatrial shunt devices, 471
  transseptal transcatheter mitral
      valve-in-valve replacement,
      312–313, *313*
atrioventricular (AV) block, 464
atrioventricular (AV) bundle,
      123–124, *124*, 126–127
ATTR *see* transthyretin cardiac
      amyloidosis
auscultation, 4–5
AV *see* arteriovenous; atrioventricular
AVA *see* aortic valve area

b
balloon angioplasty, 506–507, 508–509,
      509, *510*, 513
balloon aortic valvuloplasty (BAV),
      69–73
  acute myocardial infarction
      cardiogenic shock, 581, *582*
  balloon size, 70
  balloon types, 70
  crossing stenotic aortic valve, 70–71
  ECMO for structural
      interventions, 568
  goals and defining success, 69
  hemodynamic assistance, 72
  incidence of complications, 70
  indications and
      contraindications, 69, **70**
  low-flow, low-gradient aortic
      stenosis, 71
  post-procedure care, 72
  reducing cardiac complications of
      non-cardiac surgery, 71
  role as TAVR adjunct, 71
  stabilizing balloon during
      inflation, 71
balloon-assisted technique (BAT),
      496–497, *497*
balloon-expandable valves (BEV)
  bicuspid aortic valve, 84–86, *85*
  challenging anatomy scenarios in
      TAVR, 76–79
  clinical trials, 24–25
  conduction disturbances associated
      with TAVR, 116–117,
      119–120
  coronary artery disease, 112
  essential considerations, 64–65, *65*
  optimal selection of TAVR devices,
      51, 53–57, *54, 57*
  percutaneous pulmonary valve
      replacement, 516–517, *517*
  structural mitral valve
      interventions, 247–248
  transcatheter tricuspid valve
      devices, 359
  valve components, 63–64, *64*
  valve-in-valve TAVR, 98–99, *99*
  vascular access, 63
balloon-in-balloon (BiB) system, 517
balloon-tipped pacing catheters, 134
balloon valve fracture (BVF),
      96, 98–99

balloon valvotomy, 195
balloon valvuloplasty
    double-balloon technique, 242, 244, **245**
    Inoue technique, 242–244, *243*
    intra-procedural TEE, 223–224
    predictors of success/failure, 239–240, **241**
    structural mitral valve interventions, 239–244
    see also balloon aortic valvuloplasty; percutaneous mitral balloon valvuloplasty
bare-metal stents, 507, *508*, 509–513, **509**, *511*
Barlow's disease, 270, 273–275, *275–276*
basal hinge points, 40
BASILICA technique
    challenging anatomy scenarios in TAVR, 81–82
    coronary artery obstruction, 107, *107*
    valve-in-valve TAVR, 99, *99*
BAT *see* balloon-assisted technique
BAV *see* balloon aortic valvuloplasty; bicuspid aortic valve
berry aneurysm, 505
beta-blockers, 460
BEV *see* balloon-expandable valves
BHV *see* biological heart valves
BiB *see* balloon-in-balloon
bicuspid aortic valve (BAV)
    challenging anatomy scenarios in TAVR, 76–77
    computed tomography for TAVR planning, *41*, 47–48, *47*
    epidemiology, 12, *12*, 83
    etiology and classification, 14–15, *14*
    identification and diagnosis, 83
    morphology and classification, 83–84, *84*
    optimal selection of TAVR devices, 56
    outcomes of TAVR, 86–87
    pathologic findings, 15–16, *15–16*
    pre-dilation and post-dilation, 86
    procedural planning, 84–86, *85*
    THV sizing, 85–86, *85*
    transcatheter aortic valve replacement, 83–87
biological heart valves (BHV)

percutaneous pulmonary valve replacement, 515–516, 519
transcatheter aortic valve replacement, 33
bioprosthetic valve failure (BVF)
    pathology of valve degeneration and thrombosis, 139, 141, 146–147
    transcatheter mitral valve replacement, 305
bi-plane imaging, 218, *220*, 222
bivalirubin, 157–158
bleeding/hemorrhage
    acute pulmonary embolism, 548–550, **549**
    transcatheter aortic valve replacement, 178, *179*
    vascular access and closure for TAVR, 187
blind circulatory loop, 585
body mass index (BMI), 32
bradyarrhythmia, 125
BRAVO 3 study, 157–158
bRIGHT study, 371
bundle of His *see* atrioventricular bundle
BVF *see* balloon valve failure

C

CABG *see* coronary artery bypass graft
CAD *see* coronary artery disease
CAF *see* coronary artery fistulas
calcific aortic stenosis, 11–18
    balloon aortic valvuloplasty, 70–71
    bicuspid aortic valve, 83, 85
    challenging anatomy scenarios in TAVR, 75–76, 80
    epidemiology, 11–12, *12*, **13**
    etiology, 11
    mechanical complications of TAVR, 131
    normal aortic valve anatomy, 11
    optimal selection of TAVR devices, 53–54, 57, *57*
    pathologic findings, 12–15, *13–16*
    risk factors, 16
    underlying mechanisms of calcification, 16–17
calcific mitral valve, 247, 270
calcific peripheral disease, 172
calcium channel blockers, 460
cardiac amyloidosis, 45, *45*
cardiac arrest, 568, 571

cardiac magnetic resonance (CMR)
    coronary artery fistulas, 536
    mitral paravalvular leak, 406–407
    percutaneous pulmonary valve replacement, 516
    percutaneous treatment of aortic coarctation, 506, *507*, 512–513
    surgical tricuspid valve repair, 385
    transcatheter tricuspid valve devices, 368, **369**
cardiac output (CO)
    ECMO for structural interventions, 570
    hemodynamics in adult structural heart disease, 525–526
    shunt hemodynamics and calculations, 479, 481–482
cardiac power output (CPO), 572–573, *573*, 578–579
cardiac tamponade, 133–134, 565–566
CardiAQ-EVOQUE device, 319–320
Cardioband system, 322–323, *322*, 357–358, 372
cardiogenic shock
    acute myocardial infarction cardiogenic shock, 571–584
    ECMO for structural interventions, 568–569
    interatrial shunt devices, 471
cardiopulmonary bypass, 234
cardiopulmonary resuscitation (CPR), 568–569
Cardiovalve, 373
cardiovascular accident (CVA) *see* stroke
Carillon mitral contour system, 321, *321*
catheter-directed thrombolysis (CDL), 548–551, 553–559
caval valve implantation (CAVI)
    current and future challenges, 393, *393*
    current data, 392–393
    hemodynamics, 391, *392*
    patient selection, 391
    pre-procedural planning, 391
    rationale, 391
    severe tricuspid regurgitation, 391–394
    steps in the procedure, 391–392
    transcatheter heterotopic CAVI, 359
CDL *see* catheter-directed thrombolysis

centers of excellence, 236
CEP *see* cerebral embolic protection
CeraFlex Cribiform Septal Occluder, 494, *494*
CeraFlex Occluder, 494, *494*
cerebral embolic protection (CEP) devices
  challenging anatomy scenarios in TAVR, 77, 80
  computed tomography for TAVR planning, 44
  left atrial appendage occlusion, 452
  management of TAVR-related stroke, 157
  neuroprotection in TAVR, 163–167, *164–165*, **165–166**
CFA *see* common femoral artery
CF-LVAD *see* continuous-flow left ventricular assist devices
CHA2DS2-VASc score, 418–420, **419–420**
CHB *see* complete heart block
CHD *see* coronary heart disease
chest X-ray, 506
CHF *see* congestive heart failure
chimney technique, 100, *100*
CHOICE/SAPIEN XT study, 52–53
chordal entrapment, 266, *284*, 284
chromosomal anomalies, 505
chronic aortic regurgitation, 7
chronic structural mitral regurgitation (MR), 227, 531
CLASP TR study, 357
CLASP TR trial, 371, 374
CLEAN TAVI trial, 165–166
clopidogrel, 151, 436, 473
CLOSE trial, 485
clover lesion, 520, *521*
CMR *see* cardiac magnetic resonance
CO *see* cardiac output
COAPT trial, 212, 230, 235, 253–255, 261–262, 273, 277–278
COAST study, 512
Colibri valve, 35
collagen-based closure devices, 185
commissural alignment, 56
commissural calcification, 247
commissural lesions, 276–277
common femoral artery (CFA), 183–184

complete heart block (CHB)
  conduction disturbances associated with TAVR, 116, 120
  management of conduction disturbances post-TAVR, 124–126, 128–129
computed tomography angiography (CTA)
  acute pulmonary embolism, 555, *555*
  computed tomography for TAVR planning, 40, 41, 44–47
  coronary artery disease, 109
  left atrial appendage occlusion, 433, *434*, 438, 441, 443
  percutaneous treatment of aortic coarctation, 506, *508*, 512–513
  transcatheter aortic valve replacement, 60–61
  transcatheter tricuspid valve devices, **369**
  vascular access and closure for TAVR, 183, 184
computed tomography (CT)
  access site evaluation, 42–44, *44*
  advantages of MDCT in pre-procedural planning, 292–293
  anatomic components of mitral valve, 291, *292*
  aortic paravalvular leak closure, 397, *398*
  aortic valve annular evaluation/sizing, 40–41, *41*, 48
  aortic valve calcium score, 39–40
  balloon aortic valvuloplasty, 70
  bicuspid aortic valve, *41*, 47–48, *47*, 83, *84*
  carotid embolic protection device assessment, 44
  caval valve implantation, 391
  challenging anatomy scenarios in TAVR, 77, *78*
  complications from MitraClip procedure, *283*
  concepts and protocols for mitral CT, 293–294, *293*
  conduction disturbances associated with TAVR, 117
  coronary artery and bypass graft evaluation, 44
  coronary artery fistulas, 536, *536*
  coronary artery obstruction, 105, **105**

estimation of coplanar fluoroscopic angle, 297–298, *298*
geometry and anatomy of aorta, 41–42, *42–43*
landing zone sizing/evaluation, 294
left atrial appendage occlusion, 425–427, **426**, *427*, **428**, *432*
mechanical complications of TAVR, 132
mitral paravalvular leak, 407
mitral regurgitation, 199
myocardial extracellular volume, 45, *45*
neo-LVOT, 293–297, *294–297*
optimal selection of TAVR devices, *55*
percutaneous pulmonary valve replacement, 515
post-procedural imaging, 299, *299*
pre-procedural protocol, 39, **40**
relevant adjacent structures for TMVR, 298
reporting functional assessment and incidentals, 45
surgical tricuspid valve repair, 385
Tendyne system, *326*, 327
transapical access, 299
transcatheter aortic valve replacement, 33, 39–50, 60–61
transcatheter mitral valve replacement, 291–300, 302
transcatheter tricuspid valve devices, 354
transfemoral access, 170
transseptal access, 296–297, 298–299
transseptal puncture, 565
valve-in-valve TAVR, 97
valve-in-valve TAVR evaluation, 45–47, *46*
computer simulation, 85
conduction abnormalities
  bicuspid aortic valve, 85
  changes to ECG post-TAVR, 124
  clinical impact after TAVR, 116–117
  components of normal conduction, 123
  conduction disturbances associated with TAVR, 115–121
  incidence of disturbance in TAVR, 115–116

conduction abnormalities (*contd.*)
  intervals matched to conduction system components, 123
  management of conduction disturbances post-TAVR, 123–130
  minimization strategies, 117–120, *119–120*
  monitoring by operative stage, 124
  optimal selection of TAVR devices, 53, 54–55
  permanent pacemaker implantation, 126–129
  post-TAVR monitoring and electrophysiological assessment, 120
  predicators with TAVR, 117, *118*
  pre-operative ECG findings, 124
  procedural factors, 124
  relationship between aortic valve and conduction systems, 115, *116*
  susceptibility during TAVR implantation, 123–124, *124*
  temporary pacing, 124–126
conduit rupture, 520
congenital heart defects, 515
congestive heart failure (CHF), 258–259
continuous-flow left ventricular assist devices (CF-LVAD), 89
continuous-wave velocity profile, 366
contractile reserve, 528
CoreValve prosthesis, 587–588
  Extreme Risk study, 20
  native aortic valve regurgitation, 90–91
  optimal selection of TAVR devices, 54–55
  pathology of valve degeneration and thrombosis, 140–141, 143, *143*
  transfemoral access, 170
coronary artery access
  challenging anatomy scenarios in TAVR, 78–79, *78–79*
  computed tomography for TAVR planning, 44
  optimal selection of TAVR devices, 55–56
  transcatheter aortic valve replacement, 33
coronary artery bypass graft (CABG)

computed tomography for TAVR planning, 44
coronary artery fistulas, 538
coronary artery obstruction, 104
  optimal selection of TAVR devices, 57
  surgical techniques for mitral valve repair, 235
  surgical trials in mitral valvular disease, 228
coronary artery disease (CAD)
  assessment prior to TAVR, 109
  clinical impact on TAVR outcomes, 109
  completeness of revascularization, 111–112
  current revascularization guidelines, 113, *113*
  epidemiology, 109
  instantaneous wave-free ratio, 109–110, *110*
  management of left main disease, 111
  optimal timing for revascularization, 111
  percutaneous revascularization in TAVR, 110–113, **112**, *113*
  technical considerations for PCI post-TAVR, 112
  transcatheter aortic valve replacement, 109–114
coronary artery fistulas (CAF)
  available devices, 536, **537**
  classification, 535
  clinical presentation, 536
  coronary steal phenomenon, 535, 537–538
  diagnosis, 535–536
  incidence, 535
  indications and contraindications, 536
  outcomes, 537
  percutaneous closure, 535–540
  retrograde arterial vs. antegrade venous approach, 537, *538*
  surgical vs. percutaneous approach, 536–537
coronary artery obstruction
  BASILICA technique, 107, *107*
  challenging anatomy scenarios in TAVR, 81–82

computed tomography for TAVR planning, 46–47, *46*
delayed coronary obstruction, 103–104
  incidence, 103
  involvement of left coronary artery, 103
  mechanism of obstruction, 103, *104*
  outcomes, 104
  preparatory coronary protection, 106–107
  prevention and management in TAVR, 103–108
  prevention with TAVR, 105, **105**, *106*
  risk factors, 104–105, **105**
  symptoms, 104
  treatment, 106
  valve-in-valve TAVR, 96, **96**, 99–100, *99–100*
coronary compression, 518, *518*, 520
coronary heart disease (CHD), 230
coronary impingement, 400, *400*
coronary ostium, 42, *43*
coronary steal phenomenon, 535, 537–538
covered endovascular stents, 507, *508*, 509–513, **505**
CPO *see* cardiac power output
CPR *see* cardiopulmonary resuscitation
cryptogenic stroke, 490
CT *see* computed tomography
CTA *see* computed tomography angiography
CULPRIT-SHOCK trial, 577
cusp overlap technique, 118–119, *119–120*
CVA *see* stroke

d

DAPT *see* dual antiplatelet therapy
DaVingi TR system, 358–359, 372
DCO *see* delayed coronary obstruction
DEFENSE trial, 485
degenerative mitral regurgitation *see* primary mitral regurgitation
delayed coronary obstruction (DCO), 103–104
DENER-HTN trial, 541–542
De Vega procedure, 384
device embolization
  aortic paravalvular leak closure, 400, *400*

atrial septal defect closure, 497–498
  complications from MitraClip
    procedure, 286, *286*
  left atrial appendage occlusion,
    450–451, *451*
device migration, 489
device-related thrombus (DRT),
    282–284, 452–454, *453*, 492
diagnostic shunt study, 477–478
dialysis, 477, 482
DIC *see* disseminated intravascular
    coagulation
diffuse myxomatous degeneration
    (DMD), 270, 273–275,
    275–276
diffusion-weighted imaging (DWI), 157
digital subtraction angiography (DSA),
    178–179, *180*
diltiazem, 460
direct-acting oral anticoagulants
    (DOAC), 152, 417, 420
direct aortic access, 175–176
disseminated intravascular coagulation
    (DIC), 567–568
distal LAA thrombus, 447
DMD *see* diffuse myxomatous
    degeneration
DMR *see* primary mitral regurgitation
DOAC *see* direct-acting oral
    anticoagulants
Doppler imaging
  edge-to-edge mitral valve repair, *269*
  edge-to-edge tricuspid valve
    interventions, 349, *349*, *351*
  left atrial appendage occlusion,
    429, *430*
  mitral paravalvular leak, 403, *405*
  mitral regurgitation, 197, *197*
  transcatheter tricuspid valve devices,
    365–366, *366*
double-balloon technique, 242,
    244, **245**
double-orifice surgical repair, 228–229
double-wire technique, 413
DRT *see* device-related thrombus
DrySeal sheath, 521, *522*
DSA *see* digital subtraction
    angiography
dual antiplatelet therapy (DAPT), 435
DurAVR valve, 35
DWI *see* diffusion-weighted imaging
dyspnea

aortic stenosis, 3–4, 6
mitral stenosis, 193
optimal selection of TAVR devices,
    57, *57*

e
EAPCI *see* European Association of
    Percutaneous Cardiovascular
    Interventions
early thickening, 151–153
EBDA *see* effective balloon
    dilatation area
ECG *see* electrocardiogram
echocardiography
  aortic stenosis, 5, *5*
  bicuspid aortic valve, 83
  hemodynamics in adult structural
    heart disease, 532–533
  mitral stenosis, 194–195
  transcatheter aortic valve
    implantation, 24
  valve-in-valve TAVR, 100
  see also individual modalities
ECMO *see* extracorporeal membrane
    oxygenation
ECV *see* extracellular volume
edge-to-edge mitral valve
    repair, 257–271
  acute myocardial infarction
    cardiogenic shock, 582
  air embolism and thrombus
    formation, 282–284
  anatomical and pathophysiologic
    considerations, 214–215,
    257, 260
  calcific mitral valve, 277–278, *278*
  challenging anatomy, 273–279
  chordal entrapment, *284*, 284
  clip embolization, 286, *286*
  COAPT trial, 253–255, 261–262,
    273, 277–278
  complications from MitraClip
    procedure, 281–290
  currently available clips, 262,
    274–275, *275*
  delivery system advancement,
    265–266, *265*, *267*
  development and components
    of clip system, 257, *258*, 262, 273
  echocardiographic assessment,
    211–216, *212*, *213–215*,
    259–260, *261*

EVEREST trials, 251–253, *252*, **252**,
    260–261, 270, 275–274, **274**, 277
Heart Team, 258–259
hypertrophic cardiomyopathy,
    467–470
iatrogenic atrial septal
    defect, 288–289
iatrogenic mitral stenosis,
    287–288, *287*
incidence of vascular complications,
    281–282, *282*
indications and
    contraindications, 259
intra-procedural imaging, 217–224,
    222, 263, *265*, 266–270, *267–269*
MITRA-FR trial, 261
mitral insufficiency, 257–261
multiple clips, 269, 275, *276*, 278
myxomatous mitral valve,
    273–275, *275–276*
noncentral and commissural lesions,
    276–277, *277*
patient selection, 211–212, 259,
    273, **274**
percutaneous approach, 208, *209*,
    211–212, 260, 468–470, *469*, **469**
prevention of MitraClip
    complications, 282, **281**
procedure, 263–269, *267–269*
real-world experience and
    outcomes, 262
residual mitral
    regurgitation, 287
secondary mitral regurgitation, 278
single leaflet device attachment,
    285–286, *285*
special patient subgroups and
    considerations, 269–270
structural mitral valve
    interventions, 222
surgical techniques for mitral valve
    repair, 234–235
surgical trials in mitral valvular
    disease, 230–230
transseptal puncture, 215, *215*, 260,
    264, 282, *283*
treatment of mitral valve disease,
    317–318, **318**, 320
vascular access and closure, 263
edge-to-edge tricuspid valve
    interventions, 347–352
  challenges in TV imaging, 349

edge-to-edge tricuspid valve
interventions *(contd.)*
grading post-procedural imaging,
351, **352**
rating tricuspid regurgitation,
351, **351**
steps in TV imaging, 349–350, *350*
structures adjacent to tricuspid
valve, 348
transcatheter tricuspid valve devices,
355–357, **356**, 371
transesophageal imaging protocol,
348–349, *348–349*
vascular access, 347–348
EF *see* ejection fraction
effective balloon dilatation area
(EBDA), 244, **245**
effective blood flow, 481–482
effective orifice area (EOA)
challenging anatomy scenarios in
TAVR, 77
optimal selection of TAVR
devices, 53
Tendyne system, 325
transcatheter aortic valve
replacement, 32
effective regurgitant orifice
area (EROA)
edge-to-edge mitral valve
repair, 211–212
mitral paravalvular leak,
404–406, *405*
structural mitral valve interventions,
219, 220
transcatheter tricuspid valve devices,
355, 366, **367**
ejection fraction (EF), 5
EKOS system, 553–554, *554*, *557*
electrocardiogram (ECG)
computed tomography for TAVR
planning, 39
conduction disturbances associated
with TAVR, 116, 120
edge-to-edge mitral valve
repair, 213
left atrial appendage occlusion, 425
management of conduction
disturbances post-
TAVR, 123–129
percutaneous treatment of aortic
coarctation, 506, *506*, 514
surgical tricuspid valve repair, 385

embolic protection devices (EPD)
challenging anatomy scenarios in
TAVR, 77, 80
computed tomography for TAVR
planning, 44
left atrial appendage occlusion, 452
management of TAVR-related
stroke, 157
neuroprotection in TAVR, 163–167,
164–165, **165–166**
emergency sternotomy, 568
endocardial ischemia, 569
endothelial cells, 11
endovascular aortic repair (EVAR), 57
end systolic dimension (ESD), 8
EnVeo valve delivery system, 65, *66*
EOA *see* effective orifice area
EPD *see* embolic protection devices
EROA *see* effective regurgitant
orifice area
ESD *see* end systolic dimension
eSheath valve delivery system, 64, *65*
European Association of Percutaneous
Cardiovascular Interventions
(EAPCI), 23, *23*
EVAR *see* endovascular aortic repair
EVEREST trials, 214–215, 235,
251–253, *252*, **252**, 260–261, 270,
273–274, **274**, 277
Evolut Low Risk Trial, 25
Evolut valve platform
challenging anatomy scenarios in
TAVR, 79
conduction disturbances associated
with TAVR, 116
mechanical complications of TAVR,
134, *135*
native aortic valve
regurgitation, 90–91
optimal selection of TAVR
devices, 55–56
present generation of THVs,
34, *34*
transfemoral access, 170
valve and catheter components,
65–67, *65–66*
EVOQUE device, 373
extracellular volume (ECV), 45, *45*
extracorporeal membrane
oxygenation (ECMO)
acute myocardial infarction
cardiogenic shock, 575–576

acute pulmonary embolism,
551, 557–558
anticoagulation therapy, 567–568
ECMO for structural
interventions, 567–570
emergency procedures,
568–569
flow goals and indications, 568
inotropic management following
VA-ECMO insertion,
569, *569–570*
interatrial shunt devices, 471
patent foramen ovale, 570
surgical trials in mitral valvular
disease, 229
transaortic valve implantation/
replacement, 567–570, **567**
EXTRACT-PE trial, 550
extreme fibrotic septum, 566

f

fenestrated septum, 488–490
fibrinolytic therapy *see*
thrombolytic therapy
fibroblasts, 11
Fick equation, 478
flail mitral valve leaflets, 260, 270, 276
FLAME trial, 551
FLARE trial, 550
FlowTriever system, 550–551, 553–554,
554, 556, *557*, 558
fluoroscopy
aortic paravalvular leak closure, 397
complications from MitraClip
procedure, *286*
edge-to-edge mitral valve repair, *265*,
266, *267*, 269
left atrial appendage occlusion, 441
mechanical complications of TAVR,
134, *135*
mitral paravalvular leak, 409–410
mitral stenosis, *205*, *209*
native aortic valve regurgitation,
91, *92–93*
percutaneous treatment of aortic
coarctation, *508*
structural mitral valve interventions,
221–222, 243, 246
transcatheter mitral valve
replacement, 297–298, *298*, 303
transseptal puncture, 563
valve-in-valve TAVR, 97, *97*

vascular access and closure for
TAVR, 184
see also angiography
FMR *see* secondary mitral regurgitation
FORMA system, 344, 370–371
fossa ovalis, 561
fractional flow reserve (FFR),
109–110, *110*
free-floating thrombus, 558
functional mitral regurgitation *see*
secondary mitral regurgitation

g

Gallavardin's phenomenon, 5
genetic testing, 460
Gore CARDIOFORM Septal Occluder
(GSO), 486, 487–489, *487*, 566
Gore Septal Occluder, 494, *494*
Gorlin formula, 525
GSO *see* Gore CARDIOFORM Septal
Occluder

h

Hakki formula, 525
HALT *see* hypoattenuating leaflet
thrombosis
HAM *see* hypo-attenuation
affecting motion
HAVB *see* high-degree
atrioventricular block
HCM *see* hypertrophic cardiomyopathy
heart failure (HF)
congestive heart failure, 258–259
edge-to-edge mitral valve
repair, 253–255
interatrial shunt devices, 471–473
shunt hemodynamics and
calculations, 482
surgical tricuspid valve repair, 345
heart failure with preserved ejection
fraction (HFpEF), 471, 482
heart failure with reduced ejection
fraction (HFrEF), 253–255
Heart Team, 20–21
ECMO for structural
interventions, 567
edge-to-edge mitral valve
repair, 258–259
surgical techniques for mitral valve
repair, 236
surgical trials in mitral valvular
disease, 230

hemodynamics
acute myocardial infarction
cardiogenic shock, 572–579,
573, *575*
acute pulmonary embolism, 557–558
adult structural heart
disease, 525–533
aortic regurgitation, 7, *8*
aortic stenosis, 3–5,
525–529, *526–529*
assessment of the aortic
valve, 525–529
assessment of the mitral
valve, 529–530
balloon aortic valvuloplasty, 72
cardiac output, 525–526
caval valve implantation, 391, *392*
ECMO for structural interventions,
569, *569–570*
edge-to-edge mitral valve repair, 278
Hakki/Gorlin formula, 525
hypertrophic cardiomyopathy and
septal ablation, 532–533
MitraClip and LA pressure, 532
mitral regurgitation, 196–197, *196*,
199, 206–208, *530*, 531–532
mitral stenosis, 193–194, *194*,
203–206, 530–531, *530*
optimal selection of TAVR
devices, 52
percutaneous mitral balloon
valvuloplasty, 531
pressure waveform analysis,
527–528, *527–528*
pulmonary capillary wedge pressure,
530, *530*, 531
shunt hemodynamics and
calculations, 230, 246, 477–483
static/dynamic obstruction, 527, *527*
structural mitral valve
interventions, 243–244
surgical techniques for mitral valve
repair, 234
transcatheter aortic valve
replacement, 32–33, 529, *529*
transcatheter mitral valve
replacement, 305
transseptal transcatheter mitral
valve-in-valve replacement, 312
transvalvular gradient, 526–527, *526*
tricuspid aortic valve, 339
hemopericardium, 246

heparin
left atrial appendage occlusion,
443, 454
patent foramen ovale closure, 486
TAVR-related stroke, 157–158
heparin-induced thrombocytopenia
(HIT), 568
HF *see* heart failure
HFpEF *see* heart failure with preserved
ejection fraction
HFrEF *see* heart failure with reduced
ejection fraction
high-degree atrioventricular block
(HAVB), 124, 126, 129
high-implantation technique, 119–120
high-output heart failure, 482
high-pressure post-dilation, 98–99
HI-PIETHO trial, 548
HIT *see* heparin-induced
thrombocytopenia
horizontal aorta, 76
hybrid anterograde-retrograde
approach, *409*, 411
hypercoagulable states, 490
hyperplastic septal tissue, 566
hypertrophic cardiomyopathy
(HCM), 459–461
alcohol septal ablation, 461, 463–466,
467–470, **469**, 532–533
diagnosis, 459–460
edge-to-edge mitral valve
repair, 467–470
epidemiology, 459
genetic testing, 460
hemodynamics in adult structural
heart disease, 532–533
left ventricular outflow tract
obstruction, 459
mitral valve abnormalities,
467, *468*
percutaneous mitral valve repair
using MitraClip, 468–470,
469, **469**
permanent pacing, 461
prevention and
management, 460–461
prognosis, 459
septal myomectomy, 461, 467–468
sudden cardiac death, 459
symptoms, 460
treatment options after failed
medical therapy, 467–468

hypoattenuating leaflet thrombosis (HALT)
  clinical implications, 152–153
  pathology of valve degeneration and thrombosis, 141
  transcatheter aortic valve implantation, 26, *26*
hypo-attenuation affecting motion (HAM), 153
hypotension, 305, 529
hypoxia, 570

i

IABP *see* intra-aortic balloon pump
IABP-SHOCK trial, 572, *568*
IAS *see* interatrial septum
iASD *see* iatrogenic atrial septal defect
IASD *see* interatrial shunt devices
iatrogenic atrial septal defect (iASD)
  complications from MitraClip procedure, 288–289
  structural mitral valve interventions, 246
  transseptal puncture, 566
iatrogenic mitral stenosis, 287–288, *287*
ICD *see* intercommissural distance
ICE *see* intracardiac echocardiography
ICM *see* ischemic cardiomyopathy
IE *see* infective endocarditis
iFR *see* instantaneous wave-free ratio
iliac artery, 80
iliofemoral access, 80
iliofemoral atherosclerotic disease, 172
Impella mechanical circulatory support, 572, 573–582, *573–575*
Indigo system, 553–554, *554*, 556
infective endocarditis (IE), 139–140, *140*
inferior vena cava (IVC)
  alternative access, 178–180, *179–180*
  caval valve implantation, 391–393, *392–393*
  challenging anatomy scenarios in TAVR, 80
  complications from MitraClip procedure, 281–282, *282*
  edge-to-edge tricuspid valve interventions, 347–348
  patent foramen ovale closure, 488–489
  surgical tricuspid valve repair, 345

transcatheter tricuspid valve devices, 359, 368
tricuspid aortic valve, 339
inotropic support
  acute myocardial infarction cardiogenic shock, 572, *572*
  ECMO for structural interventions, 569, *569–570*
  surgical techniques for mitral valve repair, 234
Inoue balloon/technique, 241–244, *243*
instantaneous wave-free ratio (iFR), 109–110, *110*
Inteprid MV, 320
interatrial septum (IAS)
  atrial septal defect closure, 496–497, *496–497*
  structural mitral valve interventions, 218, 220–221, 244
  transseptal puncture, 561, *562*, 565–566
interatrial shunt devices (IASD), 471–473
  atrial septal defect, 471–473
  atrial septostomy, 471
  available devices, 472, *472*
  complications and long-term concerns, 472
  implantation steps, 472
  net shunt volume, 472
intercommissural distance (ICD), *85*
intra-annular valve design
  challenging anatomy scenarios in TAVR, 77
  transcatheter aortic valve replacement, 32
  valve-in-valve TAVR, 98–99, *99*
intra-aortic balloon pump (IABP), 72, 243
intracardiac echocardiography (ICE)
  atrial septal defect closure, 495
  interatrial shunt devices, 472
  left atrial appendage occlusion, 428–431, *429–432*, **429**, 441–443, 449
  mitral paravalvular leak, 407–409
  patent foramen ovale closure, 486
  structural mitral valve interventions, 242
intracranial aneurysm, 505
intravascular lithotripsy (IVL), 171, *171*, 172

intravascular ultrasound (IVUS), 391–392
intravenous nitroglycerin, 575
Intrepid system, 373
invasive hemodynamics
  acute myocardial infarction cardiogenic shock, 574–575
  mitral regurgitation, 197
  mitral stenosis, 195, 204–205
ischemic cardiomyopathy (ICM), 253–255
ischemic limbs, 187–188
isolated tricuspid regurgitation (TR), 338
IVC *see* inferior vena cava
IVL *see* intravascular lithotripsy
IVUS *see* intravascular ultrasound

j

jailing technique, 520, *521*
JenaValve, 34
J-Valve, 51, 90–91

k

Kansas City Cardiomyopathy Questionnaire (KCCQ), 254, 357, 371
Kay procedure, 371–372, 384

l

LAA *see* left atrial appendage
LAAO *see* left atrial appendage occlusion
LAmbre device, 433–434, 436, *437–438*, 446
LAmP *see* left atrial mean pressure
large-bore aspiration, 556, *557*
large-bore vascular access
  transcatheter aortic valve replacement, 63
  vascular access and closure for TAVR, 185, *186*, 188
large-caliber guide catheters, 106–107
Lariat/SentreHEART device, 434, 437–438
LBBB *see* left bundle branch block
LCAD *see* left ventricular assist device
LCC *see* left coronary cusp
leaflet calcification
  challenging anatomy scenarios in TAVR, 75
  edge-to-edge mitral valve repair, 270

mitral stenosis, 203, *204*
pathology of valve degeneration and thrombosis, 142–144, *145*
structural mitral valve interventions, 247
leaflet endothelialization, 141–142, *146*
leaflet tears/perforations, 145–146
leaflet thrombosis *see* valve/leaflet thrombosis
left atrial appendage (LAA), 218, 224
left atrial appendage occlusion (LAAO)
additional considerations, 420
air embolism, 451
anatomic challenges, 447, *447*
available devices, 433–439
complication prevention and management, 449–455
computed tomography/ECG-gated CT, 425–427, **426**, **427**, **428**, *432*
current US recommendations, 420, **421**
delivery system positioning, 443
device design differences, 433–434, 436–437
device embolization, 450–451, *451*
device placement, 430, 444
device-related thrombus, 452–454, *453*
device sizing, 443
device-specific characteristics, 434–436, *434*, *436–437*
device-specific considerations, 444–446, *445*
distal LAA thrombus, 447
future directions, 437–438, *438*
imaging for LAA interventions, 425–432, 441
indications for percutaneous LAAO, 417–423, 441
intra-procedural TEE/ICE, 428–432, *429–432*, **429**
patent foramen oval/atrial septal defect, 443
pericardial effusion, 449–450, 454
peri-device leaks, 452, *453*
periprocedural ischemic stroke, 451–452
pre-procedural TTE/TEE, 427, *428*, **428**
rationale, 417–418, 449
sandwich technique, 446–447, *446*
stepwise procedure, 441–444

supporting evidence, 418–420, **418–419**
technique and challenges, 441–447
vascular access, 441–443, *442*, 452
left atrial enlargement, 193
left atrial mean pressure (LAmP), 532
left bundle branch block (LBBB)
alcohol septal ablation, 463
conduction disturbances associated with TAVR, 115–117, *117*, 120
management of conduction disturbances post-TAVR, 124, 126–127, *127*
optimal selection of TAVR devices, 54–55
left coronary cusp (LCC), 119, *119–120*
left main (LM) disease, 111
left superior pulmonary vein (LSPV), 486
left-to-right shunt, 230, 246, 477–480, **481**
left ventricular assist device (LVAD)
available devices, 585, **581**
management options for post-LVAD-AI, 586, *582*
native aortic valve regurgitation, 89
pathophysiology of post-LVAD-AI, 585
prevention of post-LVAD-AI, 586
surgical trials in mitral valvular disease, 229–230
surgical tricuspid valve repair, 344–345
technical considerations, 587–588, *583*
transcatheter inverventions for aortic insufficiency, 585–588
left ventricular ejection fraction (LVEF)
computed tomography for TAVR planning, 45
conduction disturbances associated with TAVR, 116
edge-to-edge mitral valve repair, 211–212, 255, 261
hemodynamics in adult structural heart disease, 527
mitral regurgitation, 198
native aortic valve regurgitation, 89
surgical trials in mitral valvular disease, 228
Tendyne system, 328
tricuspid regurgitation, 343

left ventricular end diastolic pressure (LVEDP)
acute myocardial infarction cardiogenic shock, 574, 577
ECMO for structural interventions, 569
hemodynamics in adult structural heart disease, 529–530
left ventricular end-systolic diameter (LVESD), 89
left ventricular hypertrophy (LVH), 4
left ventricular outflow tract/obstruction (LVOT/LVOTO)
balloon aortic valvuloplasty, 70
bicuspid aortic valve, 85
challenging anatomy scenarios in TAVR, 75–77
computed tomography for TAVR planning, 39–40, 47, *47*
conduction disturbances associated with TAVR, 117
edge-to-edge mitral valve repair, 263, 467
hemodynamics in adult structural heart disease, 532–533
hypertrophic cardiomyopathy, 459, 461, 463, 465–466, *465*
intra-procedural TEE, 218, 222–223
mechanical complications of TAVR, 131, 133
optimal selection of TAVR devices, 53–54, 57
surgical techniques for mitral valve repair, 233–234
surgical trials in mitral valvular disease, 229
Tendyne system, 325–328
transcatheter aortic valve replacement, 33
transcatheter mitral valve replacement, 293–297, *294–297*, 302, 305–306, *307*
transseptal transcatheter mitral valve-in-valve replacement, 311–312, 314
lipomatous atrial septum, 488
LM *see* left main
LMWH *see* low-molecular-weight heparin
low-flow, low-gradient aortic stenosis, 5–6, 527–528, *528*

low-molecular-weight heparin
(LMWH), 454
LSPV *see* left superior pulmonary vein
LuX device, 373
LVAD *see* left ventricular assist device
LVEDP *see* left ventricular end diastolic
pressure
LVEF *see* left ventricular ejection
fraction
LVESD *see* left ventricular end-systolic
diameter
LVH *see* left ventricular hypertrophy
LVOT/LVOTO *see* left ventricular
outflow tract/obstruction

m

MAC *see* mitral annular calcification
magnetic resonance angiography
(MRA), 536
magnetic resonance imaging (MRI)
atrial septal defect closure, 495
bicuspid aortic valve, 83
challenging anatomy scenarios in
TAVR, 77, *78*
mitral paravalvular leak, 406–407
mitral regurgitation, 197
neuroprotection in TAVR, 163, 166
percutaneous pulmonary valve
replacement, 515, 516
percutaneous treatment of aortic
coarctation, 506, *507*, 512–513
tricuspid aortic valve, 338
mass obstruction, 103
MDCT *see* multidetector computed
tomography
mean arterial pressures (MAP), 569
mechanical complications of
TAVR, 131–137
annular rupture, 131–133, *132*
perforation and tamponade, 133–134
valve embolization, 135–137, *136*
valve infolding, 134–135, *135*
mechanically expandable valve
(MEV), 23–24
mechanical reperfusion
therapy, 571–572
mechanical thrombectomy (MT),
158, 550
Medtronic Intrepid valve, 331–334
available delivery systems, 332
fixation and sealing, 331
healing of the atrial space, 331, *332*

key features of Medtronic Intrepid
valve, 331, *332*
transapical delivery, 332–333, *333*
transseptal delivery, 333–334
Melody valve, 516–517
membranous septum (MS)
bicuspid aortic valve, 85
conduction disturbances associated
with TAVR, 118
management of conduction
disturbances post-TAVR,
123–124
metallic commissurotomy
technique, 241
MEV *see* mechanically
expandable valve
MI *see* myocardial infarction
MIA-T system, 359
micro-TEE, 428, **429**, 441
MIDAS approach, 118
Millipede IRIS device, 323, *323*,
358, 372
MitraClip *see* edge-to-edge mitral
valve repair
MITRA-FR trial, 212, 228, 235, 261
mitral annular calcification (MAC)
edge-to-edge mitral valve repair, 277
intra-procedural TEE, 223
mitral stenosis, 193, 195, 203
structural mitral valve
interventions, 247–248
transcatheter mitral valve
replacement, 294, 297, 303,
304, 305
mitral annuloplasty, 320–324
direct mitral annuloplasty,
322–323, *322–323*
future directions, 323–324
indirect mitral annuloplasty,
321–322, *321–322*
transcatheter devices,
320–323, *321–323*
mitral loop cerclage, 321–322, *322*
mitral paravalvular leak
adjunctive quantitative measures,
403, **404**
anatomic location, 404, *406*
available devices, **410**, 412–413
cardiac magnetic resonance
imaging, 406–407
combination imaging, 408
computed tomography, 407

defect crossing and telescoping
catheters, 411–412, **412**
device deployment, 413
grading for severity, 404–406,
404, *406*
imaging and interventional
approaches, 403–414
intracardiac
echocardiography, 407–409
negotiating uncrossable defects, 413
transcatheter closure, 408–410, *409*
transesophageal
echocardiography/3D TEE,
403–406, *405–407*, 406, 409
transthoracic echocardiography,
403, **404**
mitral regurgitation (MR), 195–200
aortic stenosis, 5
atrial vs. ventricular functional MR,
207–208, *208*
challenging anatomy, 275, 278
classification, 195–196, 211
complications from MitraClip
procedure, 281, 287
diagnosis, 197, *197*, **198**, 199
edge-to-edge mitral valve repair,
211–216, 251–255,
257–262, 269–270
etiology, 196, 198, 206
hemodynamics, 196–197, *196*,
199, 206–208
hemodynamics in adult structural
heart disease, *530*, 531–532
hypertrophic
cardiomyopathy, 467–470
mitral annuloplasty, 317–324
pathophysiology of acute vs.
chronic MR, 206
percutaneous coronary intervention,
206–207, 208, *209*
percutaneous mitral valve
interventions, 246
proportionately/disproportionately
severe SMR, 207, *207*
pulmonary capillary wedge
pressure, 206
self-expanding TMVR
systems, 332–333
structural mitral valve interventions,
218, 220–222, 224
surgical techniques for mitral valve
repair, 233–237

surgical trials in mitral valvular disease, 227–232
symptoms and physical signs, 197, 199
Tendyne system, 325
transcatheter mitral valve replacement, 305
treatment and prognosis, 198, 199–200
see also primary mitral regurgitation; secondary mitral regurgitation
mitral stenosis (MS), 193–195
classification, 239, **240**
complications, 206
complications from MitraClip procedure, 282–284, 287–288, *287*
diagnosis, 194–195, 203–204, *204*
edge-to-edge mitral valve repair, 266, 269, 277
etiology, 193, 203
hemodynamics, 193–194, *194*, 203–206
hemodynamics in adult structural heart disease, 530–531, *530*
pathophysiology, 203
percutaneous mitral balloon valvuloplasty, 203, 205–206, *205*
pulmonary capillary wedge pressure, 204–205, *204*
structural mitral valve interventions, 220–221, 223–224, 239–249
symptoms and physical signs, 193–194
treatment, 195
MITRAL trial, 248
mitral valve area (MVA)
edge-to-edge mitral valve repair, 212, 260
intra-procedural TEE, 219, 224
structural mitral valve interventions, 239, 243
mitral valve clefts, 270
mitral valve prolapse, 260, 276, *278*
MPI *see* myocardial perfusion imaging
MPR *see* multiplanar reformation
MR *see* mitral regurgitation
MRA *see* magnetic resonance angiography
MRI *see* magnetic resonance imaging
MS *see* membranous septum; mitral stenosis

MSCT *see* multislice computed tomography
MT *see* mechanical thrombectomy
multidetector computed tomography (MDCT)
structural mitral valve interventions, 223
transcatheter mitral valve replacement, 292–293
transcatheter tricuspid valve devices, 367–368, *368*, **369**
tricuspid aortic valve, 338
valve thrombosis and early thickening, 153
multiplanar reformation (MPR), 43, 46–47
multislice computed tomography (MSCT), 85–86
multivessel PCI, 580
murmur, 4–5
muscular ventricular septal defects (MVSD), 499–501, *501*
MVA *see* mitral valve area
MVSD *see* muscular ventricular septal defects
myocardial fibrosis, 45, *45*
myocardial infarction (MI)
acute myocardial infarction cardiogenic shock, 571–584
edge-to-edge mitral valve repair, 270
mitral regurgitation, 198
optimal selection of TAVR devices, 56
myocardial ischemia, 538, 574
myocardial perfusion imaging (MPI), 110
myxomatous mitral valve, 270, 275–275, *275–276*

n

National Cardiogenic Shock Initiative (NCSI), 578–581
native aortic valve regurgitation (NAVR)
challenges of TAVR, 90
clinical trials evaluating TAVR, 90–91
critical technical considerations, 91, *92–93*
epidemiology, 89
etiology, 89

indications and timing for intervention, 89
natural history and prognosis, 89
preferred type of THV, 91
recommended therapy for severe NAVR, 90
transcatheter aortic valve replacement, 89–93
native RVOT, 515, 518–519, *518–519*
NaviGate device, 373
Navitor valve, 35, *35*
NAVR *see* native aortic valve regurgitation
NCC *see* non-coronary cusp
NCSI *see* National Cardiogenic Shock Initiative
neointimal coverage, 141–142, *145–146*
neo-LVOT, 293–297, *294–297*, 302, 306
net shunt volume, 472
neuroprotection in TAVR, 163–168
challenging anatomy scenarios in TAVR, 77, 80
characteristics of dislodged debris, 164–165, *165*
clinical evidence, 165–167, **166**
computed tomography for TAVR planning, 44
future directions, 167, *171*
peri-procedural stroke, 163
rationale for embolic protection devices, 163–164, *164*, **165**
new-onset persistent left bundle branch block (NOP-LBBB), 115–117, *117*, 120, 126–127, *127*
NICM *see* nonischemic cardiomyopathy
Nicoladoni-Branham sigh, 482
Nit-Occlud Coil VSD, 502, *503*
noncentral mitral regurgitation, 276–277, *277*
non-coronary cusp (NCC), 119, *119–120*
nonischemic cardiomyopathy (NICM), 253–255
nonvalvular atrial fibrillation (NVAF), 449
NOP-LBBB *see* new-onset persistent left bundle branch block
NOTION Trial, 22–23
NVAF *see* nonvalvular atrial fibrillation
NV-TAVI trials, 100

o

Occlutech Cribiform Septal Occluder, 494, *494*
Occlutech Figulla Occluder, 494, *494–495*
open cardiac massage, 568
OPTALYSE PE trial, 556

p

PA *see* pulmonary artery
pacemakers
    bicuspid aortic valve, 86
    conduction disturbances associated with TAVR, 115–117, *117*, 120
    hypertrophic cardiomyopathy, 461
    management of conduction disturbances post-TAVR, 124–129
    mechanical complications of TAVR, 134
    optimal selection of TAVR devices, 52
    transcatheter aortic valve replacement, 33
PAD *see* peripheral artery disease
pancyclic regurgitant flow, 585
pannus formation, 141–142, *145–146*
papillary muscle sling, 235
paravalvular leakage (PVL)
    aortic paravalvular leak closure, 397–401
    bicuspid aortic valve, 84–87
    challenging anatomy scenarios in TAVR, 75–76
    mechanical complications of TAVR, 131
    mitral paravalvular leak, 403–414
    optimal selection of TAVR devices, 53, 55–56
    structural mitral valve interventions, 217, 227
    Tendyne system, 325–326, 328
    transcatheter aortic valve replacement, 31, 32–33
    transcatheter mitral valve replacement, 299, *299*, 302, 305
partial thromboplastin time (PTT), 567–568
PARTNER trials, 20–22, 24–25
    coronary artery disease, 116
    mechanical complications of TAVR, 135

pathology of valve degeneration and thrombosis, 143
    TAVR-related stroke, 155–157
    valve-in-valve interventions, 100
    valve thrombosis and early thickening, 152
PASCAL device, 344, 356–357, 371, 374
PASP *see* pulmonary artery systolic pressure
PASTA technique, 372
patent foramen ovale (PFO)
    anticoagulation therapy, 488
    atrial septal aneurysm, 485–486, 488
    available devices for closure, 485–486, *486*
    closure, 485–490
    complications of closure, 489–490
    ECMO for structural interventions, 570
    inferior vena cava filters, 488–489
    intra-procedural TEE, 218, 220
    left atrial appendage occlusion, 445
    lipomatous atrial septum, 488
    multiple atrial septal defects, 488–490
    rationale for closure, 485
    sizing closure device, 488
    structural mitral valve interventions, 243
    technique for crossing the PFO, 486
    technique for device retrieval, 488
    technique for PFO closure, 486–488
    transseptal puncture, 566
    vascular access for closure, 486, 488–489
patient–prosthesis mismatch (PPM)
    challenging anatomy scenarios in TAVR, 77, 81
    conduction disturbances associated with TAVR, 120
    optimal selection of TAVR devices, 53
    transcatheter aortic valve replacement, 31–32
    transcatheter mitral valve replacement, 305
    valve-in-valve TAVR, 95–99, **96**, *98–99*
PCI *see* percutaneous coronary intervention
PCI, coronary artery disease, 110–113, **112**, *113*

PCWP *see* pulmonary capillary wedge pressure
PDL *see* peri-device leaks
PE *see* acute pulmonary embolism; chronic pulmonary embolism; pericardial effusion
PEITHO trial, 548
percutaneous aortic paravalvular leak closure, 397–401
percutaneous coil embolization, 133
percutaneous coronary intervention (PCI)
    acute myocardial infarction cardiogenic shock, 577, 580
    challenging anatomy scenarios in TAVR, 78–79, *78–79*
    hemodynamic assessment of the mitral valve, 206–207, 208, *209*
    surgical trials in mitral valvular disease, 228
    transcatheter aortic valve replacement, 33
percutaneous edge-to-edge mitral valve repair, 208, *209*, 211–212, 260
percutaneous mitral balloon valvuloplasty (PMBV)
    hemodynamic assessment of the mitral valve, 203, 205–206, *205*
    hemodynamics in adult structural heart disease, 531
    intra-procedural TEE, 224
percutaneous mitral valve intervention
    aortic regurgitation, 246
    balloon valvuloplasty techniques, 240–244, **241**, *243*, **245**
    calcific mitral valve, 247
    complications, 244–246
    follow-up protocol, 244
    indications and contraindications in rheumatic MS, 239
    mitral stenosis, 239–247
    predictors of success/failure, 239–240, **241**
    pregnancy, 246
    repeat PMV outcomes, 247
    rheumatic MS with tricuspid regurgitation, 246–247
    treatment of mitral valve disease, 317
percutaneous pulmonary valve replacement (PPVR), 515–522
    anatomic settings, 515–516
    available valves, 516–517, *517*

complications, 520
diagnostic tests, 516
difficulties advancing the prosthesis,
    519–520, *520*
follow-up, 520
indications, 516, *516–517*
procedure, 517–518, *518*
technical innovations,
    520–521, *521–522*
type of dysfunctional RVOT, 519, *519*
percutaneous thrombectomy, 556–558
percutaneous transluminal coronary
    angioplasty (PTCA), 571
percutaneous vascular closure, 63
perforations
    left atrial appendage occlusion,
        449–450
    mechanical complications of
        TAVR, 133–134
    pathology of valve degeneration and
        thrombosis, 145–146
    vascular access and closure for
        TAVR, 187
periaortic hematoma, 131, 133
pericardial effusion (PE), 449–450, 454
peri-device leaks (PDL), 452, *453*
perimembranous ventricular
    septal defects (PMVSD),
    501–503, *502–503*
peripheral artery disease (PAD),
    169–170, *170*
periprocedural ischemic stroke
    (PIS), 451–452
permanent pacemaker
    implantation (PPI)
    bicuspid aortic valve, 86
    conduction disturbances associated
        with TAVR, 115–117, *117*, 120
    hypertrophic cardiomyopathy, 461
    management of conduction
        disturbances post-TAVR,
        126–129
    optimal selection of TAVR devices,
        52, 54–55
persistent mitral regurgitation
    (MR), 229–230
persistent systolic dysfunction, 127–128
PFO *see* patent foramen ovale
PHT *see* pulmonary hypertension
PIS *see* periprocedural ischemic stroke
PISA *see* proximal isovelocity
    surface area

Pivotal IDE trial, 356
PMBV *see* percutaneous mitral balloon
    valvuloplasty
PMR *see* primary mitral regurgitation
PMVSD *see* perimembranous
    ventricular septal defects
PORTICO IDE trial, 25–26, *26*
PPI *see* permanent pacemaker
    implantation
PPM *see* patient–prosthesis mismatch
PPVR *see* percutaneous pulmonary
    valve replacement
pre-balloon aortic valvuloplasty
    (pre-BAV), 75, 77–78
pregnancy, 246
preparatory coronary
    protection, 106–107
pressure waveform analysis,
    527–528, *527–528*
PREVENT trial, 358
primary mitral regurgitation (PMR),
    196–198, *196–197*, **198**
    complications from MitraClip
        procedure, 281
    edge-to-edge mitral valve repair, 211,
        251, 257–261
    hemodynamic assessment of the
        mitral valve, 206
    mitral annuloplasty, 317
    surgical techniques for mitral valve
        repair, 233
    surgical trials in mitral valvular
        disease, 227
progressive dyspnea, 57, *57*
progressive worsening angina, 538
prosthetic conduits, 515, 518–519
prosthetic leaflet impingement,
    400, *400*
PROTECTED study, 21
PROTECTED-TAVR trial, 157, 167
PROTECT TAVR trial, 167
proximal convergence analysis, 366
proximal isovelocity surface area
    (PISA), 197
    edge-to-edge mitral valve repair, 212
    edge-to-edge tricuspid valve
        interventions, 350
    mitral paravalvular leak,
        405–406, *405*
pseudo-aortic stenosis, 528, *528*
PTCA *see* percutaneous transluminal
    coronary angioplasty

PTT *see* partial thromboplastin time
pulmonary artery (PA) pressure, 472
pulmonary artery systolic pressure
    (PASP), 343
pulmonary capillary wedge
    pressure (PCWP)
    hemodynamic assessment of the
        mitral valve, 204–205, *204*, 206
    hemodynamics in adult structural
        heart disease, 530, *530*, 531
pulmonary embolism (PE) *see* acute
    pulmonary embolism; chronic
    pulmonary embolism
pulmonary hypertension (PHT)
    atrial septal defect closure, 493, 495
    hemodynamic assessment of the
        mitral valve, 205, 208
    mitral stenosis, 193–194
pulmonary regurgitation, *517*
pulmonary stenosis, *516*
pulmonary vascular resistance
    (PVR), 203
PVL *see* paravalvular leakage
PVR *see* pulmonary vascular resistance
pyramidal RVOT, 520, *521*

q
quadricuspid aortic valves
    (QAV), 12, *12*
quality of life (QOL), 31

r
RADIANCE-HTN trial, 542
RBBB *see* right bundle branch block
RCA *see* right coronary artery
RCC *see* right coronary cusp
RDN *see* renal denervation
reduced leaflet motion (RLM), 26, *26*
REDUCE trial, 485
renal denervation therapy
    (RDN), 541–545
    ablation systems, 542–544, *543*
    complications, 545
    first-generation trials, 541, *542*
    technique and steps, 544
renin-angiotensin-aldosterone
    blockers, 386
reperfusion therapy, 158, 571–572
residual mitral regurgitation, 287
RESPECT trial, 485
respiratory failure, 568
restricted posterior mitral valve, 270

retrograde arterial access, 537, *538*
retrograde femoral access, *409*, 411
retroperitoneal bleeding, 178, *179*, 187
REVIVAL trial, 111
rheumatic mitral stenosis, 193
   hemodynamic assessment of the
      mitral valve, 203, *204*
   structural mitral valve interventions,
      239, 246–247
right atrium (RA), 347–348
right bundle branch block (RBBB)
   alcohol septal ablation, 463
   conduction disturbances associated
      with TAVR, 117, 120
   management of conduction
      disturbances post-TAVR,
      124, 128–129
right coronary artery (RCA),
      354, 368
right coronary cusp (RCC),
      119, *119–120*
right-to-left shunt, 477–481, 566
right ventricle outflow tract (RVOT),
      515–516, *516–519*, 518–521
right ventricular ejection fraction
      (RVEF), 385
right ventricular infarction/failure, 575
right ventricular (RV) overload, 472
ring annuloplasty
   failed annuloplasty, 385–386
   outcomes and predicting results, 384
   surgical trials in mitral valvular
      disease, 229
   surgical tricuspid valve repair, 384
   transcatheter tricuspid valve devices,
      357–358, 372–373
RLM *see* reduced leaflet motion
root calcification, 85
rotational angiography, 86
RVEF *see* right ventricular ejection
      fraction
RV/LV ratio, 548–550, **549**
RVOT *see* right ventricle outflow tract

S

SAM *see* systolic anterior motion
sandwich technique, 446–447, *446*
SAPIEN valve platform
   alternative access, 175–176
   caval valve implantation, 391–392
   challenging anatomy scenarios in
      TAVR, 77, 79

conduction disturbances associated
      with TAVR, 115–116, 119–120
   native aortic valve regurgitation,
      90–91
   optimal selection of TAVR devices,
      51–53, 55–56, *55*
   PARTNER IIA/SAPIEN 3 studies, 22
   pathology of valve degeneration and
      thrombosis, 140–144, *142*, *145*
   percutaneous pulmonary valve
      replacement, 516–518,
      520–521, *522*
   present generation of THVs, 33, *34*
   transcatheter mitral valve
      replacement, 304, *305*, 320
   transcatheter tricuspid valve devices,
      373, 374
   transfemoral access, 170
   valve components, 63–65, *64–65*
SAVR *see* surgical aortic valve
      replacement
SCAI *see* Society for Cardiovascular
      Angiography and Intervention
SCD *see* sudden cardiac death
SCOUT trials, 358, 366, 374
screw-in leads, 134
SEATTLE II trial, 548, 556
secondary mitral regurgitation
      (SMR), 198–200
   complications from MitraClip
      procedure, 281
   edge-to-edge mitral valve repair,
      211–212, 251–255, 258–260, 278
   hemodynamic assessment of the
      mitral valve, 206–207, *207*
   mitral annuloplasty, 317
   surgical trials in mitral valvular
      disease, 227–228
self-expanding TMVR systems
   available delivery systems, 332
   fixation and sealing, 331
   healing of the atrial space, 331, *332*
   key features of Medtronic Intrepid
      valve, 331, *332*
   transapical delivery, 332–333, *333*
   transcatheter mitral valve
      replacement, 331–334
   transseptal delivery, 333–334
self-expanding valves (SEV)
   bicuspid aortic valve, 84–86, *85*
   challenging anatomy scenarios in
      TAVR, 76–79

clinical trials, 20, 23–26
computed tomography for TAVR
      planning, 41
conduction disturbances associated
      with TAVR, 116–117
coronary artery disease, 112
essential considerations, 66–67, *66*
left ventricular assist device-related
      AI, 587–588
mechanical complications of
      TAVR, 134–135
optimal selection of TAVR devices,
      51, 53–57, *54*
percutaneous pulmonary valve
      replacement, 520, *521*
valve and catheter components,
      65, *65–66*
valve-in-valve TAVR, 98–99, *98–99*
SENTINEL trial, 163
septal myomectomy, 461, 467–468
SEV *see* self-expanding valves
severe acute aortic regurgitation, 8–9
severe aortic regurgitation, 7, **7**
severe aortic stenosis
   balloon aortic valvuloplasty, **70**
   clinical trials, 20, 25–26
   coronary artery disease, 109–110
   management of conduction
      disturbances post-TAVR,
      127–128
   optimal selection of TAVR
      devices, 57, *57*
   TAVR-related stroke, 155–156
severe cardiomyopathy, 528
severe hypotension, 305
severe tricuspid regurgitation, 391–394
shockwave lithotripsy
   challenging anatomy scenarios in
      TAVR, 80
   transfemoral access, 171, *171*, 172
shunt hemodynamics and
      calculations, 477–483
   arteriovenous fistula for dialysis
      access, 477, 482
   basic principles and
      equations, 478–479
   bidirectional shunt, 477, 481–482
   definition and classification, 477
   diagnostic shunt study, 477–478
   heart failure, 482
   left-to-right shunt, 230, 246,
      477–480, **481**

Nicoladoni-Branham sigh, 482
right-heart catheterization and ASD closure, 479–480, **480**
right-to-left shunt, 477–481, 566
routine catheterization procedures, 478
step-up diagnostic criteria, 480–481, **481**
structural mitral valve interventions, 246
surgical trials in mitral valvular disease, 230
transseptal puncture, 566
SHV *see* superior hepatic vein
Sievers classification, 83, *84*
single leaflet device attachment (SLDA)
    complications from MitraClip procedure, 285, *284, 285*
    structural mitral valve interventions, 221, 222
sinotubular junction (STJ), 40, 42, 47, 76
sinus of Valsalva
    computed tomography for TAVR planning, 42, 46–47
    coronary artery obstruction, 103, 104
SIRS *see* systemic inflammatory response syndrome
SIV *see* surgically implanted valves
SLDA *see* single leaflet device attachment
SMR *see* secondary mitral regurgitation
Society for Cardiovascular Angiography and Intervention (SCAI), 578, 581
Society for Thoracic Surgery Predictor of Mortality (STS PROM), 20–21
SOLVE-TAVI study, 52
SPACER study, 344
SPYRAL-HTN trials, 542
stents
    coronary artery obstruction, 103
    percutaneous treatment of aortic coarctation, 507, *508,* 509–513, **505,** *511*
    valve thrombosis and early thickening, 152
STICH trial, 228
stitch phenomena, 565, 566
STJ *see* sinotubular junction
streptococcal infection, 193

stroke
    bicuspid aortic valve, 86
    challenging anatomy scenarios in TAVR, 77
    consequences of debris embolizing to brain, 163
    incidence, predictors, and impact of post-TAVR, 156–157, **156**
    left atrial appendage occlusion, 417
    management of TAVR-related stroke, 157–158
    mechanism in TAVR patients, 163
    mitral stenosis, 195
    neuroprotection in TAVR, 163–168
    pathology of valve degeneration and thrombosis, 141
    peri-procedural stroke, 163
    transcatheter aortic valve implantation, 21
    transcatheter aortic valve replacement, 155–161
    treatment recommendations, 158, *159*
    valve thrombosis and early thickening, 152
stroke volume (SV), 366, 527
structural mitral valve interventions
    balloon valvuloplasty, 223–224
    edge-to-edge mitral valve repair, 217–218, 220–222, *222*
    future directions and health system implications, 224–225
    intra-procedural TEE, 217–226
    mitral stenosis, 239–249
    percutaneous mitral valve intervention, 239–247
    transcatheter mitral valve replacement, 217–218, 220, 222–223, *223*
    transcatheter therapies for nonrheumatic mitral stenosis, 247–248
    transseptal puncture, 218, 220, *220,* 225
structural valve deterioration (SVD)
    durability of bioprosthetic valves, 146–147
    infective endocarditis, 139–140, *140*
    leaflet calcification, 142–144, *145*
    leaflet/valve thrombosis, 139–141, *142–144*

neointimal coverage and pannus formation, 141–142, *145–146*
    non-calcific causes, 145–146, *147*
    pathological insights, 139–149
    transcatheter aortic valve implantation, 22–23, *23–24*
    valve-in-valve TAVR, 96, **96**
STS PROM *see* Society for Thoracic Surgery Predictor of Mortality
STTAR trial, 359
subclavian artery access, 61–62, 185
subclinical valve thrombosis *see* hypoattenuating leaflet thrombosis
sudden cardiac death (SCD), 459
SUMMIT trial, 248, 326–328
SUNSET-sPE trial, 549
superior hepatic vein (SHV), 391
superior vena cava (SVC)
    caval valve implantation, 391–393, *393*
    edge-to-edge mitral valve repair, 264
    edge-to-edge tricuspid valve interventions, 347–348
    structural mitral valve interventions, 220
    transcatheter tricuspid valve devices, 359
    transseptal puncture, 563
supra-annular valve design
    bicuspid aortic valve, 84–85, *85*
    challenging anatomy scenarios in TAVR, 77
    transcatheter aortic valve replacement, 32
    valve-in-valve TAVR, 98–99, *98*
surgical aortic valve replacement (SAVR)
    aortic stenosis, 6
    clinical trials, 21–23
    low-surgical-risk patients, 31
    mechanical complications of TAVR, 133
    native aortic valve regurgitation, 90
    pathology of valve degeneration and thrombosis, 139–147
    stroke, 155–156, 163
surgically implanted valves (SIV), 103–106, *104*

surgical mitral valve reconstruction
  acute mitral regurgitation, 227
  clinical trials, 227–232
  complications, 229
  double-orifice surgical repair, 228–229
  guidelines for resecting, 229
  Heart Team, 230, 236
  indications for MV repair, 228
  outcomes, 235–236
  papillary muscle sling, 235
  patient selection, 233, 235
  persistent MR, 229–230
  reconstruction versus replacement,
      227–228, 233
  repair using MitraClip, 228, 234–235
  ring annuloplasty, 229
  stages of primary mitral
      regurgitation, 233
  standard surgical approaches, 234–235
  systolic anterior motion, 233–234
  techniques, 233–237
  valve-in-valve implantation, 229
  vascular access, 229
suture-based annuloplasty, 358–359,
    371–372, 384
suture-based closure devices, 185
suture bicuspidization, 354
SV *see* stroke volume
SVC *see* superior vena cava
SVD *see* structural valve deterioration
SWISS-APERO trial, 437
Symplicity HTN trials, 541
syncope, 3–4, 6
systemic hypertension, 5, 528
systemic inflammatory response
      syndrome (SIRS), *569*
systolic anterior motion (SAM)
  edge-to-edge mitral valve
      repair, 467–469
  hypertrophic cardiomyopathy, 461
  surgical techniques for mitral valve
      repair, 233–234
  surgical trials in mitral valvular
      disease, 229
  Tendyne system, 327
systolic ejection murmur, 4–5
systolic flow reversal, 366

t
tamponade, 133–134, 565–566
TAPSE *see* tricuspid annular plane
      systolic excursion

TAV *see* tricuspid aortic valve
TAVI *see* transcatheter aortic valve
      implantation
TAVR *see* transcatheter aortic valve
      replacement
TEE *see* transesophageal
      echocardiography
TEER *see* edge-to-edge mitral
      valve repair
telemetry, 125
telescoping catheters, 411–412, **412**
temporary pacemakers (TPM),
      120, 124–126
Tendyne system, 325–329
  approach to implantation, 327, *328*
  challenges and complications, 328
  clinical trials, 325–327
  components and configurations,
      325, *326*
  historical development, 325, *326*
  indications and
      contraindications, 327
  pre-procedural assessment, 327
Tetralogy of Fallot (TOF), 515
thromboembolism
  coronary artery obstruction, 103
  TAVR-related stroke, 157–158
  transseptal puncture, 566
  valve-in-valve TAVR, 100
Thrombolex system, 553–554, *554*
thrombolytic therapy,
      548–551, 553–559
thrombus formation *see* device-related
      thrombus
thrombus in transit, 558
THV *see* transcatheter heart valve
TIA *see* transient ischemic attack
TIPS *see* transjugular intrahepatic
      portosystemic shunt
tissue plasminogen activator (tPA), 158
TMG *see* transmitral gradient
TMVR *see* transcatheter mitral valve
      replacement
TOF *see* Tetralogy of Fallot
TOPCOAT trial, 548
tortuosity
  challenging anatomy scenarios in
      TAVR, 79–80
  computed tomography for TAVR
      planning, 43
  transfemoral access, 172–173, *172*
tPA *see* tissue plasminogen activator

TPM *see* temporary pacemakers
TR *see* tricuspid regurgitation
TRAIPTA system, 358, 372–373
TRALI *see* transfusion-related acute
      lung injury
transaortic access, 61–62, 175–176
transaortic pressure gradient, 5, *6*, 71
transapical access
  mitral paravalvular leak,
      409, 410–411
  self-expanding TMVR systems,
      332–333, *333*
  transcatheter aortic valve
      replacement, 61–62, 175–176
  transcatheter mitral valve
      replacement, 299, 302, 307, **308**
transaxillary access
  transcatheter aortic valve
      replacement, 61–62,
      176–177, *177*
  vascular access and closure for
      TAVR, 184–185
transcarotid access
  transcatheter aortic valve
      replacement, 61, 62,
      177–178, *178*
  vascular access and closure for
      TAVR, 184–185
transcatheter aortic valve
      implantation (TAVI)
  challenging anatomy scenarios in
      TAVR, 75–76
  clinical trials, 19–29
  CoreValve Extreme Risk study, 20
  coronary artery obstruction, 106–107
  evaluation in the United
      States, 19–20
  Evolut Low Risk Trial, 25
  future directions, 26–27
  Heart Team, 20–21
  historical development, 19
  life-long management of patients,
      26–27, *27*
  management of conduction
      disturbances post-
      TAVR, 123–124
  one-year mortality, 21–22
  PARTNER A trial, 21
  PARTNER B trial, 20
  PARTNER IIA/SAPIEN 3 studies, 22
  PARTNER III study, 24–25
  PORTICO IDE trial, 25–26, *26*

PROTECTED study, 21
REPRISE III trial, 23–24
stroke risk, 21
structural valve deterioration, 22–23, *23–24*
subclinical leaflet thrombosis, 25–26, *26*
valve-in-valve TAVR, 99
valve thrombosis and early thickening, 151–153
transcatheter aortic valve replacement (TAVR), 31–37, 59–68
acute myocardial infarction cardiogenic shock, 581
alternative access, 175–181
aortic paravalvular leak closure, 399–400
aortic regurgitation, 8
aortic stenosis, 4, 6
balloon aortic valvuloplasty, 71
bicuspid aortic valve, 83–87
challenging anatomy scenarios in TAVR, 75–82
clinical trials, 20–22, 24–25
compared with TMVR, 318–319
computed tomography for TAVR planning, 39–50
conduction disturbances associated with TAVR, 115–121
coronary access after TAVR, 33
coronary artery disease, 109–114
coronary artery obstruction, 103–108
difficult transfemoral access and bailout techniques, 169–174
durability, 32–33
ECMO for structural interventions, 567–570, **567**
future generation of THVs, 35, *35*
hemodynamics after TAVR, 32–33
hemodynamics in adult structural heart disease, 529, *525*
indications and contraindications, 59
left ventricular assist device-related AI, 586–588, *587*
life-long management of patients, 31
low-surgical-risk patients, 31
management of conduction disturbances post-TAVR, 123–130
mechanical complications, 131–137
native aortic valve regurgitation, 89–93

neuroprotection in TAVR, 163–168
optimal selection of TAVR devices, 51–58
pacemaker implantation after TAVR, 33
pathology of valve degeneration and thrombosis, 139–149
pre-procedural protocol, 59–60, **60**
present generation of THVs, 33–34, *34*
step-by-step approach, 59–60, **60–61**
stroke, 155–161
vascular access, 60–63
vascular access and closure options, 183–189
see also valve-in-valve TAVR
transcatheter edge-to-edge repair (TEER) *see* edge-to-edge mitral valve repair
transcatheter heart valve (THV)
bicuspid aortic valve, 84–87
conduction disturbances associated with TAVR, 115, 118–119
hemodynamics in adult structural heart disease, 529
mechanical complications of TAVR, 134–137, *136*
native aortic valve regurgitation, 90
optimal selection of TAVR devices, 51, 56–57
transcatheter aortic valve replacement, 31–35, *34–35*
transcatheter mitral valve replacement, 301–303
transseptal transcatheter mitral valve-in-valve replacement, 311, 314–315, *316*
valve-in-valve TAVR, 96, 99
valve thrombosis and early thickening, 151–153
transcatheter mitral annuloplasty, 320–324
direct mitral annuloplasty, 322–323, *322–323*
future directions, 323–324
indirect mitral annuloplasty, 321–322, *321–322*
transcatheter mitral valve replacement (TMVR), 301–309
advantages of MDCT in pre-procedural planning, 292–293

anatomic components of mitral valve, 291, *292*
anatomic variables, 302
anticoagulation/antiplatelet strategy, 306–307
approach for failing bioprosthetic valve, 301, *301–302*
available devices, **318**, 319–320, *319*
compared with TAVR, 318–319
complications and their management, 304–306, **306**, *307*
computed tomography, 291–300, 302
concepts and protocols for mitral CT, 293–294, *293*
contraindications, 305
echocardiography, 291–292, *292*, 302
estimation of coplanar fluoroscopic angle, 297–298, *298*
intra-procedural TEE, 217–218, 220, 222–224, *223*
landing zone sizing/evaluation, 294
neo-LVOT, 293–297, *294–297*, 302, 306
nonrheumatic mitral stenosis, 247–248
patient selection, 235
post-procedural imaging, 299, *299*
reconstruction versus replacement, 227–228, 233
relevant adjacent structures, 298
self-expanding TMVR systems, 331–334
Tendyne system, 325–329
transapical access, 299, 302, 307, **308**, 332–333, *333*
transfemoral access, 319
transseptal access, 296–297, 298–299, 302, 304, *305*, 307, **308**, 319–320, 333–334
valve-in-MAC TMVR, 297, *297*, 303, *304*, 305
valve-in-ring TMVR, 297, *297*, 302–303, 305–307
see also valve-in-valve TMVR
transcatheter tricuspid valve devices, 353–361
annular-reshaping therapies, 357
caval valve implantation, 359, 391–394
challenges, 354
future development of devices, 374, **375–378**

transcatheter tricuspid valve devices
(*contd.*)
  heterotopic devices, 359, 373
  indications for valve
    replacement, 368–369
  leaflet-directed therapies, 355–357,
    356, 370–371
  limitations of valve replacement, 374
  medical and surgical
    recommendations for TR, 353,
    365, **365**
  orthotopic devices, 373
  outcomes/complications for
    replacement devices, 370–374
  pre-procedural planning, 365–370,
    366, **367**, *368*, **369**
  recent developments, 363–381
  ring annuloplasty, 357–358, 372–373
  significance and pathophysiology
    of TR, 353
  surgical tricuspid valve repair, 354
  suture-based annuloplasty,
    358–359, 371–372
  valve-in-ring and valve-in-valve
    procedures, 386–387, *386*, *388*
  valve replacement and repair
    options, 354–355, *355*, **355**,
    370–373, *370*
transcatheter tricuspid valve-in-ring
    (TTViR) procedures,
    386–387, *386*
transcatheter tricuspid valve
    intervention (TTVI),
    343–344
transcatheter tricuspid valve-in-valve
    (TTViV) procedures, 387, *388*
transcatheter valve embolization or
    migration (TVEM),
    135–137, *136*
transcaval access
  transcatheter aortic valve
    replacement, 61–62,
    178–180, *179–180*
  vascular access and closure for
    TAVR, 185
transesophageal echocardiography
    (TEE)
  alcohol septal ablation, *465*
  aortic paravalvular leak closure,
    397, *398*
  aortic regurgitation, 9
  atrial septal defect closure, 495

balloon valvuloplasty, 223–224
bicuspid aortic valve, 85
challenging anatomy scenarios in
    TAVR, 77, *78*
complications from MitraClip
    procedure, 282–284,
    283, *285–286*
computed tomography for TAVR
    planning, 40
coronary artery fistulas,
    535–536
ECMO for structural
    interventions, 569
edge-to-edge mitral valve repair,
    212–215, *213–215*, 217–
    224, *222*, 259–260, *261*,
    263, *265*, 266–270, *267–269*,
    275, *276*, *278*, *466–467*, 467
edge-to-edge tricuspid valve
    interventions, 347, 348–350,
    348–351, **351–352**
future directions and health system
    implications, 224–225
interatrial shunt devices, 472
intra-procedural TEE for structural
    mitral valve
    interventions, 217–226
left atrial appendage occlusion,
    427–431, *428–432*, **428–429**, 433,
    435, 437, 441–443, *444*, 449,
    453, 454
mechanical complications of TAVR,
    132–134, *135*
mitral annuloplasty, 322
mitral paravalvular leak, 403–406,
    405–407, 409
mitral regurgitation, 197, 199
mitral stenosis, *204*
patent foramen ovale closure, 486
structural mitral valve
    interventions, 242
surgical techniques for mitral
    valve repair, 233–234,
    235–236
surgical tricuspid valve repair, 385
Tendyne system, *326*, 327
transcatheter mitral valve
    replacement, 217–218, 220,
    222–224, *223*, 292–293,
    294, 301–302
transcatheter tricuspid valve devices,
    354, 365–366, **367**

transseptal puncture, 218, 220, *220*,
    225, 563, 565
transseptal transcatheter mitral
    valve-in-valve replacement,
    314–315
tricuspid aortic valve, 338
ventricular septal defect closure,
    500, 502–503
transfemoral access
  abdominal aortic aneurysm,
    173, *173*
  arterial puncture technique, 183–184
  benefits, 169, 175
  calcific peripheral disease, 172
  challenging anatomy scenarios in
    TAVR, 79–80
  complications and their
    management, 185–188, **186**
  computed tomography for TAVR
    planning, 43, *44*
  delivery system size and design,
    170, *171*
  difficult access and bailout
    techniques, 169–174
  high-risk vascular anatomy, 169
  iliofemoral atherosclerotic
    disease, 172
  left atrial appendage occlusion, 441
  mitral annuloplasty, 323
  mitral paravalvular leak, *409*, 411
  peripheral artery disease,
    169–170, *170*
  pre-procedural planning, 170
  severe vascular tortuosity,
    172–173, *172*
  Shockwave intravascular lithotripsy,
    171, *171*, 172
  small vessels, 171–172
  surgical trials in mitral valvular
    disease, 229
  technology developments,
    170–171, *171*
  transcatheter aortic valve
    replacement, 60–61, 66
  transcatheter mitral valve
    replacement, 321
  ultrasound-guided vascular access,
    170–171, *171*
  vascular closure devices, 185, *186*
transfusion-related acute lung injury
    (TRALI), 567–568
transient ischemic attack (TIA)

pathology of valve degeneration and thrombosis, 141
TAVR-related stroke, 157
valve thrombosis and early thickening, 153
transjugular intrahepatic portosystemic shunt (TIPS), 482
transmitral gradient (TMG), 239
transseptal access
mitral annuloplasty, 322–323
self-expanding TMVR systems, 333–334
transcatheter aortic valve replacement, 61, 62–63
transcatheter mitral valve replacement, 296–297, 298–299, 302, 304, *305*, 307, **308**, 319–320
transseptal puncture (TSP)
available needles, 564, *564–565*
closure of interatrial communication, 566
complications, 565–566
complications from MitraClip procedure, 282, *283*
edge-to-edge mitral valve repair, 215, *215*, 260, 264, 276–277
fossa ovalis and interatrial septum, 561, *562*
imaging modalities, 565
indications for accessing left atrium, 561–562
intra-procedural TEE, 218, 220, *220*, 225
left atrial appendage occlusion, 429–431, *430–431*, 435, 441–443, *442*, 449
mitral paravalvular leak, 408–410, *409*
patent foramen ovale closure, 490
percutaneous septal occlusion, 566
site-specific access locations, 562, *563*
structural heart disease, 561–566
structural mitral valve interventions, 241, 242
technique for site-specific transseptal puncture, 562–563
transcatheter mitral valve replacement, 304
transseptal transcatheter mitral valve-in-valve replacement, 312

transseptal transcatheter mitral valve-in-valve replacement (TS MViV), 311–315
advancing the delivery system, 314
atrial septal defect, 314
atrial septostomy dilation, 312–313, *313*
baseline LVOT hemodynamics, 312
crossing mitral valve into left ventricle, 312, *313*
hemostasis at the access site, 315
inserting Edwards eSheath, 312
obstacles and bailout strategies, 315
patient preparation and room setting, 311
positioning and implanting the THV, 314, *314*
post-deployment assessment, 314
pre-dilation of mitral valve, 314
preparing the transcatheter valve, 313
pre-procedural planning, 311
transseptal puncture location, 312
vascular access, 311
transthoracic echocardiography (TTE)
aortic paravalvular leak closure, 397
aortic regurgitation, 7–8, 9
atrial septal defect closure, 494–495
balloon aortic valvuloplasty, 70
computed tomography for TAVR planning, 40
coronary artery fistulas, 535–536
edge-to-edge mitral valve repair, 211–212, *212*
left atrial appendage occlusion, 427
mitral paravalvular leak, 403
mitral regurgitation, 197, 199
percutaneous treatment of aortic coarctation, 506, *507*
transcatheter aortic valve replacement, 67
transcatheter mitral valve replacement, 291–292
transcatheter tricuspid valve devices, 365–366, **367**
tricuspid aortic valve, 338–339
ventricular septal defect closure, 495
transthyretin cardiac amyloidosis (ATTR), 45
transvalvular pressure gradient (TVPG), 99, 526–527, *526*
Trialign system, 345, 358

TriBAND study, 357–358
TRiCares device, 373
TRICAVAL study, 374
Tricento device, 373
TriCinch system, 345, 358, 374
TriClip, 344, 355–356, 371
tricuspid annular plane systolic excursion (TAPSE), 385
tricuspid annuloplasty
rationale, 383
ring annuloplasty, 357–358, 372–373, 384
surgical tricuspid valve repair, 345, 383–386
suture-based annuloplasty, 358–359, 371–372
suture-based techniques, 384
transcatheter tricuspid valve devices, 354, 357–359, 371–373
tricuspid aortic valve, 340
tricuspid aortic valve (TAV)
computed tomography for TAVR planning, 48
epidemiology, 12, *12*
pathologic findings, 12–14, *13*, 15–16
transcatheter aortic valve replacement, 83
tricuspid regurgitation (TR), 337–341
anatomic components of tricuspid valve, 337, *338*, 363, *364*
caval valve implantation for severe TR, 391–394
characteristics of severe TR, 339–340
classification, 337–338, 383
edge-to-edge tricuspid valve interventions, 347–348, *351*, **351–352**
epidemiology, natural history, and prognosis, 337, 353
etiology and pathophysiology, 343, 353, 363–364, **364**
evaluation/diagnosis, 338–339, *339*
management of tricuspid regurgitation, 340
medical and surgical recommendations, 353, 365, **365**
mortality rate for surgical repair, 343
percutaneous mitral valve intervention, 246–247
repair techniques, 344–345, *344*
signs and symptoms, 338, 365–366

tricuspid regurgitation (TR) *(contd.)*
  surgical tricuspid valve repair, 340, 343–346, 354, 383–386
  transcatheter tricuspid valve devices, 353–361, 363–381, 386–387, *386*, *388*
  when TR should be treated, 383
TRICUS study, 374
TricValve system, 373, 393, *393*
TRILUMINATE study, 344, 356, 371
triple therapy, 152
Triskele UCL valve, 35
Trisol system, 373
TS MViV *see* transseptal transcatheter mitral valve-in-valve replacement
TSP *see* transseptal puncture
TTE *see* transthoracic echocardiography
TTVI *see* transcatheter tricuspid valve intervention
TTViR *see* transcatheter tricuspid valve-in-ring
TTViV *see* transcatheter tricuspid valve-in-valve
TVEM *see* transcatheter valve embolization or migration
TVPG *see* transvalvular pressure gradient

u
UAV *see* unicuspid aortic valve
UFH *see* unfractionated heparin
ULTIMA trial, 548, 556
Ultraseal device, 433–434, 437, *438*, 446
ultrasound-assisted catheter-directed thrombolysis, 548–550, 553–554, *554*
ultrasound-guided vascular access, 80, 170
unfractionated heparin (UFH), 157–158, 443
unicuspid aortic valve (UAV)
  classification and pathology, 15–16, *16*
  epidemiology, 12, *12*

v
VA-ECMO *see* venoarterial extracorporeal membrane oxygenation

Valve Academic Research Consortium-3 (VARC3), 23, *24*
valve embolization
  mechanical complications of TAVR, 135–137, *136*
  transcatheter mitral valve replacement, 304–305
valve infolding, 134–135, *135*
valve-in-MAC (ViMAC) TMVR, 297, *297*, 303, *304*, 305
valve-in-ring (ViR) procedures
  transcatheter mitral valve replacement, 297, *297*, 302–303, 305–306
  tricuspid regurgitation, 386–387, *386*
valve-in-valve (ViV) TAVR, 95–103
  avoiding patient–prosthesis mismatch, 97–99, *98–99*
  challenging anatomy scenarios in TAVR, 81–82, *81*
  computed tomography for TAVR planning, 45–47, *46*
  coronary artery obstruction, 99–100, *99–100*, 103, 104–105, **105**, *106*
  limitations, 95–96, **96**
  mechanism of bioprosthetic valve failure, 96, **96**
  native aortic valve regurgitation, 90
  need for aortic valve-in-valve procedures, 95
  outcomes, 95
  procedural planning, 97, *97*
  tricuspid regurgitation, 387, *388*
valve-in-valve (ViV) TMVR
  complications, 305–307
  computed tomography, 295, *296–297*, 297
  fluoroscopic landmarks, 303
  intra-procedural TEE, 223, *223*
  surgical trials in mitral valvular disease, 229
  see also transseptal transcatheter mitral valve-in-valve replacement
valve/leaflet thrombosis
  clinical implications, 151–153
  pathological insights, 139–141, *142–144*
  transcatheter aortic valve implantation, 25–26, *26*

see also hypoattenuating leaflet thrombosis
valve to coronary distance (VTC), 105, *106*
valvular interstitial cells (VIC), 11
VARC3 *see* Valve Academic Research Consortium-3
vascular closure devices (VCD), 63
vasodilators, 544
vasopressor therapy, 571–572, *572*, 579, 581
VC *see* vena contracta
VCD *see* vascular closure devices
vena contracta (VC)
  edge-to-edge tricuspid valve interventions, 349, *349*, **351**
  intra-procedural TEE, 219, *219*
  transcatheter tricuspid valve devices, 365–366
  tricuspid aortic valve, 339
venoarterial extracorporeal membrane oxygenation (VA-ECMO)
  acute myocardial infarction cardiogenic shock, 575–576
  acute pulmonary embolism, 551
  ECMO for structural interventions, 567–570
  interatrial shunt devices, 471
venovenous extracorporeal membrane oxygenation (VV-ECMO), 569
ventricular decalcification, 229
ventricular functional mitral regurgitation (VFMR), 207–208, *208*
ventricular perforation, 133–134
ventricular septal defect (VSD)
  available devices for closure, 499–500, 502, *502–503*
  closure, 499–504
  complications of percutaneous closure, 501, 503
  indications and contraindications for closure, 499, 501
  mechanical complications of TAVR, 132
  muscular ventricular septal defects, 499–501, *501*

perimembranous ventricular septal defects, 501–503, *502–503*

shunt hemodynamics and calculations, 477

stepwise procedure for closure, 500, *502–503*

verapamil, 460

VIC *see* valvular interstitial cells

ViMAC *see* valve-in-MAC

ViR *see* valve-in-ring

vitamin K antagonists (VKA), 151–152, 417–420

ViV *see* valve-in-valve

VKA *see* vitamin K antagonists

VSD *see* ventricular septal defect

VTC *see* valve to coronary distance

VV-ECMO *see* venovenous extracorporeal membrane oxygenation

w

warfarin, 454

WATCHMAN device, 418–420, **421**, 433–435, 437, *438*, 444–445, *445*

WaveCrest device, 433, 437, *438*

Wilkins score, 239–240

x

x-plane imaging, 218, *220*, 222